T0343314

2011
YEAR BOOK OF
DERMATOLOGY
AND
DERMATOLOGIC
SURGERY™

The 2011 Year Book Series

Year Book of Anesthesiology and Pain Management™: Drs Chestnut, Abram, Black, Gravlee, Lien, Mathru, and Roizen

Year Book of Cardiology®: Drs Gersh, Cheitlin, Elliott, Gold, Graham, and Thourani

Year Book of Critical Care Medicine®: Drs Dellinger, Parrillo, Balk, Dorman, Dries, and Zanotti-Cavazzoni

Year Book of Dermatology and Dermatologic Surgery™: Dr Del Rosso

Year Book of Diagnostic Radiology®: Drs Osborn, Abbara, Elster, Manaster, Oestreich, Offiah, Rosado de Christenson, Stephens, and Walker

Year Book of Emergency Medicine®: Drs Hamilton, Bruno, Handly, Mullin, Quintana, and Ramoska

Year Book of Endocrinology®: Drs Schott, Apovian, Clarke, Eugster, Ludlam, Meikle, Ovalle, Schinner, Schteingart, and Toth

Year Book of Gastroenterology™: Drs Talley, DeVault, Harnois, Murray, Pearson, Philcox, Picco, and Smith

Year Book of Hand and Upper Limb Surgery®: Drs Yao and Steinmann

Year Book of Medicine®: Drs Barker, Garrick, Gersh, Khardori, LeRoith, Seo, Talley, and Thigpen

Year Book of Neonatal and Perinatal Medicine®: Drs Fanaroff, Benitz, Donn, Neu, Papile, Polin, and van Marter

Year Book of Neurology and Neurosurgery®: Drs Klimo and Rabinstein

Year Book of Obstetrics, Gynecology, and Women's Health®: Drs Dungan and Shulman

Year Book of Oncology®: Drs Arceci, Bauer, Chiorean, Gordon, Lawton, Murphy, Thigpen, and Tsao

Year Book of Ophthalmology®: Drs Rapuano, Cohen, Flanders, Hammersmith, Milman, Myers, Nelson, Penne, Pyfer, Sergott, Shields, and Vander

Year Book of Orthopedics®: Drs Morrey, Beauchamp, Huddleston, Swiontkowski, and Trigg

Year Book of Otolaryngology-Head and Neck Surgery®: Drs Sindwani, Balough, Franco, Gapany, and Mitchell

Year Book of Pathology and Laboratory Medicine®: Drs Raab, Parwani, Bejarano, and Bissell

Year Book of Pediatrics®: Dr Stockman

Year Book of Plastic and Aesthetic Surgery™: Drs Miller, Gosain, Gurtner, Gutowski, Ruberg, Salisbury, and Smith

Year Book of Psychiatry and Applied Mental Health®: Drs Talbott, Ballenger, Buckley, Frances, Krupnick, and Mack

Year Book of Pulmonary Disease®: Drs Barker, Jones, Maurer, Raza, Tanoue, and Willsie

Year Book of Sports Medicine®: Drs Shephard, Cantu, Feldman, Jankowski, Khan, Lebrun, Nieman, Pierrynowski, and Rowland

Year Book of Surgery®: Drs Copeland, Behrns, Daly, Eberlein, Fahey, Huber, Klodell, Mozingo, and Pruett

Year Book of Urology®: Drs Andriole and Coplen

Year Book of Vascular Surgery®: Drs Moneta, Gillespie, Starnes, and Watkins

2011

The Year Book of DERMATOLOGY AND DERMATOLOGIC SURGERY™

Editor-in-Chief
James Q. Del Rosso, DO, FAOCD
Dermatology Residency Director, Valley Hospital Medical Center, Las Vegas, Nevada; Clinical Professor (Dermatology), Touro University College of Osteopathic Medicine, Henderson, Nevada; JDRx Dermatology, Las Vegas Skin & Cancer Clinics, Las Vegas, Nevada, and Henderson, Nevada

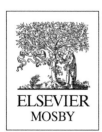

ELSEVIER
MOSBY

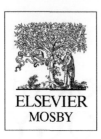

ELSEVIER
MOSBY

Vice President, Continuity: Kimberly Murphy
Editor: Stephanie Donley
Supervisor, Electronic Year Books: Donna M. Skelton
Electronic Article Manager: Emily Ogle
Illustrations and Permissions Coordinator: Dawn Vohsen

2011 EDITION

Copyright 2011, Mosby, Inc. All rights reserved.

No part of this publication may be reproduced, stored in a retrieval system, or transmitted, in any form or by any means, electronic, mechanical, photocopying, recording, or otherwise, without prior written permission from the publisher.

Permission to photocopy or reproduce solely for internal or personal use is permitted for libraries or other users registered with the Copyright Clearance Center, provided that the base fee of $35.00 per chapter is paid directly to the Copyright Clearance Center, 21 Congress Street, Salem, MA 01970. This consent does not extend to other kinds of copying, such as copying for general distribution, for advertising or promotional purposes, for creating new collected works, or for resale.

Composition by TNQ Books and Journals Pvt Ltd, India

Printed and bound by CPI Group (UK) Ltd, Croydon, CR0 4YY

Transferred to Digital Print 2011

Editorial Office:
Elsevier
Suite 1800
1600 John F. Kennedy Blvd
Philadelphia, PA 19103-2899

International Standard Serial Number: 0093-3619
International Standard Book Number: 978-0-323-08410-9

Editorial Board

Editor-in-Chief
James Q. Del Rosso, DO, FAOCD
Dermatology Residency Director, Valley Hospital Medical Center, Las Vegas, Nevada; Clinical Professor (Dermatology), Touro University College of Osteopathic Medicine, Henderson, Nevada; JDRx Dermatology, Las Vegas Skin & Cancer Clinics, Las Vegas, Nevada, and Henderson, Nevada

Associate Editors
Neal Bhatia, MD
Associate Clinical Professor, Harbor-UCLA Medical Center, Department of Dermatology, Torrance, California
Roger I. Ceilley, MD
Clinical Professor of Dermatology, The University of Iowa; Director, Mohs Micrographic Surgery and Cutaneous Oncology Fellowship, Dermatology, PC, West Des Moines, Iowa
Whitney A. High, MD, JD, MEng
Associate Professor, Dermatology and Dermatopathology, University of Colorado School of Medicine, Health Science Center, Denver, Colorado

Contributors
Andrew K. Bean, MD
Assistant Director, Mohs Micrographic Surgery and Cutaneous Oncology Fellowship, Dermatology, PC, West Des Moines, Iowa; Chief of Dermatology Section, Iowa Methodist Medical Center, Broadlawns Medical Center, Des Moines, Iowa
Susun Bellew, DO
Chief Resident (PGY-4), Valley Hospital Medical Center, Las Vegas, Nevada
Brian Berman, MD, PhD
Professor of Dermatology and Internal Medicine, Department of Dermatology and Cutaneous Surgery, University of Miami Miller School of Medicine, Miami, Florida
Sanjay Bhambri, DO
Texas Dermatology and Skin Center, PLLC, Rockwall, Texas
Elizabeth M. Billingsley, MD
Professor of Dermatology, Director, Mohs Surgery and Dermatologic Surgery, Pennsylvania State University College of Medicine, Penn State Hershey Medical Center, Hershey, Pennsylvania
Margaret M. Boyle, BS
Research Associate, Dermatoepidemiology Unit, Brown University, Providence, Rhode Island
Lloyd Cleaver, DO
Assistant Dean and Professor, Department of Internal Medicine, Division of Dermatology, A.T. Still University of Health Sciences; Program Director, Kirksville College of Osteopathic Medicine Dermatology Training Consortium; Cleaver Dermatology, Kirksville, Missouri

David E. Cohen, MD, MPH
Vice Chairman for Clinical Affairs, Director of Allergic, Occupational, and Environmental Dermatology, New York University School of Medicine, Department of Dermatology, New York, New York

David Dasher, MD
San Diego, California

Dirk M. Elston, MD
Managing Director, Ackerman Academy of Dermatopathology, New York, New York

Sheila Fallon Friedlander, MD
Clinical Professor, Pediatrics and Medicine (Dermatology), University of California San Diego School of Medicine and Children's Hospital, San Diego, California

Joseph F. Fowler, Jr, MD, FAAD
Clinical Professor of Dermatology, University of Louisville School of Medicine, Louisville, Kentucky; Assistant Clinical Professor of Occupational Medicine, University of Kentucky, Lexington, Kentucky

Brad P. Glick, DO, MPH, FAOCD
Director, Dermatology Residency, Wellington Regional Medical Center, Wellington, Florida

Michael H. Gold, MD
Medical Director, Gold Skin Care Center, Advanced Aesthetics Medical Spa, Tennessee Clinical Research Center, The Laser and Rejuvenation Center, Nashville, Tennessee; Clinical Assistant Professor, Vanderbilt University School of Medicine, Department of Dermatology, School of Nursing, Nashville, Tennessee; Visiting Professor of Dermatology, Huashan Hospital, Fudan University, Shanghai, China; No. 1 Hospital of China Medical University, Shenyang, China

Shireen Guide, MD
Pediatric Dermatology Clinical Fellow, Rady Children's Hospital, University of California, San Diego School of Medicine, San Diego, California

Sarah Hill, MD
University of California San Diego School of Medicine, San Diego, California

Kristen Hook, MD
Rady Children's Hospital, University of California San Diego School of Medicine, San Diego, California

Jessica Hsu
Medical Student, University of California San Diego School of Medicine, San Diego, California

Melinda Jen, MD
San Diego, California

Grace K. Kim, DO
Dermatology Resident (PGY-2), Valley Hospital Medical Center, Las Vegas, Nevada

Brian A. Kopitzki, DO
Fellow, Dermatology PC, West Des Moines, Iowa

Mark Lebwohl, MD
Professor and Chairman, Department of Dermatology, The Mount Sinai School of Medicine, New York, New York

Jacquelyn Levin, DO
Dermatology Resident (PGY-2), Largo Medical Center, Largo, Florida

James Leyden, MD
Emeritus Professor, University of Pennsylvania, Philadelphia, Pennsylvania

Daniel M. MacAlpine, MD, FAAD
Dermatology, PC, West Des Moines, Iowa

Catalina Matiz, MD
Medical Student, University of California San Diego School of Medicine, San Diego, California

Morgan McCarty, DO
Mohave Skin and Cancer Clinics, Dermatology Education and Research, Las Vegas, Nevada

Shawna McCarty, MD
Resident, Department of Dermatology, Loma Linda University School of Medicine, Loma Linda, California

LaVonne Meadows, MD
Resident, Department of Dermatology, Loma Linda University School of Medicine, Loma Linda, California

Neda Mehr, MD
Resident, Department of Dermatology, Loma Linda University School of Medicine, Loma Linda, California

Michael J. Messina, MD
Resident, Department of Dermatology, Loma Linda University School of Medicine, Loma Linda, California

Brent D. Michaels, DO
Dermatology Resident (PGY-3), Valley Hospital Medical Center, Las Vegas, Nevada

Saira B. Momin, DO
Dermatopathology Fellow in Mohs Micrographic Surgery, Miami, Florida

Tanya Nino, MD
Resident, Department of Dermatology, Loma Linda University School of Medicine, Loma Linda, California

Steven Purcell, DO
Chairman, Division of Dermatology, Professor of Dermatology, Philadelphia College of Osteopathic Medicine, Philadelphia, Pennsylvania; Assistant Program Director, Dermatologic Residency, Lehigh Valley Health Network/ Philadelphia College of Osteopathic Medicine, Philadelphia, Pennsylvania

Melissa Reyes, MD
San Diego, California

Ilya Reyter, MD
Procedural Dermatology Mohs Fellow, Department of Dermatology, Loma Linda University School of Medicine, Loma Linda, California

Phoebe Rich, MD
Adjunct Professor of Dermatology, Oregon Health and Science University; Private Practice, Portland, Oregon

Ted Rosen, MD
Professor of Dermatology, Baylor College of Medicine; Chief, Dermatology Services, Michael E. DeBakey VA Medical Center, Houston, Texas

Andrea Smith, MD
Resident, Department of Dermatology, Loma Linda University School of Medicine, Loma Linda, California

Jason L. Smith, MD
Northwest Georgia Dermatology, Rome, Georgia

Jeffrey Suchniak, MD
Dermatologist, Boice-Willis Clinic, Rocky Mount, North Carolina

Emil A. Tanghetti, MD
Clinical Professor, Department of Dermatology, University of California at Davis; Director, Center for Dermatology and Laser Surgery, Sacramento, California

Diane Thiboutot, MD
Professor of Dermatology, The Pennsylvania State College of Medicine, Hershey, Pennsylvania

Bruce H. Thiers, MD
Professor and Chairman, Department of Dermatology and Dermatologic Surgery, Medical University of South Carolina, Charleston, South Carolina

Abel Torres, MD, JD
Chairman, Department of Dermatology, Loma Linda University School of Medicine, Loma Linda, California

Guy Webster, MD, PhD
Clinical Professor, Department of Dermatology, Jefferson Medical College, Philadelphia, Pennsylvania

Jeffrey Weinberg, MD
Director, Clinical Research Center, Department of Dermatology, St. Luke's-Roosevelt Hospital Center, Beth Israel Medical Center; Associate Clinical Professor of Dermatology, Columbia University College of Physicians & Surgeons, New York, New York

Martin A. Weinstock, MD, PhD
Professor of Dermatology and Community Health, Brown University; Chief of Dermatology, VA Medical Center; Director, Pigmented Lesion Unit and Photomedicine, Rhode Island Hospital, Providence, Rhode Island

Adam Wiener, DO
Private Practice, Melbourne Dermatology Center, Melbourne, Florida

Joshua B. Wilson, MD
Dermatology PC, West Des Moines, Iowa

Andrea Zaenglein, MD
Associate Professor of Dermatology and Pediatrics, Penn State/Milton S. Hershey Medical Center, Hershey, Pennsylvania

Table of Contents

EDITORIAL BOARD vii

JOURNALS REPRESENTED xiii

INTRODUCTION xv

YEAR BOOK FOCUS: Skin Cancer in Asians: Part 1:
Nonmelanoma Skin Cancer 1
YEAR BOOK FOCUS: Skin Cancer in Asians: Part 2: Melanoma . . 9
YEAR BOOK FOCUS: Avoiding the Legal "Blemish": Medicolegal
Pitfalls in Dermatology. 15

STATISTICS OF INTEREST TO THE DERMATOLOGIST 31

CLINICAL DERMATOLOGY 47
1. Urticarial and Eczematous Disorders 49
2. Psoriasis and Other Papulosquamous Disorders 101
3. Bacterial and Fungal Infections. 133
4. Viral Infections (Excluding HIV Infection) 169
5. Parasitic Infections, Bites, and Infestations 179
6. Disorders of the Pilosebaceous Apparatus 181
7. Photobiology. 207
8. Collagen Vascular and Related Disorders 213
9. Blistering Disorders. 231
10. Drug Actions, Reactions, and Interactions 241
11. Drug Development and Promotion. 257
12. Miscellaneous Topics in Clinical Dermatology 265

DERMATOLOGIC SURGERY AND CUTANEOUS ONCOLOGY 311
13. Nonmelanoma Skin Cancer 313
14. Nevi and Melanoma. 371
15. Lymphoproliferative Disorders 423

16. Miscellaneous Topics in Cosmetic and Laser Surgery 429
17. Miscellaneous Topics in Dermatologic Surgery and Cutaneous
    Oncology 459

    ARTICLE INDEX 481
    AUTHOR INDEX 497

Journals Represented

Journals represented in this YEAR BOOK are listed below.
Academic Emergency Medicine
Acta Obstetricia et Gynecologica Scandinavica
Acta Paediatrica
Aesthetic Surgery Journal
Allergy American Journal of Clinical Pathology
American Journal of Epidemiology
American Journal of Gastroenterology
American Journal of Infection Control
American Journal of Medicine
American Journal of Preventive Medicine
American Journal of Public Health
American Journal of Surgical Pathology
American Surgeon
Annals of Allergy, Asthma & Immunology
Annals of Plastic Surgery
Annals of Surgical Oncology
Annals of the Rheumatic Diseases
Archives of Dermatology
Archives of Neurology
Archives of Pediatrics & Adolescent Medicine
Archives of Surgery
British Dental Journal
British Journal of Cancer
British Journal of Dermatology
British Medical Journal
Canadian Journal of Surgery
Cancer
Cancer Epidemiology, Biomarkers & Prevention
Clinical Cancer Research
Clinical Infectious Diseases
Clinical Pediatrics
Contact Dermatitis
Dermatologic Surgery
Dermatologic Therapy
Dermatology
Diabetes Care
Drugs
European Journal of Obstetrics & Gynecology and Reproductive Biology
European Journal of Radiology
European Journal of Surgical Oncology
Gynecologic Oncology
Head & Neck
International Journal of Cancer
Journal of Affective Disorders
Journal of Allergy and Clinical Immunology
Journal of Clinical Microbiology
Journal of Clinical Oncology

Journal of Clinical Psychiatry
Journal of Cutaneous Pathology
Journal of Infectious Diseases
Journal of Investigative Dermatology
Journal of Pediatrics
Journal of Rheumatology
Journal of the American Academy of Dermatology
Journal of the American Board of Family Medicine
Journal of the European Academy of Dermatology and Venereology
Journal of the National Cancer Institute
Journal of Urology
Medicine
Modern Pathology
Nephrology Dialysis Transplantation
Oral Oncology
Pediatric Dermatology
Plastic and Reconstructive Surgery
Proceedings of the National Academy of Sciences of the United States of America
Scandinavian Journal of Rheumatology
Scandinavian Journal of Urology and Nephrology
Surgery
Transplantation Proceedings
World Journal of Surgery
Wound Repair and Regeneration

STANDARD ABBREVIATIONS

The following terms are abbreviated in this edition: acquired immunodeficiency syndrome (AIDS), cardiopulmonary resuscitation (CPR), central nervous system (CNS), cerebrospinal fluid (CSF), computed tomography (CT), deoxyribonucleic acid (DNA), electrocardiography (ECG), health maintenance organization (HMO), human immunodeficiency virus (HIV), intensive care unit (ICU), intramuscular (IM), intravenous (IV), magnetic resonance (MR) imaging (MRI), ribonucleic acid (RNA), ultrasound (US), and ultraviolet (UV).

NOTE

The YEAR BOOK OF DERMATOLOGY AND DERMATOLOGIC SURGERY™ is a literature survey service providing abstracts of articles published in the professional literature. Every effort is made to ensure the accuracy of the information presented in these pages. Neither the editors nor the publisher of the YEAR BOOK OF DERMATOLOGY AND DERMATOLOGIC SURGERY™ can be responsible for errors in the original materials. The editors' comments are their own opinions. Mention of specific products within this publication does not constitute endorsement.

To facilitate the use of the YEAR BOOK OF DERMATOLOGY AND DERMATOLOGIC SURGERY™ as a reference tool, all illustrations and tables included in this publication are now identified as they appear in the original article. This change is meant to help the reader recognize that any illustration or table appearing in the YEAR BOOK OF DERMATOLOGY AND DERMATOLOGIC SURGERY™ may be only one of many in the original article. For this reason, figure and table numbers will often appear to be out of sequence within the YEAR BOOK OF DERMATOLOGY AND DERMATOLOGIC SURGERY™.

Introduction

Approximately 4 years ago, Dr Bruce Thiers approached me with the idea of becoming the Editor-in-Chief of the YEAR BOOK OF DERMATOLOGY AND DERMATOLOGIC SURGERY. He had served in that capacity for this annually distributed publication since 1998. Having accepted the position of editor of the *Journal of the American Academy of Dermatology*, Dr Thiers understandably wanted to decompress his "to-do list," as he chairs a dermatology department in South Carolina and is also editor of *Dermatologic Clinics*. In less than a heartbeat, I accepted his offer, and I have not looked back. Dr Thiers was very helpful to me during my learning-curve period, and I am thankful to him for this tremendous opportunity and his confidence in me to take on this task. The first edition under my direction as editor was the 2010 YEAR BOOK, published in July 2010, and this 2011 issue is my second.

The first step during my transition in early 2009 was to interact with Carla Holloway, who is employed by the publisher, Elsevier. After exchanging phone calls and several e-mails, we met in person for the first time in March 2009 in San Francisco at an American Academy of Dermatology meeting. Carla quickly schooled me in how to manage the YEAR BOOK Web site, where I access articles for selection and distribution to reviewers. Carla and her team have always been very dedicated to the internal management and success of this publication. More recently, Carla has passed the torch to Stephanie Donley. Stephanie has been very accessible and efficient and also has a great sense of humor, which is very welcome to a personality like mine. A touch of humor is most refreshing when working through the occasional unexpected glitches that occur on either end of the online system. At the end of the day, the Elsevier team continually ensures that all of the associate editors and contributors who write commentaries for this YEAR BOOK have a hassle-free experience when accessing assigned articles and submitting their contributions. Any honest physician will admit that many doctors require hand-holding through projects requiring Web sites, links, user ID numbers, passcodes, and other forms of the computer technology maze that Bill Gates or Steve Jobs never warned us about in advance! The team at the Elsevier "mother ship" that supports this publication behind the scenes does an outstanding job. Ruth Malwitz also assisted during the transition phase between Carla Holloway and Stephanie Donley and was very helpful.

As I started to formulate my own vision for this publication, I chose to expand the list of associate editors and contributors, a philosophy that was different from what Dr Thiers had incorporated. Bruce Thiers burned the midnight oil on many nights to do a lot of reviews himself, and he did a great job. I elected to expand the range of perspectives in the commentaries by tapping into the minds of several dermatologists who are well known as true leaders and thinkers in our specialty, including many from both academic centers and private community-based practices. As you can see from the listing of our "faculty," commentaries are provided by several household names in dermatology along with many bright and interested up-and-comers. I also recruited some seasoned dermatologists in private practice who combine academic perspectives and new advances with practical experience. These practitioners may not be as well known, as they are not "writers" or "speakers." However, this group often has the most to say that is valuable and clinically relevant, drawing on their vast experience of facing treatment challenges with many patients while also keeping up on new information. The larger number of reviewers provides a varied spectrum of perspectives and interpretations in the commentaries, with each reviewer providing his or her own unique "flavor." We do not yet have in our reviewer menu as many flavors as Baskin & Robbins, but we are working on it. Participating in this endeavor is purely a labor of love, and I am very thankful to everyone involved.

Why I Became Involved

Keeping up with scientific information that can influence the approaches we use in clinical practice is a monumental task. I had been a subscriber to the YEAR BOOK of our specialty for many years and always found myself paging through its contents after it hit my mailbox each December. I would always notice interesting articles covering a wide array of topics that would address specific subjects that I had questions about but had not yet looked into. Also, I would find myself immediately checking the statistics section, and I also wanted to see what the lead article was about. It reminded me of my junior high school and high school years, when I would get a newly released record album by The Beatles and would play it for the first time. The Beatles never disappointed me and neither did the YEAR BOOK.

As editor of this annual publication, I now have the opportunity to select from a plethora of articles in the worldwide medical literature that relate to dermatology. I try to choose for review those that seem to be most relevant and interesting. Once an article is selected, I then must match it with an individual from our roster of "all-star players" so that a meaningful commentary will ensue. Ultimately, a coach is only as good as his players. Lucky for me, I am supported by a "Dream Team!"

This Is a Group Effort ... Including at My Home Base

Thank you to everyone who has contributed to this important endeavor, both in the front-line trenches and behind the scenes. Our large cast of contributors is replete with very intelligent and busy people who could have easily said "No" but chose to contribute. For this I am very grateful.

I especially want to recognize my local professional support system; without these individuals, I would not have been able to accept this position of editor in the first place. This talented group includes previous and current dermatology residents (Sanjay Bhambri, Saira Momin, Susun Bellew, Brent Michaels, and Grace Kim), and interns (Jacquelyn Levin and Morgan McCarty) at Valley Hospital Medical Center (VHMC) in Las Vegas, Nevada. Dr Levin is now a dermatology resident in Tampa, Florida, and is a prolific writer. Dr Kim also contributed heavily to the 2010 and 2011 editions during her research fellowship with us before starting the dermatology residency program at VHMC in July 2010. As the director of this dermatology residency program, the first and only dermatology residency in the State of Nevada, I integrated YEAR BOOK article reviews into our educational process. The dermatology residents, research fellows, and selected interns with special interest in dermatology took on their YEAR BOOK responsibilities with vigor, as exemplified by the thorough nature and the high quality of their commentaries and the volume they contributed. They were not at all intimidated by the challenges of this project. For me, it was continually rewarding to see their minds develop, strengthen, and quickly progress as they regularly questioned the validity and relevance of both data and conclusions stated in publications. Additionally, it was very pleasing to see how they all grew professionally and personally, as they translated their thoughts into clear and concise written commentaries with greater confidence. What a tremendous achievement it is to acquire knowledge, learn to become a discriminating reader, and develop communication skills that can follow you over an entire lifetime.

Lastly, I want to thank Jacquelyn Levin, who contributed the Special Focus Article in the 2010 edition. Dr Levin is now a dermatology resident at Largo Medical Center, Largo, Florida, and has remained a valued contributor to this YEAR BOOK. For 2011, I am thankful for the hard work provided by Dr Susun Bellew, Dr Brent Michaels, and Dr Grace Kim, dermatology residents in our program at VHMC, and the lead authors of the 3 Special Focus Articles used in this issue.

Now, please enjoy the 2011 edition of the YEAR BOOK OF DERMATOLOGY AND DERMATOLOGIC SURGERY.

Stay healthy and happy …

James Q. Del Rosso, DO, FAOCD
Editor-in-Chief

Skin Cancer in Asians: Part 1: Nonmelanoma Skin Cancer

GRACE K. KIM, DO,[a] JAMES Q. DEL ROSSO, DO, FAOCD,[b]
AND SUSUN BELLEW, DO[c]
[a]Dermatology Research Fellow, Mohave Skin & Cancer Clinics, Las Vegas, Nevada;
[b]Dermatology Residency Director, Valley Hospital Medical Center, Las Vegas, Nevada, and
Dermatology Research Director, Mohave Skin & Cancer Clinics, Las Vegas, Nevada; and
[c]Dermatology Resident (PGY-3), Valley Hospital Medical Center, Las Vegas, Nevada

ABSTRACT

Since the 1960s, basal cell carcinoma and squamous cell carcinoma among the Caucasian population have increased 3 to 8 percent annually. Although Asians display relative protection from basal cell carcinoma and squamous cell carcinoma, incidence rates of these nonmelanoma skin cancers have been increasing over the past three decades. With changing demographics and a steady rise in the minority population in the United States, there is an increased need for further studies of cutaneous malignancies within Asian and other ethnic populations. This article reviews nonmelanoma skin cancers in the Asian population with an insight into contributing factors, such as skin type, occupation, cultural practices, and genetic components. (*J Clin Aesthetic Dermatol.* 2009;2(8):39-42.)*

Since the 1960s, basal cell carcinoma (BCC) and squamous cell carcinoma (SCC) among the Caucasian population have increased 3 to 8 percent annually.[1,2] Nonmelanoma skin cancer (NMSC) is not as extensively studied in the Asian population as it is in the Caucasian population. It has been proposed that Asians in general have skin types that protect them from NMSC.[3] Darker-skinned individuals have confirmed protection provided by increased epidermal melanin; increased melanocyte activity; and larger, more dispersed melanosomes, which can filter twice as much ulatroviolet B (UVB) radiation than lighter-skinned Caucasians.[4] Although Asians have lower incidence rates than Caucasians, NMSC is on the rise in Pacific Rim locations, such as Japan.[3] It is often difficult for many second- and third-world countries in Asia to establish uniform tumor registries in hospitals or large clinics due to logistical considerations and associated costs.[5] Many NMSC incidence rates from Asia are from locations such as Japan and Singapore because of limited financial and organizational resources in various parts of Asia.[5] In addition, Asians as a whole are

Address Correspondence To: James Q. Del Rosso, DO, FAOCD; E-mail: jqdelrosso@yahoo.com
Disclosure: Drs. Kim and Bellew report no relevant conflicts of interest. Dr. Del Rosso is a consultant, speaker, and/or researcher for Allergan, Coria, Galderma, Graceway, Intendis, Medicis, Onset Therapeutics, Obagi Medical Products, Ortho Dermatology, PharmaDerm, Quinnova, Ranbaxy, SkinMedica, Stiefel, Triax, Unilever, and Warner-Chilcott.
*Reproduced with permission from *The Journal of Clinical and Aesthetic Dermatology.*

not a homogenous population, with different regions having a wide range of skin types.[5] There are as much as 50-fold to 100-fold differences in incidence rates for BCC and SCC, even within populations of Asians with the same Fitzpatrick skin type.[6] NMSC also varies according to geographic location and latitude within countries and across the globe.[3]

RISK FACTORS AND PRECANCEROUS LESIONS

The total ozone layer has decreased over the last 20 years resulting in an increase in UVB radiation exposure.[7] UVB has been known to yield high concentrations of cyclobutane pyrimidine dimers and photoproducts in the epidermis of people with Fitzpatrick type I skin.[8] In Japan, during the last three decades, NMSC has shown a twofold increase in incidence, with Fitzpatrick skin type I being a risk factor that is of higher prevalence among rural residents.[3]

There have also been studies showing actinic keratosis (AK) as a risk factor for NMSC in Asians.[9] In recent years, AK incidence rates have been increasing among the Japanese population, as have SCC rates.[9] In Caucasians, SCCs on sun-exposed areas are sometimes found in association with AKs and usually have low metastatic potential. This is in contrast to SCCs that develop in association with AKs among the Japanese, which appear in some cases to be more biologically aggressive and metastasize more frequently.[9]

Studies strongly suggest that photoprotection, especially from sunlight, is the major preventative approach to reducing precancerous lesions, such as AKs and NMSCs in Japan.[9] In 1992, studies comparing Kasai City (34° 56′N) and Ie Island (25° 10′N) revealed that twice the dose of UVB radiation causes a threefold to fourfold higher incidence of AK with a mean prevalence rate of 203.33 and 756.26, respectively.[10] Further studies from 27 university hospitals suggest that NMSC and AK prevalence rates were approximately fivefold higher in southern parts of Japan as compared to northern Japan.[7] An increase in the latitudinal-UVB gradient has been identified as one of many factors that have contributed to NMSC rates in Japan.[3] The incidence of AK in Japan is 414 per 100,000, occurring more commonly among men that participate in outdoor activities.[11,12] The significantly higher prevalence of AKs in outdoor workers indicated that the lifetime-dose exposure of solar UV plays a key role in the development of precancerous lesions in Japan.[7] In the city of Kasai, it was found that prevalence rates of AK in males and in outdoor workers were significantly higher than females and indoor workers.[7] Use of cosmetics after 20 years of age was a protective factor for precancerous lesions and having Fitzpatrick type I skin with a history of severe sunburns during childhood were found to be important risk factors.[10]

BASAL CELL CARCINOMA

Development of BCC has been correlated with prolonged, intensive UV exposure, with BCC occurring most commonly after the fifth decade of life.[4] More than 90 percent of BCCs develop in sun-exposed areas of the head and neck region regardless of the degree of pigmentation in an individual.[4] BCC is the most common skin cancer in Caucasians, Hispanics, Chinese, and Japanese.[4] According to one study of 101 institutions in Japan from 1987 to 1996, BCC accounts for 47 percent of all cutaneous malignancies.[11] BCC rates are less in pigmented individuals because of the inherent photoprotection of melanin and the nature of melanosome dispersal.[4] The incidence of BCC per 100,000 populations is 6.4 in Chinese men; 5.8 in Chinese women; 15 to 16.5 in Japanese overall; 29.7 in Japanese residents of Kauai, Hawaii; and 26.1 in Japanese residents of Okinawa.[4] There has also been an increased trend of BCC development in Japan. The ratio of BCC to SCC in Japan in the 1960s was reported to be 1-1.4:1 as compared to the 1990s with an increased BCC:SCC ratio of 4.5:1.[13] Study results indicate that BCC incidence was higher in 1986 to 1990 compared to 1979 to 1980, while SCC rates held steady.[3] Studies were conducted in Ie Island, Okinawa, the southern part of Japan, where the annual cumulative dose of UV is assumed to be the highest in Japan.[13] There was also a higher incidence among people with outdoor occupations, such as farmers, fishermen, and laborers.[14]

NMSC is the seventh most common cancer in Singapore accounting for 9.6 per 100,000 cases among men and 8.1 per 100,000 cases among women during 1993 and 1997.[15] Singapore is situated one degree north of the equator and has a population of four million people, comprising 77 percent Chinese, 14 percent Malay, and nine percent a mixture of other races.[5] The age-standardized incidence rate (ASR) of BCC has increased at a rate of 2.8 per year among Asian residents in Singapore between 1968 and 1997.[5] Among females in Singapore, BCC accounts for 4.5 percent of all cancers in Chinese, 3.4 percent in Malays, and 2.5 percent in Asian Indians.[5] BCC incidence rates among the Chinese (Fitzpatrick skin types III-IV) were more than 2.5 times that of the Malays (Fitzpatrick skin types V-VI) and the Asian Indians (Fitzpatrick skin type VI).[16]

Similarly with Caucasians, 70 to 90 percent of BCCs occur on sun-exposed skin in Asians, thus emphasizing that photoprotection should not be ignored, even in more darkly pigmented individuals.[4] Rare BCC sites include nipple, penis, anus, groin, popliteal fossae, ankle, and scalp.[4] Other risk factors include history of radiation, scars, ulcers, arsenic ingestion, immunosuppression, trauma, albinism, and nevus sebaceus.[4] The clinical presentation and histological features of BCC in Asians include characteristics shared from darker-pigmented individuals and Caucasians.[17] Clinically, approximately 75 percent of tumors in one study of Japanese patients showed a brown- to-glossy dark pigmentation.[4] Presence of pigmented BCC may confound clinical differentiation of BCC from other skin lesions, including melanocytic neoplasms. Pigmented BCC represents 50 percent of BCCs in Asians in contrast to six percent in Caucasians.[4] The most common histopathological type of BCC in Asians is the solid (nodular) type similarly seen in Caucasians; however, the incidence of adenoid BCC is relatively higher in Asians and African-Americans compared to Caucasians.[4]

SQUAMOUS CELL CARCINOMA

SCC is the second most common skin cancer in the Chinese and Japanese.[5] SCC in the Chinese was reported to be 2.6 to 2.9 per 100,000 and has decreased 0.9 percent from 1968 to 1997.[3] SCC accounts for 30 percent of all skin cancers in Japan.[4] The male/female ratios for Chinese, Malays, and Asian Indians are 1.5 to 1.9, 1.1 to 6.2, and 0.3 to 0.9, respectively.[5] The annual incidence rates of SCC for Chinese, Malays, and Asian Indians are 2.6, 1.3, and 1.4 per 100,000 persons, respectively.[5] Among males, SCC accounts for 4.3 percent of all cancers in Chinese, 3.1 percent in Malays, and 3.2 percent of cancers in Asian Indians.[5] For SCC a small decline of 0.9 percent per year was noted in contrast to the increased rates seen in other countries, such as Australia and Canada.[5] The incidence of SCC has been reported to be 118 per 100,000 in Caucasian residents of Kauai, Hawaii, and 23 per 100,000 in Japanese residents in Kauai, Hawaii.[4] SCC is the most frequent type of malignant tumor arising in scarred skin.[17–20] According to reports, the fraction of scar carcinoma versus non-scar SCC in Japan is reported to be 31.8 and 44.0 percent, versus 1.9 and 2.5 percent in other countries.[21] In addition, the overall prognosis of scar SCC is less favorable compared to non-scar SCC.[21] The rate of recurrence of scar carcinoma was reported to be 2.53 times higher than that of non-scar SCC, with a metastasis rate ranging from 10 to 100 percent, as compared to one percent in non-scar carcinoma.[22,23] Risk factors for the development of SCC in darkly pigmented individuals are chronic scarring and areas of chronic inflammation. These risk factors have been associated with a greater potential for metastasis and are reported to occur in 20 to 40 percent of cases as compared to 1 to 4 percent in sun-induced SCC in Caucasians.[4] SCCs in Asians have a greater tendency to occur in non sun-exposed sites, with a higher potential for metastasis possibly due to advanced disease stage at the time of diagnosis.[3]

MOLECULAR PATHOGENESIS

Although environmental factors play a significant role in NMSC, molecular components have been implicated in the pathogenesis of this disease. UV-induced DNA damage in keratinocytes causes mutation, promotes the initiation step of carcinogenesis, and triggers the production of interleukin-10 (IL-10), which may contribute to tumor escape from the host immune response.[24] IL-10 production by keratinocytes or tumor infiltration cells may contribute to the immunosuppressive and anti-inflammatory effects allowing the tumor to escape from the immune response.[24] IL-10 expression has been associated with the inhibition of antitumor T-cell immune response leading to tumor growth in both melanoma and NMSC.[1] Reports demonstrate that Japanese have a low incidence of IL-10 expression (0-1%) compared to Caucasians (12-19%).[24] In addition, UV-induced DNA damage is a vital component of cutaneous carcinogenesis by producing alternations in oncogenes and tumor suppressor genes, such as p53 and patched gene, which are responsible for keratinocyte transformation.[25] Apoptosis induced by radiation or other DNA-damaging agents is controlled by the p53 suppressor gene.[26] Loss of p53 tumor suppressor gene function represents the most common genetic alteration identified in human malignancy, occurring in >50 percent of all tumors.[27] Caucasians had a reported incidence of p53 gene mutations of approximately 50 percent in BCC as compared to nine percent in Koreans and 12 percent in Japanese, thus suggesting that reasons other than UV radiation contribute to the pathogenesis of BCC.[28] Studies in Korean patients showed that either dysfunctional p53 or Bcl-2 expressions enhance skin tumor formation by suppressing apoptosis.[28] Results showed that mutations in p53 suppressor genes, BAX genes, or dysfunction of Bcl-2 protein expression could also contribute to the development of BCC.[28] Research suggests that the role of a frameshift mutation of Bax gene could be responsible for BCC formation in Asians.[29] In aggressive SCC in Asians, there have been reports of several indices that correlate with tumor behavior, such as p53 suppressor gene overexpression, decreased expression of E-cadherin and beta- catenin, and Ki-67 LI.[30] Ki-67 LI is considered to be a reliable marker for assessing the growth activity of tumors and is useful for estimating the prognosis of patients.[28] Several studies in Asians demonstrated abnormal or reduced expression of E-cadherin or B-catenin in various carcinomas and the reduction of these markers has been related to the loss of differentiation as well as to tumor invasion and metastasis.[28]

COMPARISON OF ASIANS TO OTHER COUNTRIES

Variations between ethnicities encompass a wide range of Fitzpatrick skin types, sociocultural differences, and inherent genetic variabilities. Studies revealed a three-percent increase in BCC and a 0.9-percent decline in SCC in Singapore, which is lower than other countries with fair- skinned individuals, such as Australia, Canada, and Finland.[30–32] NMSC rates vary according to ethnicities and Fitzpatrick skin types as demonstrated by rates of BCC and SCC among Japanese in Hawaii, which were 1/40 of the rates among Caucasians living in the same geographic areas.[9] In addition, the incidence rates of BCC, SCC, and SCC *in-situ* in the Japanese-American population in Kauai, Hawaii, are 12, 4, and 11 times lower, respectively, as compared to rates in Caucasian Kauaiians.[9] The incidence of BCC is twice as high among ethnic Japanese who live in Kauai, Hawaii, as compared to those living in Japan, possibly due to intense UV exposure and an emphasis on more outdoor activities in Hawaii.[9] In contrast, Caucasian Kauaiians exhibit substantially lower incidence rates of NMSC compared to Caucasian Australians, although many Kauaiians have very active outdoor lifestyles with marked exposure to intense sunlight. When evaluating geographic variability, sun exposure alone does not account for NMSC differences between ethnicities.[33] Some BCC incidence rates are increasing more quickly than SCC rates in some countries, while the reverse is true in other countries.[34] Although people have speculated that changes in sun exposure with a given race can greatly affect NMSC rates, it is important to know that variability exists based on gender, sex, tumor type, and ethnic background.[34]

DISCUSSION

General trends in the numbers of deaths from NMSC in Japan have risen since 1995.[4] It is a misconception that all Asians possess inherent relative protection from NMSC because of their skin type. It seems that NMSC development among Asians varies greatly, and solar UV exposure and Fitzpatrick skin type are useful indices to determine relative risk. Although UV radiation plays an important role in the pathogenesis of NMSC in Asians, there also seems to be other genetic and molecular components at work. It is suggested that individuals with darker skin utilize the same photoprotection precautions as recommended for individuals with lighter skin since immune surveillance is the main protection against the development of many skin malignancies.[35] It is also important to keep in mind that NMSC rates are frequently under-reported and underestimated in the Asian population due to limited resources in many countries. NMSCs in Asians are often associated with greater morbidity and mortality, necessitating increased efforts to assess risk factors in Asian individuals, to encourage periodic self examination and professional evaluation of skin, and to optimize strategies for earlier diagnosis and treatment.

References

1. Armstrong BK, Kricker A. Skin cancer. *Dermatol Clin.* 1995;13:583-594.
2. Gloster HM Jr, Brodland DG. The epidemiology of skin cancer. *Dermatol Surg.* 1996;22:217-226.
3. Ichihashi M, Naruse K, Harada S, et al. Trends in nonmelanoma skin cancer in Japan. *Recent Results Cancer Res.* 1995;139:263-273.
4. Gloster HM Jr, Neal K. Skin cancer in skin of color. *J Am Acad Dermatol.* 2006; 55:741-760.
5. Koh D, Wang H, Lee J, Chia KS, Lee HP, Goh CL. Basal cell carcinoma, squamous cell carcinoma and melanoma of the skin: analysis of the Singapore Cancer Registry data 1968-97. *Br J Dermatol.* 2003;148:1161-1166.
6. Stern RS. The mysteries of geographic variability in nonmelanoma skin cancer incidence. *Arch Dermatol.* 1999;135:843-844.
7. Naruse K, Ueda M, Nagano T, et al. Prevalence of actinic keratosis in Japan. *J Dermatol Sci.* 1997;15:183-187.
8. Ueda M, Matsunaga T, Bito T, Nikaido O, Ichihashi M. Higher cyclobutane pyrimidine dimer and (6-4) photoproduct yields in epidermis of normal humans with increased sensitivity to ultraviolet B radiation. *Photodermatol Photoimmunol Photomed.* 1996;12:22-26.
9. Takemiya M, Ohtsuka H, Miki Y. The relationship between solar keratoses and squamous cell carcinomas among Japanese. *J Dermatol.* 1990;17:342-346.
10. Araki N, Nagano T, Ueda M, et al. Incidence of skin cancers and precancerous lesions in Japanese—risk factors and prevention. *J Epidemiol.* 1999;9:S14-S21.
11. Suzuki T, Ueda M, Naruse K, et al. Incidence of actinic keratosis of Japanese in Kasai City, Hyogo. *J Dermatol Sci.* 1997;16:74-78.
12. Tada M, Miki Y. Malignant skin tumors among dermatology patients in university hospitals of Japan. A statistical survey 1971-1975. *J Dermatol.* 1984;11: 313-321.
13. Nagano T, Ueda M, Suzuki T, et al. Skin cancer screening in Okinawa, Japan. *J Dermatol Sci.* 1999;19:161-165.
14. Ishihara K. Nationwide survey of malignant skin tumors in Japan. *Skin Cancer (Tokyo).* 1994;9:7-14.

15. Chia KS, Seow A, Lee HP, et al. *Cancer Incidence in Singapore 1993-1997. Singapore Cancer Registry Report No. 5.* Singapore: Singapore Cancer Registry; 2000.
16. Fitzpatrick TB. The validity and practicality of sun-reactive skin types I through VI. *Arch Dermatol.* 1998;124:869-871.
17. Harland DL, Robinson WA, Franklin WA. Deletion of the p53 gene in a patient with aggressive burn scar carcinoma. *J Trauma.* 1997;42:104-107.
18. Treves N, Pack G. The development of cancer in burn scars: an analysis and report of thirty-four cases. *Surg Gynecol Obstet.* 1930;51:749-782.
19. Arons MS, Lynch JB, Lewis SR, Blocker TG Jr. Scar tissue carcinoma. I. A clinical study with special reference to burn scar carcinoma. *Ann Surg.* 1965;161: 170-188.
20. Jellouli-Elloumi A, Kochbati L, Dhraief S, Ben Romdhane K, Maalej M. [Cancers arising from burn scars: 62 cases]. *Ann Dermatol Venereol.* 2003;130:413-416.
21. Ueda A, Suda K, Matsumoto T, Uekusa T, Sasahara N. A clinicopathological and Immunohistochemical comparison of squamous cell carcinoma arising in scars versus non-scar SCC in Japanese patients. *Am J Dermatopathol.* 2006;28: 472-477.
22. Eroğlu A, Berberoğlu U, Berreroğlu S. Risk factors related to locoregional recurrence in squamous cell carcinoma of the skin. *J Surg Oncol.* 1996;61:124-130.
23. Crawley WA, Dellon AL, Ryan JJ. Does host response determine the prognosis in scar carcinoma? *Plast Reconstr Surg.* 1978;62:407-414.
24. Nagano T, Kunisada M, Yu X, et al. Involvement of Interleukin-10 promoter polymorphisms in nonmelanoma skin cancers: A case study in non-Caucasian skin cancer patients. *Photochem Photobiol.* 2008;84:63-66.
25. Nishigor C. Cellular aspects of photocarcinogenesis. *Photochem Photobiol Sci.* 2006;5:208-214.
26. Salazar-Onfray F. Interleukin-10: A cytokine used by tumors to escape immunosurveillance. *Med Oncol.* 1999;16:86-94.
27. Hollstein M, Sidranscky D, Vogelstein B, Harris CC. P53 mutations in human cancers. *Science.* 1991;253:49-53.
28. Cho S, Hahma JH, Hong YS. Analysis of p53 and BAX mutations, loss of heterozygosity, p53 and BCL2 expression and apoptosis in basal cell carcinoma in Korean patients. *Br J Dermatol.* 2001;144:841-848.
29. Kubo Y, Urano Y, Yoshimoto K, et al. p53 gene mutations in human skin cancers and precancerous lesions: comparison with immunohistochemical analysis. *J Invest Dermatol.* 1994;102:440-444.
30. Kaldor J, Shugg D, Young B, Dwyer T, Wang YG. Non-melanoma skin cancer: ten years of cancer-registry-based surveillance. *Int J Cancer.* 1993;53:886-891.
31. Gallagher RP, Ma B, McLean DI, et al. Trends in basal cell carcinoma, squamous cell carcinoma, and melanoma of the skin from 1973 through 1987. *J Am Acad Dermatol.* 1990;23:413-421.
32. Hannuksela-Svahn A, Pukkala E, Karvonen J. Basal cell skin carcinoma and other non-melanoma skin cancers in Finland through 1956–1995. *Arch Dermatol.* 1999;135:781-786.
33. Green A, Battistutta D, Hart V, Leslie D, Weedon D. Skin cancer in a subtropical Australian population: incidence and lack of association with occupation. The Nambour Study Group. *Am J Epidemiol.* 1996;144:1034-1040.
34. Stern R. The mysteries of geographic variability in nonmelanoma skin cancer incidence. *Arch Dermatol.* 1999;135:843-844.
35. Stephens T, Oresajo C. Ethnic sensitive skin: a review. *Cosmetics Toiletries.* 1994; 109:75-80.

Skin Cancer in Asians: Part 2: Melanoma

Susun Bellew, DO,[a] James Q. Del Rosso, DO, FAOCD,[b]
and Grace K. Kim, DO[c]

[a]Dermatology Resident (PGY-3), Valley Hospital Medical Center, Las Vegas, Nevada;
[b]Dermatology Residency Director, Valley Hospital Medical Center, Las Vegas, Nevada, and
  Dermatology Research Director, Mohave Skin & Cancer Clinics, Las Vegas, Nevada; and
[c]Dermatology Research Fellow, Mohave Skin & Cancer Clinics, Las Vegas, Nevada

ABSTRACT

The Asian population in the United States is expected to increase in the next 50 years. Concurrently, there is an overall rise in the incidence of melanoma. It is therefore crucial to obtain a better understanding of this deadly skin cancer in this minority population, as little information is currently available and prognosis remains poor. Through a review of the literature, this paper explores melanoma in the Asian population, including the most common subtype encountered, prognosis, theories on pathogenesis, and molecular biology. (J Clin Aesthetic Dermatol. 2009;2(10):34-36.)[*]

The National Cancer Institute estimates that 39,080 men and 29,640 women will be diagnosed with cutaneous melanoma (CM) in 2009.[1] It is further estimated that of those diagnosed with melanoma, 8,650 men and women will die in the United States.[1] The US census bureau projects that the Asian population will triple in the next 50 years.[2] With an overall rise in melanoma and anticipated increases in the Asian population, clinicians and patients alike must be aware of the potential for skin cancer in this minority population. Currently, there is limited available data on skin cancer in Asians, including melanoma.

CM is predominantly an ultraviolet (UV) light-induced skin cancer more commonly associated with light-skinned Caucasians than in individuals with darker skin.[3] Traditionally, clinical features associated with CM included Fitzpatrick skin types I to III with lighter color hair and eyes, an increased tendency to burn, history of multiple nevi, and strong family history of CM.[4] Therefore, it is generally recognized that CM rarely affects individuals of ethnic backgrounds other than Caucasians, including those of Asian, Indian, Hispanic, or African descent. It is believed that greater concentrations of melanin in these darker skin populations provides photoprotective activity against the carcinogenic effects of UV radiation.[3] More specifically, increased levels of melanin in darker skin tones are thought

---

Address Correspondence To: James Q. Del Rosso, DO, FAOCD; E-mail: jqdelrosso@yahoo.com

Disclosure: Drs. Bellew and Kim report no relevant conflicts of interest. Dr. Del Rosso is a consultant, speaker, and/or researcher for Allergan, Coria, Galderma, Graceway, Intendis, Medicis, Onset Therapeutics, Obagi Medical Products, Ortho Dermatology, PharmaDerm, Quinnova, Ranbaxy, SkinMedica, Stiefel, Triax, Unilever, and Warner-Chilcott.
[*]Reproduced with permission from *The Journal of Clinical and Aesthetic Dermatology*.

to allow less damage to deoxyribonucleic acid (DNA) in the lower epidermis, and more effectively prevents proliferation of UV-damaged cells via apoptosis.[3] Consequently, CM in these individuals tends to occur at anatomic locations that are not continually sun-exposed, such as the feet.

MELANOMA SUBTYPES

There are four major histological subtypes of CM. In decreasing order of frequency, they are superficial spreading melanoma (70%), nodular melanoma (15%), lentigo maligna melanoma (13%), and acral lentiginous melanoma (2-3%).[5] Acral lentiginous melanoma (ALM) is a less commonly encountered subtype with a predilection for the palms, soles, subungual region, and mucous membranes.[6] Among these sites, the plantar portion of the foot is the most common area of involvement.[7] Histologically, ALM is characterized by a distinct radial or "lentiginous" growth phase.[6] In contrast to Caucasians, ALM is the most common type of CM seen in deeply pigmented or Asian skin.[5,8] Internationally, epidemiological studies conducted in Japan during 1997 to 2001 found that ALM accounted for 47 percent of all melanomas.[9] A study of 63 Chinese people from Hong Kong diagnosed with CM reported greater than 50 percent were ALM.[10] According to reports examining ALM, the mean age at diagnosis was 62.8 years, with incidence rates increasing with advancing age.[5] Asian and Pacific Islanders exhibited the highest percentage of ALM diagnosis at Stage III.[5]

PROGNOSIS

Unfortunately, prognosis is poor in Asian patients with ALM.[7,11] The five and 10-year survival rates for patients with primary ALM without metastasis is reported to be 80.3 and 67.5 percent, respectively, compared to 91.3 and 87.5 percent, respectively ($p<.001$), for all CMs in the United States.[5] Many variables have been investigated as possible reasons for this grim prognosis. Among these, ulceration and tumor thickness were reported to be among the most significant predictors of outcome.[12,13] In fact, studies have demonstrated that non-Caucasian patients with CM consistently had thicker tumors and had more frequent ulcerations than their non-Hispanic Caucasian counterparts.[14] Such tumors are often detected at a more advanced stage, which subsequently leads to a poorer outcome. Other contributing factors may include the natural aggressive nature of ALM, unusual sites of involvement (palms and soles), and socio-economic status (SES).[15,16] An analysis of the California Cancer Registry database showed that higher SES was associated with earlier stage of tumor on presentation ($p<.0001$) and prolonged survival ($p<.0001$).[15] Further, earlier recognition and diagnosis of CM is a challenging and contributing factor. A retrospective study of plantar melanoma from 1990 to 1997 showed the mean time between initial detection of the skin lesion by the patient and the first visit with a physician was 4.8 years, and on average, an additional seven months would pass before surgical treatment was performed.[17] These results indicate that efforts need to be directed toward decreasing delays in seeking diagnosis and treatment.

PATHOGENESIS

CM is generally associated with increased exposure to UV light. However, with the predominant subtype of melanoma being in acral sites that are infrequently exposed to sunlight, one descriptive study showed no significant association between UV exposure and CM development in Asian populations.[18] This has led investigators to search for other potential causes for the development of CM in non-sun-exposed sites of the body. Previous reports indicate local trauma to acral sites as well as heavy exposure to agricultural chemicals as possible risk factors for ALM development.[19–21] In a case-controlled study of 311 CM patients in Australia and Scotland, authors found a positive association with penetrative trauma of the hands and feet with an adjusted relative risk (RR) of 5.0 and confidence interval (CI) of 3.0 to 8.6.[19] With agricultural chemical exposure the RR was reported to be 3.6 and the CI was 1.5 to 8.3.[19] A study of CM in Taiwan echoed this hypothesis as some of their farming patients worked outdoors without protection of hands and feet and subsequently were subjected to trauma in addition to being exposed to agricultural chemicals.[22] Opponents to the trauma theory state that increased trauma in acral sites is common and that CM may occur coincidentally along with the traumatic event.[23]

MOLECULAR BIOLOGY OF ALM

Molecular pathology reveals a genetically distinct pattern of alteration unique to ALM.[24] First, ALM is shown to have a greater frequency of focal gene amplifications and losses when compared to other melanoma subtypes.[24,25] Secondly, BRAF and NRAS genes encode proteins that are a part of the mitogen-activated protein kinase (MAPK) pathway, which is responsible for the proliferation and differentiation of cells.[26] It is hypothesized that mutations in the BRAF gene may be one of the early events in the pathogenesis of some CMs. In fact, BRAF mutations are seen in two thirds of CM with much of the remainder having NRAS mutations.[26] In contrast, studies indicate that ALM has low frequency of BRAF mutations and high levels of NRAS mutations, although the reasons for this remain unclear.[26] Therefore, recent reports searched for alternative pathways that might mediate tumor formation in ALM. Studies from Taiwan suggest an over expression of Ankyrin repeat-rich membrane spanning (ARMS) as a possible pathogenic mechanism for ALM by inhibiting apoptosis of the cancerous cell via regulation of the MEK/ERK signaling pathway.[27]

DISCUSSION

CM is a relatively rare occurrence in the Asian population compared to fair-skinned populations. Limited data are available on skin cancer in Asians, including information on prevalence rates on CM in different Asian populations. Research shows that ALM is the most common subtype found in Asian populations in the United States as well as in many native Asian countries, such as China and Japan. Asians diagnosed with CM were more likely to have thicker tumors with an advanced disease state at time of presentation ultimately resulting in poorer overall prognosis and greater morbidity and mortality. There is evidence that delays in seeking diagnosis and treatment are major contributing factors. As a result, educational efforts should be put in motion to decrease delays in diagnosis. Skin cancer is no longer attributed solely to fair-skinned individuals with light-colored hair and eyes. Skin cancer has a new face, and that face is multicultural. Increasing awareness about CM in both Caucasian and non-Caucasian populations may facilitate early diagnosis and treatment, and ultimately will save lives.

References

1. National Cancer Institute. Surveillance epidemiology and end result (SEER) STAT fact sheets—melanoma of the skin. http://seer.cancer.gov/statfacts/html/melan.html. Accessed July 2009.
2. US Census Bureau News. More diversity, slower growth. http://www.census.gov/Press-Release/www/releases/archives/population/001720.html. Accessed July 2009.
3. Yamaguchi Y, Beer JZ, Hearing VJ. Melanin mediated apoptosis of epidermal cells damaged by ultraviolet radiation: factors influencing the incidence of skin cancer. *Arch Dermatol Res.* 2008;300:S43-S50.
4. Byrd-Miles K, Toombs EL, Peck GL. Skin cancer in individuals of African, Asian, Latin-American, and American-Indian descent: differences in incidence, clinical presentation, and survival compared to Caucasians. *J Drugs Dermatol.* 2007;6:10-16.
5. Bradford PT, Goldstein AM, McMaster ML, Tucker M. Acral lentiginous melanoma: incidence and survival patterns in the United States, 1986-2005. *Arch Dermatol.* 2009;145:427-434.
6. Reed RJ. *New Concepts in Surgical Pathology of the Skin.* New York, NY: John Wiley & Sons; 1976. 89–90.
7. Cormier JN, Xing Y, Ding M, et al. Ethnic differences among patients with cutaneous melanoma. *Arch Intern Med.* 2006;166:1907-1914.
8. Bristow IR, Acland K. Acral lentiginous melanoma of the foot and ankle: a case series and review of the literature. *J Foot Ankle Res.* 2008;1:11.
9. Ishihara K, Saida T, Otsuka F, Yamazaki N. Statistical profiles of malignant melanoma and other skin cancers in Japan: 2007 update. *Int J Clin Oncol.* 2008;13:33-41.
10. Luk NM, Ho LC, Choi CL, Wong KH, Yu KH, Yeung WK. Clinicopathological features and prognostic factors of cutaneous melanoma among Hong Kong Chinese. *Clin Exp Dermatol.* 2004;29:600-604.
11. Jemal A, Murray T, Ward E, et al. Cancer statistics, 2005. *CA Cancer J Clin.* 2005;55:10-30.
12. Balch C, Soong SJ, Gershenwald JE, et al. Prognostic factors analysis of 17,600 melanoma patients: validation of the American Joint Committee on Cancer melanoma staging system. *J Clin Oncol.* 2001;19:3622-3634.
13. Wells KE, Reintgen DS, Cruse CW. The current management and prognosis of acral lentiginous melanoma. *Ann Plast Surg.* 1992;28:100-103.
14. Hemmings DE, Johnson DS, Tominaga GT, Wong JH. Cutaneous melanoma in a multiethnic population: is this a different disease? *Arch Surg.* 2004;139:968-973.
15. Zell JA, Cinar P, Mobasher M, Ziogas A, Meyskens FL Jr, Anton-Culver H. Survival for patients with invasive cutaneous melanoma among ethnic groups: the effects of socioeconomic status and treatment. *J Clin Oncol.* 2008;26:66-75.
16. Jeffreys M, Sarfati D, Stevanovic V, et al. Socioeconomic inequalities in cancer survival in New Zealand: the role of extent of disease at diagnosis. *Cancer Epidemiol Biomarkers Prev.* 2009;18:915-921.

17. Franke W, Neuman NJ, Ruzicka T, Schulte KW. Plantar malignant melanoma—a challenge for early recognition. *Melanoma Res*. 2000;10:571-576.
18. Eide MJ, Weinstock MA. Association of UV index, latitude, and melanoma incidence in nonwhite populations—US Surveillance, Epidemiology, and End Results (SEER) Program, 1992 to 2001. *Arch Dermatol*. 2005;141:477-481.
19. Green A, McCredie M, MacKie R, et al. A case-control study of melanomas of the soles and palms (Australia and Scotland). *Cancer Causes Control*. 1999;10:21-25.
20. Coleman WP 3rd, Loria PR, Reed RJ, Krementz ET. Acral lentiginous melanoma. *Arch Dermatol*. 1980;116:773-776.
21. Phan A, Touzet S, Dalle S, Ronger-Savlé S, Balme B, Thomas L. Acral lentiginous melanoma: a clinicoprognostic study of 126 cases. *Br J Dermatol*. 2006;155:561-569.
22. Chang JW, Yeh KY, Wang CH, et al. Malignant melanoma in Taiwan: a prognostic study of 181 cases. *Melanoma Res*. 2004;14:537-541.
23. Kaskel P, Kind P, Sander S, Peter RU, Krähn G. Trauma and melanoma formation: a true association? *Br J Dermatol*. 2000;143:749-753.
24. Curtin JA, Fridlyand J, Kageshita T, et al. Distinct sets of genetic alterations in melanoma. *N Engl J Med*. 2005;353:2135-2147.
25. Bastian BC, Kashani-Sabet M, Hamm H, et al. Gene amplifications characterize acral melanoma and permit the detection of occult tumor cells in the surrounding skin. *Cancer Res*. 2000;60:1968-1973.
26. Saldanha G, Potter L, DaForno P, Pringle JH. Cutaneous melanoma subtypes show different BRAF and NRAS mutation frequencies. *Clin Cancer Res*. 2006;12:4499-4505.
27. Liao YH, Hsu SM, Huang PH. ARMS depletion facilitates UV irradiation induced apoptotic cell death in melanoma. *Cancer Res*. 2007;67:11547-11556.

Avoiding the Legal "Blemish": Medicolegal Pitfalls in Dermatology

BRENT D. MICHAELS, DO, JD, JAMES Q. DEL ROSSO, DO, FAOCD,
AND SAIRA B. MOMIN, DO
Valley Hospital Medical Center, Las Vegas, Nevada

ABSTRACT

In today's legal environment, it is unlikely that a physician will complete a medical career without being introduced to the legal system in some way. Despite this, medical education often does not incorporate a basic teaching of general legal principles, and many physicians are left unaware of some of the important legal aspects of practicing medicine. The purpose of this article is to provide a background of the essential legal principles of a malpractice action as well as review the fundamentals of the legal process, provide published caselaw of prior dermatological pitfalls, and ultimately, provide suggestions to better prepare the dermatologist to practice medicine. (*J Clin Aesthetic Dermatol.* 2009;2(12):35-43.)[*]

Throughout the first year of law school, a favorite question of legal professors is, "Can the party sue?" The answer is always the same—yes. Anyone can sue and for just about any reason. Although this may be somewhat of an unrealistic position, the underlying message of this statement should not be overlooked—dermatologists do get sued. Even though dermatologists enjoy lower malpractice rates than many other specialists, they are not exempt from medical malpractice actions. It is therefore essential for dermatologists to become familiar with the basic mechanism of a legal malpractice action and to educate themselves on some of the more common legal pitfalls in practice.

This article addresses the basic concepts of a malpractice action as well as reviews important legal concepts, such as informed consent. In addition, this article discusses actual legal cases that have found both in favor of and against dermatologists and the alleged negligent medical basis of those actions. Finally, suggestion points are provided throughout the article for how practicing dermatologists can better prepare themselves to hopefully avoid a lawsuit.

Address Correspondence To: James Q. Del Rosso, DO, FAOCD; E-mail: jqdelrosso@yahoo.com

Disclosure: Drs. Michaels, Del Rosso, and Momin report no relevant conflicts of interest. Dr. Michaels previously was employed as a Deputy Attorney General for the Nevada Attorney General's Office.

Disclaimer: While informative lessons can be learned from this article, dermatologists who have any legal question or concern should always consult with an attorney before taking any action. Moreover, readers should also be aware that the law and legal standards may not only vary from case to case, but also from jurisdiction to jurisdiction.

[*]Reproduced with permission from *The Journal of Clinical and Aesthetic Dermatology.*

WHAT IS THE PROCEDURAL PROCESS BEHIND A LAWSUIT?

The procedural process of a lawsuit is an area of law often not understood and usually an area that formulates many questions. While this article is not intended to provide the entire nuts and bolts of the legal system, the authors will begin by addressing the basic "skeleton" of the legal process—from filing the complaint to trial.

The conception of a lawsuit starts with the filing of what is known as a complaint. Under the complaint, the plaintiff (patient) will list just that—his or her "complaints," which are referred in legal terms as the plaintiff's "causes of action." Under the causes of action, the plaintiff will also list the allegations and facts that purportedly support his or her claims. Generally, in a negligence malpractice action, a plaintiff has two years to file the complaint from the time the patient knew or should have known of the negligent action, although this timeframe may vary depending on the jurisdiction in which the complaint is filed. If the plaintiff fails to file the complaint within this timeframe, he or she is generally barred from bringing suit against a physician (under the concept of the statute of limitations).

Once the complaint is filed, it often has to be served on the physician within 180 days. Personal service is required on the physician or his or her agent or designee by a process server. After service is properly made, an "answer" will need to be prepared by the physician within 20 days. Thus, expeditious contact should be made with the malpractice carrier so that the complaint can be referred to an attorney for assistance. Once the attorney files the requisite pleadings, a discovery conference will eventually be set, and a discussion of the discovery timeframes will be established as well as the needed discovery modalities. Discovery is a broad term that can be thought of as the time allotted to gather the facts and evidence necessary to support each party's claims and defenses. Discovery includes such items as interrogatories (written questions that are answered by the physician and reviewed by the lawyer), requests for production of documents (a list of documents that the patient would like the physician to provide), and depositions. Depositions are familiar to most, and comprise a series of questions asked by an opposing lawyer to the patient, physician, witness, or expert witnesses under oath—usually conducted at a law office or court reporter's office. During the discovery process, various motions by either party may be filed for a variety of reasons. Once discovery is finalized, the next phase is the trial. From start to finish, a lawsuit can take up to five years or more, although most are generally completed within a shorter timeframe. However, if served, dermatologists should anticipate exercising patience as there is no guarantee of a specific timeframe. Noting that not all jurisdictions are the same, this is a very general overview of the procedural process of a lawsuit.

WHAT COMPRISES THE BASICS OF A NEGLIGENCE MALPRACTICE ACTION?

Most often a dermatologist will be sued for malpractice based on a negligence cause of action. In order for a patient to recover for a negligence action against a dermatologist, four basic elements must be established (and proven by a preponderance of the evidence) in every case. Those elements include the following: 1) a duty owed to the patient; 2) a breach of that duty owed; 3) the breach of the duty owed was the cause (both actual and proximate cause) of the patient's injuries; and 4) the patient must show damages as a result of the physician's actions.

A duty owed to the patient is established by the presence of the physician-patient relationship and the requirements of a physician in this fiduciary relationship. A physician's duty requires that he or she provide the same standard of care as other dermatologists in good standing so as to protect the patient from unreasonable risk or harm. A duty owed can be thought of as the obligation the dermatologist owes to his or her patient to always have the patient's best interest in mind and to utilize the skill and knowledge of a competent dermatologist in implementing services to the patient.

Once a duty owed is established, a breach of the duty must be shown to have existed. A breach stems from a dermatologist failing to perform an action that he or she had a duty to do. In other words, his or her actions fell below the standard of care expected of a competent dermatologist in good standing. A simple example of this is the failure to provide proper informed consent to a patient by not, for instance, disclosing the important risks of a treatment.

In addition, a patient must also show the breach caused the patient's injuries. A way of thinking about causation is that it is not only the actual cause of the patient's injuries (i.e., if the physician had not failed to check the patient's drug allergies, the patient would not have taken the sulfa medication and developed Stevens Johnson Syndrome—SJS), but also the proximate cause of the patient's injuries (i.e., whether the injuries that occurred were "foreseeable" as a result of the physicians actions).

Finally, the patient must show damages. A patient might argue that it was negligent to prescribe a penicillin-based antibiotic because of a noted penicillin allergy in his or her history; however, the patient takes the medication and suffers no adverse reaction. While it may have been a breach of the physician's duty to the patient to provide the antibiotic, no damages ensued and so the patient would likely not have a viable negligence action against the physician.

All of these elements must be proven to sustain a *prima facie* case of negligence. Once a plaintiff has presented evidence to support his or her *prima facie* case, it is up to the dermatologist's lawyer to provide a convincing defense to interrupt any notion by the jury that the allegations have been proven by a preponderance of the evidence.

INFORMED CONSENT

Before some common causes of dermatology mishaps and errors that have introduced dermatologists to the legal system are discussed, informed consent must be addressed. The doctrine of informed consent is a common basis for malpractice lawsuits. In its basic form, the doctrine of informed consent is that a physician will obtain consent from a patient, absent an emergency, before treating or operating on the patient.[1,2] This doctrine implies that it is the duty of a doctor to disclose pertinent information to a patient. The implied consent doctrine can be found under statute in most states. Caselaw is prevalent on this issue.

In Nevada, the lead author's home state, Nevada Revised Statute 41A.110 provides the framework for obtaining informed consent and is likely similar in nature to other states, and thus will be used for discussion. Under Nevada's implied consent statute, medical consent is obtained if the physician has explained to the patient in general terms, without specific details, the procedure to be undertaken, the alternative methods of treatment, and the general nature and extent of the risks involved without enumerating such risks, and the physician has obtained a signature for the same.[3] This statute only provides the general framework for when implied consent has been obtained, but unfortunately, the statute cannot provide specific details as to whether the physician, for example, indeed provided adequate alternative methods of treatment for a malignant melanoma or provided the appropriate risk factors for the procedure in treating this malignancy.

In most jurisdictions, including Nevada, the standard for when informed consent has been established is under a "professional" standard, which states that the physician has a duty to disclose information that a reasonable dermatologist would disclose.[4] This standard must be determined by expert testimony regarding the custom and practice of the particular field.[4] Thus, dermatologists should ensure the patient is adequately informed and uncertainties are discussed.

A good piece of advice for any dermatologist is to take the time to discuss the treatment as well as alternatives and risks/benefits involved in the treatment, then ask the patient if he or she has any questions. While some offices have preprinted forms for procedures, it is important to review these forms to ensure that they contain the necessary elements for informed consent. Dermatologists should not just allow patients to read the form and sign it without explaining the consent form to them and ensuring the patients' questions are answered. After meeting with the patient, the dermatologist should consider documenting in the medical record that the treatment, alternatives, and risks were discussed (in addition to the signed form)—to ensure that he or she in fact reviewed the information with the patient. Although generally not an issue in dermatology offices, a brief assessment should also be made to make certain the patient has the capacity to formulate an informed decision.

A HYPOTHETICAL CASE ILLUSTRATION DEMONSTRATING THE CONCEPT OF NEGLIGENCE AND INFORMED CONSENT

To provide a case illustration of the above concepts, consider a patient who presents to a dermatology office with a history of intravenous (IV) drug abuse. The patient's diagnosis is psoriasis and the patient is interested in tumor necrosis factor alpha (TNF-α) inhibitor treatment after attempting other failed modalities. The first potential pitfall for the physician is failing to review the patient's history. During the history, the physician should check important information, such as the patient's medical history, social history, and drug allergies. In this case, it would reveal that the patient has a history of IV drug abuse—a potential high risk for tuberculosis (TB) infection. Next, a discussion of the risks and benefits and alternative treatments should be discussed. An explanation of the risk of developing disseminated TB in a patient with latent TB when using a TNF-α inhibitor is clearly mandated by a physician's duty to disclose and obtain complete informed consent for treatment.

Next, the physician should offer purified protein derivative (PPD) testing for possible latent TB. The argument in a negligence action would be whether requiring testing for TB before providing TNF-α inhibitor therapy is the standard of care now in dermatology (and thus not providing testing is a breach of the physician's duty). While testing does not currently appear to be written as mandatory in the package inserts for some of the biologic agents used to treat psoriasis, it is recommended when prescribing a TNF-α inhibitor. Testing is also mentioned in a black box warning. Although published caselaw against a physician was not found on the issue of the standard of care, all dermatologists should avoid becoming the named defendant defining this issue. With patients in a high-risk group such as this, dermatologists should consider offering testing not only before treatment, but also yearly to monitor for changes.

What happens to the IV drug-abusing patient who is later found to have disseminated TB and was not offered testing? Aside from the duty of informed consent and TB testing, the other remaining elements are causation and damages. If a plaintiff can show disseminated TB, damages will be proven. The additional question to be answered is whether the TNF-α inhibitor is the proximal cause of the patient's disseminated TB or might the patient have already had disseminated TB prior to therapy. The likely inference in this scenario is not in the physician's favor. Thus, by providing the benefits and risks of treatment and ensuring testing before treatment, the physician not only protects the patient, but also protects his or her interests by establishing the patient's current state of health before treatment as well as assuring that the appropriate medications are given and informed consent obtained. Importantly, all of these precautions will help the physician avoid the rigor of a lawsuit.

WHAT IS THE CURRENT LEGAL ENVIRONMENT OF DERMATOLOGY?

Dermatologists undoubtedly enjoy lower malpractice rates than many other specialties.[5] However, the premiums paid by dermatologists, as with other specialists, have trended upward in past years. In a recent survey, it was noted that premiums increased by 24.4 percent in 2003 and 16.7 percent in 2004.[6] Dermatologists in the past have also been found to avoid the brunt of litigation dollars against physicians. In a study reviewing closed claims against physicians from 1975 to 1978, only 0.7 percent of total paid claims were attributed to dermatologists, even though dermatologists accounted for 1.4 percent of all practicing physicians.[6] To put this in perspective, however, this study was performed before the increase in dermatological cosmetic procedures and the advent of isotretinoin and newer medications, such as biologics.

The Physicians' Insurance Association of America (PIAA) has compiled information on medical claims against dermatologists, among other specialties. According to PIAA data from 1985 to 2001, the most prevalent "medical misadventure" was operative procedures on the skin (289 claims), followed by malignant neoplasms (93 claims) and malignant melanoma (77 claims).[7] The most common medical diagnosis involved in malpractice claims was malignant neoplasms, followed by acne and dyschromia.[8] In addition, in an article by Read and Hill[7] wherein they reviewed both Westlaw and Lexis searches (the major caselaw computerized reporters) of legal cases in combination with jury verdict searches, the authors found that the most common conditions forming the basis of reported claims involved melanoma, followed by malignant neoplasms of the skin, then acne, and cosmetic procedures.[7] Interestingly, adverse reactions to medications only comprised two of the cases found or less than one percent of the total cases. The lead author's review of Westlaw of reported cases in the past five years also revealed the misdiagnosis and treatment of neoplasms as a common basis of lawsuits.

Ultimately, the common trend of these similar litigated issues may simply be due to the larger percentage of these conditions seen in dermatology and thus comprise a larger percentage of the cases filed. The bottom line, however, is that lawsuits against dermatologists tend to involve similar litigated issues of the past. While there is no way to completely avoid lawsuits in dermatology, lessons can certainly be learned from past cases in an attempt to avoid these errors.

PITFALLS AND ERRORS—PUBLISHED CASELAW OF PHYSICIAN MALPRACTICE ACTIONS

Cases involving prescription medications. One of the areas involving potential litigation in medicine involves prescription medications—and dermatology is no exception. Although Read and Hill reported that adverse reactions to oral medications are not a large percentage of the reported legal cases and claims, filed lawsuits over prescription medications have occurred and will likely continue to occur especially in light of future advances in medications, such as biologics and the future litigation over such issues as isotretinoin side effects. As such, a review of prior caselaw involving prescription medication errors is important. The caselaw presented here is provided to illustrate a few of the common medication writing errors, but it is also presented in order to provide insight as to what might be legally expected from a dermatologist when writing prescription medicines.

As a general rule, physicians must exercise reasonable care in prescribing medications. It cannot be emphasized enough that a thorough review of the patient's history be conducted prior to prescribing medications—most notably history, such as pregnancy/last menstrual period and drug allergies. Reviewing patient history might seem obvious, but there is ample caselaw on this issue.[9] It is unlikely a court will sympathize with a physician who writes a prescription medication in ignorance of a patient's listed medication allergy. Not surprisingly, in Baylis,[10] a physician was held liable for an anaphylactic reaction a patient suffered from cephalexin when a prior allergic reaction to cephalexin was written in the chart and the nurse was told by the patient of a penicillin allergy.[10] In Walsted,[11] a physician was found liable for prescribing ampicillin when an allergic reaction to penicillin had been listed in a previous hospital record.[11] Ultimately, if a drug reaction is listed anywhere (from present or past visit) in the chart, the physician will likely be held responsible for any harm. Thus, as most physicians do—all dermatologists should write patient allergies clearly on the front of the chart and ensure that the allergies are updated on every visit.

There are situations in which physicians were able to avoid liability for allergic reactions. In Tangoro,[12] a patient brought suit for developing anaphylactic shock secondary to penicillin. The patient was asked about prior allergies to penicillin, but reported no adverse reactions and appropriately, the court found in favor of the physician. In the case of Regan v. Gore,[13] the patient testified that she verbally informed the physician that she was allergic to sulfa medication. The patient was given a sulfa medication and developed a stroke. However, there was no notation in the chart indicating the patient was allergic to sulfa (only codeine), and the physician and nurse both testified that it was standard practice to document allergies. The court found in favor of the physician noting that given it was the physician's inveterate policy to document allergies to medications and only codeine was written, it was reasonable for the jury to find the patient had only informed the physician about an allergy to codeine and not sulfa.[13] The important suggestion here is to ensure that it is common protocol to document all hypersensitivities/allergies to medications in your practice. Moreover, allergy testing before prescribing medication has been held by at least one court to be unnecessary. In Slack,[14] expert witnesses testified regarding the impracticability of testing for possible drug reactions in advance of treatment and how it is economically unfeasible to test all patients for possible adverse drug reactions.[14] The court held in favor of the physician and found the physician was not negligent for failing to test the plaintiff prior to prescribing the medication.

In addition to allergies, the question has arisen as to what adverse effects a physician has a duty to disclose concerning a prescribed medication. Unfortunately, there is no absolute guideline on this issue. Some cases appear to suggest that the more "rare" or "remote" side effects may not require disclosure by the physician. In Watkins,[15] the patient was prescribed quinacrine (Atabrine, an anti-malarial drug) by his dermatologist for the treatment of discoid lupus erythematosus (DLE).[15] The patient was warned of the possibility of his skin turning yellow, and eventually developed exfoliative dermatitis. On the issue of adequately warning the patient about side effects of the drug, the district court found that "the physician was not required, under recognized standard of acceptable professional practice in medical profession and specialty of dermatology, to warn the patient about rare side effects of the drug and the physician did warn about common side effects." This was supported by the appellate court that further held that "[u]nder the recognized standard in the medical profession and the specialty of dermatology, [the physician] was not required to warn [the patient] about rare side effects including exfoliative dermatitis and erythema multiforme."

In Akers,[16] the patient brought a malpractice action after developing cataracts secondary to the long-term use of potent topical corticosteroids for psoriasis.[16] The appellate court supported the district court's findings in favor of the physician. The court noted that the patient was informed of the material risks involved with the treatment of potent topical corticosteroids, and even though the physician did not warn of the risk of cataracts, the court noted that there was a dispute among the experts as to whether cataracts were a known risk. The court also noted that while there was disagreement regarding the length of use and potency levels, there was expert testimony that the treatment met the standard of care. Further, in Woods,[17] a dermatologist had provided a course of gold injection therapy for DLE. The patient developed jaundice from hepatitis caused by the course of treatment. In finding for the physician, the court noted that through the testimony, it was not the customary standard of practice to inform the patient of all the risks involved, nor to recite the symptoms. Also in Bullock,[18] the patient was prescribed quinacrine (Atabrine) for DLE and developed liver dysfunction. The patient alleged the physician failed to warn of possible liver dysfunction and thus, informed consent was not obtained. The court noted that the patient must prove the risk is inherent in the medical procedure undertaken so as to influence a reasonable person's decision to consent. In finding in favor of the physician, the court found that liver dysfunction was not a material risk of taking quinacrine (Atabrine).

In contrast, the patient in Bowman[19] brought a negligence claim against a dermatologist who prescribed methoxsalen (Oxsoralen, Valeant Pharmaceuticals, Aliso Viejo, California) for a chronic skin condition. The patient, while using Oxsoralen, suffered second- and third-degree burns after being out in the sun too long. It was found that the physician did not warn of the danger of burns with the drug and the package insert as well as the Physician's Desk Reference (PDR) advised of the drug's potential to cause severe burns.

Which adverse effects need to be disclosed depends on the type of medication, and the extent of information required to be disclosed legally may change depending on the jurisdiction in which the dermatologist resides. With the advent of the information superhighway and personal digital assistants (PDAs), an argument can be made that more may be expected of today's physician including informing the patient of the more significant common adverse effects. For example, in a patient taking doxycycline, it would be important to warn of photosensitivity, and with sulfonamide (sulfa) medication, the physician should warn the patient of the risks of SJS and toxic epidermal necrolysis (TEN), but possibly not a remote adverse effect, such as aseptic meningitis, absent any known predisposing condition. The more information the physician gives the patient, the better for both the physician and the patient. Whatever information is required can change from case to case and depends on the requisite standard of care in the jurisdiction.

In emergent situations, some courts found it justified for failing to warn the patient of remote adverse effects. In Shinn,[20] a patient was given phenytoin for seizures and was not warned of the possibility of SJS. The court held that in a life-threatening circumstance in which the treatment administered resulted in adverse affects that were rare, a physician may not be liable for failing to obtain informed consent. In Niblack,[21] a court found in favor of a physician who treated a patient with dexamethasone for pseudotumor cerebri. The patient later developed aseptic necrosis. The physician failed to warn against the possibility of aseptic necrosis. In holding for the physician, the court found that the risk of aseptic necrosis was only a remote possibility in comparison to the immediate likelihood of the patient developing permanent loss of vision or life. With this noted, there are not a vast number of day-to-day dermatological emergencies and thus, in a clinical situation for a nonemergency, care should be taken to warn of potential common and significant adverse effects. The severity of disease and necessity for treatment also has been a reason to excuse a duty to warn of an adverse effect. In Jackson,[22] the patient had a positive PPD test and was given isoniazid (INH) for treatment, but was not told of the risk of possible hepatitis, which the patient later developed. The court found in favor of the physician and noted that a reasonable person in the patient's position would have consented to INH treatment even with the knowledge of the risk of hepatitis.

If a dermatologist decides to utilize a medication for a purpose other than indicated on the manufacturer's package insert or as noted in the PDR, the use of the medication should be viewed as an acceptable application of the medication by competent physicians in the dermatology community. Even if it is common dermatology practice to use a medication in some other manner that is not approved by the US Food and Drug Administration (FDA) and is not provided for by the PDR or package insert and the patient later develops an adverse reaction, it should be noted that some courts have gone as far as to hold that information contained in a PDR or a manufacturer's package insert as *prima facie* evidence of a physician's standard of care.[23] In other jurisdictions, this information is merely some evidence of a physician's standard of care, and in yet another, it has been determined to have no legal significance.[24] In many jurisdictions, however, it is likely that the expert's testimony will be what is relied on to determine the medical community's accepted application of a medication, while a PDR or a manufacturer's package insert, if admitted, will be used as supplemental evidence of this standard. For example, in Morlino,[25] the court found that the PDR did not establish the standard of care in a negligent malpractice action against a physician for prescribing an antibiotic to a pregnant patient; instead, the court found the PDR and package insert could be used as additional evidence only if supported by expert testimony.[25] In Hogle v. Hall,[26] a dermatologist was found liable in district court after prescribing isotretinoin (Accutane) to a pregnant patient.[26] The district court found that the physician had failed to follow guidelines appearing in the PDR for Accutane.

Proper monitoring of adverse effects is also an important issue. This is especially true for dermatological medications. Examples of when dermatologists have found themselves liable have involved drugs such as Accutane and oral and topical corticosteroids. In Cooper,[27] a dermatologist was found to have breached the standard of care when he prescribed dexamethasone (Decadron) for recurrent dishydrotic eczema that was found to be prescribed in excessive doses for excessive periods of time and without appropriate monitoring. The patient eventually developed avascular necrosis that required hip replacement surgery. In Moyer,[28] two consecutive physicians prescribed Accutane to a patient. The patient's triglyceride and cholesterol levels were increased before Accutane was prescribed and had been "high" at only one point after treatment. The patient eventually developed cardiac disease requiring quadruple bypass surgery and sued for malpractice suggesting a negligent connection between the prescribed Accutane and the cardiac disease. The case was ultimately dismissed based on statute of limitations issues, but not before a lengthy lawsuit.

There are several suggestions to reduce risk based on the above caselaw. Several of the suggestions are often commonsense approaches to treating the patient, but unfortunately, are not always carried out. To begin with, dermatologists need to be familiar with common and potentially significant adverse effects of medications. There are not many clinical dermatological emergencies, so some time should be taken to inform patients of potentially common adverse effects before providing the medication. Dermatologists must also always check the patient's history before prescribing a medication for the particulars, such as allergies, pregnancy, and significant past medical history. Such questions, as well as documenting and reviewing the answers, do not take a significant amount of time and should become rote practice. Also, dermatologists must become familiar with routine testing standards for medications and stay ahead of the changes that may be made to those standards. For example, if prescribing a TNF-α inhibitor, perform a PPD not only before treatment, but also consider possibly yearly testing. The patient's expert witness may just testify that this is the standard and a jury may be persuaded by such testimony. Additionally, documentation is important. Although testimony will be provided at trial, it is better to assume that the four corners of the medical record are what will be presented as having occurred during the visit. If, for example, a dermatologist informed a patient about the risks of a medication, the dermatologist should document that he or she in fact did so.

Cases involving diagnosis and treatment of skin disease. As with prescription medications, the lack of informed consent also applies to procedures and is a potential legal snare for dermatologists. The possibility for error can occur in such areas as failing to warn of the risks involved in a procedure, failing to discuss alternatives, and making representations regarding the outcome of a procedure, to name a few.[29] While in a limited review of cases, the jury and courts have been relatively sympathetic to the physician's position, this is not to say dermatologists have never had to compensate a patient for wrongdoing as discussed below.

In regard to failing to warn of the possible risks involved in a procedure, one example is a suit that was brought against a physician whose nurse had caused three disfiguring, permanent scars after draining acne cysts. The jury found that there was no liability even though the physician and nurse failed to obtain proper informed consent regarding the risks of the procedure, since even if the risks were provided, a reasonably prudent person in the patient's position would not have declined the procedure.[30] Nonetheless, even though this physician was able to avoid liability, it is better practice to ensure that the physician sees all patients before a procedure is performed, no matter how trivial it may seem, and ensure that the important risks are explained as well as document what the patient has agreed to.

In addition to failing to enumerate risks, some physicians have been sued for representing more than they could deliver. Cosmetic dermatological procedures are a potentially viable area for these types of errors, but are equally applicable to general dermatological procedures as well. In the Lerner matter, the patient alleged the physician made various representations as to the success of his tattoo- removal procedure, such as "Don't worry. The operation is a simple thing to do."[31] The patient later developed unsightly scars. The physician was found to have described the nature of the operation performed and he testified that he performed the procedure according to the proper and approved practice. The court found in favor of the physician and held the doctor is not a guarantor of good results. The court dismissed the case, without evidence that the doctor guaranteed a good result. However, in Korman,[32] the patient brought a negligence claim against the physician for extreme scarring she developed after breast surgery, despite a consent form signed by the patient acknowledging the risk of scarring and despite the physician discussing on prior visits that the likelihood of scarring was possible.[32] It was noted that when the patient asked about the risks of scarring from her breast reduction surgery, the physician informed the patient not to "worry about it, I've done hundreds of these" and "I think that you'll be happy with the results." Given the findings, the court set aside summary judgment in favor of the physician. The valuable lesson here is to frankly discuss the treatment and risks, but not to minimize a potentially significant risk, even if it is unlikely to occur or is an outcome that has not yet occurred in your practice. Dermatologists should keep within the informed consent form and the risks delineated therein that are acknowledged by the patient. By downplaying the risks or suggesting a guarantee of success, physicians may be perceived as misrepresenting the procedure to induce the patient to undergo the procedure, should a poor result occur.

Cases involving cosmetic dermatological procedures continue to be a common basis for lawsuits. Lawsuits have included matters from fillers to tattoo removals. For example, in Beckwith,[33] a patient brought an action against a physician who used an "infrared coagulator device" for tattoo removal. The patient later developed burns and full-thickness skin necrosis. The patient alleged the physician's use of the infrared coagulator fell below the standard of care and the physician should have instead used an ultra-short pulsed neodymium-doped yttrium aluminium garnet (Nd:YAG) laser. The physician initially prevailed on a motion to dismiss, but the appellate court later reversed the district court order and remanded the matter back for further proceedings. In another cosmetic case, the patient in Osburn[34] brought a medical malpractice action against a physician after the patient sustained facial eruptions and swelling after silicone injections to the face. The above cases are only a few examples of issues that have arisen in cosmetic dermatology. There are, of course, many more cases involving cosmetic matters, and given the rise in cosmetic procedures, it is likely that more malpractice actions involving cosmetic dermatology will continue to present in courts.[35,36]

Physicians have also been exposed to lawsuits for failing to diagnose a skin lesion as well as for issues surrounding treatment decisions. As we previously noted, the most common conditions forming the basis of negligence claims have been malignant neoplasms, including melanoma. In Dible,[37] a physician was sued for erroneously diagnosing a basal cell carcinoma (BCC) as a squamous cell carcinoma (SCC) as well as for failing to inform the patient of a viable alternative to radiation therapy.[37] After diagnosis, the patient was referred for radiation therapy, rather than for what the patient alleged was a safer, more effective alternative therapy—Mohs micrographic surgery. In holding for the physician, the court found that not only did the physician rely on the pathology report from other physicians in making the diagnosis (whose reports did not fall below the standard of care), but that radiation is a recognized therapy for both BCC and SCC.

There are several recent cases involving lawsuits for failing to timely diagnose and treat neoplasms. In Dunn,[38] a dermatologist was sued for not diagnosing an SCC in a timely manner. In Nichols,[39] a physician was sued for removing a "spot" without the lesion being sent for pathology review. The "spot" recurred and another physician diagnosed the condition as melanoma. The key lesson here is any lesion removed should be sent for pathology interpretation. In yet another case, a physician was sued for failing to identify and treat a skin lesion that was thought to be a sebaceous cyst. This "cyst" was found later to be a malignant fibrous histiocytoma.[40] Another case involved a plastic surgeon who was sued for a biopsied lesion that was diagnosed as melanoma *in situ*.[41] The physician had failed to report the findings to the patient after the biopsy results were obtained. The patient never received follow-up care for the malignancy and the patient eventually died a few years later. In Lawrinson,[42] a dermatologist biopsied a lesion that turned out to be a Merkel cell tumor. The results of the biopsy were known before the follow-up visit. On the follow-up visit, the lesion was larger and more erythematous, but on that visit and the subsequent visit, the dermatologist informed the patient the lesion was healing well. By the third visit, the dermatologist indicated he did not know what to do and so the patient went to another dermatologist who sent the patient for surgery. The patient had most of the left side of his face removed. In total, the patient was subject to approximately a two-month delay before the surgery. The patient argued that this delay resulted in a much larger portion of the face being removed and undergoing radiation treatment. The physician argued lack of causation as the patient would have had to undergo the same treatment even if treatment was begun two months prior. The appellate court agreed with the jury's determination in support of the patient, noting that the patient likely suffered more injury due to the delay, than if he would have had surgery two months earlier.

In regard to choice of treatment options, the courts have ruled in support of dermatologists in several opinions when choosing which treatment to employ for a dermatological condition. In Akers,[16] the court found in favor of a dermatologist who used long-term potent topical corticosteroids in the treatment of psoriasis. The court determined that although there was a disagreement regarding the length of use of the potent topical corticosteroid, there was expert testimony to establish that the treatment met the accepted standard of care. In Thompson,[43] a dermatologist was sued for using cryosurgery for skin cancer on the patient's nose on separate occasions over an 11-month period. Despite the cryosurgery treatment, the condition worsened and eventually resulted in the loss of the patient's nose, which required reconstructive surgery. The court found, through the expert's testimony, that the use of cryosurgery was not inappropriate and even though a better alternative may have been employed, ruled in favor of the dermatologist. In Roberts,[44] the court found in favor of the physician who had treated the patient at three months of age for a capillary hemangioma on the cheek with dry ice to the lesion. The patient eventually developed scar tissue. The court found that there was no medical evidence that the treatment administered was in any manner improper, and that the treated lesion, even though having healed with scarring, healed in the usual and expected manner. In yet another matter involving a physician's proper selection of treatment, a physician was sued for removing a capillary hemangioma surgically rather than simply monitoring the lesion.[45] The patient was an infant and developed a capillary hemangioma on the side of the leg near the knee. The physician determined that surgery was appropriate as the lesion had steadily grown and was ulcerating. After surgery, the patient eventually developed extensive scarring along the leg. The patient's expert testified that the physician performed the surgery unnecessarily. Ultimately, the case was found to be a "battle of the experts" and the jury resolved the conflict in favor of the physician.

Poor performance in the carrying out of a procedure has subjected a dermatologist to a negligence judgment where the dermatologist dropped acid on healthy tissue while attempting to remove warts, and the patient suffered burns and scarring.[46] In Machacek,[47] a dermatologist treated a wart on the eyelid of a patient with topical cantharidin-podophyllin liquid. The patient later developed a 40-percent corneal abrasion/chemical burn. The patient sued alleging that the dermatologist should have referred the patient to a specialist because the removal of a wart on the lid margin was outside the physician's area of expertise. The patient also sued the physician for using cantharidin-podophyllin liquid on the face despite warnings from the manufacturer and for allowing the medication to get into the patient's eye. The jury found in favor of the dermatologist and determined her care did not fall below the applicable standard of care. In Hines,[48] a patient sued for negligence on the basis of the removal of a dermatofibroma. The patient argued that an excessive amount of skin was removed during a surgical excision, which resulted in highly visible scarring. This case was also resolved in favor of the dermatologist.

There are several observations to be gained based on the above cases. Again, dermatologists must properly inform their patients of the treatment, the alternatives, and risks involved. For example, if cryotherapy is to be used, the dermatologist needs to inform the patient of potential hypopigmentation or hyperpigmentation without attempting to minimize the risks or guarantee a better outcome than is absolutely certain. Also, dermatologists need to correlate their pathology findings with their clinical findings. If there is some question regarding the diagnosis, dermatologists should not hesitate to obtain an additional pathology reading before implementing treatment. On the other hand, if the diagnosis is certain and requires timely action, dermatologists should not unnecessarily delay treatment or wait for a future follow- up visit that may be scheduled months later. They should make efforts to ensure the patient is seen in an approprtiate timeframe. If a patient cannot come to the office for any reason or the patient creates the delay, the dermatologist must document this as well as his or her attempt to reach the patient, for this may be considered a factor for contributory negligence on the part of the patient should a lawsuit arise. Further, dermatologists must understand the various treatment modalities and ensure that they are within the dermatology community standards. A dermatologists must also always review the patient's chart, including past medical history (such as cardiac history), allergies, pregnancy, social history, and current medications (such as recent antibiotics and anticoagulation therapy), to avoid overlooking simple, but potentially important and dangerous consequences. Moreover, the physician must document his or her interaction with the patient, including diagnosis and treatment. If the patient refuses a course of treatment or is nonadherent with medication or follow-up visits, the dermatologist should document those encounters in a professional manner. Finally, although the details are outside the purview of this article, physicians who manage their own practices must take the time to become reasonably familiar with the basics of the law governing healthcare and business practice, as it not only relates to patients, but also to employees. Dermatologists should familiarize themselves with Medicare changes, the Health Insurance Portability and Accountability Act (HIPPA), the Family Medical Leave Act (FMLA), the Fair Labor Standards Act (FLSA), Title VII (dealing with discrimination/harassment issues), the American with Disabilities Act (Titles I and III), and the Age Discrimination in Employment Act (ADEA). Seminars are often given on these areas of law and contacting the local State Bar Office in your community is a good place to start to find this information.

Finally, there is an abundance of medicolegal issues that cannot all be addressed in the framework of this article. Moreover, the issues that have been may not only vary from case to case, but also state to state. The only certainty is that the law is ever changing. Thus, as always, dermatologists who have any legal questions or concerns, should consult an attorney before taking action.

CONCLUSION

Many dermatologists will become familiar with the legal process during their careers. Dermatologists should become familiar with the law and keep current on the trending legal issues involving not only dermatologists, but also physicians in general. Knowledge of the law and of prior litigated issues is a good way to avoid becoming the party to a suit. Dermatologists should always keep current on the advances in dermatology and always keep the best interests of the patient in mind. These simple rules will prove beneficial to any dermatologist attempting to avoid the legal system.

References

1. 61 Am Jur 2d, Physicians, Surgeons and Other Healers §§152-161 (1981).
2. Frantz LB. Annotation, Modern status of views as to general Measure of physician's duty to inform patient of risks of proposed treatment. *Am Law Rep ALR 3rd Cases Annot.* 1978;88:1008-1044.
3. Nev Rev Stat §41A.110.
4. *Smith v Cotter*, 107 Nev 267, 810 P2d 1204 (1991).
5. Resneck JS Jr. Trends in malpractice premiums for dermatologists: results of a national survey. *Arch Dermatol.* 2006;142:337-340.
6. Altman J. The National Association of Insurance Commissioners (NAIC) Medical Malpractice Closed Claim Study 1975-1978. A review of dermatologic claims. *J Am Acad Dermatol.* 1981;5(6):721-725.
7. Read S, Hill HF 3rd. Dermatology's malpractice experience: clinical settings for risk management. *J Am Acad Dermatol.* 2005;53:134-137.
8. Elston DM, Taylor JS, Coldiron B. Patient safety: Part I. Patient safety and the dermatologist. *J Am Acad Dermatol.* 2009;61:179-190.
9. Linda A. Sharp, Annotation, Malpractice: Physician's Liability for Injury or Death Resulting from Side Effects of Drugs Intentionally Administered to or Prescribed for Patient, 47 A.L.R.5th 433 (1997).
10. *Bayles v Lourdes Hospital, Inc.*, 805 SW2d 122 (Ky 1991).
11. *Walstad v University of Minnesota Hospitals*, 442 F2d 634 (8th Cir 1971).
12. *Tangoro v Matansky*, 231 Cal App 2d (2nd Dist 1964).
13. *Regan v Gore*, 670 So2d 268 (La App 3d Cir 1996).
14. *Slack v Fleet*, 242 So2d 650 (La App 1970).
15. *Watkins v United States*, 482 F Supp 1006 (MD Tenn 1980).
16. *Akers v Levitt*, Ohio App LEXIS 300 (Ohio App. 1992).
17. *Woods v Pommerening*, 44 Wash2d 867, 271 P2d 705 (1954).
18. *Bullock v Sasso*, Tex App LEXUS 602 (1998).
19. *Bowman v Songer*, 820 P2d 1110 (Colo 1991).

20. *Shinn v St. James Mercy Hospital*, 675 F Supp 94 (WD NY 1987).
21. *Niblack v United States*, 438 F Supp 383 (DC Colo 1977).
22. *Jackson v State*, 428 So2d 1073 (La App 1983).
23. *Mulder v Parke Davis & Co.*, 181 NW2d 882 (Minn 1970).
24. *Ramon v Farr*, 770 P2d 131 (Utah 1989); *Grassis v Retik*, 521 NE2d 411(1988).
25. *Morlino v Medical Center of Ocean County*, 12 NJ 563, 706 A2d 721 (1998).
26. *Hogle v Hall*, 112 Nev 599, 916 P2d 814(1996).
27. *Cooper v Bronx Cross County Medical Group*, 259 AD2d 410, 687 NYS2d 156 (1999).
28. *Moyer v Three Unnamed Physicians from Marion County and Delaware County, Indiana*, 845 NE2d 252 (2006).
29. Jay M. Zitter, Annotation, Malpractice in Treatment of Skin Disease, Disorder, Blemish, or Scar, 19 A.L.R.5th 563 (1994).
30. *Hoffson v Orentreich*, 543 NYS2d 242 (1989).
31. *Lerner v Huber*, 139 NYS2d 549 (1955).
32. *Korman v Mallin*, 858 P2d 1145 (Alaska 1993).
33. *Beckwith v White*, 285 SW2d 56 (2009).
34. *Osburn v Goldman*, 603 SE2d 695 (2004).
35. Orentreich D, Jones D. Liquid injectable silicone. In: Carruthers J, Carruthers A, eds. *Soft Tissue Augmentation*. Philadelphia, PA: Saunders Elsevier; 2005:78-91.
36. Nev Rev Stat § 202.248.
37. *Dible v Vagley*, 612 A2d 493 (1992).
38. *Dunn v Schultz*, 873 NYS2d 233 (2008).
39. *Nichols v Gross*, 653 SE2d 747 (2007).
40. *Zemaitis v Spectrum Health*, 2006 WL 890064 (Mich App).
41. *Cochran v Bowers*, 617 SE2d 563 (2005).
42. *Lawrinson v Bartruff*, 600 So2d 22 (1992).
43. *Thompson v Griffith*, Tenn App LEXIS 791(1988).
44. *Roberts v Gale*, 139 SE2d. 272 (1964).
45. *Dabros v Wang*, 611 NE2d 1113 (1993).
46. *Reichert v Barbera*, 601 So2d 902 (1992).
47. *Machacek v Cole*, 2005 WL 1738728 (Minn App).
48. *Hines v Silos-Badalamenti*, 2006 WL 2933944 (NJ Super AD).

Statistics of Interest to the Dermatologist

MARTIN A. WEINSTOCK, MD, PhD, AND MARGARET M. BOYLE, BS
Brown University Dermatoepidemiology Unit, Providence, Rhode Island

Morbidity and Mortality

Table 1 Reportable Infectious Diseases, United States
Table 2 HIV/AIDS: Geographic Distribution
Table 3 AIDS: Cumulative Cases, United States
Table 4 Deaths from Selected Causes, United States
Table 5 Cancer Incidence, United States
Table 6 Melanoma: Incidence and Mortality, United States
Table 7 Melanoma: Five-Year Relative Survival
Table 8 Contact Dermatitis, Belgium

Health Care Delivery in the United States

Table 9 Dermatology Trainees
Table 10 Diplomates of the American Board of Dermatology
Table 11 Physicians Certified in Dermatologic Subspecialties
Table 12 Dermatologic Outpatient Care
Table 13 Health Insurance Coverage
Table 14 Health Insurance Coverage by Family Income
Table 15 Health Maintenance Organization Market Penetration
Table 16 National Health Expenditures
Table 17 Expenditure for Consumer Advertising of Prescription Products, United States

Miscellaneous

Table 18 American Academy of Dermatology Skin Cancer Screening Program
Table 19 Leading Dermatology Journals

TABLE 1.—New Cases of Selected Reportable Infectious Diseases in the United States

	1940	1950	1960	1970	1980	1990	2000	2010*
AIDS	***	***	***	***	***	41,595	40,758	34,247**
Anthrax	76	49	23	2	1	0	1	0
Congenital Rubella	***	***	***	77	50	11	9	0
Congenital Syphilis	***	***	***	***	***	3,865	529	213
Diphtheria	15,536	5,796	918	435	3	4	1	0
Gonorrhea	175,841	286,746	258,933	600,072	1,004,029	690,169	358,995	280,555
Hansen's Disease	0	44	54	129	223	198	91	57
Lyme Disease	***	***	***	***	***	***	17,730	27,895
Measles	291,162	319,124	441,703	47,351	13,506	27,786	86	61
Plague	1	3	2	13	18	2	6	2
Rocky Mountain Spotted Fever	457	464	204	390	1,163	651	495	155
Syphilis (primary and secondary)	***	23,939	16,145	21,982	27,204	50,223	5,979	12,164
Toxic-Shock Syndrome (staphylococcal)	***	***	***	***	***	322	135	73
Toxic-Shock Syndrome (streptococcal)	***	***	***	***	***	***	***	155
Tuberculosis#	102,984##	121,742##	55,494	37,137	27,749	25,701	16,377	11,181
U.S. Population (millions)	132	151	179	203	227	249	281	309

Key:
*For 52 weeks ending January 1, 2011. Case counts for reporting year 2010 are provisional and subject to change.
**Estimated numbers resulted from statistical adjustment that accounted for reporting delays, but not for incomplete reporting. U.S. subtotal (not dependent areas).
***Data not available.
#Reporting criteria changed in 1975.
##Data include newly reported active and inactive cases.

Sources:
Centers for Disease Control and Prevention: Summary of Provisional Cases of Notifiable Diseases, United States, 2010. *Morbidity and Mortality Weekly Report* 59(52):1704-1717, 2011.
Centers for Disease Control and Prevention: *HIV Surveillance Report, 2009.* Vol. 21. Atlanta: U.S. Department of Health and Human Services, Centers for Disease Control and Prevention, Division of HIV/AIDS Prevention, National Center for HIV/AIDS, Viral Hepatitis, STD, and TB Prevention, February 2011. http://www.cdc.gov/hiv/topics/surveillance/resources/reports/.
Centers for Disease Control and Prevention: Trends in Tuberculosis, United States 2010. *Morbidity and Mortality Weekly Report* 60(11):333-337, 2011.
U.S. Census Bureau, Population Division: Preliminary Annual Estimates of the Resident Population for the United States, Regions, States, and Puerto Rico: April 1, 2000 to July 1, 2010. Release Date: February, 2011.
Centers for Disease Control and Prevention: Summary of Notifiable Diseases, United States, 2000. *Morbidity and Mortality Weekly Report* 49(518&52):1167-1174,2001.
Centers for Disease Control and Prevention: Annual Summary 1994:Reported morbidity and mortality. *Morbidity and Mortality Weekly Report* 1994:43(53):(70-71].
Centers for Disease Control and Prevention: Annual Summary 1984:Reported morbidity and mortality. *Morbidity and Mortality Weekly Report* 33:124-129, 1986.

TABLE 2.—Estimates of HIV/AIDS, 2009

Region	Adults and Children Living with HIV	Adults and Children Newly Infected with HIV	Adult Prevalence (15-49 years) (%)	AIDS-Related Deaths Among Adults and Children
Sub-Saharan Africa	20.9-24.2 million	1.6-2.0 million	4.7-5.2	1.1-1.5 million
Middle East and North Africa	400,000-530,000	61,000-92,000	0.2-0.3	20,000-27,000
South and South-East Asia	3.7-4.6 million	240,000-320,000	0.3-0.3	230,000-300,000
East Asia	560,000-1.0 million	48,000-140,000	0.1-0.1	25,000-50,000
Oceania	50,000-64,000	3,400-6,000	0.2-0.3	<1,000-2,400
Central and South America	1.2-1.6 million	70,000-120,000	0.4-0.6	43,000-70,000
Caribbean	220,000-270,000	13,000-21,000	0.9-1.1	8,500-15,000
Eastern Europe and Central Asia	1.3-1.6 million	110,000-160,000	0.7-0.9	60,000-95,000
Western and Central Europe	720,000-910,000	23,000-40,000	0.2-0.2	6,800-19,000
North America	1.2-2.0 million	44,000-130,000	0.4-0.7	22,000-44,000
Total	33.3 million	2.6 million	0.8%	1.8 million
	31.4-35.3 million	2.3-2.8 million	0.7-0.8	1.6-2.1 million

Source:
Global Report: UNAIDS Report on the Global AIDS Epidemic, 2010, Joint United Nations Programme on HIV/AIDS (UNAIDS) World Health Organization (WHO), 2010.

TABLE 3.—AIDS Cases by Age Group and Exposure Category, and Cumulative Totals Through 2009, United States

	2008 Estimated** No.	Totals 2009 Estimated** No.	Cumulative* Estimated** No.
Male adult or adolescent exposure category			
Male-to-male sexual contact	16,469	17,005	529,908
Injection drug use	3,303	3,012	186,318
Male-to-male sexual contact and injection drug use	1,706	1,580	77,213
Heterosexual contact	3,949	3,832	72,183
Other***	185	158	12,744
SUBTOTAL	25,612	25,587	878,366
Pediatric exposure category (<13 years at diagnosis)			
Perinatal	35	12	8,640
Other****	5	1	807
SUBTOTAL	40	13	9,448
TOTAL#	34,755	34,247	1,108,611

Key:
*From the beginning of the epidemic through 2009.
**Estimated numbers resulted from statistical adjustment that accounted for reporting delays, and missing risk-factor information, but not for incomplete reporting.
***Includes hemophilia, blood transfusion, perinatal exposure, and risk factor not reported or identified.
****Includes hemophilia, blood transfusion, and risk factor not reported or identified.
#Because column totals for estimated numbers were calculated independently of the values for the subpopulations, the values in each column may not sum to the column total.
Source:
Centers for Disease Control and Prevention: *HIV Surveillance Report*, 2009;Vol. 21. Atlanta: U.S. Department of Health and Human Services, Centers for Disease Control and Prevention, Division of HIV/AIDS Prevention, National Center For HIV/AIDS, Viral Hepatitis, STD, and TB Prevention. February, 2011. http://www.cdc.gov/hiv/topics/surveillance/resources/reports/.

TABLE 4.—Selected Causes of Death, United States, 1997, 2007, and 2008*

Cause of Death	Number of Deaths 1997	2007	2008
Malignant melanoma	7,238	8,461	8,643
Infections of the skin	870	1,834	**
Motor vehicle traffic accidents	42,340	42,031	**
Accident involving animal being ridden	76	101	**
Accidental drowning and submersion	3,561	3,443	3,549
Victim of lightning	58	46	**
Homicide and legal intervention	19,846	18,773	18,217
All cancer	539,577	562,875	566,137
All causes	2,314,245	2,423,712	2,472,699

Key:
*Data for 2008 are preliminary.
**The preliminary number of deaths for this cause is not available.
Source:
National Center for Health Statistics, Division of Vital Statistics, personal communication, June, 2011.

TABLE 5.—Annual Percent Change in Cancer Incidence in the United States

Top 20 Highest Incidence Sites	Annual Percent Change 1992–2008	1975–1991
Thyroid	5.6	0.8
Liver and Intrahepatic Bile Duct	3.4	3.0
Melanoma of the skin	2.6	3.7
Kidney and Renal Pelvis	2.4	2.4
Pancreas	0.7	−0.2
Non-Hodgkin Lymphoma	0.5	3.6
Hodgkin Lymphoma	0.3	0.4
Esophagus	0.2	0.7
Urinary Bladder	0.1	0.6
Myeloma	0	1.2
Corpus Uteri	0	−2.1
Leukemia	−0.1	0.1
Brain and Other Nervous System	−0.3	1.2
Breast	−0.4	2.2
Lung and Bronchus	−0.8	1.5
Oral Cavity and Pharynx	−0.9	−0.6
Ovary	−1.1	0.0
Stomach	−1.5	−1.5
Colon and Rectum	−1.5	−0.1
Prostate	−1.5	4.9
All sites	−0.4	1.3

Notes:
SEER 9 registries.
Rates are per 100,000 and age-adjusted to the 2000 US Standard Population (19 age groups–Census P25-1130) standard. Rates are for invasive cancers only.
Sources:
Surveillance Research Program, National Cancer Institute SEER*Stat Software (www.seer.cancer.gov/seerstat) version 7.0.4.

Surveillance, Epidemiology, and End-Results (SEER) Program, (www.seer.cancer.gov) SEER*Stat Database: Incidence-SEER 18 Regs+ Arizona Indians, November 2010 Sub (1990-2008 varying)<Katrina/Rita Population Adjustment> Linked to County Attributes–Total U.S., 1969-2009 Counties, National Cancer Institute DCCPS, Surveillance Research Program, Cancer Statistics Branch, released January 2011, based on the November 2010 submission.

Howlader N, Noone AM, Krapcho M, Neyman N, Aminou R, Waldron W, Altekruse SF, Kosary CL, Ruhl J, Tatalovich Z, Cho H, Mariotto A, Eisner MP, Lewis DR, Chen HS, Feuer EJ, Cronin KA, Edwards BK (eds). SEER Cancer Statistics Review, 1975-2008, National Cancer Institute. Bethesda, MD, http://seer.cancer.gov/csr/1975-2008/, based on November 2010 SEER data submission, posted to the SEER web site, 2011.

TABLE 6.—Melanoma Incidence and Mortality Rates, United States

Year	Incidence*	Mortality**
1973	6.8	1.9
1974	7.2	2.1
1975	7.9	2.1
1976	8.2	2.2
1977	8.9	2.3
1978	9.0	2.3
1979	9.6	2.4
1980	10.5	2.3
1981	11.1	2.4
1982	11.2	2.5
1983	11.1	2.5
1984	11.4	2.5
1985	12.8	2.6
1986	13.3	2.6
1987	13.7	2.6
1988	12.9	2.6
1989	13.7	2.7
1990	13.8	2.8
1991	14.6	2.7
1992	14.8	2.7
1993	14.6	2.7
1994	15.6	2.7
1995	16.4	2.7
1996	17.3	2.8
1997	17.7	2.7
1998	17.9	2.8
1999	18.3	2.6
2000	18.9	2.7
2001	19.6	2.7
2002	19.2	2.6
2003	19.4	2.7
2004	20.5	2.7
2005	22.2	2.7
2006	21.8	2.7
2007	21.4	2.7
2008	22.5	—

Key:
—Data not available.
*SEER 9 areas. Rates are per 100,000 and are age-adjusted to the 2000 US Standard population (19 age groups- Census P25-1130) standard.
**National Center for Health Statistics public use data file for the total US. Rates per 100,000 and age-adjusted to the 2000 U.S. standard population. (19 age groups – Census P25-1130) standard.
Sources:
Surveillance Research Program, National Cancer Institute SEER*stat Software (www.seer.cancer.gov/seerstat) version 7.0.3.
Surveillance, Epidemiology, and End-Results (SEER) Program, (www.seer.cancer.gov) SEER*Stat Database: Incidence-SEER 9 Regs Research Data, November 2010 Sub (1973-2008)<Katrina/Rita Population Adjustment> Linked to County Attributes–Total U.S.,1969-2009 Counties, National Cancer Institute DCCPS, Surveillance Research Program, Cancer Statistics Branch, released April 2011, based on the November 2010, submission.
Surveillance, Epidemiology, and End-Results (SEER) Program, SEER* Stat Database:Mortality-All COD, Total US (1969-2007)<Katrina/Rita Population Adjustment>-Linked to County Attributes–Total U.S., 1969-2007 Counties, National Cancer Institute DCCPS, Surveillance Research Program, Cancer Statistics Branch, released May 2010. Underlying mortality data provided by the National Center for Health Statistics (www.cdc.gov/nchs).
Howlader N, Noone AM, Krapcho M, Neyman N, Aminou R, Waldron, W, Altekruse SF, Kosary CL, Ruhl J, Tatalovich Z, Cho H, Mariotto A, Eisner MP, Lewis DR, Chen HS, Feuer EJ, Cronin KA, Edwards BK (eds). *SEER Cancer Statistics Review: 1975-2008,* National Cancer Institute. Bethesda, MD, http://seer.cancer.gov/csr/1975-2008/, based on November 2010 SEER data submission posted to the SEER website, 2011.

TABLE 7.—Melanoma Five-Year Relative Survival

Year	Whites	Blacks
By Year at Diagnosis		
1960-63*	60%	—
1970-73*	68%	—
1975-77+	82%	58%
1978-80+	83%	60%
1981-83+	83%	62%
1984-86+	86%	70%
1987-89+	88%	79%
1990-92+	89%	62%
1993-95+	90%	68%
1996-2000+	92%	73%
2001-2007+	93%	73%
By Stage at Diagnosis (2001-2007)**		
Local	98%	94%
Regional	62%	41%
Distant	15%	25%

Key:
—Insufficient data.
*Rates are based on the End Results data from a series of hospital registries and one population-based registry.
+Rates are from the SEER 9 registries. Rates are based on follow-up of patients into 2008.
**Rates are from the SEER 17 registries. Rates are based on follow-up of patients into 2008.
Notes:
Relative survival is the observed survival divided by the survival expected in a demographically similar subgroup of the general population.
Survival estimates among blacks are imprecise due to small numbers of cases observed.
Source:
Howlader N, Noone AM, Krapcho M, Neyman N, Aminou R, Waldron, W, Altekruse SF, Kosary CL, Ruhl J, Tatalovich Z, Cho H, Mariotto A, Eisner MP, Lewis DR, Chen HS, Feuer EJ, Cronin KA, Edwards BK (eds). *SEER Cancer Statistics Review: 1975-2008,* National Cancer Institute. Bethesda, MD, http://seer.cancer.gov/csr/1975-2008/, based on November 2010 SEER data submission posted to the SEER website, 2011.

TABLE 8.—Contact Dermatitis in Belgium: Proportion of Positive Patch Tests to Standard Chemicals in 261 Patients With at Least 1 Positive Reaction (Among 479 Patients Tested in 2010)

1.	Nickel sulphate	39.5%
2.	Fragrance mix I	19.6%
3.	Fragrance mix II	15.0%
4.	Paraphenylenediamine	13.0%
5.	Cobalt chloride	11.4%
6.	Balsam of Peru	11.2%
7.	Colophonium	9.8%
8.	Wool alcohols	7.1%
9.	Potassium dichromate	7.0%
10.	Methyl(chloro)isothiazolinone	6.7%
11.	Hydroxyisohexyl-3-cyclohexene carboxaldehyde	6.7%
12.	Methyldibromo glutaronitrile	5.9%
13.	Thiuram mix	4.7%
14.	Formaldehyde	4.0%
15.	Budesonide	3.5%
16.	Tixocortol pivalate	2.8%
17.	Isopropyl-phenylparaphenylenediamine	2.8%
18.	Mercapto mix	2.4%
19.	Mercaptobenzothiazole	2.4%
20.	Epoxy resin	2.0%
21.	Benzocaine	2.0%
22.	Paratertiarybutylphenol-formaldehyde resin	1.6%
23.	Neomycin sulphate	1.2%
24.	Sesquiterpene lactone mix	1.2%
25.	Quaternium-15	0.8%
26.	Primin	0.4%
27.	Clioquinol	0.0%
28.	Paraben mix	0.0%

(From Goossens A., University Hospital, Katholieke Universiteit Leuven, Belgium, personal communication, January 2011.)

TABLE 9.—Dermatology Trainees in the United States

Year Residency to be Completed	Male Residents	Female Residents	Unknown	Total
MD Programs				
2011	144	258		402
2012	144	249		393
2013	157	248		405
2014	4	8		12
2015		1		1
DO Programs				
2011	11	25		36
2012	13	17	2	32
2013	14	26		40

Source:
American Academy of Dermatology, personal communication, April, 2011.

TABLE 10.—Diplomates Certified by the American Board of Dermatology from 1933-2010

Decade Totals (Inclusive Dates)	Average Number Certified per Year
1933–1940	69
1941–1950	74
1951–1960	76
1961–1970	112
1971–1980	247
1981–1990	271
1991–2000	295
2001–2010	340
TOTAL 1933 through 2010	14,719

Individual Year Totals	Actual Number Certified
1999	286
2000	283
2001	305
2002	309
2003	307
2004	329
2005	352
2006	319
2007	342
2008	377
2009	385
2010	379

Source:
The American Board of Dermatology, Inc., personal communication, March, 2011.

TABLE 11.—Physicians Certified in Dermatologic Subspecialties

A. Physicians Certified for Special Qualification in Dermatopathology, 1974-2010
Average Number Certified Per Year

Year	Dermatologists	Pathologists	Total
1974–1975	108	44	302
1976–1980	54	49	515
1981–1985	37	34	351
1986–1990	11	14	125
1991–1995	20	20	196
1996–2000	14	32	227
2001–2005	15	46	306
2006–2010	31	49	403
Actual Number Certified			
2006	32	37	69
2007	26	50	76
2008	27	54	81
2009	28	51	79
2010	41	57	98
Total Number Certified 1974 through 2010	1124	1304	2428

B. Dermatologists Certified for Special Qualification in Clinical and Laboratory Dermatological Immunology, 1985-2010

Year	Number Certified
1985	52
1987	16
1989	22
1991	15
1993	5
1997	5
2001	6
Total 1985 through 2010	121

C. Dermatologists Certified for Special Qualification in Pediatric Dermatology

Year	Number Certified
2004	90
2006	41
2008	31
2010	33
Total 2004 through 2010	195

Notes:
No special qualification examination for Dermatopathology was administered in 1992, 1994, and 1996.
No special qualification examination in Clinical and Laboratory Dermatological Immunology was administered in 1986, 1988, 1990, 1992, 1994, 1995, 1996, 1998, 1999, 2000, or since 2002.
Special qualification in Pediatric Dermatology began in 2004. No special qualification examination in Pediatric Dermatology was administered in 2005, 2007 or 2009.
Source:
American Board of Dermatology and American Board of Pathology, personal communication, March, 2011.

TABLE 12.—Visits to Non-Federal Office-Based Physicians in the United States, 2008

	Type of Physician Dermatologist Number of Visits (1000's)	Percent	Other Number of Visits (1000's)	Percent	All Physicians Number of Visits (1000's)	Percent
Diagnosis						
Acne vulgaris	3,985	11.6	*	*	5,330	0.6
Eczematous dermatitis	2,284	6.6	6,483	0.7	8,767	0.9
Warts	1,608	4.7	2,162	0.2	3,770	0.4
Skin cancer	2,429	7.1	1,809	0.2	4,239	0.4
Psoriasis	1,660	4.8	*	*	2,008	0.2
Fungal infections	*	*	1,997	0.2	2,375	0.3
Hair disorders	736	2.1	*	*	1,295	0.1
Actinic keratosis	3,547	10.3	*	*	4,046	0.4
Benign neoplasm of the skin	2,566	7.4	*	*	3,326	0.4
All disorders	34,483	100.0	921,486	100.0	955,969	100.0

*Figure suppressed due to small sample size.
Figures may not add to totals because of rounding.
Source:
Centers for Disease Control and Prevention, National Center for Health Statistics, 2008 National Ambulatory Medical Care Survey, personal communication, March, 2011.

TABLE 13.—Health Insurance Coverage of the United States Population, 2009

	Children 1-17 Years	Adults 18-64 Years	Adults 65 Years and Over
Individually Purchased Insurance	5%	6%	27%
Employment-based Coverage	56%	59%	34%
Public Insurance, All types	37%	21%	94%
Medicaid	34%	17%	9%
No Health Insurance	10%	19%	2%

Note:
Some individuals have both public and private insurance, so the numbers will not add to 100%.
Sources:
Fronstin P, "Sources of Health Insurance and Characteristics of the Uninsured: Analysis of the March 2010 Current Population Survey." *EBRI Issue Brief,* No. 347. Employee Benefit Research Institute, Washington DC, September, 2010.
DeNavas-Walt, Carmen, Bernadette D. Proctor, and Jessica C. Smith, U.S. Census Bureau, Current Population Reports, P60-238, *Income, Poverty, and Health Insurance Coverage in the United States: 2009.* U.S. Government Printing Office, Washington, DC, 2010.

TABLE 14.—Nonelderly Population With Selected Sources of Health Insurance, by Family Income, 2009

Yearly Family Income Level	Employment-Based Coverage %	Individually Purchased %	Public %	Uninsured %	Total %
under $10,000	11	4	49	36	100
$10,000-$19,999	17	5	45	35	100
$20,000-$29,999	34	6	34	31	100
$30,000-$39,999	50	6	26	25	100
$40,000-$49,999	61	7	20	19	100
$50,000-$74,000	72	7	14	15	100
$75,000 and over	84	7	8	8	100
Total	59	6	21	19	100

Note:
Details may not add to totals because individuals may receive coverage from more than one source.
Source:
Fronstin P, "Sources of Health Insurance and Characteristics of the Uninsured: Analysis of the March 2010 Current Population Survey." *EBRI Issue Brief,* No. 347. Employee Benefit Research Institute, Washington DC, September, 2010.

TABLE 15.—Health Maintenance Organization (HMO) Market Penetration in the United States, July 1, 2010

HMO Penetration in Region

Pacific	39%
Northeast	30%
Mid-Atlantic	30%
Mountain	22%
East North Central	21%
South Atlantic	21%
West North Central	14%
East South Central	13%
West South Central	11%

HMO Penetration Top Ten Most Highly Penetrated Metropolitan Statistical Areas

Vallejo-Fairfield, CA	70%
Sacramento-Arden-Arcade-Roseville, CA	57%
Santa Rosa-Petaluma, CA	57%
Madison, WI	55%
Leominster-Fitchburg-Gardner, MA	55%
Oakland-Fremont-Hayward, CA	54%
Worcester, MA-CT	54%
Napa, CA	54%
Honolulu, HI	53%
Stockton, CA	52%

Source:
2010 HealthLeaders-Interstudy Publications, *Managed Care Census,* Nashville, TN, personal communication, May, 2011.

TABLE 16.—National Health Expenditure Amounts: Selected Calendar Years

Spending Category	1980	1990	(Billions of Dollars) 2000	2005	2008	2019*
Total National Health Expenditures	246	696	1,310	1,983	2,339	4,483
Health Services and Supplies	234	670	1,262	1,852	2,181	4,170
Personal Health Care	215	609	1,138	1,655	1,952	3,709
Hospital Care	102	254	417	608	718	1,375
Professional Services	67	217	425	622	731	1,371
Physician and Clinical Services	47	158	289	422	496	882
Other Professional Services	4	18	39	56	66	124
Dental Services	13	32	61	86	101	180
Other Personal Health Care	3	10	37	62	68	185
Nursing Home and Home Health	20	65	126	178	203	400
Home Health Care	2	13	32	53	65	154
Nursing Home Care	18	53	94	125	138	246
Retail Outlet Sale of Medical Products	26	73	171	276	300	564
Prescription Drugs	12	40	122	217	234	458
Other Medical Products	14	33	49	59	66	106
Durable Medical Equipment	4	11	18	24	27	43
Other Non-Durable Medical Products	10	23	31	36	39	63
Program Administration and Net Cost of Private Health Insurance	12	40	81	145	160	320
Government Public Health Activities	7	20	44	59	69	140
Investment	12	26	48	139	158	313
Research+	6	13	29	42	44	91
Structures and Equipment	7	14	19	98	114	222

Key:
*Projected values. The health spending projections were based on the 2008 version of the National Health Expenditures (NHE) released in January, 2010.
+Research and development expenditures of drug companies and other manufacturers and providers of medical equipment and supplies are excluded from research expenditures. These research expenditures are implicitly included in the expenditure class in which the product falls, in that they are covered by the payment received for that product.
Note:
Numbers may not add to totals because of rounding.
Source:
Centers for Medicare and Medicaid Services, Office of the Actuary, March, 2011.

TABLE 17.—Spending on Consumer Advertising of Prescription Products, United States

Year	(Annual Dollars in Millions)
2010	4,174
2009	4,571
2008	4,412
2007	4,905
2006	4,745
2005	4,132
2004	4,084
2003	3,082
2002	2,514
2001	2,479
2000	2,150*
1999	1,590
1998	1,173
1997	844
1996	595
1995	313
1994	242
1993	165
1992	156
1991	56
1990	48
1989	12

*Estimated.
Source:
Kantar Media, Copyright 2011. Magazine Publishers of America, Inc., personal communication, April, 2011.

TABLE 18.—Results of the American Academy of Dermatology Skin Cancer Screening
Program 1985-2010

Year	Number Screened	Basal Cell Carcinoma	Suspected Diagnosis Squamous Cell Carcinoma	Malignant Melanoma
1985	32000	1056	163	97
1986	41486	3049	398	262
1987	41649	2798	302	257
1988	67124	4457	474	435
1989	78486	6266	761	593
1990	98060	7959	1069	872
1991	102485	8110	1193	1062
1992	98440	8403	1280	1054
1993	97553	7067	1068	2465*
1994	86895	6908	1235	1010
1995	88934	7503	1317	1353
1996	94363	8713	1656	1399
1997	99554	8730	1685	1469
1998	89536	6687	1308	1078
1999	89916	5790	1136	635
2000	65854	5074	1053	653
2001	70562	5192	1102	642
2002	64492	4733	1009	692
2003	70692	4481	1032	489
2004	71243	4891	1165	760
2005	82532	5659	1411	794
2006	85272	6354	1649	876
2007	90484	6193	1852	883
2008	88249	5746	1739	749
2009	92977	6179	1928	906
2010	92996	6329	2152	957
Total	2,081,834	154327	31137	22442

Key:
*Number of cases included melanoma, "rule out melanoma," and lentigo maligna.
Source:
American Academy of Dermatology: *2010 Skin Cancer Screening Statistics*, March, 2011.

TABLE 19.—Leading Dermatology Journals

Journal	Total Citations in 2009	Number of Articles Published in 2009	Impact Factor
Journal of Investigative Dermatology	20245	269	5.5
Journal of the American Academy of Dermatology	17472	251	4.1
British Journal of Dermatology	17207	373	4.3
Archives of Dermatology	11875	152	4.8
Contact Dermatitis	5413	82	3.6
Dermatologic Surgery	5080	279	2.3
International Journal of Dermatology	4631	239	1.2
Dermatology	4524	135	2.7
Burns	4075	166	2.0
Acta Dermato-Venereologica	3556	76	3.0
Clinical and Experimental Dermatology	3279	381	1.6
Journal of the European Academy of Dermatology	3090	168	2.8
Journal of Cutaneous Pathology	2858	220	1.5
American Journal of Dermatopathology	2508	139	1.3
Experimental Dermatology	2503	126	3.2
Pigment Cell Melanoma Research	2362	55	4.3
Archives of Dermatological Research	2304	90	1.8
Wound Repair and Regeneration	2293	100	2.8
Journal of Dermatological Science	2173	88	3.7
Pediatric Dermatology	2156	193	1.0
Mycoses	1886	71	1.4
Clinical Dermatology	1849	71	3.1
Cutis	1838	82	1.0
Journal of Dermatology	1824	93	1.0
Melanoma Research	1779	56	2.1

Source:
Journal Citation Reports Web Version 2009:JCR, Science Edition, June, 2010, Philadelphia: Thomson Reuters. March, 2011.

CLINICAL DERMATOLOGY

1 Urticarial and Eczematous Disorders

5-Methoxypsoralen plus ultraviolet (UV) A is superior to medium-dose UVA1 in the treatment of severe atopic dermatitis: a randomized crossover trial

Tzaneva S, Kittler H, Holzer G, et al (Med Univ of Vienna, Austria)

Br J Dermatol 162:655-660, 2010

Background.—Ultraviolet (UV) A1 and psoralen plus UVA (PUVA) are effective treatment options for severe atopic dermatitis (AD); however, their relative efficacy has not yet been determined in a head-to-head study.

Objectives.—To compare UVA1 and oral 5-methoxypsoralen (5-MOP) plus UVA with respect to efficacy, tolerability and duration of response in patients with severe generalized AD.

Methods.—Forty patients were included in this randomized observer-blinded crossover trial. The patients received either 15 exposures to medium-dose UVA1 as the first treatment and, in cases of relapse, another 15 exposures to 5-MOP plus UVA as the second treatment, or vice versa. All patients were followed until 12 months after discontinuation of the last treatment. The SCORAD score was determined by a blinded investigator at baseline, after 10 and 15 treatments each and during the follow-up period. In addition, all adverse events were recorded during the whole study period.

Results.—Twenty-three patients completed the crossover treatment. Both phototherapies resulted in clinical improvement; however, PUVA reduced the baseline SCORAD score to a significantly greater extent than UVA1 (mean ± SD 54·3 ± 25·7% vs. 37·7 ± 22·8%; $P = 0·041$). The median length of remission was 4 weeks (interquartile range 4−12) after UVA1 and 12 weeks (interquartile range 4−26) after PUVA therapy ($P = 0·012$).

Conclusions.—PUVA provides a better short- and long-term response than medium-dose UVA1 in patients with severe AD.

▶ This study demonstrates the superior efficacy of psoralen plus ultraviolet A (PUVA) therapy with 5-methoxypsoralen over UVA1 in the treatment of atopic dermatitis. Because UVA1 and narrow-band UVB are felt to be equally efficacious, one can assume that if a patient fails narrow-band UVB, the next step of therapy would be PUVA. Unfortunately, in the United States, 8-methoxypsoralen has not been available for an extended period of time. This fact argues strongly in favor of legalizing the reimportation of unavailable drugs by United States manufacturers.

E. A. Tanghetti, MD

A 6-month follow-up study of 1048 patients diagnosed with an occupational skin disease
Mälkönen T, Jolanki R, Alanko K, et al (Finnish Inst of Occupational Health (FIOH), Helsinki, Finland; et al)
Contact Dermatitis 61:261-268, 2009

Background.—Occupational skin diseases (OSDs) often have considerable medical and occupational consequences. Previous data on prognostic factors have been derived from studies with fairly small sample sizes.

Objectives.—To determine the medical and occupational outcome in 1048 patients diagnosed with OSD at the Finnish Institute of Occupational Health and to identify the prognostic risk factors for the continuation of OSD.

Methods.—Patients examined in 1994–2001 filled out a follow-up questionnaire 6 months after the diagnosis. Data on atopy, contact allergies, and occupation were analysed.

Results.—Six months after the diagnosis the skin disease had healed in 27% of the patients. The OSD had cleared up in 17% of those with no changes at work, and in 34% of those who had changed their job/occupation. The best clearing had occurred in the patients with contact urticaria (35%), whereas the healing of allergic (27%) and irritant (23%) contact dermatitis was similar. The risk factors for continuing occupational contact dermatitis (OCD) were no changes in work, age >45 years, food-related occupations, respiratory atopy, and male sex.

Conclusions.—The healing of OSD was associated with discontinuation of the causative exposure. A change in work and the presence of easily avoidable work-related allergies were associated with a good prognosis.

▶ Occupational skin diseases (OSDs) can severely debilitate people. This is a study examining risk factors and prognostic factors in 1048 patients diagnosed with OSD in 1994-2001 with follow-up questionnaires 6 months post-diagnosis. Results revealed that 85% of patients had hand dermatitis. The diagnosis was based on clinical examination, patch test, and prick test results. The 3 main diagnoses that patients were required to have were allergic contact dermatitis (ACD) confirmed by patch testing, irritant contact dermatitis (ICD), and contact urticaria (CU). Patients were not allowed to have multiple diagnoses, which could have affected the results since patients may have concomitant ACD and ICD. Contact allergy was detected more in 85% of women and in 65% of men. During the 6-month follow-up, one-fourth of the patients had been on sick leave because of their skin disease. Patients with chromate allergy and those in food exposure-related jobs were most frequently on sick leave.

After the 6-month follow-up, the healing of OSD was considerably worse in patients who continued without any change in their work (17% healed) compared with those who changed work (33% healed). The risk factors for continuing OSD were no change in work, age > 45 years, food exposure-related occupations, respiratory atopy, and male gender. Limitations to this study were that it was performed in a single institution and a patient's recall bias for completion of questionnaires. There was also a short 6-month follow-up period. Also, different countries have different restrictions on contact allergens in the work place, and global multicenter studies in different countries are needed to examine the risk and prognosis of OSD. To add, this study only examined occupation-related allergens and did not consider possible allergen exposure at home or in other nonwork locations as inciting agents to OSD. In conclusion, change in work and avoidance of work-related allergens correlated with better prognosis.

J. Q. Del Rosso, DO

G. K. Kim, DO

A randomized controlled trial in children with eczema: nurse practitioner vs. dermatologist
Schuttelaar MLA, Vermeulen KM, Drukker N, et al (Univ of Groningen, the Netherlands)
Br J Dermatol 162:162-170, 2010

Background.—We hypothesized that a nurse practitioner would improve the quality of life of a child with eczema more than a dermatologist because of a structured intervention and more consultation time.

Objectives.—To compare the level of care by nurse practitioners with that by dermatologists in children with eczema.

Methods.—New referrals aged ≤ 16 years with a diagnosis of eczema were recruited. In a randomized, parallel-group study with a follow-up period of 1 year, 160 participants were randomized either to conventional care from a dermatologist or to care from a nurse practitioner. The primary outcome measure was change in quality of life at 12 months, as assessed by the Infants' Dermatitis Quality of Life Index (IDQOL) for children aged ≤ 4 years, and by the illustrated version of the Children's Dermatology Life Quality Index (CDLQI) for children aged 4—16 years. Secondary outcomes were changes in IDQOL and CDLQI at 4 and 8 months, family impact of childhood atopic dermatitis (Dermatitis Family Impact Questionnaire, DFI), eczema severity (objective SCORAD) and patient satisfaction (Client Satisfaction Questionnaire-8, CSQ-8) at 4, 8 and 12 months.

Results.—The mean IDQOL in the dermatologist group improved significantly from 11·6 [SD 8·1; 95% confidence interval (CI) 9·0—14·2] at the baseline to 5·6 (SD 3·9; 95% CI 4·3—7·0) at 12 months with a mean change from the baseline of −6·5 (SD 6·6; 95% CI −14·2 to

$-8 \cdot 9$; $P < 0 \cdot 001$). The mean IDQOL in the nurse practitioner group improved significantly from $10 \cdot 7$ (SD $4 \cdot 9$; 95% CI $9 \cdot 1 - 12 \cdot 3$) at baseline to $5 \cdot 7$ (SD $5 \cdot 4$; 95% CI $4 \cdot 0 - 7 \cdot 5$) at 12 months with a mean change from the baseline of $-4 \cdot 9$ (SD $5 \cdot 5$; 95% CI $-6 \cdot 8$ to $-3 \cdot 0$; $P < 0 \cdot 001$). The between-groups difference was $(-)1 \cdot 7$ (95% CI $-4 \cdot 6$ to $1 \cdot 2$; $P = 0 \cdot 26$). The mean CDLQI in the dermatologist group improved significantly from $12 \cdot 1$ (SD $6 \cdot 3$; 95% CI $9 \cdot 9 - 14 \cdot 2$) at baseline to $5 \cdot 6$ (SD $4 \cdot 2$; 95% CI $4 \cdot 2 - 7 \cdot 1$) at 12 months with a mean change from the baseline of $-5 \cdot 9$ (SD $6 \cdot 0$; 95% CI $-8 \cdot 0$ to $-3 \cdot 9$; $P < 0 \cdot 001$). The mean CDLQI in the nurse practitioner group improved significantly from $10 \cdot 0$ (SD $4 \cdot 4$; 95% CI $8 \cdot 5 - 11 \cdot 4$) at the baseline to $4 \cdot 9$ (SD $3 \cdot 5$; 95% CI $3 \cdot 7 - 6 \cdot 1$) at 12 months with a mean change from the baseline of $-5 \cdot 2$ (SD $4 \cdot 0$; 95% CI $-6 \cdot 6$ to $-3 \cdot 8$; $P < 0 \cdot 001$). The between-groups difference was $(-)0 \cdot 7$ (95% CI $-3 \cdot 3$ to $1 \cdot 7$; $P = 0 \cdot 55$). The between-groups comparison was not significant for the IDQOL and the CDLQI at baseline or 4, 8 and 12 months. Both treatment groups showed significant improvement in DFI and objective SCORAD at 12 months. The between-groups comparison was not significant at baseline or 4, 8 and 12 months. Significantly higher satisfaction levels were observed at 4, 8 and 12 months in the nurse practitioner group.

Conclusions.—The level of care provided by a nurse practitioner in terms of the improvement in the eczema severity and the quality of life outcomes was comparable with that provided by a dermatologist. In addition, the parents were more satisfied with the care that was provided by a nurse practitioner.

▶ With essentially every article, there is going to be a bias by an author that the reader needs to evaluate critically. With an article written by nurse practitioners (NPs) to evaluate practice performance compared with a physician specialist, the first paragraph should ideally set a positive tone for a common goal in approaching patient care. Instead, this article opens with this inflammatory generalization: "The dermatologist focuses primarily on the diagnosis and treatment and does not have enough time for the education of children and parents managing eczema. Moreover, dermatologists are not necessarily very good at assessing the degree of disability that patients experience because of their eczema." When I read a general statement like this, even though it is referenced from an obscure article from 2002, I take a step back and ask if that applies to me and my colleagues simply because this article is making global statements from a narrow focus of exposure.

In a true clinical setting, where the nursing staff or physician extender is just as involved with the patients' well-being as the clinician, it seems hard to believe that most dermatologists are simply throwing prescriptions at our patients with eczema without taking into consideration how much quality of life is affected. But then, are we truly asking how many sleepless nights from scratching there are or what the patient has had to sacrifice, such as swimming? I am not sure an advanced nursing degree separates a medical assistant from taking a similar history, but it does not compare with the fundamental science of immunology and pharmacology that dermatology training provides to benefit the patient, hardly an education that an NP is given in training from nursing school. Nor is the assumption that dermatologists focus on diagnosis and treatment and not on other aspects of patient management substantiated.

Of course, later in the article, it is disclosed that the source of the funding for the article came from The Healthcare Efficiency Research Programme of the University Medical Center, Groningen in the Netherlands. So now we have a purpose for the propaganda and self-promotion expressed by this article, especially when we read, "The aim of the NP is to reinforce the belief in the parents' own abilities with regard to controlling the eczema by teaching and counseling parents to collect systematically information on the eczema symptoms of their child, to interpret the severity and course of the eczema based on this information and to start ointment therapy according to these symptoms (self-control)."

In addition, the focus of the article presents itself to be a justification to substitute NPs for dermatologists to contain health care costs. Paradoxically, even though at lower costs "the time investment by the NP is almost twice that by the dermatologist," which is a point that hardly signals efficiency, the authors point to the salary costs for the dermatologist, which they state are about 3 times as high as those for the NP. In a socialized health care environment such as the Netherlands, costs might be more of a concern compared with quality of care. But when the author states, "Although the salary costs of the NPs are lower, NPs may order more tests and use other services more, which in turn may reduce such possible cost savings..." then we have to question the validity of the point.

Is it the goal of the author to reprimand dermatologists for doing an incomplete job and threaten replacement by publishing a biased study on quality and efficiency? Or are we not doing enough for our patients and using our own time and ancillary staff to educate patients with eczema on more than just the application of therapy? This is up to the reader to decide, but the concept of possible replacement of dermatologists by physician extenders with less training definitely need not be ignored. Unfortunately, the author chose to introduce a theme of competition rather than cooperation among health care providers to best serve patients, which, independent of nationality, will not resonate well with all readers and is based on accusation without substantiation.

N. Bhatia, MD

A study of matrix metalloproteinase expression and activity in atopic dermatitis using a novel skin wash sampling assay for functional biomarker analysis
Harper JI, Godwin H, Green A, et al (Great Ormond Street Hosp for Children, London UK; et al)
Br J Dermatol 162:397-403, 2010

Background.—Atopic dermatitis (AD) is a chronic inflammatory skin condition that is characterized by a defective skin barrier. Despite the well-recognized role of proteases in skin barrier maintenance, relatively little is known of the contribution made by matrix metalloproteinases (MMPs) to the inflammatory process in AD.

Objectives.—To test a simple, novel *ex vivo* bioassay technique in an analysis of the MMPs present in wash samples taken from the skin surface of patients with AD.

Methods.—Saline wash samples were collected from eczematous and unaffected areas of the skin of patients with AD and from the skin of normal controls. Wash samples were analysed for their MMP content using a functional peptide cleavage assay, gelatin zymography and an antibody array.

Results.—Using a functional substrate cleavage assay, skin wash samples from AD lesions were shown to contain 10- to 24-fold more MMP activity than those from normal control skin ($P < 0 \cdot 02$) and fivefold more than those from unaffected AD skin ($P < 0 \cdot 05$); this activity was inhibited by a broad-spectrum MMP inhibitor Ro 31-9790. Gelatin zymography and antibody array analysis revealed substantial levels of MMP-8 (neutrophil collagenase) and MMP-9 (92-kDa gelatinase) in AD skin wash samples as well as lower levels of MMP-10 (stromelysin 2) and tissue inhibitor of metalloproteinases (TIMP)-1 and TIMP-2; low levels of MMP-1 (fibroblast collagenase), MMP-3 (stromelysin 1) and TIMP-4 were also detected.

Conclusions.—A simple skin wash technique suitable for the quantitative and functional analysis of biomolecules in AD is described. Using this method we show that MMPs, and in particular MMP-8 and MMP-9, represent an important potential component of the pathology of AD. The method is expected to prove useful in advancing our understanding of AD and in identifying biomarkers for the evaluation of new therapies.

▶ Atopic dermatitis (AD) is a multifactorial disease that is now being recognized as a disease of skin barrier. Matrix metalloproteinases (MMPs) have been associated with inflammation, and their expression with inflammatory cells has been well established. However, the link between AD and MMP upregulation or downregulation has not been evaluated. This is a study of 15 patients with AD and 17 normal controls, with saline wash samples collected from eczematous and unaffected areas. In a comparative analysis, active AD lesions, unaffected AD skin, or normal control samples showed significantly more activity in active lesions when compared with non-AD skin or control samples. Skin wash samples from AD lesions contained 10- to 24-fold more activity of specific MMPs as compared with normal control skin ($P < .02$) and 5-fold more than those from unaffected AD skin ($P < .05$). This study revealed that MMP-8 (neutrophil collagenase) and MMP-9 were increased 22-fold and 26-fold, respectively, and dominate a mixture of MMPs that are detectable on the skin surface in acute AD. There was also a small (< 2-fold) increase in the levels of MMP-1 and MMP-3 (stromelysin 1). There was no difference in MMP-2 or MMP-13 (collagenase 3) observed in this study. Limitations of this study include the following: (1) it was a single-center study and (2) other skin conditions of patients were not discussed. Although MMP-8 and

MMP-9 were significantly elevated in this study, these MMPs may also be elevated in other skin conditions, suggesting a possible bystander effect as opposed to participation in the pathogenesis of AD. They may also have other functions in the skin that are still not revealed and may not be specific to AD flares. However, specific MMP elevations may be a marker for certain cascades of inflammation and may have clinical implications, which can be targeted by certain medications.

J. Q. Del Rosso, DO

G. K. Kim, DO

Allergenic potential of *Arnica*-containing formulations in *Arnica*-allergic patients
Jocher A, Nist G, Weiss JM, et al (Univ Med Ctr Freiburg, Germany; Hosp Bad Cannstatt, Germany; Univ of Ulm, Germany; et al)
Contact Dermatitis 61:304-306, 2009

Contact allergies to *Arnica* are usually attributed to sesquiterpene lactones (SL), which may also have some anti-inflammatory properties (1,2). *Arnica* allergies are either induced by contact with *Arnica* flowers, with other SL-containing Compositae species, or with a particular *Arnica*-containing topical preparation. The question arises whether sensitization to *Arnica* is detectable by a commercially available *Arnica* patch test formulation or it is explained by the SL within it. To address this issue we performed patch tests in patients with a previously documented *Arnica* allergy with commercial *Arnica* patch test preparations, topical pharmaceutical preparations containing *Arnica*, or pure *Arnica*-specific SL.

▶ The *Arnica* plant is occasionally allergenic, and extracts used in topical skin-care formulations may also cause allergic contact dermatitis (ACD). Sesquiterpene lactones (SLs) in plants of the Compositae family, including *Arnica*, are a family of substances that are often responsible for ACD. It would be helpful for clinicians to be able to patch test (PT) to a few SLs for screening and identify allergy to Compositae plants, instead of having to test to a multitude of separate, individual plants. This report discusses 8 patients with positive PTs to various *Arnica* components who are retested to a panel of SLs and 7 *Arnica* extracts. Unfortunately, there was a wide variability in reactions to the various allergens. The commercial PT material for *Arnica* produced by 1 German company (Hermal) and ether extracts from the *Arnica* flower were the best screening allergens, but both failed to react in 3 of the 8 subjects. When ACD resulting from Compositae plants, including *Arnica*, is suspected, testing with a wide range of commercial allergens and actual plant materials gives the greatest accuracy.

J. F. Fowler, Jr, MD

Association of the *toll-like receptor 2* A-16934T promoter polymorphism with severe atopic dermatitis

Oh D-Y, Schumann RR, Hamann L, et al (Institut für Mikrobiologie und Hygiene, Berlin, Germany; et al)
Allergy 64:1608-1615, 2009

Background.—Atopic dermatitis (AD) is a chronic inflammatory skin disease with a multifactorial pathogenesis and increasing incidence in the Western world. A genetically determined defective function of pattern recognition receptors such as toll-like receptors (TLRs) has been proposed as a candidate mechanism in the pathogenesis of AD.

Aim.—To study the impact of genetic predisposition of five genes encoding for pattern recognition-related molecules for the phenotype of AD.

Methods.—We examined nine different single-nucleotide polymorphism (SNP) frequencies in the genes encoding TLR1, -2, -4, -9 and the adapter molecule TIRAP by PCR with subsequent melting curve analysis in a case-control cohort of 136 adult AD patients and 129 age and gender matched non-atopic, healthy individuals. TLR2-expression and -function in cells from genotyped individuals were analysed.

Results.—For the SNPs examined, similar genotype frequencies were found in both groups. In a subgroup of patients suffering from severe AD (SCORAD > 50), a significantly increased representation of the A-allele in position -16934 of the *tlr2* gene was present ($P = 0.004$). Constitutive *tlr2* mRNA expression in peripheral monocytes was independent of this *tlr2* promoter SNP. Stimulation assays indicated that IL-6, but not TNF-α secretion following TLR2 stimulation is reduced in homozygous *tlr2*-16934-A allele carriers.

Conclusion.—These data indicate that TLR2 is relevant for the phenotype of severe AD in adults.

▶ Cytokine release and inflammation are in part regulated by the activation of toll-like receptors (TLRs) located on the cell surface. The effect of single-nucleotide polymorphisms (SNPs) of *tlr* genes on the development of certain inflammation-mediated conditions (ie, asthma, hay fever, and rhinoconjunctivitis) has been studied. This study noted that an increased frequency of the A-allele (instead of the normal T) in position 16934 of the *tlr2* gene was found in patients with severe atopic dermatitis (AD). The secretion of interleukin 6 (IL-6) was also increased in those with the A-allele at position 16934. This study is important as it may have discovered a protective role of the T-allele at position 16934 of *tlr2* against the development of severe forms of AD. The pathogenesis of AD is multifactorial, and this study provides innovative information regarding the genetic alterations that may underlie the condition.

B. Berman, MD, PhD

Contact allergy to allergens of the TRUE-test (panels 1 and 2) has decreased modestly in the general population

Thyssen JP, Linneberg A, Menné T, et al (Univ of Copenhagen, Hellerup, Denmark; Univ of Copenhagen, Denmark; et al)
Br J Dermatol 161:1124-1129, 2009

Background.—The prevalence of contact allergy in the general population is nearly 20%.

Objectives.—This study aimed to monitor the development of contact allergy to allergens from the TRUE-test (panels 1 and 2) between 1990 and 2006.

Methods.—Two random samples of adults from the general population in Copenhagen, Denmark, were invited to participate in a general health examination including patch testing. In 1990 and 2006, we patch tested and questioned 543 and 3460 adult Danes. Patch test readings were performed on day 2 only.

Results.—The overall prevalence decreased significantly from $15 \cdot 5\%$ in 1990 to $10 \cdot 0\%$ in 2006, mainly as a result of a decrease in thimerosal allergy from $3 \cdot 4\%$ to $0 \cdot 8\%$. Furthermore, the prevalence of cobalt allergy and rubber-related allergens decreased from $1 \cdot 1\%$ to $0 \cdot 2\%$ and from $1 \cdot 5\%$ to $0 \cdot 2\%$, respectively. Stratification by sex and age group revealed decreasing prevalences of contact allergy in all male age groups and in young and middle-aged female age groups (18—55 years) whereas increasing prevalences were observed among older women (56—69 years). The diverging trend observed in women was probably explained by a cohort effect due to a change in the prevalence of nickel allergy following the Danish regulation on nickel exposure.

Conclusions.—Although the overall prevalence of contact allergy decreased in the general population, frequent contact allergens such as fragrance mix II and methyldibromo glutaronitrile were not tested. Thus, contact allergy remains prevalent in the general population.

▶ Most of the data generated by researchers regarding prevalence of positive patch test reactions come from patients who present with eczematous dermatitis. This selection bias makes it difficult to extrapolate this information to the general public to estimate prevalence of contact allergy. This report from Denmark summarizes data gathered from patch testing unselected persons at 2 time points, 16 years apart. It gives us 2 important bits of information, but there is an important flaw that must be considered. The important information is that 10% of Danes in 2006 had 1 positive patch test or more and that this number was quite a bit lower than in 1996 when 15% were positive. The main problem is that testing was done only with the TRUE test (TT). This is a fine system, as far as it goes, but contained only 23 allergens and no newer allergens that have been recognized since the early 1990s. Estimates range that the TT system misses some 30% to 70% of all potential allergic reactions. Given this and the fact that older allergens may be less commonly available for exposure today, the data are really hard to feel comfortable with. I would say, in fact, there is probably no real difference from 1996 to today, if more allergens were evaluated. In addition, readers in the United States must remember that allergen positivity rates vary widely from country to country, so even this flawed information is not transferable to the experience in the United States.

J. F. Fowler, Jr, MD

Delay in medical attention to hand eczema: a follow-up study
Hald M, on behalf of the Danish Contact Dermatitis Group (Univ of Copenhagen, Hellerup, Denmark; et al)
Br J Dermatol 161:1294-1300, 2009

Background.—Hand eczema often runs a chronic course but early medical intervention may be assumed to improve the prognosis.

Objectives.—To follow patients with hand eczema for 6 months after seeing a dermatologist to investigate if delay in medical attention would impair the prognosis.

Methods.—Study participants were 333 patients with hand eczema from nine dermatological clinics in Denmark. Severity of hand eczema was assessed by the patients at baseline and at the 6-month follow up using a self-administered photographic guide. Additional information was obtained by self-administered questionnaires.

Results.—Median patient delay (defined as the period from onset of symptoms until seeing a general practitioner) was 3 months [interquartile range (IQR) $1 \cdot 5 - 8 \cdot 0$]. The median healthcare delay (defined as the period from the first visit to a general practitioner until seeing a dermatologist) was 3 months (IQR 1—8). In a logistic regression model, the odds ratio of a poor prognosis increased by a factor of $1 \cdot 11$ [95% confidence interval (CI) $1 \cdot 02 - 1 \cdot 21$] per month of patient delay and by $1 \cdot 05$ (95% CI $1 \cdot 00 - 1 \cdot 10$) per month of healthcare delay.

Conclusions.—A poorer prognosis of hand eczema was associated with longer delay before medical attention.

▶ Most physicians would probably assume that the longer a patient delays treatment, the more likely it will be that treatment will be more difficult and/or less effective. This nicely done study shows exactly that. A delay in seeing a dermatologist of over 6 months was associated with a worsened scenario. One weakness of the study is that obviously patient recall was relied upon for the duration and severity of symptoms at onset because by definition the patients were not seen at that time. However, the study was adequately powered and controlled to compensate at least partially for this. Given the continued movement toward socialism in the American health care system, delays of this sort will probably become commonplace in the United States. Chronic hand eczema is such a potentially serious condition, from a standpoint of ability to work and quality of life, that any delay would seem to be problematic.

J. F. Fowler, Jr, MD

Effects of nonsedative antihistamines on productivity of patients with pruritic skin diseases
Murota H, Kitaba S, Tani M, et al (Osaka Univ, Suita, Japan)
Allergy 65:924-932, 2010

Background.—Although allergies are a recognized cause for reduced performance socially and at work, skin diseases are not. However, pruritic skin diseases have the potential to disrupt work productivity, classroom effectiveness, and daily activities. Their impact and the effect of antihistamines in reducing that impact were assessed.

Methods.—Two hundred six patients (mean age 52 years) with pruritic skin diseases participated in the study. No medical attention was given to the patients for 1 week at baseline, then patients received treatment determined by the physician. Both nonsedative (fexofenadine and loratadine; 74 patients) and sedative (all others; 121 patients) antihistamines were given. Eleven patients received only topical medications. The Skindex-16 instrument was used to assess the effects of the skin diseases on patients' quality of life (QOL). Itch sensation magnitude was determined using a visual analog scale (VAS) from 0 to 100. The Work Productivity-Activity Impairment-Allergy Specific (WPAI-AS) instrument was used to assess overall work and daily life productivity. Patients self-administered these instruments at baseline and 1 month after treatment began.

Results.—The impairment scores for overall productivity for the workplace, classroom, and daily life activity were 39.3%, 45.0%, and 42.3%, respectively. The various disease groups (including dermatitis/eczema, urticaria, atopic dermatitis, and pruritus cutaneous) showed no differences at baseline. After 1 month of treatment, itch intensity was reduced significantly in patients taking antihistamines but not affected by the topical treatments. The nonsedative and sedative antihistamines performed comparably with respect to itch relief. However, the nonsedative antihistamines reduced the impairment in overall work and daily activity productivity whereas the sedative antihistamines did not improve either measure.

Conclusions.—The WPAI-AS scores were negatively affected by pruritic diseases. Sedative antihistamines did not improve on this situation even though they were able to reduce itchiness. Maintaining patient productivity should be considered a new goal in treating pruritic skin diseases. The best results in this respect are achieved with nonsedative antihistamines.

▶ Antihistamines have been used in the past to help patients with symptoms of pruritus and to help improve quality of life (QOL) in many individuals. This is a study of 206 males and 93 females with a variety of pruritic skin diseases (eg, dermatitis/eczema, urticaria, atopic dermatitis) evaluating the effects of antihistamines on the intensity of pruritus and QOL. Patients were also allowed to continue their topical medications while they participated in the study. The 2 medications that were used which were considered nonsedatives were fexofenadine (n = 72) and loratadine (n = 2), and all other medications used were considered as sedatives. The effects of pruritic skin diseases on QOL were measured using the Skindex-16, and the daily productivity was assessed by the Work Productivity-Activity Impairment-Allergy Specific (WPAI-AS) instrument. These measurements were assessed at baseline and at 1 month after treatment was initiated. This study revealed that pruritic skin diseases negatively impacted WPAI-AS scores compared with baseline. In addition, at the end of the study, there was no significant difference between disease groups identified. Itch intensity was reduced significantly ($P < .001$) by antihistamine therapy, and the effects of nonsedative and sedative antihistamines on itch intensity were similar. Sedative antihistamines did not increase or affect productivity but did decrease itch and Skindex-16 measures. Impairment in overall work productivity and daily activity were reduced significantly by nonsedative antihistamines, whereas sedative antihistamines failed to improve either measure. However, this study did not control for other factors that may have affected work productivity, such as other disease processes, medications, and unidentified external factors. Also, patients were able to continue their other topical medications, which may have an effect on pruritus. Also, there were no controls for these patients and therefore it may be difficult to evaluate if pruritus and work productivity are statistically different as compared with a control group (nondiseased patients). To note, nonsedatives and sedatives did not significantly impair productivity with school or work. This study revealed that clinicians should be aware not to overestimate the benefits of sedative antihistamines on work productivity if based on intensity of pruritus and QOL values, and there may be rationale to switch to nonsedative antihistamines in some cases. However, the lack of control of troublesome pruritus in individual cases may warrant a switch in the type of antihistamine used.

J. Q. Del Rosso, DO

G. K. Kim, DO

Fragrance contact allergic patients: strategies for use of cosmetic products and perceived impact on life situation
Lysdal SH, Johansen JD (Univ of Copenhagen, Denmark)
Contact Dermatitis 61:320-324, 2009

Background.—Fragrance ingredients are a common cause of contact allergy. Very little is known about these patients' strategies to manage their disease and the effect on their daily lives.

Objectives.—To investigate if patients with diagnosed fragrance contact allergy used scented products, how they identified tolerated products, and if fragrance allergy affected their daily living.

Method.—One hundred and forty-seven patients diagnosed with fragrance contact allergy in a 20-month period were included and received a postal questionnaire concerning the subjects of the study. One hundred and seventeen (79.6%) replied.

Results.—In total, 53/117 (45.3%) responded that they had found some scented products that they could tolerate. Thirty-seven (31.6%) had not tried to find any scented products and 26 (22%) had tried but could not find any. The methods most often used were trying different products and reading the ingredient label. Of the total respondents, 17.1% reported sick-leave due to fragrance allergy and 45.3% found that fragrance allergy significantly affected their daily living.

Conclusion.—Many patients with fragrance contact allergy succeeded in finding some scented products, which they could tolerate, e.g. by use of ingredient labelling, but a significant proportion had continued skin problems. Almost half of the patients perceived that fragrance allergy significantly affected their daily lives.

▶ This is a very useful report, indicating the extent to which our patients with fragrance allergy need to alter their lifestyle and personal care product usage. The prevalence of fragrance allergy, as determined by positive patch tests to various fragrance chemicals and mixes, ranks in the top 5 of all causes of contact allergy in the United States and Europe. Consequently, we often have to recommend fragrance avoidance to our allergic patients. Other potential allergens in personal care products can be identified by the patient easily by reading the package labeling. In the United States, however, the 1200 or more fragrance ingredients that may be found in such products are listed simply by the word fragrance or sometimes parfum. In Europe, new labeling laws require the listing of 20 or so individual fragrance chemicals. But even there, many others can be allergens and will not be listed separately. Therefore, patients must usually use a trial-and-error method for finding the fragrance-containing products that they can tolerate. In this report, about half of the patients eventually were able to find some products with fragrance that they could tolerate. In contrast, about one-fifth could not and about one-third did not even try. This article gives us useful numbers to tell our patients when we discuss with them the likelihood or their ability to find tolerable fragrance-containing products.

J. F. Fowler, Jr, MD

Hairdressers with dermatitis should always be patch tested regardless of atopy status
O'Connell RL, White IR, Mc Fadden JP, et al (St Thomas' Hosp, London, UK)
Contact Dermatitis 62:177-181, 2010

Background.—Allergic contact dermatitis is common in hairdressers because of their exposure to chemicals used in hair dyes and permanent wave solutions. Atopic individuals are known to have a higher prevalence of leaving the profession due to morbidity associated with hand eczema.

Objectives.—To assess which chemicals are responsible for allergic contact dermatitis in hairdressers and whether the prevalence is the same according to atopy status.

Methods.—A total of 729 hairdressers who had been patch tested were retrospectively identified. Allergic reactions to relevant allergens from the extended European baseline series and hairdressing series were analysed against history of atopic eczema.

Results.—Of the total, 29.9% of patients had a current or past history of atopic eczema. The most frequent positive allergens from the European baseline series were nickel sulfate (32.1%) and *p*-phenylenediamine (19.0%) and from the hairdressing series were glyceryl monothioglycolate (21.4%) and ammonium persulfate (10.6%). There was no significant difference between people with or without a history of atopic eczema, except for fragrance mix I and nickel sulfate.

Conclusions.—We present findings from the largest cohort of hairdressers patch tested from a single centre. It is necessary to patch test hairdressers with dermatitis, regardless of a history of atopy. Strategies to reduce prevalence of allergic contact dermatitis are required.

▶ This article doesn't have any surprises but is valuable because of the size of the population base. Many hairdressers (HDs) develop either irritant or allergic hand dermatitis (or both), and often this leads to a career change. These authors found that allergens that are common in the general patch-tested population are also common in HDs, such as metals, fragrances, formaldehyde, preservatives, and rubber. However, the prevalence of some of these was higher in the HD group than we usually see in general. In addition, as expected, specific cosmetic allergens were frequent in the HD group: para-phenylenediamine (dye), glyceryl thioglycolate (perm), and ammonium persulfate (bleach). Interestingly, both atopics and nonatopics had relatively similar rates of patch-test reactivity. It would have been a very valuable addition to the study if the authors had determined what proportion of patients had to leave the cosmetology field due to their eczema, but that was not the focus of this article. In HDs, as in anyone with chronic hand eczema, patch testing is absolutely critical for proper diagnosis and optimal therapy. This is true, regardless of the morphology of the eczematous eruption or atopic status of the patient.

J. F. Fowler, Jr, MD

Histamine H_4 receptor antagonist ameliorates chronic allergic contact dermatitis induced by repeated challenge
Seike M, Furuya K, Omura M, et al (Sagami Women's Junior College, Sagamihara, Kanagawa, Japan; et al)
Allergy 65:319-326, 2010

Background.—The present study observed effects of the histamine H_4 receptor on chronic allergic contact dermatitis induced by repeated challenge in mice.

Methods.—Acute contact dermatitis was induced by single epicutaneous challenge of 2,4,6-trinitro-1-chlorobenzene (TNCB) to the ear. Chronic allergic contact dermatitis was developed by repeated epicutaneous challenge using TNCB on the dorsal back skin. H_4 receptor antagonist

JNJ7777120 was administered to wild-type mice, while H_4 receptor agonist 4-methylhistamine was administered to histidine decarboxylase (HDC) $(-/-)$ mice that synthesized no histamine.

Results.—HDC $(-/-)$ mice did not differ phenotypically from HDC $(+/+)$ mice, and H_4 receptor antagonist/agonist did not have clinical effects in terms of acute contact dermatitis reactions. H_4 receptor antagonist ameliorated skin eczematous lesions induced by repeated TNCB challenge in HDC $(+/+)$ mice. On the contrary, H_4 receptor agonist exacerbated skin lesions exclusively in HDC $(-/-)$ mice. Application of H_4 receptor agonist induced migration of mast cells and eosinophils in skin lesions, and H_4 receptor antagonist suppressed these changes. H_4 receptor was immuno-histochemically detected on mast cells in eczematous lesions. Levels of interleukin (IL)-4, -5, and -6 in lesions were decreased, whereas levels of interferon-γ and IL-12 were increased by H_4 receptor antagonistic activity. Serum Immunoglobulin E levels rapidly increased with repeated challenge, but decreased with H_4 receptor antagonist.

Conclusion.—Because chronic allergic contact dermatitis is developed by H_4 receptor stimulation, H_4 receptor antagonists might represent new candidate drugs for treating chronic allergic contact dermatitis.

▶ Antihistamines in clinical usage for the treatment of eczemas are directed toward blocking H_1 receptors to reduce itching. Their usefulness in treating symptoms is fairly low, although they are much more useful in controlling symptoms of allergic upper airway disease. The sedating antihistamines are primarily useful by inducing drowsiness, rather than by their direct effect on the skin. H_1-blocking antihistamines do not have a measurable effect on lesions of allergic contact dermatitis (ACD) or on patch testing. These investigators have targeted a different histamine pathway, through antagonism of H_4 recep-tors. At least in the mouse model, they have shown reduced development of ACD following allergen exposure. They have also shown a reduction in infiltra-tion of mast cells and eosinophils into ACD lesions. It is unclear whether the observed reduction in ACD severity (reduced mouse ear swelling) is a direct effect of the treatment or is because of reduced itching and scratching of the area. In either case, further evaluation in humans of the blockade of the H_4 receptor may be useful in treating the symptoms of eczemas.

J. F. Fowler, Jr, MD

Impaired TLR-2 expression and TLR-2-mediated cytokine secretion in macrophages from patients with atopic dermatitis
Niebuhr M, Lutat C, Sigel S, et al (Hannover Med School, Germany; Univ of Konstanz, Germany)
Allergy 64:1580-1587, 2009

Background.—In many patients with atopic dermatitis (AD), the disease is complicated by their enhanced susceptibility to bacterial skin infections, especially with *Staphylococcus aureus*. The pattern recognition receptor toll-like receptor (TLR)-2 recognizes components of *S. aureus*, for example, lipoteichoic acid (LTA) and peptidoglycan (PGN) and, therefore, might be crucial in the pathogenesis and flare-ups of AD.

Objective.—To investigate TLR-2 expression and cytokine secretion in macrophages from patients with AD compared to healthy controls upon TLR-2 stimulation with PGN, LTA and Pam3Cys.

Methods.—Macrophages were cultivated from highly purified peripheral blood monocytes of AD patients and nonatopic healthy controls and stimulated with PGN, LTA and Pam3Cys in a time and dose—dependent manner. Afterwards, TLR-2 expression and cytokine secretion were measured on protein and mRNA level. TLR-1 and TLR-6 expression were investigated on the mRNA level. Immunohistochemical stainings from punch biopsies were performed to investigate TLR-2 expression in skin macrophages.

Results.—We could clearly show that macrophages from patients with AD expressed significantly less TLR-2, whereas the expression pattern of TLR-1 and TLR-6 were not altered. Macrophages had a reduced capacity to produce pro-inflammatory cytokines such as IL-6, IL-8 and IL-1β after stimulation with TLR-2 ligands.

Conclusion.—Our findings clearly show an impaired TLR-2 expression and functional differences of TLR-2-mediated effects on macrophages of AD patients compared to healthy controls which might contribute to the enhanced susceptibility to skin infections with *S. aureus* in AD.

▶ Understanding the mechanism of how disease is created allows the potential to apply therapies to the targets necessary to modify the disease process and alleviate the symptoms and control the progression. In atopic dermatitis, our conventional therapies and traditional approaches are directed to controlling flares, reducing symptoms, such as itch, and more recently, protecting the barrier of the skin. The genetic predispositions of patients with atopic dermatitis that lead to epidermal defects (ie, imbalances in ceramides and other phospholipids in both lesional and nonlesional skin) and immune responses from T helper 2—induced immunity are the major driving forces of pathogenesis. New understanding of toll-like receptor (TLR) activity, specifically TLR-2, and the antigenic processing of bacterial peptidoglycans and lipoteichoic acids may have potential applications for therapy for the process of atopic dermatitis. The TLR-2 pathway and role of the nuclear binding oligomerization domain receptor are gaining a lot of attention in the treatment of acne for similar reasons. TLR-2 has been shown to have response elements to vitamin D and interactions with LL-37 cathelicidins, so it is possible that we may soon be incorporating therapy against these targets in atopic dermatitis and not just treating the itch.

N. Bhatia, MD

Increased expression of glucocorticoid receptor β in lymphocytes of patients with severe atopic dermatitis unresponsive to topical corticosteroid

Hägg PM, Hurskainen T, Palatsi R, et al (Univ of Oulu and Clinical Res Ctr, Finland)
Br J Dermatol 162:318-324, 2010

Background.—Variable response to topical glucocorticoid therapy occurs in the treatment of severe atopic dermatitis (AD). Glucocorticoid receptor (GR)-β does not bind glucocorticoids but antagonizes the activity of the classic GRα, and could thus account for glucocorticoid insensitivity.

Objectives.—To investigate GRα and GRβ mRNA and protein expression in lymphocytes of patients with AD before and after treatment with topical corticosteroids.

Methods.—Blood was collected from 11 healthy donors, 10 patients with mild AD and 13 patients with severe AD. mRNA was isolated from peripheral blood mononuclear cells. Expression of GRα and GRβ mRNA was determined by reverse transcriptase–polymerase chain reaction and quantitated. Expression of the GRs was confirmed by Western blot analysis.

Result.—The expression of GRα mRNA was detected in all subjects. GRβ mRNA was detected in four out of 11 healthy volunteers, five out of 10 patients with mild AD and 11 out of 13 patients with severe AD. The incidence of GRβ mRNA expression was higher in patients with severe AD (85%) than in patients with mild AD (50%), and significantly higher than in healthy volunteers (36%, $P = 0.033$). Four of the 13 patients with severe AD showed a $3.3–13.2$-fold increase in the expression of GRβ mRNA during a 2-week treatment with topical corticosteroids. In these patients the response to topical corticosteroids was poor.

Conclusions.—Expression of GRβ is increased during topical corticosteroid treatment in the lymphocytes of patients with AD and, in particular, glucocorticoid-insensitive AD is associated with increased expression of GRβ.

▶ Atopic dermatitis (AD) is a common chronic inflammatory skin disease with topical glucocorticoids often being used as first-line agents for treatment. Glucocorticoid receptor (GR) expression has undergone limited study in patients with AD. This is a study of patients with mild AD (n = 10) and severe AD (n = 13) investigating GRα and GRβ messenger RNA (mRNA) and protein expression in lymphocytes of patients with AD before and after treatment with topical corticosteroids, compared with 11 healthy controls. The clinical severity of AD was determined by use of the Eczema Area and Severity Index (EASI) score. The sex, serum immunoglobulin E level, blood eosinophil count, and EASI score before and after a 2-week treatment period with a topical corticosteroid were noted. The expression of GRα mRNA was detected in all patients (both healthy and AD). However, GRβ mRNA was detected in 4 (36%) out of 11 healthy volunteers, 5 (50%) of 10 patients with mild AD, and 11 (85%) of 13 patients with severe AD. It was observed more in severe AD (85%)

than in mild AD (50%) and significantly higher than in healthy volunteers (36%, $P = .033$). Four of the 13 patients with severe AD showed a 3.3- to 13.2-fold increase in the expression of GRβ mRNA during the 2-week treatment with a topical corticosteroid. These patients had a poor clinical response to topical corticosteroids (EASI score decreased by < 8%). None of the 13 patients showed a minor increase or a notable change in the expression of GRβ mRNA (0-2.9 fold) during the 2-week treatment. The increase in expression of GRβ in the development of glucocorticoid-resistant forms of AD may be significant in terms of response to treatment and optimal selection of therapy. A limitation of this study was that concurrent medical conditions of the patients were unknown. This may be relevant because other inflammatory conditions may elevate GRβ and GRα, including false elevations. To add, GRβ and GRα were detected in whole blood, which may be different from a localized lymphocytic response. Also, expression of these receptors is limited in this study only to the use of topical corticosteroids, and results may change with systemic corticosteroids or possibly other therapeutic agents. The relative potency and/or chemical class of the prescribed topical corticosteroids was not differentiated in this study, as receptor expression may be different with different corticosteroid agents. A treatment duration of longer than 2 weeks may also change expression of lymphocyte receptors. In this study, the expression of GRβ mRNA increased during topical corticosteroid treatment in lymphocytes of patients with AD and may signify the presence of glucocorticoid-insensitive AD.

J. Q. Del Rosso, DO

G. K. Kim, DO

Low-dose cyclosporine A therapy increases the regulatory T cell population in patients with atopic dermatitis
Brandt C, Pavlovic V, Radbruch A, et al (Deutsches Rheuma-Forschungszentrum, Berlin, Germany; et al)
Allergy 64:1588-1596, 2009

Background.—Atopic dermatitis (AD) is a T cell dependent chronic relapsing inflammatory skin disorder successfully treated with cyclosporine A (CsA). Clinical observations indicate that even low-dose CsA therapy is successful in severely affected AD patients. We studied the impact of low-dose CsA therapy on the ability of T helper cells to be activated, and examined whether regulatory T (Treg) cells are increased in these patients.

Methods.—Peripheral T cells were activated in a whole blood sample and interleukin-2 producing cells were measured by intracellular cytokine staining. Regulatory T cells were analyzed by intracellular FoxP3 staining. Regulatory T cells ($CD4^+CD25^+CD127^{low}$) and effector T cells ($CD4^+CD25^-CD127^+$) were sorted by flow cytometry and used for suppression assays.

Results.—A group of AD patients treated with low-dose CsA had a significantly larger Treg cell population than a healthy control subject group. In individual patients, onset of low-dose CsA therapy reduced the ability of T cells to be activated to 42 ± 18% ($P < 0.005$) and significantly increased Treg cells, both in absolute numbers (1.6-fold change) and frequencies (1.7-fold change). Treg cells from AD patients showed similar suppressive capacities as Treg cells from healthy donors. Furthermore, Treg cells from AD patients had skin homing properties.

Conclusion.—Our results indicate that the therapeutic effect of low-dose CsA therapy in AD patients might be not only mediated by the inhibition of T cell hyperactivity but also by an increased population of Treg cells.

▶ Atopic dermatitis (AD) is a chronic, eczematous, inflammatory skin disease. Past reports have noted systemic cyclosporine A (CsA) therapy as an effective treatment option for severe refractory AD. CsA is an immunosuppressive drug interfering with T-cell receptor signaling, which inhibits the expression of cytokines such as interleukin-2 (IL-2) and the proliferation of T cells. This is a study examining systemic CsA treatment and the role of T regulatory (Treg) cells and their effects on T helper cells in response to low-dose CsA therapy in patients with AD. Subjects that were included were 12 untreated patients with AD. Twenty patients with AD were treated with low-dose CsA therapy and compared with 17 healthy age- and sex-matched controls. T cells in whole blood samples and IL-2—producing cells were measured by intracellular cytokine staining. Treg cells and effector T cells were also analyzed. AD was monitored by the severity scoring of atopic dermatitis (SCORAD) score. The SCORAD index was monitored before onset of CsA and during low-dose CsA treatment. SCORAD was significantly reduced by CsA compared with baseline (53.1 vs 27.2, $P < .005$). Absolute numbers of IL-2—producing $CD3^+$ T cells from patients with AD under CsA therapy were lower compared with those from healthy controls and AD subjects ($P < .005$). The authors identified significantly higher frequencies of CLA^+ T cells in patients with AD without (14.4, $P < .005$) and with low-dose CsA therapy (13.5, $P > .05$) compared with healthy control subjects. Patients with AD treated with low-dose CsA for at least 3 weeks had significantly higher frequencies for FoxP3 expressing T cells than healthy subjects ($P < .005$). This revealed that low-dose CsA treatment induces Treg cells in vivo by measuring $FoxP3^+$ T cells before and after the onset of CsA therapy. Furthermore, the authors found that Treg cells from patients with AD had skin homing properties. Side effects and adverse events with patients on low-dose CsA were not discussed, although many of the patients were on CsA therapy ranging from 20 to 40 weeks. It may also be interesting to note if these patients had a lower incidence of cutaneous lymphoma because there is inhibition of T-cell activity with low-dose CsA. In conclusion, low-dose CsA therapy may inhibit hyperactivation of T cells by allergens or superantigens directly by the inhibition of cytokine production and indirectly by enhanced numbers of functional $FoxP3^+$ Treg cells.

J. Q. Del Rosso, DO

G. K. Kim, DO

Maternal Asthma, its Control and Severity in Pregnancy, and the Incidence of Atopic Dermatitis and Allergic Rhinitis in the Offspring

Martel M-J, Beauchesne M-F, Malo J-L, et al (Université de Montréal, Québec, Canada; Hôpital du Sacré-Cœur de Montréal, Québec, Canada; et al)
J Pediatr 155:707-713, 2009

Objective.—To evaluate the relationship between maternal asthma, its level of control and severity during pregnancy, and atopic dermatitis (AD) and allergic rhinitis (AR) incidence in children.

Study Design.—A cohort of 26 265 singletons born to mothers with and without asthma (1990–2002) was constituted by use of 3 Quebec databases. Mothers with asthma had to have received ≥1 diagnosis and ≥1 prescription for asthma 2 years before or during pregnancy. Asthma control and severity during pregnancy was based on validated indexes. ICD-9 codes 691 and 477 allowed us to identify cases of AD and AR.

Results.—Maternal asthma during pregnancy was associated with an increased AD risk (adjusted hazard ratio: 1.11, 95% confidence interval: 1.02-1.21), but not of AR (adjusted hazard ratio: 1.04, 95% confidence interval: 0.91-1.20) in children. Asthma control and severity were not associated with either outcome. Maternal AR and intranasal corticosteroid use during pregnancy increased the risk of childhood AR by 70% and 45%.

Conclusions.—Children of mothers with asthma or AR during pregnancy should be closely monitored to diagnose and treat AD and AR as early as possible.

▶ After reading this cohort study, performed in the setting of a socialized health care model with a very credible number of participants screened, I am left with 1 question: So now what? Dermatologists have been trained to screen for the atopic diathesis in affected family members, to monitor for symptoms associated with atopy developing in childhood, and to incorporate a multidisciplinary approach with allergists to ensure comprehensive care. The concept of the atopic march and the potential for patients with atopic dermatitis to develop asthma or allergic rhinitis later in childhood led to closer monitoring of symptoms and more aggressive management strategies.[1,2] Now the authors tell us that mothers who required government-provided health care possibly had different outcomes than "women and children from higher income families" and "are underrepresented in this study population, because they are mostly covered by private insurance for their medications." Is this testimony to the concept of approaching patients differently because of their health care coverage or is this a statement of how different socioeconomic groups fail to respond to adherence to treatment and ignore the outcomes? So now what?

What does this mean to a society where more patients every year qualify for state or federal health plans that do not pay for the higher level care that these patients might need for complete management or for more screening? The authors state that "it may be more difficult to generalize the results to children born in families of higher socioeconomic status," yet hasn't it been determined that the atopic diathesis syndromes are diseases of the middle and upper classes?

Even more concerning about the authors' findings is the role of adherence by the pregnant mothers to a treatment plan and the outcomes that affect the child. In the results section there is the observation that "the incidence of AR was statistically significantly increased if the child had previously been diagnosed with AD or asthma, had filled at least 1 antibiotic prescription up to 6 months after birth, if its mother had filled INS and antibiotics prescriptions during pregnancy, if she had consulted an obstetrician and had more than 16 prenatal visits." Because most children are not allowed to fill prescriptions on their own, especially at 6 months of age, it is an important indicator when, even in a social health care model, noncompliance can significantly impact the incidence of a condition that, as per the authors' hypothesis, might not have to pass through to the next generation.

I think the information here is very thorough and comprehensive and provides some excellent retrospective insight, but when a cohort study is inherently handcuffed by the bias of its patient group, it is hard to accept some of the outcomes, to no fault of the authors. And now when I see my next atopic patient or a pregnant mother with atopy, still I am left to ask, "So now what?"

N. Bhatia, MD

References

1. Ker J, Hartert TV. The atopic march: what's the evidence? *Ann Allergy Asthma Immunol.* 2009;103:282-289.
2. Spergel JM. Epidemiology of atopic dermatitis and atopic march in children. *Immunol Allergy Clin North Am.* 2010;30:269-280.

Methotrexate: a useful steroid-sparing agent in recalcitrant chronic urticaria
Perez A, Woods A, Grattan CEH (St Thomas' Hosp, London, UK)
Br J Dermatol 162:191-194, 2010

Background.—Reports of methotrexate for chronic urticaria are anecdotal.

Objectives.—To assess the effectiveness of methotrexate in steroid-dependent chronic urticaria, its impact on steroid reduction and any differences in response between patients with and without functional autoantibodies.

Methods.—A retrospective case-note review of 16 patients with steroid-dependent chronic urticaria treated with methotrexate was carried out. Ten patients had chronic ordinary/spontaneous urticaria (CU), including three with associated delayed-pressure urticaria; four patients had normo-complementaemic urticarial vasculitis (UV); and two patients had idiopathic angio-oedema without weals. Median disease duration before methotrexate was 48·5 months (range 12–164). All were unresponsive to antihistamines and second-line agents, except prednisolone. Eleven were assessed for autoimmune urticaria with the basophil histamine release assay $(n = 5)$, autologous serum skin test $(n = 5)$ or both $(n = 1)$. Response to methotrexate was scored: no benefit; some benefit (fewer weals and symptomatic improvement but no steroid reduction); considerable benefit (improvement with steroid reduction); or clear (no symptoms, off steroids but on antihistamines).

Results.—Twelve of 16 patients (eight CU, three UV, one idiopathic angio-oedema) responded. Three showed some benefit, seven considerable benefit and two cleared. Four of eight responders and three out of three nonresponders showed evidence of functional autoantibodies. The dose to achieve a steroid-sparing effect was 10–15 mg weekly (cumulative dose range 15–600 mg, median 135 mg). Methotrexate was well tolerated.

Conclusions.—Methotrexate may be a useful treatment for steroid-dependent chronic urticaria. Functional autoantibodies do not correlate with response. The beneficial effects of methotrexate may be anti-inflammatory and immunosuppressive. It may therefore benefit chronic urticaria independently of the pathogenic mechanism, whether autoimmune or not.

▶ Perez et al report an interesting treatment consideration regarding chronic urticaria. There are no previous reports on the use of methotrexate for chronic urticaria; however, this study documents a reportable benefit from methotrexate as a third-line therapy. Given that these patients were previously oral corticosteroid dependent before the study but were able to subsequently decrease or eliminate oral corticosteroids after using methotrexate, this study provides some potentially promising data on an alternative treatment for oral corticosteroid–dependent urticaria. The usual weekly methotrexate dose given in the study was between 10 and 15 mg. With this dose, 12 of 16 patients reported benefit from methotrexate use, in addition to being able to reduce their oral corticosteroid regimen. While 16 patients is certainly a limited number and the study itself is retrospective, this type of reported benefit certainly shows an encouraging alternative to oral corticosteroids in the treatment of chronic urticaria. In all, Perez et al provide an interesting insight into a potentially beneficial treatment consideration and, hopefully, into one that will be subject to a larger prospective study in the future.

B. D. Michaels, DO

J. Q. Del Rosso, DO

Nickel allergy in patch-tested female hairdressers and assessment of nickel release from hairdressers' scissors and crochet hooks
Thyssen JP, Milting K, Bregnhøj A, et al (Univ of Copenhagen, Denmark)
Contact Dermatitis 61:281-286, 2009

Background.—Hand eczema as well as nickel contact allergy is prevalent among hairdressers. Recently, two female hairdressers were diagnosed with nickel contact allergy-related hand eczema following prolonged skin contact with scissors and crochet hooks used during work.

Objectives.—To determine the proportion of hairdressers' scissors and crochet hooks that released an excessive amount of nickel and to determine the prevalence of nickel allergy among patch-tested female hairdressers.

Materials.—Random hairdressers' stores in Copenhagen were visited. The dimethylglyoxime (DMG) test was used to assess excessive nickel release. The prevalence of nickel allergy among female hairdressers from the database at Gentofte Hospital was compared with the prevalence of nickel allergy among other consecutively patch-tested dermatitis patients.

Results.—DMG testing showed that 1 (0.5%; 95% CI = 0 − 2.0) of 200 pairs of scissors and 7 (53.8%; 95% CI = 26.0 − 82.0) of 13 crochet hooks released an excessive amount of nickel. The prevalence of nickel allergy was higher among middle-aged and older female hairdressers than among young female hairdressers.

Conclusions.—The prevalence of nickel allergy was lower among young hairdressers in comparison to older hairdressers. This may possibly be a result of the European Union (EU) Nickel Directive or a consequence of a decreased use of nickel-releasing work tools in salons. When nickel allergic hairdressers present with hand eczema, their work tools should be investigated for nickel release.

▶ Nickel allergy is generally regarded as the most common patch test reaction in epidemiologic studies of allergic contact dermatitis evaluated with patch testing. Consequently, the sensitized population and those at potential risk represent a large force of individuals in the workplace. Governmental intervention, particularly in Europe, regulates the exposure of individuals to nickel in metal items found in activities of routine daily living and work. These regulations serve to potentially reduce the sensitization rate of at-risk individuals and control the expression of the allergic reactions in those who are already sensitive. Hand dermatitis is an obvious target of investigation because the hands are the most readily used body site to manipulate objects and to use tools. Controversy exists regarding the epidemiologic association of nickel allergy and hand dermatitis; however, the negative effect of nickel exposure on the hands of sensitized individual has little room for debate. Clinicians are often reticent to aggressively counsel the patient with nickel allergy to assess their nickel exposure through home-based methods, such as the dimethylglyoxime test. It is probably still quite important to encourage this level of attentiveness because metal tools will variably and unpredictably release nickel in direct contact with the operator's hands.[1]

D. E. Cohen, MD, MPH

Reference

1. O'Connell RL, White IR, Mc Fadden JP, White JM. Hairdressers with dermatitis should always be patch tested regardless of atopy status. *Contact Dermatitis.* 2010;62:177-181.

Patch testing in patients treated with systemic immunosuppression and cytokine inhibitors

Wee JS, White JML, McFadden JP, et al (St Thomas' Hosp, London, UK)
Contact Dermatitis 62:165-169, 2010

Background.—Currently, there is little data available on the reliability of patch testing in patients taking immunosuppressive agents other than systemic corticosteroids.

Objectives.—We present data from 38 patients who were patch tested whilst taking various immunomodulating agents to determine if positive reactions can be elicited.

Patient/Materials/Methods.—Between September 2006 and May 2009, 38 patients attending the St John's Institute of Dermatology were patch tested whilst taking immunosuppressive agents including azathioprine, ciclosporin, infliximab, adalimumab, etanercept, methotrexate, mycophenolate mofetil, and tacrolimus.

Results.—Positive patch test reactions of varying degrees and significance were elicited in: 2 of 10 patients on azathioprine; 5 of 11 patients on ciclosporin; 1 patient on ciclosporin and Fumaderm®; 1 patient on infliximab; 1 patient on infliximab and methotrexate; 1 of 2 patients on adalimumab; 1 patient on etanercept and methotrexate; 3 of 4 patients on methotrexate; 1 of 3 patients on mycophenolate mofetil; and 1 patient on mycophenolate mofetil and tacrolimus. Negative patch test reactions occurred in 1 patient on azathioprine and ciclosporin; 1 patient on infliximab and azathioprine; and 1 patient on mycophenolate and ciclosporin.

Conclusions.—Positive patch test reactions can be elicited in patients taking azathioprine, ciclosporin, infliximab, adalimumab, etanercept, methotrexate, mycophenolate mofetil, and tacrolimus. However, it remains unclear what effect these immunosuppressive drugs may have on suppressing allergic patch test reactions and further studies should be carried out to determine the reliability of testing in these circumstances.

▶ Patch testing is the gold standard diagnostic test for the detection of the etiologic agents responsible for the pathogenesis of the quintessential clinical form of delayed-type hypersensitivity: allergic contact dermatitis. The complex orchestration of Langerhans cells and presumably T helper type 1 lymphocytes requires the elaboration of many cytokines for the elicitation, propagation, and subsequent elimination of the inflammatory response. Treatments for this disease include many types of immunomodulatory agents delivered both topically and systemically, which serve to foil the inflammatory response and sever some component of the inflammatory cascade. At times, clinical scenarios arise in which patients who would benefit from diagnostic patch testing are required to continue some form of systemic immunosuppression. Such situations may include the ongoing suppression of autoimmune disease, prevention of rejection of transplanted organs, or the containment of an overwhelming inflammatory dermatosis, without which testing would be even more problematic. The use of concomitant immunosuppression medications ought to, and probably does, influence the interpretation of patch test readings, although the elicitation of at least some test reactions is possible under these suppressive conditions.[1]

D. E. Cohen, MD, MPH

Reference

1. Rosmarin D, Gottlieb AB, Asarch A, Scheinman PL. Patch-testing while on systemic immunosuppressants. *Dermatitis*. 2009;20:265-270.

Patch testing with benzoyl peroxide: reaction profile and interpretation of positive patch test reactions
Ockenfels H-M, Uter W, Lessmann H, et al (Klinikum Hanau, Hanau, Germany; Friedrich Alexander Univ, Erlangen, Germany; Univ of Göttingen, Germany)
Contact Dermatitis 61:209-216, 2009

Background.—Patch testing with benzoyl peroxide 1% pet. frequently leads to (weak) positive reactions, often with uncertain clinical relevance.

Objectives.—To describe the pattern of patch tests reactions to benzoyl peroxide and to identify patients at risk of a positive reaction.

Methods.—Retrospective analysis of data from the Information Network of Departments of Dermatology (IVDK), 1992–2007.

Results.—Benzoyl peroxide 1% pet. was tested in 29 758 patients. Weak positive reactions (erythema, infiltration, possibly papules) occurred in 6.5%, and strong positive reactions (erythema, infiltration, vesicles) in 1.3%. According to logistic regression analysis, strong positive reactions to benzoyl peroxide were associated with leg or face dermatitis, work as dental technicians, young age and being female. Patients with atopic dermatitis had a significantly increased risk of weak positive reactions only.

Conclusions.—Our analysis confirms that benzoyl peroxide 1% pet. is a problematic patch test preparation. Hence, clinical relevance of reactions to benzoyl peroxide has to be assessed very carefully. Patients with atopic dermatitis are particularly prone to irritant reactions to benzoyl peroxide. True allergic reactions may occur in dental technicians and following the treatment of leg ulcers with highly concentrated benzoyl peroxide in past. In contrast, widely used acne treatments with benzoyl peroxide seems to sensitize only rarely.

▶ Benzoyl peroxide (BP) is known to be a strong irritant and may cause individuals to be sensitized. BP is frequently used by dental technicians as well as for leg ulcers and orthopedic cements. The concentrations are higher than those used in the topical medications for acne vulgaris. BP is patch tested at 1% in petrolatum. However, patch testing produces many weakly positive reactions because BP can be an irritant. This is a retrospective analysis of 29 758 patients tested with BP 1% petrolatum during the years 1992-2007. Ages ranged from

12 to 84 years, with mean and median age of 47 years. In this 16-year study, there were more women patients (63.4% vs 58.6%), patients with occupational dermatitis (22.8% vs 20.9%), atopics (18.3% vs 14.0%), patients with face dermatitis (11.8% vs 9.1%), and patients younger than 40 years (39.8% vs 35.2%) who tested positive to the patch test. There was a constant decline of the percentage of positive reactions (5.8%) in 2003-2007 than in previous years (7.8%-8.8%). Additionally, there was a constant decline in the percentage of positive test reactions from 8.7% to 6.9% with age. Age range of 34 to 47 years and leg dermatitis increased the risk of strong positive reactions only, while atopic dermatitis and facial dermatitis were risk factors for weak positive reactions only. Limitations to this study were that the registry was not able to differentiate between those who were exposed to lower concentrations of BP (ie, acne topical medications) compared with those who were exposed to higher concentrations of BP. In addition, the investigators did not state if the patch test was open or closed, which can also affect the results. Also, the location of the patch test was not discussed and may react differently on different locations of the skin, causing false-positive reactions. Ideally, patch tests should be done on locations the agent is frequently in contact with to achieve more accurate results. Also, the authors did not comment on whether patients with atopic dermatitis had been controlled while the patch tests were being administered or whether patch tests were done on previous dermatitis locations. The authors were also not able to assess if patients were previously exposed to BP in the form of a cement-fixed endoprosthesis at the time of the patch testing. They stated that they found reactions to be indicative of irritant and not allergic without adequate description of controls or providing multiple controls to confirm irritant reactions. In conclusion, the authors state that BP 1% petrolatum is a problematic patch test and those with atopic dermatitis may be at a greater risk.

J. Q. Del Rosso, DO
G. K. Kim, DO

Predicting risk for early infantile atopic dermatitis by hereditary and environmental factors
Wen H-J, Chen P-C, Chiang T-L, et al (Natl Cheng Kung Univ, Tainan, Taiwan; Natl Taiwan Univ, Taipei; et al)
Br J Dermatol 161:1166-1172, 2009

Background.—Hereditary and environmental factors contribute to the occurrence of atopic dermatitis (AD). However, the interaction of these two factors is not totally understood.

Objectives.—To evaluate the early risk factors for infantile AD at the age of 6 months and to develop a predictive model for the development of AD.

Methods.—In 2005, a representative sample of mother and newborn pairs was obtained by multistage, stratified systematic sampling from the Taiwan national birth register. Information on hereditary and environmental risk factors was collected by home interview when babies were 6 months old. Multivariate regression analysis was applied to determine the risk factors for AD in the infants.

Results.—A total of 20 687 pairs completed the study satisfactorily. AD was diagnosed in 7·0% of 6-month-old infants by physicians. Parental asthma, atopic dermatitis and allergic rhinitis, and maternal education levels were risk factors for AD in infants. Among environmental factors, fungus on walls at home and renovation/painting in the house during pregnancy were significantly associated with early infantile AD. Using these factors, the probability of having infantile AD was estimated and grouped into low, high and very high. With five runs of tests in mutually exclusive subsets of this population, the likelihood of AD for 6-month-old infants was consistent in all the groups with the predictive model. The highest predicted probability of AD was 70·1%, among boys with maternal education levels > 12 years, both parents with AD, renovation and painting of the house during pregnancy and fungus on walls at home. The lowest probability was 3·1%, among girls with none of the above factors.

Conclusions.—This investigation provides a technique for predicting the risk of infantile AD based on hereditary and environmental factors, which could be used for developing a preventive strategy against AD, especially among those children with a family history of atopy.

▶ The Taiwan Birth Cohort Study was created to better understand the effects of social and environmental factors on the growth and health of children in Taiwan. The Department of Health started a nationwide birth register in 2000, mandating all medical institutions that delivered infants to report demographic and vital statistics of all newborns. The sampling population was based on government divisions and regional fertility rates and in total, enrolled 24 200 pairs of mothers and newborns. The study used home interviews completed at 6 months, 18 months, and 3 years of age and included questionnaires collecting information on demographics, history of atopic diseases in parents, home environmental conditions (incense burning, presence of carpets, pets, fungus on walls, painting/home renovation during pregnancy, and presence of cockroaches), birth order, breastfeeding, vaccination status, and infant health. The article describes the genetic and environmental risk factors in Taiwan that may play an early role in the development of atopic dermatitis (AD).

This project successfully gathers data representing the general population of Taiwan. In total, 20 687 singleton infant-mother pairs were included in the analysis to develop a predictive model for development of AD in infants at 6 months of age in Taiwan. The Taiwanese data that correlate with worldwide data include positive associations between infantile AD and the sex of the baby, parental history of atopy, and a higher level of parental education. Of the environmental factors queried, the presence of fungus on walls in the home and renovation or painting in the home during the pregnancy showed the strongest predictive effect for infantile AD. The findings of this study support what we already know regarding the genetic factors associated with AD and adds the important aspect of environmental factors. Although the environmental factors identified in the Taiwanese cohort were not stratified by severity or duration of exposure, they are factors that may be present in most countries and thus relevant to most of the world's population.

This study brings us a step closer in understanding how to advise pregnant mothers who are concerned about AD in their children, either from having a previous child affected or because of a family history of atopy. Advising pregnant mothers to avoid certain allergens, which may affect the fetal immune system, could possibly be a simple way to curb the development of infantile AD. However, confirmation of these findings will be necessary before large-scale interventions take place. It would be helpful to have a more detailed questionnaire capturing specific chemical exposures or laboratory confirmation of types of fungus or chemicals present within homes to clarify the positive associations with infantile AD. The study has taken a large step forward in the assessment of early factors that may predispose individuals to infantile AD. Further research investigating the interactions during fetal development, the mother's exposure during pregnancy, and the development of infantile AD is warranted and has the potential to greatly impact the prevalence of the disease.

M. Reyes Merin, MD
S. Fallon Friedlander, MD

Prevalence of nickel and cobalt allergy among female patients with dermatitis before and after Danish government regulation: A 23-year retrospective study
Thyssen JP, Johansen JD, Carlsen BC, et al (Univ of Copenhagen, Denmark)
J Am Acad Dermatol 61:799-805, 2009

Background.—An increased prevalence of nickel allergy prompted the Danish government to prohibit excessive nickel release (ie, >0.5 μg nickel/cm²/wk) from consumer products in 1990. Concomitant allergy to nickel and cobalt is often observed among patients with dermatitis, probably as a result of cosensitization.

Objectives.—The study investigated the development of nickel and cobalt allergy among Danish female patients with dermatitis tested between 1985 and 2007. This was done to examine whether Danish nickel regulation has reduced the prevalence of nickel allergy and to examine whether the prevalence of cobalt allergy has increased as a result of the nickel regulation.

Methods.—A retrospective analysis of all patch test data from our database was performed (n = 10,335). Comparisons were made using a chi-square test for trend. Logistic regression analyses were used to test for associations.

Results.—The prevalence of nickel allergy decreased significantly among those aged 5 to 30 years from 27.6% in 1985 to 16.8% in 2007 ($P_{trend} < .002$) but increased among those aged 31 to 49 years from

21.3% to 33.8% in the same period ($P_{trend} < .001$). The median age was significantly higher among patients with isolated cobalt allergy than among patients with nickel allergy ($P < .001$).

Limitations.—No information on causative exposures was available.

Conclusions.—Nickel allergy decreased among young female patients with dermatitis between 1985 and 2007 whereas it increased among older patients, probably as a result of a cohort effect. The prevalence of cobalt allergy remained relatively unchanged.

▶ Nickel is one of the most common allergens detected in patch-tested patients. In fact, nickel was recently named the "Contact Allergen of the Year" by the North American Contact Dermatitis Society in 2008. This ubiquitous metal is found in widely available objects, such as zippers, eye glasses, belt buckles, jewelry, keys, and cell phones to name a few. Moreover, some common foods are also implicated with containing high levels of nickel. The rising trend in nickel allergies prompted the government in Denmark to initiate legislation dictating nickel release from consumer products in 1990. Subsequently, a retrospective study was performed on Danish females with dermatitis between 1985 and 2007. As expected, there was a decrease in nickel allergy during this time but only in the youngest age group (5-30 years). As stated by authors, the increase in prevalence of nickel allergy for older patients may be explained by a cohort effect as they most likely were sensitized before the implementation of this regulation. In addition, older patients are more likely to own older products saved before 1990. Further, no significant difference in cobalt allergy was found.

S. Bellew, DO

J. Q. Del Rosso, DO

Shoe contact dermatitis from dimethyl fumarate: clinical manifestations, patch test results, chemical analysis, and source of exposure
Giménez-Arnau A, Silvestre JF, Mercader P, et al (Universitat Autònoma, Barcelona, Spain; Hosp General Universitario, Alicante, Spain; Hosp General Universitario Morales Meseguer, Murcia, Spain; et al)
Contact Dermatitis 61:249-260, 2009

Background.—The methyl ester form of fumaric acid named dimethyl fumarate (DMF) is an effective mould-growth inhibitor. Its irritating and sensitizing properties were demonstrated in animal models. Recently, DMF has been identified as responsible for furniture contact dermatitis in Europe.

Objective.—To describe the clinical manifestations, patch test results, shoe chemical analysis, and source of exposure to DMF-induced shoe contact dermatitis.

Patients, Materials, and Methods.—Patients with suspected shoe contact dermatitis were studied in compliance with the Declaration of

Helsinki. Patch test results obtained with their own shoe and the European baseline series, acrylates and fumaric acid esters (FAE), were recorded according to international guidelines. The content of DMF in shoes was analysed with gas chromatography and mass spectrometry.

Results.—Acute, immediate irritant contact dermatitis and non-immunological contact urticaria were observed in eight adults and two children, respectively. All the adult patients studied developed a delayed sensitization demonstrated by a positive patch testing to DMF $\leq 0.1\%$ in pet. Cross-reactivity with other FAEs and acrylates was observed. At least 12 different shoe brands were investigated. The chemical analysis from the available shoes showed the presence of DMF.

Conclusion.—DMF in shoes was responsible for severe contact dermatitis. Global preventive measures for avoiding contact with DMF are necessary.

▶ Dimethylfumarate (DMF) has been responsible for an epidemic of allergic contact dermatitis (ACD), primarily in Europe, with some reports from Canada. The initial reports demonstrated that furniture manufactured in the Far East was usually the culprit. DMF is a mold inhibitor that was placed in small packets within the furniture before transport to the west. It is highly volatile and therefore penetrated the furniture fabrics easily. It is also a very potent allergen, with positive patch tests reported down to levels of 0.0001%. Hundreds of reports of severe ACD, often bullous, from simply sitting on the affected furniture, have been published. Most recently, a few reports of ACD from DMF in clothing and shoes manufactured in the Far East have surfaced. This report is the most detailed one regarding shoe ACD. An interesting finding is that apparently DMF cross-reacts with acrylates, which are also common sensitizers in adhesives, inks, and plastics.

J. F. Fowler, Jr, MD

Sites of dermatitis in a patch test population: hand dermatitis is associated with polysensitization
Carlsen BC, Andersen KE, Menné T, et al (Copenhagen Univ Hosp Gentofte, Niels Andersens Vej, Hellerup, Denmark; Univ of Southern Denmark, Odense)
Br J Dermatol 161:808-813, 2009

Background.—Sites of dermatitis in larger series of contact allergic patients are rarely reported. Increased risk of polysensitization has been linked only to stasis dermatitis and leg ulcers. However, a large proportion of polysensitized individuals may have dermatitis in other skin areas.

Objectives.—To examine the site of dermatitis at time of first appearance in contact allergic individuals with special focus on the distribution of dermatitis in polysensitized individuals and to examine if widespread dermatitis is more frequent in polysensitized than in single/double-sensitized patients.

Methods.—A matched case—control study was carried out including 394 polysensitized and 726 single/double-sensitized patients who responded to a postal questionnaire. All subjects were recruited from a hospital patch test population.

Results.—The hands were the most frequent and the anogenital region was the least frequent skin area affected with dermatitis. Dermatitis on the hands/wrists [odds ratio (OR) 1·58], in the armpits (OR 1·56) and on the back (OR 1·91) was positively associated with polysensitization. The hands were the only skin area with dermatitis which maintained the association to polysensitization in two subpopulations consisting of, respectively, individuals with and without atopic eczema. Dermatitis on the scalp was negatively associated with polysensitization (OR 0·66) primarily for individuals without atopic eczema. The dermatitis did not seem to be more widespread in polysensitized compared with single/double-sensitized patients.

Conclusions.—Special awareness in patients with hand dermatitis seems justified either to prevent development of multiple contact allergies or to document polysensitization as an aetiological factor.

▶ The evaluation of the patients suspected for contact dermatitis by patch testing has a limited set of outcome scenarios: negative: 1 or 2 positive reactions, or polysensitization to multiple related or unrelated allergens. Needless to say, the potential number of permutations that can occur in the positive patch test patient group is nearly limitless. The literature provides data with regard to the sites of dermatitis and the epidemiologic relationship to specific allergens and allergen groups. Because the hands are expectedly the most commonly exposed body site with regard to occupational and environmental exposure, the potential for polysensitization is great in the at-risk individual. Debate still exists regarding the role of a concomitant atopic diathesis in the expected rate of allergic sensitization, as it relates to body site. Regardless, patch testing provides an important tool in the diagnosis of patients with hand dermatitis, and the resultant data are important to heed to prevent initial or further sensitization in those suffering from the incapacitating impact of hand dermatitis.

D. E. Cohen, MD, MPH

Staphylococcus aureus and hand eczema severity
Haslund P, Bangsgaard N, Jarløv JO, et al (Univ of Copenhagen, Denmark; et al)
Br J Dermatol 161:772-777, 2009

Background.—The role of bacterial infections in hand eczema (HE) remains to be assessed.

Objectives.—To determine the prevalence of Staphylococcus aureus in patients with HE compared with controls, and to relate presence of S. aureus, subtypes and toxin production to severity of HE.

Methods.—Bacterial swabs were taken at three different visits from the hand and nose in 50 patients with HE and 50 controls. Staphylococcus aureus was subtyped by spa typing and assigned to clonal complexes (CCs), and isolates were tested for exotoxin-producing S. aureus strains. The Hand Eczema Severity Index was used for severity assessment.

Results.—Staphylococcus aureus was found on the hands in 24 patients with HE and four controls ($P < 0\cdot001$), and presence of S. aureus was found to be related to increased severity of the eczema ($P < 0\cdot001$). Patients carried identical S. aureus types on the hands and in the nose in all cases, and between visits in 90% of cases. Ten different CC types were identified, no association with severity was found, and toxin-producing strains were not found more frequently in patients with HE than in controls.

Conclusions.—Staphylococcus aureus was present on hands in almost half of all patients with HE, and was significantly related to severity of the disease. This association indicates that S. aureus could be an important cofactor for persistence of HE.

▶ Hand eczema (HE) is a multifactoral disease often characterized by frequent relapses. Past studies have suggested that *Staphylococcus aureus* colonization in atopic dermatitis (AD) may be a major exacerbating factor, but there are few studies examining the severity of disease with concomitant colonization. This prospective study sought to determine the prevalence of *S aureus* involving the hands and nares of patients with HE and assessed the potential correlation of staphylococcal colonization with HE severity. There were 50 HE subjects and 50 control subjects with bacterial swabs taken from hand and nose at 3 different visits. *S aureus* was also subtyped and assigned to clonal complexes (CCs), and isolates were tested for exotoxin-producing *S aureus* strains. *S aureus* was found in significantly more HE patients, with 24/50 HE patients affected and 4/50 controls affected ($P < .001$). To add, the presence of *S aureus* was found to correlate with disease severity of HE ($P < .001$) as assessed using the Hand Eczema Severity Index. Also, patients carried identical *S aureus* types on the hands and nares in all cases and in 90% of follow-up visits. Authors also found no association with severity of HE correlating with toxin-producing strains of *S aureus* as compared with controls. No specific clonal complexes were related to HE, and toxin-producing strains were not found more frequently in patients with HE compared with controls. Patients with *S aureus* hand colonization had significantly greater HE severity as compared with subjects without *S aureus* colonization of the hands. The high frequency of *S aureus* in patients with HE and its correlation with severity would indicate that *S aureus* is an important cofactor for persistence of the disease and may be important in HE morbidity. Limitations included small sample size, a 20% dropout rate at visit 2, and a 50% dropout rate at visit 3. However, there was no difference between patients and dropouts according to the authors. It was concluded that patients with HE presenting with no clinical signs of infection were colonized with *S aureus* in 50% of cases, and presence of *S aureus* was correlated with severity of HE. In future studies, it would be interesting to include treatment addressing *S aureus* eradication and correlation with disease severity and therapeutic response in HE patients.

J. Q. Del Rosso, DO
G. K. Kim, DO

Th17/Tc17 infiltration and associated cytokine gene expression in elicitation phase of allergic contact dermatitis

Zhao Y, Balato A, Fishelevich R, et al (Univ of Maryland School of Medicine, Baltimore; Univ of Naples, Italy)
Br J Dermatol 161:1301-1306, 2009

Background.—Allergic contact dermatitis (ACD) is a typical delayed-type hypersensitivity to sensitizing haptens mediated by T cells. Th1/Tc1 cells are currently considered to be the primary effectors in ACD. There is little information concerning the role played in ACD in humans by Th17/Tc17 cells, a recently defined subpopulation of effector T cells.

Objectives.—In the present report we attempted to characterize Th17/Tc17 cells in the infiltrates of the skin in the elicitation phase of ACD.

Methods.—Th17 as well as Th1/Th2 cytokine gene expression was examined by semiquantitative real-time polymerase chain reaction in paired samples of positive patch test biopsies and normal skin from 11 patients allergic to nine different allergens. The *in situ* characterization of interleukin (IL)-17-producing cells was carried out using anti-RORC and anti-T-cell subset antibodies by double immunofluorescence.

Results.—Compared with normal paired skin samples, gene expression of transcription factor for human Th17 cells, RORC, and Th17-related cytokines IL-17A, IL-17F and IL-23 was significantly increased in positive patch test biopsies. The mRNA for interferon-γ and IL-4 was also increased. In the dermal infiltrates, about 20% of the infiltrating cells were IL-17-producing cells as they expressed RORC, and such RORC-expressing cells were detected in both CD4+ ($\sim$30%) and CD8+ ($\sim$20%) subsets.

Conclusions.—This is the first demonstration of Th17/Tc17 cells in the elicitation phase of human ACD, showing that they are a regular participant in the immunopathology of this common allergic reaction regardless of the nature of the triggering allergen.

▶ In recent years, the proinflammatory cytokine IL-23 has been found to share a common p40 subunit with IL-12 and contribute to the development of a new effector T-helper-cell lineage (ie, Th17) from naïve T cells, characterized by the production of proinflammatory cytokines such as IL-17A, IL-17F, IL-21, and IL-22. Th17 cells have been associated with immune reactions against extracellular bacterial and fungal infections as well as with several autoimmune conditions such as psoriasis, rheumatoid arthritis, and other autoimmune diseases. These conditions, previously thought to be in part mediated by

IL-12-dependent interferon-gamma-producing Th1 cells, are being reclassified as Th17. This study demonstrated, in humans, that allergic contact dermatitis, another predominantly Th1-mediated condition, seems to be additionally associated with Th17 and related cytokines, confirmed by the significant increase in the gene expression of cytokines from Th1, Th2, and Th17 cells restricted to positive patch test sites, compared with normal skin. In addition, mRNA for the human retinoic acid receptor-related orphan nuclear receptor C (RORC), the characteristic Th17 master transcription factor, was also significantly increased in positive patch test sites compared with normal skin. Interestingly, in 2 positive sites from 1 case, as the severity of the reaction increased, there was an increase in IL-17 mRNA expression and a decrease in interferon-gamma and IL-4 gene expression. The immunochemistry results confirmed the presence of CD3+, CD4+, and CD8+/RORC+/Th17 cells predominantly detected among the superficial dermal perivascular patches but not in the epidermis or healthy skin samples. This study describes new immunopathological aspects of allergic contact dermatitis with potential therapeutic implications. Clinical trials targeting Th17-derived cytokines might be the next step to prove this therapeutic concept in allergic contact dermatitis.

B. Berman, MD, PhD

The additive value of patch testing with patients' own products at an occupational dermatology clinic
Slodownik D, Williams J, Frowen K, et al (Occupational Dermatology Res and Education Centre, Victoria, Australia; Monash Med Centre, Clayton, Victoria, Australia; et al)
Contact Dermatitis 61:231-235, 2009

Background and Objectives.—Patch testing with commercially available kits detects only 70–80% of relevant allergens in patients with contact dermatitis. This is not ideal, especially when occupational issues are being evaluated. This study analyses our data regarding reactions to patients' own products.

Methods.—In a 5-year period, 1532 patients were assessed in our occupational dermatology clinic.

Results.—We found that 101 patients (6.6%) reacted to their own samples. In 20 (1.3%) cases, reacting to their own samples was the only clue for detecting the responsible allergen. In 59 (3.9%) cases, testing with their own samples reinforced their reactions to commercial allergens.

Conclusions.—We found the overall additive value of testing with patients' own products to be 5.2%. This is not a low proportion considering the 20–30% false negative rate when patch testing. Patch testing with patients' own samples, appropriately diluted should be undertaken whenever possible.

▶ It has long been recognized that better diagnostic accuracy of contact dermatitis ensues with increasing number of allergens patch tested. This is especially true when dealing with occupational allergens that may not be present on a standard screening series. This report indicates that over 100 patients in a 5-year period had positive patch tests to substances that were brought in from the workplace. Although many occupations and exposures were involved, coolant fluids, adhesives, and personal protective gear were among the most common substances giving positive patch tests. However, patch testing items brought in by a patient must be tested with care. In general, substances that are intended for prolonged skin contact, such as cosmetics, coolant fluids, and gloves, can be tested safely. Items intended to be avoided or rinsed off, such as soaps, shampoos, acids, alkalis, and organic solvents, should not be patch tested under occlusion unless they are diluted properly. Otherwise a false-positive irritant reaction is likely. When in doubt, a literature review may reveal proper test concentrations. Unknown substances should not be patch tested. When properly done, a positive patch test to a workplace allergen is extremely helpful in documenting occupational causation of allergic contact dermatitis.

J. F. Fowler, Jr, MD

The association between hand eczema and nickel allergy has weakened among young women in the general population following the Danish nickel regulation: results from two cross-sectional studies
Thyssen JP, Linneberg A, Menné T, et al (Univ of Copenhagen, Denmark; et al)
Contact Dermatitis 61:342-348, 2009

Background.—An association between nickel contact allergy and hand eczema has previously been demonstrated. In 1990, Denmark regulated the extent of nickel release in the ear-piercing process as well as nickel release from consumer products.

Objectives.—This study aimed to evaluate the effect of the Danish nickel regulation by comparing the prevalence of concomitant nickel allergy and hand eczema observed in two repeated cross-sectional studies performed in the same general population in Copenhagen.

Materials.—In 1990 and 2006, 3881 18−69 year olds completed a postal questionnaire and were patch tested with nickel. Data were analysed by logistic regression analyses and associations were expressed as odds ratios (ORs) with 95% confidence intervals (CIs).

Results.—The prevalence of concomitant nickel contact allergy and a history of hand eczema decreased among 18−35-year-old women from 9.0% in 1990 to 2.1% in 2006 ($P < 0.01$). The association between nickel contact allergy and a history of hand eczema decreased in this age group between 1990 ($OR = 3.63$; $CI = 1.33−9.96$) and 2006 ($OR = 0.65$; $CI = 0.29−1.46$). Among older women, no significant changes were observed in the association between nickel contact allergy and hand eczema.

Conclusions.—Regulatory control of nickel exposure may have reduced the effect of nickel on hand eczema in the young female population.

▶ The increasing prevalence of nickel allergies prompted the Danish government to initiate strict standards for nickel release in consumer products in 1990. Additional reports support a strong correlation between nickel allergies and hand eczema. Therefore, authors sought to examine if decrease in nickel exposure due to the regulation would subsequently decrease prevalence of hand eczema. Patients were evaluated via postal questionnaires and patch testing with nickel. As a portion of the study is dependent on self-administered questionnaires, it may be subject to responder bias. In fact, the survey asks subjects to self-diagnose themselves with hand eczema following a description of the dermatosis. It is unclear whether selected individuals would understand medical terminology, such as "vesicles or exudation." Nevertheless, the results support other findings of the Danish nickel regulation impacting nickel allergy in young females and, subsequently, decreasing prevalence of hand eczema. No statistically significant changes were observed in older women, and that may be due to cohort effect.

S. Bellew, DO

J. Q. Del Rosso, DO

The effectiveness of levocetirizine and desloratadine in up to 4 times conventional doses in difficult-to-treat urticaria
Staevska M, Popov TA, Kralimarkova T, et al (Med Univ, Sofia, Bulgaria, UK; et al)
J Allergy Clin Immunol 125:676-682, 2010

Background.—H_1-antihistamines are first line treatment of chronic urticaria, but many patients do not get satisfactory relief with recommended doses. European guidelines recommend increased antihistamine doses of up to 4-fold.

Objective.—To provide supportive evidence for the European guidelines.

Methods.—Eighty tertiary referral patients with chronic urticaria (age range, 19-67 years) were randomized for double-blind treatment with levocetirizine or desloratadine (40/40). Treatment started at the conventional daily dose of 5 mg and then increased weekly to 10 mg, 20 mg, or 20 mg of the opposite drug if relief of symptoms was incomplete. Wheal and pruritus scores, quality of life, patient discomfort, somnolence, and safety were assessed.

Results.—Thirteen patients became symptom-free at 5 mg (9 levocetirizine vs 4 desloratadine), compared with 28 subjects on the higher doses of 10 mg (8/7) and 20 mg (5/1). Of the 28 patients nonresponsive to 20 mg desloratadine, 7 became symptom-free with 20 mg levocetirizine. None of the 18 levocetirizine nonresponders benefited with 20 mg desloratadine. Increasing antihistamine doses improved quality of life but did not increase somnolence. Analysis of the effect of treatment on discomfort caused by urticaria showed great individual heterogeneity of antihistamine responsiveness: $\sim 15\%$ of patients were good responders, $\sim 10\%$ were nonresponders, and $\sim 75\%$ were responders to higher than conventional antihistamine doses. No serious or severe adverse effects warranting discontinuation of treatment occurred with either drug.

Conclusion.—Increasing the dosage of levocetirizine and desloratadine up to 4-fold improves chronic urticaria symptoms without compromising safety in approximately three quarters of patients with difficult-to-treat chronic urticaria.

▶ Chronic urticaria (CU) is defined as the presence of pruritus and wheals with or without angioedema for greater than 6 weeks' duration. Symptoms can often be debilitating for the patient, as CU can disrupt sleep patterns and activities of daily living. Adding to the frustration, 80% to 90% of patients with CU have no identifiable cause.[1] During the third International Consensus Meeting, guidelines were established for the management of urticaria.[2] The newer second-generation H_1-antihistamines (eg, cetirizine, desloratadine, fexofenadine, levocetirizine, and loratadine) are considered first-line agents that are less sedating than the previous generation. If patients do not respond to the conventional dosage, it is recommended to increase the dose up to 4-fold. If patients are nonresponders to the increased dosage, second-line therapy may be added to the existing anti-histamine treatment. This randomized double-blinded study aimed to provide supportive evidence for the European guidelines. In fact, results indicate that 75% of patients responded well to 4-fold increases in the 2 antihistamines studied (levocetirizine and desloratadine) without concomitant increase in somnolence or untoward side effects. More specifically, of the 2 drugs studied, levocetirizine was found to be more effective in treatment of CU compared with desloratadine.

S. Bellew, DO

J. Q. Del Rosso, DO

References

1. Sheikh J. Autoantibodies to the high-affinity IgE receptor in chronic urticaria: how important are they? *Curr Opin Allergy Clin Immunol.* 2005;5:403-407.
2. Zuberbier T, Bindslev-Jensen C, Canonica W, et al. EAACI/GA2LEN/EDF guideline: management of urticaria. *Allergy.* 2006;61:321-331.

The Histamine H_4 Receptor Mediates Inflammation and Pruritus in Th2-Dependent Dermal Inflammation
Cowden JM, Zhang M, Dunford PJ, et al (Johnson & Johnson Pharmaceutical Res & Development, LLC, San Diego, CA)
J Invest Dermatol 130:1023-1033, 2010

The role of histamine H_4 receptor (H_4R) was investigated in a T-helper type 2 (Th2)-cell-mediated mouse skin inflammation model that mimics several of the features of atopic dermatitis. Treatment with two specific H_4R antagonists before challenge with FITC led to a significant reduction in ear edema, inflammation, mast cell, and eosinophil infiltration. This was accompanied by a reduction in the levels of several cytokines and chemokines in the ear tissue. Upon *ex vivo* antigen stimulation of lymph nodes, H_4R antagonism reduced lymphocyte proliferation and IL-4, IL-5, and IL-17 levels. One explanation for this finding is that lymph nodes from animals dosed with the H_4R antagonist, JNJ 7777120, contained a lower number of FITC-positive dendritic cells. The effect of H_4R antagonism on dendritic cell migration *in vivo* may be an indirect result of the reduction in tissue cytokines and chemokines or a direct effect on chemotaxis. In addition to anti-inflammatory effects, JNJ 7777120 also significantly inhibited the pruritus shown in the model. Therefore, the dual effects of H_4R antagonists on pruritus and Th2-cell-mediated inflammation point to their therapeutic potential for the treatment of Th2-mediated skin disorders, including atopic dermatitis.

▶ The authors used a contact dermatitis model for atopic dermatitis (AD) in this study in light of the T-helper type 2 (Th2) pattern of cytokine responses elicited being similar to those obtained during early stages of AD. The involvement of this newly identified histamine receptor (ie, histamine H_4 receptor [H_4R]) in other inflammatory and allergic conditions has recently been demonstrated. Potentially relevant mechanisms related to H_4R antagonists include the reduction of Th2 proinflammatory cytokines directly decreasing tissue edema and indirectly reducing tissue levels of mast cells and eosinophils; the reduction of antigen + dendritic cells in the draining lymph nodes, probably because of the reduction of cytokines mediating the migration of dendritic cell or Langerhans cell from the skin to the lymph node; and the reduction of pruritus, probably indirectly by decreasing inflammation and decreasing interleukin-31 (recently linked to pruritus in AD) or directly by affecting sensory neurons. Of interest, H_4R antagonists' anti-inflammatory antipruritic effects seem to be superior to that of histamine H_1 receptor in the Th2-dependent model of skin inflammation. This study confirms, at least partially, the involvement of H_4R in the skin and particularly in AD and suggests the potential of H_4R in becoming an important target for the treatment of this condition.

B. Berman, MD, PhD

The importance of propolis in patch testing—a multicentre survey
Rajpara S, Wilkinson MS, King CM, et al (Aberdeen Royal Infirmary, UK; Leeds General Infirmary, UK; Royal Liverpool and Broadgreen Hosps NHS Trust, UK; et al)
Contact Dermatitis 61:287-290, 2009

Background.—Propolis is widely used in 'natural' cosmetics, remedies, and over-the-counter products. The incidence of propolis allergy is increasing, and cross-reaction with fragrance mix I (FMII), colophonium, and *Myroxylon pereirae* can occur.

Objectives.—To find out the prevalence and clinical relevance of positive patch tests to propolis and assess cross-reactions with *Myroxylon pereirae*, colophonium, FMI, and beeswax.

Methods.—Two thousand eight hundred and twenty-eight subjects in 10 UK centres were patch tested with propolis and beeswax. Generic data were acquired from British Contact Dermatology Society (BCDS) database and further relevant information was requested by survey of participating centres.

Results.—The prevalence of propolis allergy was 1.9% (55/2828). Out of these 55 subjects, only 4 (7.2%) were allergic to beeswax, 22 (40%) to *Myroxylon pereirae*, 15 (27.2%) to colophonium, and 6 (10.9%) to FMI. Additional data for 41 propolis allergic subjects were collected by questionnaire. Hands were the most common sites of involvement, and cosmetics were the most common source of contact. Eight out of 12 subjects reported improvement in eczema following avoidance of propolis.

Conclusions.—Propolis is an important allergen of increasing frequency and its inclusion in BCDS baseline series is appropriate. Cross-sensitivity to beeswax is rare.

▶ Propolis, also called bee glue, is produced by bees while constructing their hives. It occurs naturally in close proximity to beeswax. It has been used in a variety of cosmeceutical products. In the United States it is most often found in lip-care products. This large multicenter report from the United Kingdom shows the incidence of allergy to propolis about 2% in the tested subjects. This is almost identical to the prevalence in reports from North America, making it an allergen of significant importance. This report further tells us that usually beeswax is not allergenic in these patients. In contrast, cross-reaction often occurs with another common allergen used to detect the fragrance sensitivity—*Myroxylon pereirae* (formerly called Balsam of Peru). In this report, hands were the most common location of dermatitis, followed by face. Other reports implicate propolis commonly in cheilitis. Patients suspected to have allergy to skin-care products and cosmeceuticals, especially those with lip, facial, or hand dermatitis, should be tested with this allergen.

J. F. Fowler, Jr, MD

Therapeutic Hotline: Treatment of prurigo nodularis and lichen simplex chronicus with gabapentin

Gencoglan G, Inanir I, Gunduz K (Med Faculty of Celal Bayar Univ, Manisa, Turkey)
Dermatol Ther 23:194-198, 2010

Psychocutaneous conditions are frequently encountered in dermatology practice. Prurigo nodularis and lichen simplex chronicus are two frustrating conditions that are classified in this category. They are often refractory to classical treatment with topical corticosteroids and antihistamines. Severe, generalized exacerbations require systemic therapy. Phototherapy, erythromycine, retinoids, cyclosporine, azathiopurine, naltrexone, and psychopharmacologic agents (pimozide, selective serotonin reuptake inhibitor antidepressants) were tried with some success. Here five cases with lichen simplex chronicus and four cases with prurigo nodularis, who responded well to gabapentin, are presented.

▶ Both prurigo nodularis (PN) and lichen simplex chronicus (LSC) are 2 disease entities that may likely be similar in etiology in some cases and are often challenging to manage. Both are characterized by intense pruritus and scratching and/or picking at localized areas of skin, and psychogenic factors may often play a dominant role. However, pruritus is not always reported as initiating the desire to scratch or pick at an area, especially in PN. This is a study of 9 patients (4 with PN and 5 with LSC) who were treated with gabapentin. The mean age of the patients was 44.8 years with papules and nodules existing for 2 to 20 years. Lesions were only on extremities in 3 patients, and the other 6 patients had truncal involvement also. All patients were previously treated with antihistamines, corticosteroids, phototherapy, and antidepressants. The patients were started on gabapentin 300 mg/d and the dosage was increased to 900 mg/d, with intensity of pruritus evaluated every month. Although patients had at least a partial remission after 2 months, the study did not have a standardized scale to assess pruritus. Total treatment period ranged from 4 to 10 months, and the patients were followed 3 months afterward. One weakness of this study was the short follow-up period. It was unknown if patients had recurrent disease after discontinuation of the drug. There was no control group in this study. Also, an optimal treatment period was not discussed, and some patients may have benefited from a longer course of therapy. There was also no mention of a washout period, and it was unknown whether patients were on other therapies, which may have affected results. However, this report suggests that gabapentin may be added to our armamentarium for treatment of recalcitrant LSC and PN. Although larger controlled studies need to be done in the future, gabapentin may be promising.

J. Q. Del Rosso, DO

G. K. Kim, DO

Topical treatment of perianal eczema with tacrolimus 0·1%
Schauber J, Weisenseel P, Ruzicka T (Ludwig-Maximilians Univ, Munich, Germany)
Br J Dermatol 161:1384-1386, 2009

Background.—Perianal eczema is an inflammatory skin disease with a high prevalence in most industrialized countries. As general practitioners and dermatologists frequently see patients with perianal eczema the need for efficient, fast and safe therapies is high. Topical calcineurin inhibitors such as tacrolimus (FK506) ameliorate cutaneous inflammation and associated pruritus in an array of inflammatory dermatoses.

Objectives.—To investigate the effect of topical tacrolimus in perianal eczema.

Methods.—Twenty-four patients with perianal eczema were treated with tacrolimus 0·1% ointment twice daily on the affected skin area for 2 weeks.

Results.—All returning patients showed clinical improvement as assessed by macroscopic appearance and clinical score (modified SCORAD index).

Conclusions.—In this short-term trial we demonstrate that topical tacrolimus 0·1% is safe, efficient and well tolerated in patients with perianal eczema irrespective of the underlying cause.

▶ Perianal eczema has been traditionally treated with topical glucocorticosteroids. However, patients risk known side effects, such as skin atrophy with chronic glucocorticosteroid use, especially in intertriginous areas. Therefore, alternative treatment options are sought and this 24-patient pilot trial looks at another option: topical calcineurin inhibitors. Specifically, patients were given topical tacrolimus 0.1% ointment applied twice daily to the affected area for 2 weeks. All patients had symptoms related to perianal eczema for at least 4 weeks before treatment. Of the 24 patients, 19 showed clinical improvement as evidenced by reduction in inflammation and erythema seen clinically and with modified Severity Scoring of Atopic Dermatitis index score (clinical score). Five patients were lost to follow-up and excluded from data. Tacrolimus was well tolerated, with the exception of mild burning at the start of the treatment. Limitations of the study include the small number of patients studied and short duration of treatment. Topical calcineurin inhibitors such as tacrolimus may be a good alternative choice to topical corticosteroid use.

S. Bellew, DO

J. Q. Del Rosso, DO

Treatment with a barrier-strengthening moisturizing cream delays relapse of atopic dermatitis: a prospective and randomized controlled clinical trial
Wirén K, Nohlgård C, Nyberg F, et al (ACO HUD NORDIC AB, Upplands Väsby, Sweden; Läkarhuset Fruängen, Sweden; Danderyd Hosp AB, Stockholm, Sweden; et al)
J Eur Acad Dermatol Venereol 23:1267-1272, 2009

Background.—Standard treatment of atopic dermatitis (AD) is based on topical glucocorticosteroids or calcineurin inhibitors to treat flares combined with moisturizer treatment to alleviate dry skin symptoms. Patients with AD have an abnormal skin barrier function, and strategies for reducing the risks for eczema would be to repair the barrier or prevent barrier dysfunction.

Objectives.—The objective of this study was to explore the time to relapse of eczema during a 26-week maintenance treatment with a urea containing moisturizer compared to no treatment (neither medical nor nonmedicated preparations) after successful clearing of atopic lesions. The moisturizer has previously been shown to improve skin barrier function.

Methods.—Patients applied betamethasone valerate (0.1%) on eczematous lesions during a 3-week period. Those with cleared eczema entered a 26-week maintenance phase, applying the moisturizer or left the previously affected area untreated. Upon eczema relapse, patients were instructed to contact the clinic and to have the relapse confirmed by the investigator.

Results.—Fifty-five patients entered the study and 44 patients were included in the maintenance phase (22 using moisturizer twice daily and 22 using no treatment). Median time to relapse for patients treated with moisturizer was > 180 days (duration of the study) compared with 30 days for the no-treatment group. Sixty-eight per cent of the patients treated with the moisturizer and 32% of the untreated patients remained free from eczema during the observation period.

Conclusions.—Maintenance treatment with a barrier-improving urea moisturizer on previous eczematous areas reduced the risk of relapse to approximately one third of that of no treatment.

▶ This is a randomized controlled, parallel-group, prospective, multicenter study conducted at 5 dermatology outpatient clinics in Sweden. This study included 55 Caucasians (18-65 years) diagnosed with atopic dermatitis (AD). The severity of eczema was graded with a score of at least 6 according to the Atopic Dermatitis Severity Index. Patients applied 0.01% betamethasone valerate (BV) cream to the lesions for 3 weeks. After this 3-week period, patients were randomized into either a no-treatment control group or urea moisturizer group for 26 weeks postclearance for areas only treated with BV. Patients allocated to the treatment group were instructed to apply the moisturizer on the identified area twice daily, whereas the control group had to abstain from using any topical formulation on the area. However, control patients were allowed to treat other parts of the body with other topical preparations. Transepidermal water loss (TEWL) was also measured throughout the study for both groups. TEWL was not significantly different for the 2 treatment arms ($P > .05$). In the maintenance therapy, 68% of patients treated with moisturizer and 32% of untreated patients experienced no relapse in eczema during the 180 days of observation. The median time to relapse of the patients treated with the moisturizer was > 180 days compared with 30 days in the control group. There was a significant difference in the time to relapse of AD during the maintenance phase ($P < .01$) with a hazard ratio of 3.2, indicating that patients using the moisturizer experienced a one-third reduction in the risk of relapse as compared with patients using no treatment. The results also indicated a 53% relative risk reduction and a 36% absolute risk reduction at the 26-week time point associated with maintenance moisturizer use. One limitation of this study was that it was conducted only in Sweden and results may vary with other geographic locations, seasons according to humidity, and populations. Additionally, all patients were Caucasian. Another study limitation was that moisturizer use was restricted to a specified target site for evaluation, with the same results not necessarily applicable to widespread application. The vulnerability to eczema may vary between body areas, with certain areas being more prone to relapse. Also, with clearance of AD after BV treatment, with complete absence of prior eczematous sites, how could one be sure that patients remembered previously affected areas accurately? In conclusion, maintenance treatment with a urea-based moisturizer may reduce the risk of relapse in patients with AD after initial topical corticosteroid therapy, although studies evaluating results with widespread moisturizer application are needed.

J. Q. Del Rosso, DO

G. K. Kim, DO

A pilot study of emollient therapy for the primary prevention of atopic dermatitis
Simpson EL, Berry TM, Brown PA, et al (Oregon Health and Science Univ, Portland)
J Am Acad Dermatol 63:587-593, 2010

Background.—Prevention strategies in atopic dermatitis (AD) using allergen avoidance have not been consistently effective. New research reveals the importance of the skin barrier in the development of AD and possibly food allergy and asthma. Correcting skin barrier defects from birth may prevent AD onset or moderate disease severity.

Objective.—We sought to determine the feasibility of skin barrier protection as a novel AD prevention strategy.

Methods.—We enrolled 22 neonates at high risk for developing AD in a feasibility pilot study using emollient therapy from birth.

Results.—No intervention-related adverse events occurred in our cohort followed up for a mean time of 547 days. Of the 20 subjects who remained in the study, 3 (15.0%) developed AD, suggesting a protective effect when compared with historical controls. Skin barrier measurements remained within ranges seen in normal-appearing skin.

Limitations.—No conclusions regarding efficacy can be made without a control group.

Conclusions.—Skin barrier repair from birth represents a novel and feasible approach to AD prevention. Further studies are warranted to determine the efficacy of this approach.

▶ The development of atopic dermatitis (AD) is increasingly being linked to primary defects in the epidermal barrier. In fact, often the severity of disease parallels the extent of barrier permeability dysfunction.[1] This study focuses on the prevention of AD signs and symptoms by attempting to correct skin barrier defects from birth with the application of emollients. Infants who were at high risk for development of AD were included in this study, and cetaphil cream (an oil-in-water petrolatum-based cream) was applied to the skin immediately after bathing. At the conclusion of the study, 3 of 20 subjects developed AD. Limitations of the study include no control group for comparison and the small number of subjects involved. With the chronic nature of AD, clinicians are always seeking alternative therapies to long-term topical corticosteroid use because of its associated side effects. Therefore, emphasis on the barrier dysfunction is a prudent novel approach. Future investigations involving application of the newer physiologic barrier repair creams may be warranted, as there are reported differences in barrier recovery after application of nonphysiologic (ie, petrolatum) versus complete physiologic lipid mixtures containing ceramides, cholesterol, and fatty acids in the proper ratio.[2]

S. Bellew, DO
J. Q. Del Rosso, DO

References

1. Elias PM, Schmuth M. Abnormal skin barrier in the etiopathogenesis of atopic dermatitis. *Curr Opin Allergy Clin Immunol.* 2009;9:437-446.
2. Elias PM. Physiologic lipids for barrier repair in dermatology. In: Draelos Z, ed. *Procedures in Cosmetic Dermatology. Cosmeceuticals.* Elsevier; 2005:63-70.

Prednisolone vs. ciclosporin for severe adult eczema. An investigator-initiated double-blind placebo-controlled multicentre trial
Schmitt J, Schäkel K, Fölster-Holst R, et al (Technical Univ Dresden, Fetscherstr, Germany; Christian Albrecht Univ Kiel, Germany; et al)
Br J Dermatol 162:661-668, 2010

Background.—Patients with severe eczema frequently receive systemic glucocorticosteroids. The efficacy of prednisolone and other steroids, however, has never been evaluated appropriately. A meta-analysis indicated that ciclosporin is the best evaluated systemic treatment for eczema.

Objectives.—To investigate the comparative efficacy of prednisolone and ciclosporin for severe eczema.

Methods.—In an investigator-initiated double-blind randomized multicentre trial, adults with severe eczema (objective SCORAD ≥ 40 and Dermatology Life Quality Index ≥ 10) were randomly allocated to receive prednisolone (initial dose $0\cdot5$-$0\cdot8$ mg kg^{-1} daily) for 2 weeks followed by placebo for 4 weeks or ciclosporin ($2\cdot7$-$4\cdot0$ mg kg^{-1} daily) for 6 weeks and followed for another 12 weeks. Concomitant treatment included a moderately potent topical steroid, emollients, and continuation of antihistamines. Primary endpoint was the proportion of patients with stable remission, i.e. $\geq 50\%$ SCORAD improvement under active treatment and no flare ($\geq 75\%$ of baseline SCORAD) during follow-up. Sample size calculation indicated that 66 patients were needed to see clinically relevant differences between groups. Analysis was by intention-to-treat (ClinicalTrials.gov Identifier: NCT00445081).

Results.—Because of unexpectedly high numbers of withdrawals due to significant exacerbations of eczema (*n* = 15/38) an independent data monitoring and safety board proposed early study termination. Thirty-eight patients were randomized and analysed. Stable remission was achieved in one of 21 patients receiving prednisolone compared with six of 17 patients treated with ciclosporin (*P* = 0·031).

Conclusions.—Ciclosporin is significantly more efficacious than prednisolone for severe adult eczema. Despite its frequent use in daily practice, prednisolone is not recommended to induce stable remission of eczema.

▶ The clinician treating adult patients with moderate to severe eczematous dermatitis often elicits a history of multiple courses of systemic corticosteroids (CSs). This class of drugs is readily used by both dermatologists and general medical practitioners to control acute flares of the dermatitis; however, few data exist about their efficacy or ability to control disease activity after the drugs are discontinued. Increasing interest regarding the use of nonsteroidal systemic immunomodulatory agents has been evidenced by the publication of case reports, case series, and small clinical trials. While CSs have an irreplaceable role in the management of acute or paroxysmal flares of disease activity, their role in the long-term control of eczema remains dubious. Cyclosporine and other nonsteroidal drugs should be considered with greater alacrity for the control of this difficult and life-altering dermatosis.[1,2]

D. E. Cohen, MD, MPH

References

1. Amor KT, Ryan C, Menter A. The use of cyclosporine in dermatology: part I. *J Am Acad Dermatol.* 2010;63:925-946.
2. Ryan C, Amor KT, Menter A. The use of cyclosporine in dermatology: part II. *J Am Acad Dermatol.* 2010;63:949-972.

Effectiveness of skin protection measures in prevention of occupational hand eczema: results of a prospective randomized controlled trial over a follow-up period of 1 year

Kütting B, Baumeister T, Weistenhöfer W, et al (Friedrich-Alexander Univ of Erlangen-Nuremberg, Germany)

Br J Dermatol 162:362-370, 2010

Background.—We recently found a very low adherence to a generally recommended skin protection regimen in a sample of 1355 metalworkers.

Objectives.—The present study assessed the effectiveness of skin protection as presently recommended, especially the differential contribution of skin care and skin protection, to the prevention of occupational hand eczema.

Methods.—Of 1355 metalworkers screened, 1020 male volunteers, all fit for work, were recruited for a prospective intervention study with four arms (skin care, skin protection, both combined, and control group, i.e. no recommendation). The study was performed from winter 2006/2007 to spring 2008, following each subject for up for 12 months. Both hands were examined using a quantitative skin score, and a standardized personal interview was performed three times. The change of the objective skin score from baseline to 12 months was used as primary outcome measure.

Results.—After 12 months 800 subjects were included (78·4% of those recruited). The compliance to follow the randomized measure depended on the recommended measure and ranged from 73·7% to 88·7%. While in the control group a significant deterioration was found, the largest and significant improvement was noted in the group following the generally recommended skin protection programme (skin care + skin protection) followed by skin protection alone as second best.

Conclusions.—The generally recommended skin protection regimen seems to provide effective prevention of occupational skin disease. Therefore, the compliance to follow the skin protection regimen, especially the use of skin protection, should be enhanced.

▶ Hand dermatitis is a particularly vexing condition in the clinician's office. Not only is therapy challenging, the determination of a cause can be quite confounding. In addition to potential allergen exposure through activities of routine daily living and work, irritants are commonly involved in producing and perpetuating the problem. While personal protection and proper skin care have often been touted by the clinician, little investigative work has been carried out to determine the magnitude of the effects of protection versus proper skin care. Patients should understand that not only are personal protective devices and equipment important to use, the concurrent use of emollients and gentle skin cleanser may augment the preventative effect and potentially avert a debilitating condition of dermatitis on the hands.

D. E. Cohen, MD, MPH

Natural moisturizing factor components in the stratum corneum as biomarkers of filaggrin genotype: evaluation of minimally invasive methods
Kezic S, Kammeyer A, Calkoen F, et al (Univ of Amsterdam, the Netherlands; Bioskin, Berlin, Germany)
Br J Dermatol 161:1098-1104, 2009

Background.—The carriers of loss-of-function mutations in the filaggrin gene (*FLG*) have reduced levels of natural moisturizing factor (NMF) in the stratum corneum. The concentration of NMF components which are formed by filaggrin protein breakdown in the stratum corneum might therefore be useful as a biomarker of the *FLG* genotype.

Objectives.—To investigate the feasibility of different sampling methods for the determination of two NMF components, 2-pyrrolidone-5-carboxylic acid (PCA) and urocanic acid (UCA), in the stratum corneum as biomarkers for the *FLG* genotype.

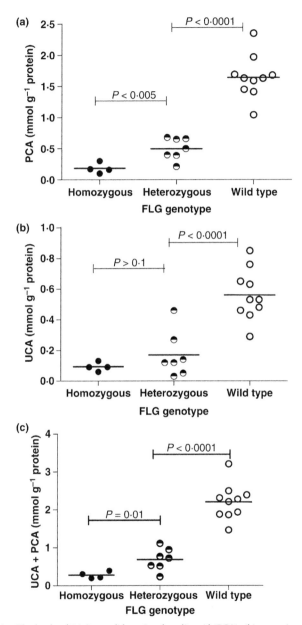

FIGURE 1.—The levels of (a) 2-pyrrolidone-5-carboxylic acid (PCA), (b) urocanic acid (UCA) and (c) the sum of UCA and PCA levels obtained by tape stripping normalized for protein amount. (Reprinted from Kezic S, Kammeyer A, Calkoen F, et al. Natural moisturizing factor components in the stratum corneum as biomarkers of filaggrin genotype: evaluation of minimally invasive methods. *Br J Dermatol.* 2009;161:1098-1104, with permission from the British Association of Dermatologists.)

Methods.—PCA and UCA from the stratum corneum were sampled by using a tape stripping technique and an extraction technique using skin patches containing potassium hydroxide (KOH). The concentrations of PCA and UCA were measured by high-performance liquid chromatography. Eleven carriers of an *FLG* mutation and 10 individuals wild type for the two most common *FLG* mutations (R501X and 2282del4) were included in the study.

Results.—The most significant difference between the *FLG* genotypes was found for PCA sampled by the tape stripping technique. The mean values of PCA obtained by the tape stripping technique were, respectively, $0 \cdot 18$, $0 \cdot 50$ and $1 \cdot 64$ mmol g^{-1} protein in homozygous (or compound heterozygous), heterozygous and wild-type genotypes ($P < 0 \cdot 005$ homozygous vs. heterozygous; $P < 0 \cdot 0001$ heterozygous vs. wild type). The tape stripping technique showed less intrasubject variation compared with the KOH patches, in particular when the concentrations of UCA and PCA on the tape strips were normalized for protein amount.

Conclusions.—The concentration of PCA in the stratum corneum collected by tape stripping showed it to be a feasible biomarker of the *FLG* genotype (Fig 1).

▶ This article provides evidence from a small sample of individuals with filaggrin mutations that high-performance liquid chromatography analysis of stratum corneum obtained by tape stripping may be useful in the diagnosis of this common disorder associated with icthyosis vulgaris, dry skin, and an increased risk of atopic disease. Hydrolysis of filaggrin results in a mixture of amino acids that have water-binding properties and was named natural moisturizing factor (NMF). NMF is a part of the story of how skin maintains an optimal level of hydration required for normal enzymatic activity for breakdown of corneodesmosomes and desquamation. If normal hydration is not present, desquamation is inhibited and the stratum corneum thickens and with reduced hydration, tissue stiffness leads to microfissures and flaky rough skin. Pyrrolidone carboxylic acid and urocanic acid are the major constituents of NMF, and their levels were found to be lower than controls (Fig 1). This method offers promise, but as the authors correctly point out, the specificity and sensitivity need to be investigated in a larger group of patients.

J. Leyden, MD

Treatment of episodes of hereditary angioedema with C1 inhibitor: serial assessment of observed abnormalities of the plasma bradykinin-forming pathway and fibrinolysis
Joseph K, Tholanikunnel TE, Kaplan AP (Med Univ of South Carolina, Charleston)
Ann Allergy Asthma Immunol 104:50-54, 2010

Background.—Hereditary angioedema (HAE) is typically the result of a deficiency of C1 inhibitor (C1-INH) with gene defects that lead to diminished plasma levels or the production of a dysfunctional protein. Replacement therapy with C1-INH has been shown to be effective in ameliorating episodes of swelling. We have reported elevated baseline levels of bradykinin, C4a, and plasmin-α_2—antiplasmin complexes in the plasma of patients with HAE compared with the plasma of healthy controls. The production of factor XII fragment on in vitro activation of plasma with HAE has also been observed.

Objective.—To perform serial assessment of abnormalities of the bradykinin-forming pathway and fibrinolysis in patients with HAE after treatment of episodes of swelling with intravenous C1-INH.

Methods.—We obtained samples of plasma from 9 patients with HAE at a quiescent period (baseline), during an attack of swelling, and at 1, 4, and 12 hours after termination of an infusion of C1-INH. Factor XIIa, kallikrein, and plasmin were each measured by cleavage of synthetic substrates specific for each item.

Results.—Each enzyme was strikingly elevated at baseline compared with the levels in pooled healthy plasma, and there was a progressive decline of activity to normal for factor XIIa and plasmin. Kallikrein decreased in 7 of the 9 patients at 1 hour and then decreased in all patients. Bradykinin levels were elevated at the outset in all patients, increased prominently during an attack of swelling, decreased to baseline after 1 hour, and then decreased toward normal by 4 and 12 hours.

Conclusion.—The plasma levels of factor XIIa, kallikrein, and bradykinin decreased when measured serially subsequent to the infusion of nanofiltered C1-INH.

▶ The authors provide an excellent synopsis of the pathophysiology of hereditary angioedema and the rationale for the selected treatment in this study. C1 inhibitor (C1-INH) deficiency results in elevated bradykinin, which mediates angioedema in these patients. These patients also have elevated levels of cleavage product C4a (and therefore diminished C4 levels), elevated plasmin-α_2-antiplasmin complexes, and elevated factor XII fragment. There is sufficient evidence to presuppose that providing purified C1-INH replacement therapy would result in decreased plasma levels of these markers, thus providing justification for a novel treatment approach for these patients.

The authors also provide a good explanation of why certain markers, such as kallikrein, were selected for quantification. Quantification of the dosage of intravenous C1-INH treatment would be useful for practitioners and the period of time of administration from the onset of symptoms for each patient. Several study limitations are considered by the authors; however, despite small sample size and variability of gene expression in the patient population, the results demonstrate substantial differences pre- and posttreatment.

This study provides compelling evidence for intravenous C1-INH therapy in patients with hereditary angioedema in the acute care setting. Clinical correlations would be appreciated and photographs of edema remission, if this was noted. Further studies assessing the efficacy of C1-INH in augmenting bradykinin levels in patients with acquired C1-INH deficiency, as well as prevention studies as mentioned, would be interesting and would also provide legitimate expansions on this discussion.

B. Berman, MD, PhD

Antibiotic use in infancy and symptoms of asthma, rhinoconjunctivitis, and eczema in children 6 and 7 years old: International Study of Asthma and Allergies in Childhood Phase III
Foliaki S, the International Study of Asthma and Allergies in Childhood Phase III Study Group (Massey Univ, Wellington, New Zealand; et al)
J Allergy Clin Immunol 124:982-989, 2009

Background.—Phase III of the International Study of Asthma and Allergies in Childhood measured the global prevalence of symptoms of asthma, rhinoconjunctivitis, and eczema in children.

Objective.—To investigate the associations between the use of antibiotics in the first year of life and symptoms of asthma, rhinoconjunctivitis, and eczema in children 6 and 7 years old.

Methods.—Parents or guardians of children 6 and 7 years old completed written questionnaires on current symptoms and possible risk factors. Prevalence odds ratios (ORs) were estimated by using logistic regression.

Results.—A total of 193,412 children from 71 centers in 29 countries participated. Reported use of antibiotics in the first year of life was associated with an increased risk of current asthma symptoms (wheezing in the previous 12 months) with an OR (adjusted for sex, region of the world, language, and per capita gross national income) of 1.96 (95% CI, 1.85-2.07); this fell to 1.70 (1.60-1.80) when adjusted for other risk factors for asthma. Similar associations were observed for severe asthma symptoms (OR, 1.82; 95% CI, 1.67-1.98), and asthma ever (OR, 1.94; 95% CI, 1.83-2.06). Use of antibiotics in the first year of life was also associated, but less strongly, with increased risks of current symptoms of rhinoconjunctivitis (OR, 1.56; 95% CI, 1.46-1.66) and eczema (OR, 1.58; 95% CI, 1.33-1.51).

Conclusion.—There is an association between antibiotic use in the first year of life and current symptoms of asthma, rhinoconjunctivitis, and eczema in children 6 and 7 years old. Further research is required to determine whether the observed associations are causal or are a result of confounding by indication or reverse causation.

▶ This study investigates whether there is a strong association between antibiotic use in the first year of life and symptoms of asthma, rhinoconjunctivitis, and eczema. Strengths of this study include large number of subjects involved ($N = 193\,412$ children) with geographic diversity (29 countries), different environmental backgrounds, and varying socioeconomic status. A cross-sectional study of randomly chosen children aged 6 to 7 years old and 13 to 14 years old was performed. Results via parent-answered questionnaires for the younger age group yielded a positive association between antibiotic use in the first year of life and current symptoms of asthma, rhinoconjuctivitis, and eczema, although the latter 2 variables were to a lesser extent.

Although this is a well-done, large, multicountry, multicentered study, there are apparent limitations to this investigation as well. First, results are subject to recall bias as parents were expected to remember retrospectively if their child had antibiotics in their first year or not. Second, depending on their education, socioeconomic status, or access to health care, subjects may not know what medicines were given and some may not have access to antibiotics at all. In addition, it is not clear whether observed associations were causal or a result of confounders. Further research is needed.

S. Bellew, DO

J. Q. Del Rosso, DO

2 Psoriasis and Other Papulosquamous Disorders

Antinuclear antibodies associate with loss of response to antitumour necrosis factor-α therapy in psoriasis: a retrospective, observational study
Pink AE, Fonia A, Allen MH, et al (King's College London, UK)
Br J Dermatol 162:780-785, 2010

Background.—An increasing number of patients with severe psoriasis are failing to respond to antitumour necrosis factor (TNF)-α therapy (etanercept, infliximab and adalimumab).

Objectives.—We observed that many of these patients developed antinuclear antibodies (ANA) and antidouble-stranded DNA (anti-dsDNA) antibodies while on treatment prompting us to investigate whether their development is associated with anti-TNF treatment failure.

Methods.—All patients with psoriasis who had received anti-TNF therapies were identified and their blood results and treatment histories were obtained from electronic patient records and case notes.

Results.—A total of 97 patients had been treated with anti-TNF agents (60 were on their first agent, 22 had been on and stopped one agent, nine had been on and stopped two agents and six had been on and stopped all three agents). ANA developed in 17% of patients on their first treatment, 54% of patients who had failed one treatment, 78% of patients who had failed two treatments and 83% of patients who had failed all three treatments. Anti-dsDNA antibodies developed in 2%, 27%, 33% and 83% of patients from the same respective groups. Significantly, the antibodies developed before treatment had failed with all three agents and their development was not related to the total time that patients had been on anti-TNF therapy.

Conclusions.—This study suggests that the development of ANA and anti-dsDNA antibodies on anti-TNF treatment may act as a marker of forthcoming treatment failure. Large-scale prospective studies are required to assess the importance of this observation.

▶ Anti—tumor necrosis factor (TNF) therapy has been a major advancement in the treatment of psoriasis, but what has been persistently perplexing is that some individuals either fail to respond to therapy or begin to show initial improvement and then become treatment resistant. Formation of antibodies to the drug itself has been shown to be involved in some cases but may not explain every case. This retrospective observational study looked at 97 patients from 1 clinic in England during a 5-month period and compared the rate of autoantibody formation in individual patients with treatment failure while having been on 1, 2, or all 3 anti-TNF-α therapies (infliximab, adalimumab, and etanercept) at some time. Only 6 patients had a positive antinuclear antibody (ANA) prior to starting therapy; all of them were TNF-α therapy naïve. The data reveal that the patients who have failed more treatments showed an increasing tendency to develop ANAs and anti–double-stranded DNA (dsDNA) antibodies while on therapy and that the duration of time spent while on therapy was not relevant to their formation. The authors propose that because the antibodies were formed prior to failing therapy, not after, the new-onset ANA/anti-dsDNA antibodies formed while patients are on anti-TNF therapy may be a marker for impending treatment failure.

While this information is enlightening, it raises the question as to how clinically relevant it is. Many patients who failed treatment did not develop autoantibodies, and several of the patients who demonstrated ANAs prior to therapy continued to demonstrate them without diminishment of treatment response. It is well established that the ANA test is nonspecific and can exist in a small percentage of normal individuals. The authors propose that anti-TNF therapy can lead to T-cell/monocyte apoptosis, thereby exposing the immune system to more nuclear material than normal and that this may explain the increased incidence of ANAs in some patients. While finding elevated autoantibodies in our patients with psoriasis may be of some interest and may eventually lead to the discovery of more specific irregularities that might explain the failure rate, it is not likely to change treatment decisions. I suspect that most practitioners would continue to choose intervention strategies based primarily on the clinical response and would only find information regarding ANAs to be of academic interest. More specific tests for antibodies to the drugs themselves would of course be more practically relevant, should they ever become available.

J. M. Suchniak, MD

Comparison of two etanercept regimens for treatment of psoriasis and psoriatic arthritis: PRESTA randomised double blind multicentre trial
Sterry W, Ortonne J-P, Kirkham B, et al (Charité Univ Medicine, Berlin, Germany; Hôpital de l'Archet, Nice, France; NIHR Biomed Res Centre at GStT, London; et al)
BMJ 340:c147, 2010

Objectives.—To compare the efficacy over 12 weeks of two different etanercept regimens in treating the skin manifestations of psoriasis in patients who also have psoriatic arthritis and to evaluate efficacy and safety over an additional 12 weeks of open label etanercept treatment.

Design.—Randomised double blind multicentre outpatient study.

Setting.—98 outpatient facilities in Europe, Latin America, and the Asia Pacific region.

Participants.—752 patients with both psoriasis (evaluated by dermatologists) and psoriatic arthritis (evaluated by rheumatologists).

Interventions.—During the blinded portion of the study, participants were randomised to receive etanercept 50 mg twice weekly (n=379) or 50 mg once weekly (n=373) for 12 weeks by subcutaneous injection. All participants then received open label etanercept 50 mg once weekly for 12 additional weeks, while remaining blinded to the regimen.

Main Outcome Measures.—The primary efficacy end point was the proportion of participants achieving "clear" or "almost clear" on the physician's global assessment of psoriasis at week 12. Secondary efficacy analyses included psoriasis area and severity index, American College of Rheumatology responses, psoriatic arthritis response criteria, and improvement in joint and tendon disease manifestations.

Results.—At week 12, 46% (176/379) of participants receiving etanercept 50 mg twice weekly achieved a physician's global assessment of psoriasis of "clear" or "almost clear" compared with 32% (119/373) in the group treated with 50 mg once weekly (P<0.001). In contrast, an equally high percentage of participants in both groups achieved psoriatic arthritis response criteria (77% (284/371) in the twice weekly/once weekly group versus 76% (282/371) in the once weekly/once weekly group). Participants treated with 50 mg twice weekly/once weekly had greater mean reductions from baseline in the psoriasis area and severity index at week 12 compared with those who received 50 mg once weekly/once weekly (71% *v* 62%, P<0.001), with less difference at week 24 (78% *v* 74%, P<0.110). Joint and tendon disease manifestations improved from baseline in both groups to a similar extent. No new safety signals were seen in either etanercept treatment group, and no significant difference in the safety profiles was observed.

Conclusions.—In participants with active psoriasis and psoriatic arthritis, initial treatment of the psoriasis with etanercept 50 mg twice weekly may allow for more rapid clearance of skin lesions than with 50 mg once weekly. A regimen of 50 mg once weekly seems to be appropriate for treatment of joint and tendon rheumatic symptoms. The choice of regimen should be determined by the clinical needs of the individual patient.

Trial Registration.—Clinical trials NCT00245960.

▶ The results of this study are not surprising to those clinicians familiar with the data and clinical activity of etanercept. The study demonstrates that significant differences in skin responses were seen at week 12 between the 50 mg twice weekly/once weekly and 50 mg once weekly/once weekly dosages. At week twelve, 46% (176/379) of the participants receiving etanercept 50 mg twice weekly achieved a physician global assessment of psoriasis of clear or almost clear compared with 32% (119/373) in the group treated with 50 mg once weekly (*P* < .001). In contrast, efficacy for psoriatic arthritis was similar. An equally high percentage of participants in both groups achieved psoriatic arthritis response criteria 77% (284/371) in the twice weekly/once weekly group versus 76% (282/371) in the once weekly/once weekly group. Both regimens achieved significant improvement from baseline in skin, joint, and entheseal disease components at week 24. There was no significant safety difference between the 2 groups. These results are consistent with the profile of etanercept and only help to confirm this profile.

J. Weinberg, MD

Early skin biopsy is helpful for the diagnosis and management of neonatal and infantile erythrodermas
Leclerc-Mercier S, Bodemer C, Bourdon-Lanoy E, et al (Université René-Descartes, Paris V, France; et al)
J Cutan Pathol 37:249-255, 2010

Background.—Erythrodermas are often life-threatening conditions in infants. Determination of the underlying cause is crucial. Microscopic changes in adult erythroderma lack specificity.

Objective.—To determine if an early skin biopsy is helpful for the diagnosis of neonatal and infantile erythroderma.

Methods.—Seventy-two patients admitted for erythroderma in the first year of life were retrospectively included. One hundred and eleven skin biopsies (12-year period) were examined by 3 pathologists blinded to the clinical diagnosis, and classified into atopic dermatitis, immunodeficiency (ID), psoriasis, Netherton syndrome (NS), ichthyosis, other. From year 2000, LEKTI antibody was performed when NS was suspected. Pathological diagnosis was then compared with clinical diagnosis.

Results.—The final diagnosis was made in 69.3% of the cases. In 57.6%, pathological diagnosis was in accordance, and in 11.7%, it was in accordance, but other diagnosis had also been proposed. For ID, sensitivity and specificity were 58.5 and 98.5%, respectively. Before year 2000, NS was frequently misdiagnosed with psoriasis, but with the use of LEKTI antibody, sensitivity and specificity were 100%.

Conclusion.—Skin biopsy is helpful for etiologic diagnosis of early erythroderma of infancy, particularly in ID and NS, the most severe diseases. Consequently, these results justify an early systematic skin biopsy for a better and earlier management.

▶ The object of this article is to determine the usefulness of early biopsy in patients presenting with neonatal and infantile erythrodermas. I think that this is a very clinically relative article, which indicates that the major differential for neonatal and infantile erythrodermas is atopic dermatitis, immunodeficiency, psoriasis, Netherton syndrome, ichthyosis, and few other disorders. The pathologists were blinded as to the clinical diagnosis (slides were read blindly). The final diagnosis was made in 63% of the patients. In 57.6%, pathologic diagnosis was in accordance, and in 11%, it was in accordance but other diagnoses had been proposed. This article nicely demonstrated the objectives and the diagnostic criteria for early skin biopsies with the pathologic diagnostic criteria and the evaluation of patients presenting with neonatal and infantile erythrodermas. This is a research article where 72 patients were admitted with erythrodermas in the first year of life and were retrospectively included; 111 skin biopsies over a 12-year period were examined by 3 individual pathologists blinded to the clinical diagnosis and were classified into the major differential diagnosis for erythrodermas. This is very valid and very useful information for a practicing dermatologist. The conclusions appear to be valid, and the references are well documented. The methods are sound, and the interpretation of the biopsies appears to be appropriate. This is an article that should be required reading for anyone who sees neonatal and infantile patients.

Prior to 2000 many patients with Netherton syndrome were frequently misdiagnosed with psoriasis, but with the use of the lymphoepithelial kazal type inhibitor antibody, sensitivity and specificity were 100%. This study shows that the early skin biopsy diagnosis is helpful in the etiologic diagnosis and management of erythrodermas on the basis of the results of this study. The proposal of a decision tree would be helpful in evaluating patients with these sometimes challenging clinical presentations.

L. Cleaver, DO

Effective treatment of psoriasis with etanercept is linked to suppression of IL-17 signaling, not immediate response TNF genes

Zaba LC, Suárez-Fariñas M, Fuentes-Duculan J, et al (Rockefeller Univ, NY)
J Allergy Clin Immunol 124:1022-1030, 2009

Background.—TNF inhibitors have revolutionized the treatment of psoriasis vulgaris as well as psoriatic and rheumatoid arthritis and Crohn disease. Despite our understanding that these agents block TNF, their complex mechanism of action in disease resolution is still unclear.

Objective.—To analyze globally the genomic effects of TNF inhibition in patients with psoriasis, and to compare genomic profiles of patients who responded or did not respond to treatment.

Methods.—In a clinical trial using etanercept TNF inhibitor to treat psoriasis vulgaris (n = 15), Affymetrix gene arrays were used to analyze gene profiles in lesional skin at multiple time points during drug treatment (baseline and weeks 1, 2, 4, and 12) compared with nonlesional skin. Patients were stratified as responders (n = 11) or nonresponders (n = 4) on the basis of histologic disease resolution. Cluster analysis was used to define gene sets that were modulated with similar magnitude and velocity over time.

Results.—In responders, 4 clusters of downregulated genes and 3 clusters of upregulated genes were identified. Genes downmodulated most rapidly reflected direct inhibition of myeloid lineage immune genes. Upregulated genes included the stable dendritic cell population genes CD1c and CD207 (langerin). Comparison of responders and nonresponders revealed rapid downmodulation of innate IL-1β and IL-8 sepsis cascade cytokines in both groups, but only responders downregulated IL-17 pathway genes to baseline levels.

Conclusion.—Although both responders and nonresponders to etanercept inactivated sepsis cascade cytokines, response to etanercept is dependent on inactivation of myeloid dendritic cell genes and inactivation of the T_H17 immune response.

▶ Tumor necrosis factor (TNF) was discovered in 1976 as a factor that killed tumor cells. Subsequently, it was found to play a pivotal role in innate immunity and induce expression of multiple cytokines. Ultimately, TNF was found to play a role in inflammatory bowel disease, rheumatoid arthritis, and psoriasis. Over the past decade, TNF-α antagonists have been approved for the treatment of inflammatory bowel disease, rheumatoid arthritis, and psoriasis. Etanercept, one of the earliest TNF-α antagonists, is a fusion protein that blocks soluble TNF-α. It is effective in the treatment of psoriasis, psoriatic arthritis, and rheumatoid arthritis.

Etanercept was used to treat 15 patients with psoriasis, and skin biopsies were taken at baseline at weeks 1, 2, 4, and 12. At the end of 12 weeks, patients were divided into responders (11 patients) or nonresponders (4 patients). RNA was extracted from the skin biopsies, and tissue gene expression was analyzed by Affymetrix microarrays. In responders, myeloid lineage immune genes were downregulated as were interleukin (IL)-17 genes, resulting in inactivation of the T helper 17 (T_H17) immune response.

It should not be surprising that etanercept, a drug that is effective for psoriasis, would downregulate the T_H17 immune response. Most recently, ustekinumab, a monoclonal antibody that targets the p40 component of IL-12 and IL-23, has been introduced for the treatment of psoriasis. Its success has been attributed to its blocking a newly implicated group of cells, the T_H17 cells, which are thought to lead to the development of psoriatic plaques. This study reinforces the recent emphasis on T_H17 cells in the pathogenesis of psoriasis and points out that etanercept, a TNF antagonist, also results in improvement of psoriasis by inactivation of T_H17 immune responses.

M. Lebwohl, MD

Effectiveness and retention rates of methotrexate in psoriatic arthritis in comparison with methotrexate-treated patients with rheumatoid arthritis
Lie E, van der Heijde D, Uhlig T, et al (Diakonhjemmet Hosp, Oslo, Norway; et al)
Ann Rheum Dis 69:671-676, 2010

Objective.—To examine the effectiveness and 2-year retention rates of methotrexate (MTX) in MTX naïve patients with psoriatic arthritis (PsA).

Methods.—Data on 430 patients with PsA participating in an ongoing longitudinal observational multicentre study in Norway were analysed. 1218 MTX naïve patients with rheumatoid arthritis (RA) from the same study served as a reference population. Assessments included measures of disease activity (28 joint counts, acute phase reactants), health status and utility scores. Six-month effectiveness data were compared both by crude analyses and with adjustments for age, sex and the respective baseline values. Two-year drug survival was compared by Kaplan—Meier and Cox regression analyses.

Results.—After 6 months of MTX treatment, both patients with PsA and those with RA improved in most disease activity measures and patient reported outcomes. In the adjusted analysis, patients with PsA tended to have less improvement, but changes were in the same range as in patients with RA. Two-year retention rates of MTX therapy in patients with PsA and RA were 65% and 66%, respectively, with only minor differences in reported reasons for discontinuation. Lower age, longer disease duration and higher Modified Health Assessment Questionnaire (MHAQ) score and patient global assessment were independent predictors of MTX termination within the first 2 years of treatment.

Conclusion.—In this real-life study, MTX treatment was associated with improvement in disease activity and health-related quality of life in patients with PsA after 6 months of treatment. Retention rates of MTX were similar in PsA and RA.

▶ There are many articles documenting the effectiveness of methotrexate for the treatment of psoriatic arthritis, but there are few data on retention rates. How many patients who start on methotrexate for psoriatic arthritis are still taking the drug 2 years later? Beginning December 2000, five Norwegian rheumatology departments collaborated in a prospective, multicenter, longitudinal observational study of adults with inflammatory arthropathies who were started on disease-modifying antirheumatic drugs (DMARDs). Patients were examined at baseline and at 3, 6, and 12 months and yearly thereafter. Four thousand seven hundred ninety-two patients were included, and the completeness of the register has been an impressive 85%. This article reports data on 430 patients with psoriatic arthritis and 1218 patients with rheumatoid arthritis who were newly started on methotrexate. Patients were assessed for 28 swollen and tender joints counts, erythrocyte sedimentation rate, C-reactive protein, physician's global assessment using visual analog scales, patients' assessment of joint pain, fatigue and global disease, Modified Health Assessment Questionnaire, Medical Outcome Study 36-Item Short Form Health Survey (SF-36), and an interesting tool derived from the SF-36 called the SF-6D with scores ranging from 0 (dead) to 1 (perfect health).

Patients with psoriatic arthritis had somewhat less improvement than patients with rheumatoid arthritis in response to methotrexate therapy. Two-year retention rates for methotrexate therapy, however, were similar between the 2 groups: 65% were still on methotrexate for psoriatic arthritis, and 66% were still on methotrexate for rheumatoid arthritis at 2 years. During the first

6 months of therapy, 17% of patients with psoriatic arthritis and 17% of patients with rheumatoid arthritis discontinued therapy. In both groups, 47% stopped methotrexate as a result of adverse events, 28% stopped the drug because of lack of efficacy in psoriatic arthritis and 30% for lack of efficacy in rheumatoid arthritis. In contrast, lack of efficacy was the main reason for discontinuation between months 6 and 12; 51% of discontinuations in the patients with psoriatic arthritis were for lack of efficacy in that time period compared with 53% in the patients with rheumatoid arthritis. Of the adverse effects that resulted in discontinuation, nausea and elevated liver function tests were most common.

The data in this article provide excellent insights into the efficacy and tolerability of methotrexate over 2 years. There are a number of factors that should be considered when reviewing these data. Differences in medical practice, insurance, and cultures between Norway and the United States have an impact on methotrexate therapy and side effects of methotrexate therapy. For example, obesity increases the likelihood of developing hepatic fibrosis as does alcohol ingestion.[1] Different insurance coverage of medications between Norway and the United States may result in differences in prescription patterns of methotrexate. If biologic therapies are more easily obtained, the threshold for switching from methotrexate to those therapies may be lower. Differences between rheumatologists and dermatologists in their approach to methotrexate therapy should also be considered. Most rheumatologists seldom obtain liver biopsies in patients on methotrexate, whereas the most recent methotrexate guidelines for dermatologists call for periodic liver biopsies in patients with risk factors for hepatic fibrosis, such as obesity.[2] Nevertheless, the data in this article should be of interest to any practitioners prescribing methotrexate.

M. Lebwohl, MD

References

1. Rosenberg P, Urwitz H, Johannesson A, et al. Psoriasis patients with diabetes type 2 are at high risk of developing liver fibrosis during methotrexate treatment. *J Hepatol.* 2007;46:1111-1118.
2. Kalb RE, Strober B, Weinstein G, Lebwohl M. Methotrexate and psoriasis: 2009 National Psoriasis Foundation Consensus Conference. *J Am Acad Dermatol.* 2009;60:824-837.

Effectiveness of adalimumab in treating patients with active psoriatic arthritis and predictors of good clinical responses for arthritis, skin and nail lesions
Van den Bosch F, Manger B, Goupille P, et al (Univ Hosp, Ghent, Belgium; Universität Erlangen/Nürnberg, Germany; Université François Rabelais, Tours, France; et al)
Ann Rheum Dis 69:394-399, 2010

Objectives.—To evaluate the effectiveness of adalimumab in patients with psoriatic arthritis (PsA) and identify predictors of good clinical response for joint and skin lesions.

Methods.—Patients received adalimumab 40 mg every other week in addition to standard therapy in this prospective, 12-week, open-label, uncontrolled study. Four definitions of good clinical response were used: ≥50% improvement in American College of Rheumatology response criteria (ACR50), good response according to European League Against Rheumatism (EULAR) guidelines, a ≥3-grade improvement in Physician Global Assessment of psoriasis (PGA) and a ≥50% improvement in the Nail Psoriasis Severity Index (NAPSI). Response predictors were determined by logistic regression with backward elimination (selection level was 5%).

Results.—Of 442 patients, 94% completed 12 weeks of treatment. At week 12, 74%, 51% and 32% of the patients had achieved ACR20, 50 and 70, respectively; 87% and 61% experienced moderate and good responses according to EULAR criteria, respectively. The percentage of patients with PGA results of "clear/almost clear" increased from 34% (baseline) to 68%. The mean NAPSI score was reduced by 44%. No new safety signals were detected. A lower Health Assessment Questionnaire Disability Index (HAQ-DI) score, greater pain assessment, male sex and absence of systemic glucocorticoid therapy were strongly associated with achievement of ACR50 and good response according to EULAR criteria. In addition, greater C-reactive protein concentration and polyarthritis predicted ACR50, and non-involvement of large joints predicted a good response according to EULAR criteria.

Conclusions.—Adalimumab was effective in patients with PsA. Lower impairment of physical function, greater pain, male sex and no systemic treatment with glucocorticoids were factors that increased the chance of achieving a good clinical response.

▶ The goal of this study was to evaluate the effectiveness of adalimumab in patients with psoriatic arthritis (PsA) and identify predictors of good clinical response for joint and skin lesions. The authors found that patients with long-term active PsA experienced clinically important improvement in arthritis, psoriasis, and psoriatic nail disorder. Low impairment of physical function, greater pain, greater C-reactive protein concentration, polyarthritis without inflammation of large joints, previous treatment with >2 disease-modifying antirheumatic drugs, no systemic treatment with glucocorticoids, and male sex were factors that increased the chance of achieving substantial clinical improvements. Studies such as this are important because they provide data regarding factors that may influence optimal response to a biologic agent. While many of the factors are not relevant to dermatologists, they still provide data to consider when making therapeutic decisions.

As per the authors, this was the first study that has investigated the effect of adalimumab on nail psoriasis. After the relatively short treatment duration of 12 weeks, the median reduction in Nail Psoriasis Severity Index score was 57%. Clearance of psoriasis of the nails was increasing in those patients who continued adalimumab up to week 20.

J. Weinberg, MD

Efficacy and safety of mycophenolate mofetil for lichen planopilaris
Cho BK, Sah D, Chwalek J, et al (Palo Alto Med Foundation, Mountain View, CA; Palo Alto Med Foundation, Fremont, CA; Kaiser Med Group, Union City, CA; et al)
J Am Acad Dermatol 62:393-397, 2010

Background.—Lichen planopilaris (LPP) is a chronic inflammatory disorder that causes permanent scalp hair loss and significant patient discomfort.

Objectives.—We sought to determine the efficacy and safety of mycophenolate mofetil (MMF) for treatment of LPP in patients who had failed prior topical, intralesional, or oral anti-inflammatory medications such as hydroxychloroquine or cyclosporine.

Methods.—We conducted a retrospective chart review of 16 adult patients with LPP treated with at least 6 months of MMF in an open-label, single-center study from 2003 to 2007. Subjective and objective end points were quantified using the LPP Activity Index (LPPAI) and scores before and after treatment were assessed using a paired t test. Adverse events were monitored.

Results.—Patients who completed treatment with MMF had significantly decreased signs and symptoms of active LPP despite having failed multiple prior therapies (P < .005). Five of 12 patients were complete responders (LPPAI score decreased>85%), 5 of 12 patients were partial responders (LPPAI score decreased 25%-85%), and two of 12 patients were treatment failures (LPPAI score decreased<25%). Four patients withdrew from the trial because of adverse events.

Limitations.—Retrospective analysis and small sample size were limitations.

Conclusions.—MMF was effective at reducing the signs and symptoms of active LPP in 83% of patients (10 of 12) who had failed multiple prior treatments after at least 6 months of treatment.

▶ As noted by the article, current treatments for lichen planopilaris (LPP) are based mainly on case reports or case series. This study sought to determine the efficacy of mycophenolate mofetil (MMF) for the treatment of LPP in patients who have failed other treatment modalities. The results of the study are promising. Of the 12 patients who completed the study, 10 patients were found to have a complete or partial response of their active LPP to MMF after at least 6 months of treatment. Again, it should be recognized that these same patients had failed other treatments including topical, intralesional, or oral anti-inflammatory medications such as hydroxychloroquine or cyclo-sporine. This represents an 83% response rate. Although the results are promising, there is still a limitation to the study. Namely, the size of the study included only 16 patients, 4 of whom withdrew from the study secondary to adverse events. However, it must be recognized that a small sample size is based on the relative rarity of LPP. Ultimately, however, the result of this study shows a potentially promising treatment for recalcitrant LPP and hopefully will be the subject of an additional or even larger study in the future.

B. D. Michaels, DO

J. Q. Del Rosso, DO

Epidemiology and comorbidity of psoriasis in children
Augustin M, Glaeske G, Radtke MA, et al (Univ Clinics of Hamburg, Germany; Univ of Bremen, Germany; et al)
Br J Dermatol 162:633-636, 2010

Background.—Psoriasis is a common disease affecting all age groups. In contrast to adult psoriasis, only few studies on the epidemiology of childhood psoriasis have been published.

Objectives.—Assessment of prevalence and comorbidities of juvenile psoriasis in Germany based on health insurance data.

Methods.—Data were collected from a database of about 1·3 million nonselected individuals from a German statutory health insurance organization which covers all geographical regions. Individuals with psoriasis were identified by ICD-10 codes applied to all outpatient and inpatient visits. The present analysis consists of all patients who were enlisted throughout the year 2005. The diagnosis of psoriasis was registered whenever there was at least one documented patient contact using code L40 and subcodes. Comorbidities were also evaluated by ICD-10 diagnoses.

Results.—In total, 33 981 patients with the diagnosis of psoriasis were identified. The prevalence in 2005 was 2·5%. The total rate of psoriasis in children younger than 18 years was 0·71%. The prevalence rates increased in an approximately linear manner from 0·12% at the age of 1 year to 1·2% at the age of 18 years. The overall rate of comorbidity in subjects with psoriasis aged under 20 years was twice as high as in subjects without psoriasis. Juvenile psoriasis was associated with increased rates of hyperlipidaemia, obesity, hypertension, diabetes mellitus, rheumatoid arthritis and Crohn disease.

Conclusions.—Psoriasis is a common disease in children. Like in adults, it is associated with significant comorbidity. Increased attention should be paid to the early detection and treatment of patients affected.

▶ Psoriasis is one of the most common inflammatory disorders of skin in children; however, epidemiologic data in this age group are limited. Recent studies indicate that psoriasis does not have a dual peak in age of onset as was once thought. More specifically, the incidence of pediatric psoriasis has been shown to rise with increasing age.[1] In fact, this study found an almost linear increase in prevalence rates with age. In total, 33 981 insured German patients with psoriasis in 2005 were identified and of those, 0.71% of children younger than 18 years were affected. In addition, pediatric patients with psoriasis were found to have increased risk of hyperlipidemia, obesity, hypertension, diabetes mellitus, rheumatoid arthritis, and Crohn disease compared with unaffected children. These results suggest that physicians should more carefully examine young patients with psoriasis for associated comorbidities.

This article states that medical records obtained for this study were mainly from office-based general practitioners and only a few dermatologists. This may be a limitation, as psoriasis can be misdiagnosed by nondermatologists because it may be mimicked by other skin diseases. In addition, the severity of psoriasis was not mentioned as a variable in the study. Also, all evaluated patients were from Germany, and therefore, results may not be generalized to other population groups.

S. Bellew, DO

J. Q. Del Rosso, DO

Reference

1. Tollefson MM, Crowson CS, McEvoy MT, Maradit Kremers H. Incidence of psoriasis in children: a population-based study. *J Am Acad Dermatol.* 2009;62: 979-987.

Extent and Clinical Consequences of Antibody Formation Against Adalimumab in Patients With Plaque Psoriasis
Lecluse LLA, Driessen RJB, Spuls PI, et al (Univ of Amsterdam, the Netherlands; Radboud Univ Nijmegen Med Ctr, the Netherlands)
Arch Dermatol 146:127-132, 2010

Objectives.—To investigate the extent antibodies to adalimumab are formed in patients with plaque psoriasis and whether these antibodies have clinical consequences. Also, to examine the relationship between antibodies to adalimumab and adalimumab trough titers.

Design.—Prospective observational cohort study.

Setting.—Two Dutch dermatology departments in university hospitals.

Patients.—All consecutive patients starting a regimen of adalimumab for chronic plaque psoriasis. Patients were screened and fulfilled the Dutch reimbursement criteria for adalimumab to treat psoriasis.

Intervention.—Adalimumab treatment (per label).

Main Outcome Measures.—The titer of antibodies to adalimumab, the adalimumab trough concentration, and the Psoriasis Area and Severity Index at weeks 12 and 24.

Results.—Antibodies to adalimumab were detected in 13 of 29 patients (45%) during 24 weeks of treatment. Differences in response rates among patients with low, high, and no titers of antibodies to adalimumab were significant at weeks 12 and 24 ($P = .04$ and $P < .001$, respectively). The median adalimumab trough concentrations varied significantly among patients with low, high, and no titers of antibodies to adalimumab (1.30 [range, 0.01-5.50], 0.0 [range, 0.0-0.0], and 9.6 [range, 0.0-22.6] mg/L, respectively; $P < .001$). At week 24, the median adalimumab trough concentrations also differed significantly among good responders, moderate responders, and nonresponders (9.7 [range, 0.0-22.6], 8.9 [range, 3.2-12.6], and 0.0 [range, 0.0-13.3] mg/L, respectively; $P = .01$).

Conclusion.—Antibodies to adalimumab are associated with lower serum adalimumab trough concentrations and with nonresponse or loss of response to adalimumab in patients with plaque psoriasis.

▶ This study recapitulates what prescribers of adalimumab see clinically. The quantification of adalimumab antibody titers correlated well with the Psoriasis Area Severity Index data. Moreover, the concomitant use of traditional immunosuppressants by 4 patients, either lowering or preventing adalimumab antibody production, supports the validity of the antibody test. In theory, B-cell production of the adalimumab antibody would be inhibited by the use of traditional immunosuppressants (ie, prednisone and methotrexate, as in this study).

The authors were also able to demonstrate undetectable trough concentrations of adalimumab in patients with high adalimumab antibody titers and correlate these findings with poor clinical disease response to adalimumab. Interestingly, patients who had been treated with etanercept previously developed adalimumab antibodies at a much more frequent rate (12/13, 92%) as compared with those in the study who had not (8/16, 50%). This finding is definitely worth further investigation. Even though a small sample population, the methods and results of this study are legitimate and contribute to our fund of knowledge as dermatologists.

B. P. Glick, DO, MPH

T. J. Singer, DO

A. Wiener, DO

Guidelines of care for the management of psoriasis and psoriatic arthritis: Section 5. Guidelines of care for the treatment of psoriasis with phototherapy and photochemotherapy
Menter A, Korman NJ, Elmets CA, et al (Baylor Univ Med Ctr, Dallas, TX; Univ Hosps Case Med Ctr, Cleveland, OH; Univ of Alabama at Birmingham; et al)
J Am Acad Dermatol 62:114-135, 2010

Psoriasis is a common, chronic, inflammatory, multisystem disease with predominantly skin and joint manifestations affecting approximately 2% of the population. In this fifth of 6 sections of the guidelines of care for psoriasis, we discuss the use of ultraviolet (UV) light therapy for the treatment of patients with psoriasis. Treatment should be tailored to meet individual patients' needs. We will discuss in detail the efficacy and safety as well as offer recommendations for the use of phototherapy, including narrowband and broadband UVB and photochemotherapy using psoralen plus UVA, alone and in combination with topical and systemic agents. We will also discuss the available data for the use of the excimer laser in the targeted treatment of psoriasis. Finally, where available, we will summarize the available data that compare the safety and efficacy of the different forms of UV light therapy.

▶ More treatments have been developed for psoriasis over the past decade than for all the rest of dermatologic conditions. Yet 1 of our oldest treatments, phototherapy with ultraviolet B (UVB), remains a viable treatment option in the armamentarium of therapies used for psoriasis. This fifth of 6 sections on Guidelines for Care of Psoriasis reviews all the forms of phototherapy used for psoriasis, including broadband UVB, narrowband UVB, psoralen + ultraviolet A (PUVA), the excimer laser, and even a brief section on Grenz rays.

The guidelines start out with general principles and point out that a minimum body surface area of 10% has been used as a prerequisite for phototherapy, although patients with severe disease affecting more limited body surface areas (such as the palms and soles) might also be candidates for phototherapy. Targeted therapy, such as the excimer laser, and Grenz rays are of course applied to more localized body surface areas. Variations on phototherapy, including the Goeckerman regimen and the Ingram regimen, are discussed.

The guidelines point out some features that are easily forgotten. For example, a complete history and physical examination should be performed to exclude conditions like lupus erythematosus or xeroderma pigmentosum. Patients with photosensitivity disorders or on photosensitizing medications must be screened before phototherapy. Those with a history of melanoma, with atypical moles, with nonmelanoma skin cancers, or on immunosuppressive medications must also be evaluated before phototherapy. The guidelines review a number of special circumstances that arise in phototherapy, including pediatric use, phototherapy during pregnancy, home UV-B, and combination therapies with topical agents, systemic agents, and biologic therapies. The combination of UV-B and PUV-A is briefly discussed.

The guidelines are noteworthy for their discussion of a number of controversial issues in phototherapy. The question of carcinogenicity of narrowband UV-B is discussed with a review of studies suggesting that narrowband UV-B could be carcinogenic, while others suggest that it is not. Likewise, the controversy over combining UV-B with topical corticosteroids is addressed in some detail. Where evidence is lacking, such as in the combination of phototherapy with biologic therapies, the authors point out the absence of good studies at the present time.

M. Lebwohl, MD

Inverse relationship between contact allergy and psoriasis: results from a patient- and a population-based study
Bangsgaard N, Engkilde K, Thyssen JP, et al (Univ of Copenhagen, Denmark; et al)
Br J Dermatol 161:1119-1123, 2009

Background.—An inverse association between contact allergy and autoimmune diseases has been suggested. Psoriasis is an autoimmune disease and it has been debated whether contact allergy is less prevalent among patients with psoriasis. Previous studies have shown conflicting results.

Objectives.—To examine a possible association between contact allergy and psoriasis in two conceptually different epidemiological studies.

Patients and Methods.—Two study populations were included: (i) a clinic-based register linkage study population, achieved by record linking information from the Danish National Hospital Registry identifying patients with psoriasis with information on contact allergy from a comprehensive patch test database of 15 641 patients; and (ii) a population-based cross-sectional study population organized in 1990, 1998 and 2006 and obtained by random samples from the Danish Central Personal Register. Information was obtained by questionnaire and patch testing of 4989 subjects.

Results.—An inverse association was found between a psoriasis diagnosis and a positive patch test in both studies. The odds ratio for a person with a psoriasis diagnosis of having a positive patch test was, adjusted for sex and age, $0·58$ [95% confidence interval (CI) $0·49-0·68$] and $0·64$ (95% CI $0·42-0·98$), respectively, in the two studies.

Conclusions.—The finding of an inverse association between psoriasis and contact allergy may express opposite immunological mechanisms and calls for additional research in this field.

▶ There continues to be a controversy regarding the relative ease or difficulty of psoriatic patients to become sensitized to classic contact allergens. Past studies have demonstrated an unusually great range in the prevalence of positive reactions to patch-tested chemicals via routine methods in patients with psoriasis. Under controlled circumstances, psoriatic patients may react less vigorously to allergens like dinitrochlorobenzene compared with nonpsoriatic patients. From a clinical perspective, the diagnosis of psoriasis and contact dermatitis may be more difficult to differentiate in contradistinction to classical descriptions of both diseases. Dermatitis of the palms may present in such an ambiguous way that only with the presence of classic stigmata of the disease in other locations can the diagnosis be readily rendered. In this study, accomplished through 2 retrospective means, the odds of diagnosis of allergic contact dermatitis were inversely associated with the diagnosis of psoriasis. While this may be of consequence to populations at large with either disease, the mere possibility of the disorders coexisting should remind us to be cognizant of the issue when diagnosing and treating patients with inflammatory skin disease.

D. E. Cohen, MD, MPH

Narrowband ultraviolet B therapy in psoriasis: randomized double-blind comparison of high-dose and low-dose irradiation regimens
Kleinpenning MM, Smits T, Boezeman J, et al (Radboud Univ Nijmegen Med Centre, the Netherlands)
Br J Dermatol 161:1351-1356, 2009

Background.—Ultraviolet (UV) B phototherapy is an established treatment option for psoriasis. The optimum dosage regimen still has to be determined. Within-subject comparisons do not take into account the systemic effects of UVB phototherapy. The area of the body treated with low-dose UVB may benefit from the systemic effects of the site treated with a higher UVB dose.

Objectives.—To study the time to clearance in patients with psoriasis in a randomized controlled trial, in which patients were treated with narrowband UVB in either a high-dose or a low-dose regimen.

Methods.—One hundred and nine patients were randomized to a high-dose regimen (group 1) or to a low-dose regimen (group 2). Patients of group 1 and 2 were irradiated with 40% and with 20% incremental doses, respectively, three times weekly. Psoriasis Area and Severity Index (PASI) was measured at baseline and at every 4-week control visit. Treatment was stopped in cases of clearance (90% reduction of baseline PASI).

Results.—No significant differences were found in the number of patients achieving clearance. The high-dosage scheme resulted in four fewer treatments with no significant differences in cumulative UV dose, although more protocol adjustments were required in the beginning of the study because of erythema. After 3 months a significantly better clinical outcome was seen after high-dose UVB therapy.

Conclusions.—High-dose UVB therapy results in fewer treatments with better long-term efficacy, with cost-effective benefits for hospital and patients. Therefore UVB phototherapy in a high-dose regimen for psoriasis is recommended. However, a protocol adjustment in the second week with a high-dose regimen is desirable to prevent erythema.

▶ The goal of successful phototherapy for psoriasis is to treat patients as quickly and effectively as possible, while minimizing the risk of toxicity such as burning. The objective of this report was to study the time to clearance in patients with psoriasis in a randomized controlled trial, in which patients were treated with narrowband ultraviolet B (UVB) in either a high-dose or a low-dose regimen. The high-dosage scheme resulted in 4 fewer treatments, with no significant differences in cumulative UV dose. However, more protocol adjustments were required in the beginning of the study because of erythema. The authors concluded that high-dose UVB therapy results in fewer treatments with better long-term efficacy, with cost-effective benefits for hospital and patients. UVB phototherapy in a high-dose regimen for psoriasis is preferred with a protocol adjustment after 4 irradiations to prevent erythema. In an era of rising patient costs for phototherapy, this information is of note when planning a treatment regimen.

J. Weinberg, MD

No Increased Risk of Cancer after Coal Tar Treatment in Patients with Psoriasis or Eczema
Roelofzen JHJ, Aben KKH, Oldenhof UTH, et al (Radboud Univ Nijmegen Med Centre, The Netherlands; et al)
J Invest Dermatol 130:953-961, 2010

Coal tar is an effective treatment for psoriasis and eczema, but it contains several carcinogenic compounds. Occupational and animal studies have shown an increased risk of cancer after exposure to coal tar. Many dermatologists have abandoned this treatment for safety reasons, although the risk of cancer after coal tar in dermatological practice is unclear. This large cohort study included 13,200 patients with psoriasis and eczema. Information on skin disease and treatment, risk factors, and cancer occurrence was retrieved from medical files, questionnaires, and medical registries. Proportional hazards regression was used to evaluate differences in cancer risk by treatment modality. Patients treated with coal tar were compared with a reference category of patients treated with dermatocorticosteroids (assumed to carry no increased cancer risk). The median exposure to coal tar ointments was 6 months (range 1−300 months). Coal tar did not increase the risk of non-skin malignancies (hazard ratio (HR) 0.92; 95% confidence interval (CI) 0.78−1.09), or the risk of skin cancer (HR 1.09; 95% CI 0.69−1.72). This study has sufficient power to show that coal tar treatment is not associated with an increased risk of cancer. These results indicate that coal tar can be maintained as a safe treatment in dermatological practice.

▶ Coal tar is a mixture of thousands of compounds including polycyclic aromatic hydrocarbons, such as benzopyrene and benzanthracene, which are well-known carcinogens. Indeed, the first cancer attributed to occupational exposure was squamous cell carcinoma of the scrotum described in 1775 by Percivall Pott in chimney sweeps exposed to tar. This study involved a retrospective review of medical records at 3 large hospitals in the Netherlands. The study was started in 2003, and the investigators looked at patients diagnosed with psoriasis or eczema between 1960 and 1990. Patients had to have visited dermatologists at least 3 times to be included, as the authors wanted to ensure that the skin disease was sufficiently severe to require treatment. Ultimately, 13 200 patients with psoriasis and eczema were included. Patients treated with coal tar had a median exposure of 6 months with a range of 1 to 300 months. They were compared with patients treated with topical corticosteroids who were presumed to not have an increased risk of cancer. Compared with topical corticosteroids, coal tar did not increase the risk of skin cancer (hazard ratio, 1.09; 95% confidence interval, 0.69-1.72) or other cancers (hazard ratio, 0.92; 95% confidence interval, 0.78-1.09). This study is particularly timely given a lawsuit in California that resulted in a requirement that companies making coal tar products should place a statement warning that the product contains chemicals known to the State of California to cause skin cancer. The study reinforces an older long-term study of patients treated for psoriasis and eczema with tar and UVB at the Mayo Clinic.[1] That study also did not show an increase in skin cancers.

M. Lebwohl, MD

Reference

1. Pittelkow MR, Perry HO, Muller SA, Maughan WZ, O'Brien PC. Skin cancer in patients with psoriasis treated with coal tar. A 25-year follow-up study. *Arch Dermatol.* 1981;117:465-468.

Once-Weekly Administration of Etanercept 50 mg Improves Patient-Reported Outcomes in Patients with Moderate-to-Severe Plaque Psoriasis
Reich K, Segaert S, Van de Kerkhof P, et al (Dermatologikum, Hamburg, Germany; Univ Hosp Sint-Rafaël, Leuven, Belgium; Univ Hosp, Nijmegen, The Netherlands; et al)
Dermatology 219:239-249, 2009

Objective.—To assess baseline patient-reported outcomes (PROs) and PRO improvement in patients with psoriasis administered etanercept 50 mg once weekly (QW).

Methods.—Adult patients with moderate-to-severe plaque psoriasis participated in a 12-week, double-blind, controlled trial in which they received etanercept 50 mg QW (n = 96) or placebo QW (n = 46), followed by a 12-week, open-label extension in which they received etanercept 50 mg QW (etanercept-etanercept, n = 90; placebo-etanercept, n = 36). Patients completed the Dermatology Life Quality Index (DLQI), EuroQoL-5D (EQ-5D) and Functional Assessment of Chronic Illness Therapy-Fatigue (FACIT-F) at baseline and subsequent study visits.

Results.—At baseline, DLQI and EQ-5D scores indicated significant quality of life (QoL) impairment, and FACIT-F scores suggested more fatigue than in the general population. At week 12, etanercept 50 mg QW provided statistically significantly (p < 0.05) and clinically meaningfully greater improvement in DLQI and EQ-5D utility scores than placebo, but not in FACIT-F scores. After 24 weeks of etanercept, the mean DLQI suggested psoriasis had a small effect on QoL, while EQ-5D and FACIT-F scores were comparable to population norms.

Conclusions.—Patients with moderate-to-severe psoriasis entered this trial with serious PRO impairment. At week 12, etanercept 50 mg QW provided significant QoL improvements compared with placebo. After

24 weeks of etanercept, the patients' serious PRO impairment had largely abated.

▶ Etanercept has proven effective for plaque psoriasis in large, double-blinded, placebo-controlled trials. Two dosage regimens have been approved in the United States. One dosage regimen is 50 mg administered subcutaneously twice per week for 12 weeks, which is then followed by 50 mg subcutaneously weekly thereafter. Alternatively, studies have shown that 50 mg administered subcutaneously weekly from the beginning ultimately results in similar outcomes by week 24 when compared with the regimen that starts with 2 doses per week. The main advantage of the latter regimen is that patients improve more quickly.

The authors performed a double-blinded, placebo-controlled trial in which patients received etanercept 50 mg weekly for 12 weeks or placebo. The 12-week placebo-controlled period was followed by a 12-week open-label extension in which all patients were treated with 50 mg of etanercept weekly. The Dermatology Life Quality Index (DLQI), EuroQoL-5D (EQ-5D), and Functional Assessment of Chronic Illness Therapy-Fatigue (FACIT-F) were performed throughout the study. At week 12, there was a statistically significant improvement in DLQI and EQ-5D scores compared with placebo. FACIT-F scores were not significantly improved. By week 24, the impairment of patient-reported outcomes found at baseline had largely improved.

Previous studies have shown that quality of life scores mirror clinical improvement in patients with psoriasis. Therefore, it should not be surprising that the quality of life scores studied in this report improved with etanercept therapy. It is only surprising that the FACIT-F score did not improve with therapy. In a previous study of etanercept 50 mg twice weekly, a statistically significant improvement in fatigue was reported at week 12,[1] and the differences reported are not necessarily because of the different dosages studied, but rather the differences in the incidences of psoriatic arthritis in the population studied. This report found an incidence of psoriatic arthritis in 11% of placebo patients and 16% of etanercept-treated patients. In contrast, the study by Tyring et al[1] found psoriatic arthritis in 33% of placebo patients and 35% of etanercept-treated patients. Nevertheless, the previously demonstrated utility of etanercept in improving quality of life of patients with psoriasis was confirmed in this study.

M. Lebwohl, MD

Reference

1. Tyring S, Gottlieb A, Papp K, et al. Etanercept and clinical outcomes, fatigue, and depression in psoriasis: double-blind and placebo-controlled randomized phase III trial. *Lancet.* 2006;367:29-35.

Patients with moderate-to-severe psoriasis recapture clinical response during re-treatment with etanercept
Ortonne J-P, Taïeb A, Ormerod AD, et al (Univ of Nice-Sophia Antipolis, France; Hôpital Saint Andre, Bordeaux, France; Aberdeen Royal Infirmary, Scotland; et al)
Br J Dermatol 161:1190-1195, 2009

Background.—Patients with psoriasis experience remission and gradual reappearance of erythematous and scaly plaques and require individualized treatment over time. A goal of psoriasis treatment is to provide optimal efficacy with a flexible therapeutic regimen that may include treatment pauses.

Objectives.—To determine whether patients receiving initial treatment with etanercept who then pause therapy would subsequently recapture response during re-treatment.

Patients and Methods.—A *post-hoc* analysis of 226 patients with moderate-to-severe psoriasis from a large multicentre trial was performed. Patients had received etanercept 50 mg twice weekly subcutaneously until a target clinical response had been achieved, then had paused treatment and eventually relapsed. They were then re-treated with etanercept 25 mg twice weekly. The number of patients recapturing a Physician Global Assessment (PGA) of psoriasis rating of ≤ 2 (clear, almost clear or mild) on first re-treatment was assessed. Patient satisfaction during the initial treatment and first re-treatment period was also determined.

Results.—A total of 187 (83%) patients recaptured the target clinical response of a PGA of ≤ 2 after re-treatment. The majority of patients [219 of 226 (97%)] reported satisfaction with etanercept re-treatment. No new safety concerns emerged during re-treatment.

Conclusions.—In this *post-hoc* analysis, patients with psoriasis who were re-treated with etanercept 25 mg twice weekly effectively recaptured clinical responses that patients found satisfactory. A flexible treatment option is available to dermatologists and patients for individualized care.

▶ Psoriasis is a chronic debilitating disorder marked by remissions and relapses. Although traditional treatment options involve topical corticosteroid use, patients with more severe plaque psoriasis may eventually require the use of biologic therapy. This randomized, open-label, multicenter trial investigates whether patients who responded favorably to etanercept then paused treatment would recapture that response with retreatment. Two hundred twenty-six patients with moderate-to-severe plaque psoriasis received etanercept 50 mg twice weekly until a Physician Global Assessment (PGA) of ≤2 (clear, almost clear, mild) was achieved. These patients paused treatment, subsequently relapsed, and then restarted etanercept 25 mg twice weekly. One hundred eighty-seven (83%) patients were able to recapture clinical response of PGA ≤2. A paused dose regimen may be beneficial for patients wanting to pause therapy for the summer, in preparation for surgery, for illness, or for pregnancy. Limitations of the study as mentioned by the authors include a relatively small number of patients in the study, and the PGA rating of mild may vary in clinical assessment.

S. Bellew, DO

J. Q. Del Rosso, DO

Predictive Factors of Eczema-Like Eruptions among Patients without Cutaneous Psoriasis Receiving Infliximab: A Cohort Study of 92 Patients

Esmailzadeh A, Yousefi P, Farhi D, et al (Tenon Hosp, Paris, France; Tarnier Hosp, Paris, France; et al)
Dermatology 219:263-267, 2009

Background.—Anti-tumor-necrosis-factor-α agents are limited by their side effects. Eczema is one of the most frequent adverse reactions affecting quality of life.

Objective.—To assess potential predictive risk factors for eczema in patients receiving infliximab.

Methods.—We conducted a prospective cohort study including patients treated with infliximab for a variety of disorders with the exception of cutaneous psoriasis. Clinical features were compared among patients with and without eczema under therapy.

Results.—92 consecutive patients were included; 15 developed eczema after the initiation of infliximab. In univariate analyses, a personal history of atopic symptoms was the only predictive factor for the occurrence of eczema (odds ratio = 3.6). Sex, age, principal diagnosis, dose and duration of infliximab and concomitant use of other immunosuppressors had no influence on the occurrence of eczema.

Conclusions.—A personal history of atopic symptoms is predictive of eczema under infliximab. Specific information should be provided to atopic patients starting such a treatment.

▶ The goal of this study was to assess potential predictive risk factors for eczema in patients receiving infliximab. The authors conducted a prospective cohort study, including patients treated with infliximab for a variety of disorders, with the exception of psoriasis. Of the 92 patients included, 15 developed an eczematous eruption after the initiation of infliximab. In univariate analyses, a personal history of atopic symptoms was the only predictive factor for the occurrence of eczema (odds ratio = 3.6). Eczema is not one of the more common conditions we observe in our psoriasis patients treated with infliximab. The authors note that there is a trend in their study, suggesting that under infliximab therapy, patients with rheumatoid arthritis therapy are more at risk of developing eczema. The major limitations of this study are the small sample size and the fact that those with a history of atopy may develop eczema in the absence of infliximab. Therefore, it is difficult to assess causality of infliximab in this population. Nevertheless, eczema-like eruptions are a potential side effect of infliximab to consider, especially in those with rheumatoid arthritis.

J. Weinberg, MD

Prurigo nodularis: systematic analysis of 58 histological criteria in 136 patients
Weigelt N, Metze D, Ständer S (Univ of Münster, Germany)
J Cutan Pathol 37:578-586, 2010

Background.—To date, there has been no systematic investigation of the detailed histological features of prurigo nodularis (PN) in a large cohort of patients.

Methods.—This retrospective study includes skin biopsies of 136 patients (63 males, 73 females; mean age: 58.38 years) with PN.

Results.—Highly characteristic for PN is the presence of thick compact orthohyperkeratosis; the hairy palm sign (folliculosebaceous units in non-volar skin in conjunction with a thick and compact cornified layer, like that of volar skin); irregular epidermal hyperplasia or pseudoepithelioma-tous hyperplasia; focal parakeratosis; hypergranulosis; fibrosis of the papillary dermis with vertically arranged collagen fibers; increased number of fibroblasts and capillaries; a superficial, perivascular and/or interstitial inflammatory infiltrate of lymphocytes, macrophages and, to a lesser extent, eosinophils and neutrophils. For comparison, histological findings in 45 patients (18 males, 27 females; mean, 55.64 years) with lichen simplex (LS) were studied. PN and LS, both of them scratch-induced, had 50 of 58 (86.2%) histological features in common.

Conclusions.—PN revealed a characteristic histological pattern. Absence of pseudoepitheliomatous hyperplasia or nerve fiber thickening, however, does not rule out the histological diagnosis of PN. A correlation of clinical and histological findings is necessary to reliably distinguish between PN and LS.

▶ This article attempts to "delineate the precise histological pattern of prurigo nodularis." Ultimately, the analysis shows that there is a wide spectrum of histopathological findings in prurigo nodularis. In addition, the analysis shows quite an overlap of histopathological findings between prurigo nodularis and lichen simplex.

This is a retrospective analysis of 136 cases of prurigo nodularis and 45 cases of lichen simplex. The authors did define several histopathological features, which "may be considered as highly characteristic for prurigo nodularis..." Although the analysis is interesting, it does not add critical new information to the field of dermatology or dermatopathology. This article primarily substantiates previously documented or suspected knowledge of prurigo nodularis and lichen simplex.

S. M. Purcell, DO

Randomized, double-blind, placebo-controlled evaluation of the efficacy of oral psoralen plus ultraviolet A for the treatment of plaque-type psoriasis using the Psoriasis Area Severity Index score (improvement of 75% or greater) at 12 weeks

Sivanesan SP, Gattu S, Hong J, et al (Pittsburgh Univ, PA; Univ of California, Irvine; Univ of California, San Francisco; et al)
J Am Acad Dermatol 61:793-798, 2009

Background.—Psoralen plus ultraviolet A (PUVA) for the treatment of psoriasis has never been evaluated using the Psoriasis Area Severity Index (PASI) in a randomized, double-blind, placebo-controlled trial. The lack of such data limits our capacity to estimate PUVA's efficacy relative to other treatment options that are available today.

Objectives.—The purpose of this study was to evaluate the efficacy of PUVA therapy for patients with plaque-type psoriasis.

Methods.—This study involved 40 patients with psoriasis; 30 received PUVA and 10 received UVA with placebo. PASI scores were assessed at baseline and every 4 weeks thereafter for 12 weeks.

Results.—By nonresponder imputation, 60% (18 of 30) in the PUVA group achieved 75% or more improvement in PASI score after 12 weeks of treatment compared with 0% (0 of 10) in the UVA plus placebo group ($P < .0001$). Using intent to treat with last observation carried forward analysis, 63% (19 of 30) in the PUVA group achieved 75% or more improvement in PASI score compared with 0% (0 of 10) in the UVA plus placebo group ($P < .0001$). By per protocol analysis, 86% (18 of 21) in the PUVA group as compared with 0% (0 of 7) in the UVA plus placebo group reached 75% or more improvement in PASI score after 12 weeks ($P < .0001$).

Limitations.—The study was relatively small with only 40 patients enrolled and 28 patients who completed the protocol. Further studies that involve head-to-head comparison of PUVA with other treatment modalities are needed. Nonresponder imputation, last observation carried forward with intent to treat, and per protocol analyses each have separate advantages and limitations when determining clinical significance.

Conclusions.—This study supports the observation that PUVA is a highly efficacious treatment for chronic plaque psoriasis.

▶ This article nicely demonstrates the use of psoralen plus ultraviolet A (PUVA) for the treatment of psoriasis. The efficacy has always been known, but not demonstrated with conventional Psoriasis Area Severity Index scores. The main limitation of this therapy is the use in patients who have skin types I-III. This group clearly has issues with skin cancers that preclude its safe use for long-term therapy. However, patients with skin types IV-VI are a different story. An increased skin cancer incidence has not been demonstrated in this group of patients. PUVA is much more convenient than UVB therapy and should again be reconsidered in patients of color.

E. A. Tanghetti, MD

Recent Trends in Systemic Psoriasis Treatment Costs

Beyer V, Wolverton SE (Indiana Univ School of Medicine, Indianapolis)
Arch Dermatol 146:46-54, 2010

Objectives.—To analyze the current total cost of systemic therapy for psoriasis and to compare annual trends in the cost of both generic and brand-name therapies with trends in the Consumer Price Index—Urban since 2000.

Design.—A cost model was developed that includes costs for prescription drugs, office visits, and suggested laboratory tests and monitoring procedures. Annual trends in psoriasis drug costs from 2000 through 2008 were analyzed by calculating the percentage change in the average wholesale price from the previous year; these values were compared with changes in the yearly Consumer Price Index—Urban values.

Setting.—The United States.

Main Outcome Measures.—Total annual costs for systemic psoriasis therapies and trends in cost compared with the trends in Consumer Price Index—Urban values (equivalent to inflation).

Results.—Current total annual costs for systemic psoriasis therapies ranged from $1197 (methotrexate) to $27 577 (alefacept, two 12-week courses). Trends in the average wholesale price of brand-name psoriasis therapies from 2000 through 2008 demonstrate an average increase of 66% (range, −24% to +316%); thus, costs of several brand-name psoriasis drugs greatly outpaced the rates of inflation for all items and all prescription drugs.

Conclusions.—Despite the higher monitoring costs associated with traditional systemic therapies, annual costs of biologics exceed those of other available therapies. Current trends demonstrate that systemic psoriasis therapy costs are increasing at a much higher rate compared with general inflation.

▶ Biologic therapies have been of great benefit in our treatment of psoriasis. However, one of the barriers to usage of the drugs has been the high costs associated with them. The analyses of this study were developed to answer 2 questions—First, what is the current, direct cost of systemic therapy for psoriasis? Second, what is the trend in these costs relative to general inflation? The authors found that trends in the average wholesale price of brand-name psoriasis therapies from 2000 to 2008 demonstrated an average increase of 66%. Therefore, costs of several brand-name psoriasis drugs greatly outpaced the rates of inflation for all items and all prescription drugs. They concluded that the current trends demonstrate an increase in systemic psoriasis therapy costs at a much higher rate compared with general inflation. In this era of rising health care costs, this is certainly problematic, as coverage of expensive drugs is restricted and costs are passed on to patients. Cost considerations will be a major factor in the treatment of psoriasis in the foreseeable future.

J. Weinberg, MD

Paediatric psoriasis - narrowband UVB treatment

Zamberk P, Velázquez D, Campos M, et al (Hospital General Universitario Gregorio Marañón, Madrid, Spain)
J Eur Acad Dermatol Venereol 24:415-419, 2010

Narrowband UV-B is a safe and efficacious option for the treatment of adult psoriasis. However, the use of this therapy has been limited in children due to its long-term carcinogenic potential. It has proven to be an adequate alternative in patients whose condition is refractory to topical treatment.

Aims.—To evaluate the efficacy and short-term safety of narrowband UV-B in the treatment of paediatric psoriasis, and to compare our results with those obtained in other studies on paediatric psoriasis.

Materials and Methods.—Over a period of 2 years and 4 months, we administered narrowband UV-B to 20 children diagnosed with psoriasis that was refractory to topical therapy. The therapeutic response was measured using the Psoriasis Area and Severity Index (PASI).

Results.—Between August 2005 and December 2007, 20 children received narrowband UV-B. Their median age was 13 years (range, 5–17 years), and the median initial PASI score was 8.25 (2.7–22.2). A median of 28 (10–59) sessions was required to achieve clearance, reaching almost complete or total remission (median final PASI) in all but two patients. Six patients required a new therapeutic course because of relapse, and the mean duration of remission was 8 months (4–18). No patients experienced severe adverse events during therapy, and only one discontinued treatment, for unrelated reasons.

Discussion and Conclusion.—Narrowband UV-B for the treatment of paediatric psoriasis has received little attention in the literature. This treatment has been limited in children because of its potential long-term carcinogenic effects, and most information has been extrapolated from adults. Nevertheless, narrowband UV-B phototherapy is an effective and well-tolerated therapeutic alternative in paediatric patients with severe psoriasis.

▶ Pediatric therapeutics, whether device or drug, is a neglected area in dermatology. This study, though retrospective, does provide added evidence that narrowband ultraviolet B treatments are safe and effective in the pediatric population.

E. A. Tanghetti, MD

Standards for genital protection in phototherapy units

Abdulla FR, Breneman C, Adams B, et al (Univ of Cincinnati Med Ctr, OH; Univ of Illinois, Urbana; College of Medicine, Cincinnati, OH; et al)
J Am Acad Dermatol 62:223-226, 2010

Background.—Phototherapy is a useful therapy for many dermatologic disorders and is known for its low side-effect profile. However, one potential notable side effect is genital skin cancer. Unfortunately, no standards for genital protection currently exist for this preventable complication. Patients treated with phototherapy may already have a decreased quality of life because of their primary dermatologic disorder. Development of squamous cell carcinoma of the genitalia may certainly further affect the quality of life.

Objective.—The objective was to determine which readily available materials afford the best photoprotection of the male genitalia.

Methods.—Seven common materials used in phototherapy units for genital protection were placed over ultraviolet (UV) B and UVA monitors and placed in broadband UVB, narrowband UVB, and UVA full-body units. The percentage of light blocked was then calculated.

Results.—Blue and white cotton underwear, blue surgical towels, an athletic supporter with or without a cup, and the psoralen plus UVA pouch provided acceptable means of genital protection; however, surgical masks did not.

Limitations.—Only the most commonly used materials were tested in the phototherapy units. The materials were not of a single material type or similar masses. In addition, only one of each type of full-body phototherapy unit was used to obtain the data.

Conclusion.—Although a polyester composition provides better UV protection, factors such as low porosity and higher mass are intrinsic to decreasing the amount of UV penetration of any fabric. Of the commonly used objects, surgical masks do not provide sufficient protection to the genital area.

▶ If you are a male undergoing phototherapy with ultraviolet B, ultraviolet A (UVA), or psoralen plus UVA, it is imperative to cover your genital region. Most commonly used blocking devices worked well, with the exception being a surgical mask that did allow significant transmittance of UV light. The athletic support with a cup seemed to provide the best protection against UV exposure.

E. A. Tangetti, MD

The Risk of Stroke in Patients with Psoriasis
Gelfand JM, Dommasch ED, Shin DB, et al (Univ of Pennsylvania School of Medicine, Philadelphia)
J Invest Dermatol 129:2411-2418, 2009

Psoriasis is a chronic Th-1 and Th-17 inflammatory disease. Chronic inflammation has also been associated with atherosclerosis and thrombosis. The purpose of this study was to determine the risk of stroke in patients with psoriasis. We conducted a population-based cohort study of patients seen by general practitioners participating in the General Practice Research Database in the United Kingdom, 1987–2002. Mild psoriasis was defined as any patient with a diagnostic code of psoriasis, but no history of systemic therapy. Severe psoriasis was defined as any patient with a diagnostic code of psoriasis and a history of systemic therapy consistent with severe psoriasis. The unexposed (control) population was composed of patients with no history of a psoriasis diagnostic code. When adjusting for major risk factors for stroke, both mild (hazard ratio (HR) 1.06, 95% confidence interval (CI) 1.0−1.1) and severe (1.43, 95% CI 1.1−1.9) psoriasis were independent risk factors for stroke. The excess risk of stroke attributable to psoriasis in patients with mild and severe disease was 1 in 4,115 per year and 1 in 530 per year, respectively. Patients with psoriasis, particularly if severe, have an increased risk of stroke that is not explained by major stroke risk factors identified in routine medical care.

▶ There is a growing literature concerning the comorbidities associated with psoriasis, including cardiovascular disease, obesity, and metabolic syndrome. However, there is a paucity of data examining the risk of stroke in patients with psoriasis. The purpose of this study was to determine the risk of stroke in patients with psoriasis. The authors conducted a population-based cohort study of patients seen by general practitioners participating in the General Practice Research Database in the United Kingdom, 1987-2002. The results of this study showed that patients with severe psoriasis have a 44% increased risk of stroke. The risk of stroke in patients with psoriasis was not explained by both common and rare major risk factors for stroke as identified in routine medical practice, suggesting that psoriasis may be an independent risk factor for stroke. Patients who were classified as having mild psoriasis had a statistically significant increased risk of stroke; however, this association was very modest and of limited clinical significance for the individual patient. On the basis of the study data, a patient with mild psoriasis has an excess risk of stroke attributable to psoriasis of 1 in 4115 per year, whereas a patient with severe psoriasis has an excess risk of stroke attributable to psoriasis of 1 in 530 per year. The authors concluded that patients with psoriasis, particularly if severe, have an increased risk of stroke that is not explained by the major stroke risk factors identified in routine medical care. Therefore, stroke is another comorbidity to consider in the patient with psoriasis, and those at risk should be counseled and given proper medical referrals accordingly.

J. Weinberg, MD

Treatment of scalp psoriasis with clobetasol-17 propionate 0.05% shampoo: a study on daily clinical practice
Bovenschen HJ, Van de Kerkhof PCM (Dept of Dermatology, Nijmegen, The Netherlands)
J Eur Acad Dermatol Venereol 24:439-444, 2010

Background.—Safety and clinical effectiveness of clobetasol-17 propionate 0.05% shampoo have been shown in patients with scalp psoriasis.

Aim.—First, to evaluate treatment satisfaction, user convenience safety and effectiveness of clobetasol-17 propionate 0.05% shampoo treatment in daily clinical practice. Second, to identify subgroup variables that may predict treatment success or failure.

Methods.—A total of 56 patients with scalp psoriasis were treated with short-contact clobetasol-17 propionate 0.05% shampoo once daily for 4 weeks. Data on treatment satisfaction, user convenience, safety and effectiveness were assessed on a 7-point Likert scale using postal questionnaires. Subgroup analyses were performed to identify variables that may predict treatment outcome.

Results.—A total of 41 patients returned both questionnaires (73%). Positive treatment satisfaction and user convenience were reported by 66% and 79% of patients respectively. Patient-rated indicators for disease severity improved by 39–46% ($P < 0.05$%). No major side-effects were reported. Subgroup analyses did not reveal any statistically significant patient variable that may predict treatment outcome. However, a tendency towards improved treatment satisfaction was observed in patients who had received fewer topical antipsoriatic treatments previously ($P > 0.05$).

Conclusions.—Short-contact treatment with clobetasol-17 propionate 0.05% shampoo has high user convenience and patient satisfaction rates. Moreover, the treatment is well-tolerated and efficacious from patients' perspective. Subgroup analyses did not reveal factors predicting treatment outcome, although treatment success tended to be more evident in patients who had received fewer treatments previously.

▶ There are considerable numbers of patients who have scalp psoriasis in those afflicted with psoriasis elsewhere on their body, and some present with scalp involvement alone. High-potency topical corticosteroids for scalp psoriasis have been demonstrated to be effective in patients. However, patient compliance is low for the topical treatment of scalp psoriasis because some products may not be easy to use because of presence of hair or are formulated in a messy formulation. This is a cross-sectional study to evaluate treatment satisfaction and user convenience, with patients reporting safety and effectiveness of clobetasol-17 propionate 0.05% shampoo in daily clinical practice. Treatment consists of short-contact clobetasol-17 propionate 0.05% shampoo every day once daily for 15 minutes on scalp skin with dry hair. Then patients were instructed to rinse off the shampoo after 15 minutes. Researchers also administered questionnaires on clinical effectiveness, current signs and symptoms, user convenience, patient satisfaction, and side effects of the medication. A total of 56 patients with scalp psoriasis were recruited at the outpatient department. Six patients (17%) used concomitant systemic antipsoriatic medications. A total of 34 of 41 patients (83%) had previously used topical medication for scalp psoriasis. Overall, 79% of patients reported a positive user convenience of clobetasol-17 propionate 0.05% shampoo. A total of 66% of patients rated the treatment as satisfactory after 4 weeks. The severity of symptoms significantly declined after treatment ($P < .05$). There were no major side effects other than mild skin irritation. There were no statistically significant differences that were observed between these patients and patients without any systemic antipsoriatic treatment with respect to user convenience, patient satisfaction, effectiveness, or safety. There was no significant difference in user convenience between the separate products; however, there was a preference in favor of clobetasol-17 propionate shampoo. The authors concluded that clobetasol-17 propionate shampoo treatment once daily for 4 weeks in a short-contact regimen is more convenient for the user with high treatment satisfaction noted (compared with coal tar shampoo, desoximethasone emulsion 0.25%, betamethsone valerate lotion, clobetasol-17 propionate lotion, calcipotriol/betamethsone dipropionate gel, calcipotriol lotion, and hydrocortisone-17 butyrate). Overall, treatment satisfaction was rated positive in 66% of patients. This study evaluated patient-reported variables in contrast to other studies to measure efficacy. There was no significant correlation of baseline characteristics of scalp psoriasis and treatment responses that were identified, and this study was not able to identify subtypes of scalp psoriasis that were most eligible for treatment with clobetasol-17 propionate shampoo. Authors did not observe significant differences between mild, moderate, or severe scalp psoriasis. Limitations to this study were that it was retrospective in design, and because of the small sample size, the authors were unable to identify differences for subgroup analyses. This was a study using subjective patient reporting, and therefore, investigator efficacy data were not included. In conclusion, the authors found that clobetasol-17 propionate 0.05% shampoo short-contact treatment has a high user convenience rating and a high rate of treatment satisfaction.

J. Q. Del Rosso, DO

G. K. Kim, DO

Treatment of severe, recalcitrant, chronic plaque psoriasis with fumaric acid esters: a prospective study
Wain EM, Darling MI, Pleass RD, et al (St Thomas' Hosp, London, UK)
Br J Dermatol 162:427-434, 2010

Background.—Fumaric acid esters (FAE) are used in Germany as a first-line systemic treatment for chronic plaque psoriasis, with proven efficacy and low toxicity. Their use in the U.K. is variable, and they remain unlicensed. Consequently, efficacy and safety data from U.K. patients is limited and their place in the psoriasis treatment armamentarium is unclear.

Objectives.—To examine the efficacy and safety of FAE in a prospective cohort of U.K. patients with severe, treatment-recalcitrant, chronic plaque psoriasis.

Methods.—A single-centre, open, nonrandomized, prospective study was performed in a regional referral centre for patients with severe psoriasis. Outcomes were measured by the Psoriasis Area and Severity Index (PASI), Dermatology Life Quality Index (DLQI), blood investigations and adverse events monitoring.

Results.—Eighty patients were recruited. Fifty-nine per cent were taking a concomitant oral antipsoriatic agent; 20% achieved a PASI-50, 8% a PASI-75 and 4% a PASI-90 on intention-to-treat analysis at 3 months with an overall, statistically significant, reduction in PASI from $13 \cdot 9 \pm 9 \cdot 0$ to $11 \cdot 3 \pm 9 \cdot 2$ ($P < 0 \cdot 0001$). At 3 months, lymphopenia was seen in 33% of the cohort with significantly lower counts in patients responsive to FAE ($P = 0 \cdot 008$). In addition, by 3 months, 36% of concomitant antipsoriatic medication had been stopped and 25% of doses had been reduced without loss of disease control. Side-effects (most commonly diarrhoea, abdominal pain and flushing) were reported by 74% of patients resulting in cessation of FAE in 36%.

Conclusions.—FAE is a useful alternative treatment option in patients with severe, treatment-resistant, chronic plaque psoriasis and can allow dose reduction, and subsequent cessation, of other, potentially more toxic agents.

▶ This study was of fair quality. The trial was a single-center, open-label, non-randomized, prospective study performed in a regional referral center and included 80 patients. The length of the study was 5 years; however, less than half of the study patients remained after 1 year, and only 4 remained in the study after 4 years.

The authors' objective was to examine the efficacy and safety of fumaric acid esters (FAEs) in a prospective cohort of patients in the United Kingdom with severe, treatment-recalcitrant, chronic plaque psoriasis. This objective was challenging to meet, given a single small group of participants with a significant long-term discontinuation rate.

The study limitations, therefore, commence with a small sample size. The long-term data had very few patients to assess both the efficacy and overall safety. The patient population chosen, however, is the most difficult of psoriasis patient populations, and one might generally have expected respondent numbers to be low. A Psoriasis Area Severity Index (PASI) 50 of 20% is a low number and far below the present-day benchmark of PASI 75 for systemic agents under study, such as biologics. Moreover, more concerning is that 74% of patients reported adverse events, although none were serious. Another major limitation is the absence of a direct population comparison with placebo or perhaps another agent. One would assume that patients in a trial might be more compliant and receive more optimal care than previously administered.

The potential for an alternative treatment, particularly an oral agent, to our already impressive psoriasis armamentarium is always welcome. However, the availability of FAEs, their cost, and their side-effect profile may make this class of psoriasis agents a potentially challenging group to implement. With this said, it is clear that the potential role of FAEs in psoriasis management is intriguing and therefore deserves further study in the United States.

B. P. Glick, DO, MPH

A. Wiener, DO

T. J. Singer, DO

Ustekinumab improves health-related quality of life in patients with moderate-to-severe psoriasis: results from the PHOENIX 1 trial
Lebwohl M, Papp K, Han C, et al (Mount Sinai School of Medicine, NY; Waterloo and Univ of Western Ontario, London, Ontario, Canada; Johnson & Johnson Pharmaceutical Services, Horsham, PA; et al)
Br J Dermatol 162:137-146, 2010

Background.—PHOENIX 1 was a phase III, randomized, double-blind, placebo-controlled study that demonstrated the long-term efficacy and safety of ustekinumab in patients with moderate-to-severe psoriasis.

Objectives.—To assess the effect of ustekinumab maintenance therapy on health-related quality of life (HRQoL) in PHOENIX 1 patients.

Patients and Methods.—Patients ($n = 766$) were randomized to receive ustekinumab 45 mg ($n = 255$) or 90 mg ($n = 256$) at weeks 0 and 4 and every 12 weeks thereafter, or placebo ($n = 255$) at weeks 0 and 4 with crossover to ustekinumab at week 12. Ustekinumab-randomized patients achieving at least 75% improvement in Psoriasis Area and Severity Index (PASI) 75 at weeks 28 and 40 were re-randomized at week 40 to continue ustekinumab or be withdrawn until loss of therapeutic effect. HRQoL was assessed using the SF-36 and Dermatology Life Quality Index (DLQI).

Results.—At baseline, more than 97% had a DLQI > 1 and the average DLQI was > 10, indicating a significant impact on patients' HRQoL. Significantly greater proportions of patients receiving ustekinumab 45 and 90 mg achieved a normalized DLQI score ($\le$ 1) compared with placebo (53.2%, 52.4% and 6.0%, respectively, both $P < 0.001$) at week 12 and achieved a clinically meaningful improvement (increase of at least five points) in SF-36 physical (23.1%, 33.7% and 15.6%) and mental (25.5%, 31.3% and 14.8%) component summary scores. At week 12, changes in individual DLQI and SF-36 domains were significantly better in each ustekinumab group vs. placebo ($P < 0.001$). The magnitude of improvement across SF-36 scales was greatest for the bodily pain and social functioning domains. Improvements in HRQoL were sustained with maintenance ustekinumab therapy through at least 1 year. Regression analysis showed that, after adjustment for improvement in PASI or Physician's Global Assessment (PGA), ustekinumab-treated patients demonstrated significant improvements in DLQI.

Conclusions.—Ustekinumab improves HRQoL in patients with moderate-to-severe psoriasis. Patient-reported outcomes measured a treatment effect beyond that indicated by clinical measures.

▶ Agents that block interleukin (IL)-12/IL-23 have proven to be highly effective in the treatment of psoriasis. Ustekinumab is a human monoclonal antibody that blocks the p40 component of IL-12 and IL-23 and is the first such agent to be approved for the treatment of psoriasis. PHOENIX 1 was the title given to the first pivotal trial that led to the approval of ustekinumab. The impact of psoriasis on a patient's quality of life was evaluated using the Dermatology Life Quality

Index (DLQI). The DLQI is a 10-item questionnaire that assesses disease impact on day-to-day symptoms and activities of the preceding week. Each question has a score from 0 to 3. Thus, the total score can range from 0 (no effect) to 30 (great effect on quality of life). General health-related quality of life (HRQoL) was evaluated with the Short Form (SF-36), another questionnaire that has physical and mental components. On the latter scale, higher scores indicate a better HRQoL.

Patients achieving Psoriasis Area and Severity Index 75 at weeks 28 and 40 were rerandomized at week 40 to either continue on ustekinumab or be treated with placebo until loss of therapeutic effect.

Seven hundred sixty-six patients were enrolled in this double-blinded placebo-controlled study. They were randomized to receive ustekinumab 45 mg or 90 mg at baseline 4 weeks later and every 12 weeks thereafter or placebo at baseline and 4 weeks later with crossover to ustekinumab at week 12.

The average DLQI at baseline was higher than 10. At week 12, DLQI scores less than 1 were achieved by 53.2% of those receiving 45 mg of ustekinumab, 52.4% in the 90-mg group, and 6% in the placebo group, a difference that was highly statistically significant. Improvement of at least 5 points in the SF-36 was likewise achieved by significantly more patients in the active groups than the placebo group. Improvements in quality of life persisted in patients who were maintained on ustekinumab therapy for at least 1 year.

It should not be surprising that a drug that effectively treats psoriasis would result in marked improvement in quality of life. Those improvements should mirror the improvements seen in psoriasis.

M. Lebwohl, MD

3 Bacterial and Fungal Infections

A double-blind, randomized, placebo-controlled, dose-finding study of oral pramiconazole in the treatment of pityriasis versicolor

Faergemann J, Todd G, Pather S, et al (Sahlgrenska Univ Hosp, Göteborg, Sweden; Groote Schuur Hosp, Cape Town, South Africa; Univ Cape Town, South Africa; et al)

J Am Acad Dermatol 61:971-976, 2009

Background.—Pramiconazole is a broad-spectrum triazole antifungal with potential for oral treatment of pityriasis versicolor.

Objective.—We sought to assess the efficacy and tolerability of 5 doses of pramiconazole relative to placebo.

Methods.—This was a randomized, multicenter, double-blind, placebo-controlled, 28-day, dose-finding study. A total of 147 patients were randomized to treatment with placebo or one of 5 doses of pramiconazole; treatment lasted for 3 consecutive days. Efficacy was based on mycological response, severity of clinical signs and symptoms, and the Investigator Global Assessment of lesion clearance.

Results.—A statistically significant ($P < .001$) dose-dependent effect was observed. When compared with placebo, a significant response ($P < .05$) was obtained for all but the lowest single dose of pramiconazole. There were no serious, treatment-related adverse events or other safety concerns.

Limitations.—The follow-up period was limited to 1 month after treatment onset.

Conclusions.—Pramiconazole is a well-tolerated and effective treatment for pityriasis versicolor and the most effective treatment regimen in this study included 200 or 400 mg taken once, and 200 mg taken once daily for 2 or 3 days.

▶ Pityriasis versicolor (PV) is a common recurrent infectious disorder of the skin due to the mycelial form of the lipophilic yeast of *Malassezia* spp. Currently, PV is treated with topical and oral antifungal agents. In vitro studies have indicated that oral pramiconazole is active against yeast such as *Malassezia* spp, *Candida* spp, and dermatophytes. The objective of this study was to describe the efficacy and tolerability of 5 different dosing regimens of pramiconazole in comparison with placebo. This was a randomized, multicenter, double-blinded, placebo-controlled, 28-day, dose-finding study of 147 patients with

PV. Those who were excluded were immunocompromised and previously on topical corticosteroid treatments. All cases were confirmed microscopically by positive potassium hydroxide (KOH) preparation results consistent with the presence of PV. Effective treatment was defined as a negative KOH microscopy and either erythema, desquamation, or pruritus scores of 0. Statistically significant comparisons between the active treatments and placebo were observed at day 28 for all treatments except pramiconazole 100 mg once (single dose) in the evaluations of complete cure ($P < .013$). Statistically significant ($P < .001$) dose-dependent efficacy was observed. The most common adverse effects were diarrhea and nausea, with the highest being in the 100 mg once group (34.6%). In this study, 200 mg or 400 mg taken once and 200 mg taken once daily for 2 to 3 days were shown to be an effective treatment of PV. A limitation to this study was the short follow-up period. Those who have PV usually have a chronic course, and future studies are needed to assess whether patients can safely use the suppressive dosage regimens of oral pramiconazole long-term without associated side effects or drug interactions. Head-to-head comparative studies with topical agents are also needed. In conclusion, oral pramiconazole appears to be well tolerated and an effective treatment of PV; however, it is not clear based on these data whether it provides any advantages over other currently used oral therapies for PV.

J. Q. Del Rosso, DO

G. K. Kim, DO

Antibody-mediated enhancement of community-acquired methicillin-resistant *Staphylococcus aureus* infection
Yoong P, Pier GB (Brigham and Women's Hosp, Boston, MA)
Proc Natl Acad Sci U S A 107:2241-2246, 2010

Community-acquired infections caused by methicillin-resistant *Staphylococcus aureus* (MRSA) expressing the Panton-Valentine leukocidin (PVL) are rampant, but the contribution of PVL to bacterial virulence remains controversial. While PVL is usually viewed as a cytotoxin, at sublytic amounts it activates protective innate immune responses. A leukotoxic effect might predominate in high inoculum studies, whereas protective proinflammatory properties might predominate in settings with lower bacterial inocula that more closely mimic what initially occurs in humans. However, these protective effects might possibly be neutralized by antibodies to PVL, which are found in normal human sera and at increased levels following PVL$^+$ *S. aureus* infections. In a low-inoculum murine skin abscess model including a foreign body at the infection site, strains deleted for the *pvl* genes replicated more efficiently within abscesses than isogenic PVL$^+$ strains. Coinfection of mice at separate sites with isogenic PVL$^+$ and PVL$^-$ MRSA abrogated the differences in bacterial burdens, indicating a systemic effect on host innate immunity from production of PVL. Mice given antibody to PVL and then infected with seven different PVL⁺ strains also had significantly higher bacterial counts in abscesses compared with mice given nonimmune serum. Antibody to PVL had no effect on MRSA strains that did not produce PVL. In vitro, antibody to PVL incapacitated PVL-mediated activation of PMNs, indicating that virulence of PVL⁺ MRSA is enhanced by the interference of PVL-activated innate immune responses. Given the high rates of primary and recurring MRSA infections in humans, it appears that antibodies to PVL might contribute to host susceptibility to infection.

▶ This is an important and potentially significant study regarding the likely enhancement of community-acquired methicillin-resistant *Staphylococcus aureus* (CA-MRSA) infection as a result of acquired antibodies that are reactive with CA-MRSA expressing the Panton-Valentine leukocidin (PVL). Under high inoculation levels, PVL is generally considered a cytotoxin. However, based on the authors' research with mouse models, they found that under low inoculation levels (sublytic amounts), the body produces proinflammatory protective effects against the bacteria. However, in PVL-positive CA-MRSA strains, the immune system will also generate a high level of antibodies against PVL. This was noteworthy because what they found was that these antibodies may actually offset the body's protective proinflammatory effects against PVL-positive CA-MRSA infections. Namely, these antibodies likely impair the process through which immune cells are activated and thus may actually increase the bacterial burden. What was also notable was that their findings suggested that these high levels of antibodies to PVL may actually promote reinfection. In addition, they further noted that given their findings, caution should be used when considering the value of immunization against PVL because of the potential of the enhanced virulence associated with the antibody. Overall, the article was well written and researched. Additional research on this issue may be necessary; however, the findings of the study certainly provide an important background on understanding the virulence of PVL-positive CA-MRSA infections and their effects on the immune system.

B. D. Michaels, DO

J. Q. Del Rosso, DO

Bacterial colonization of chronic leg ulcers: current results compared with data 5 years ago in a specialized dermatology department
Körber A, Schmid EN, Buer J, et al (Univ of Essen, Germany)
J Eur Acad Dermatol Venereol 24:1017-1025, 2010

Background.—In nearly every chronic wound different bacteria species can be detected. Nevertheless, the presence of such microorganisms is not necessarily obligatory associated with a delayed wound healing. But from this initially unproblematic colonization an infection up to a sepsis can arise in some patients. The aim of our clinical investigation was to analyse the spectrum of microbial colonization of patients with a chronic leg ulcer in our specialized dermatological outpatient wound clinic, and to compare them with the results of comparable data already collected 5 years ago.

Objectives.—In our retrospective investigation the results of bacteriological swabs were documented in 100 patients with a total of 107 chronic leg ulcers. All patients visited the specialized wound outpatient clinic, Department of Dermatology, University of Essen in Germany.

Methods.—A total of 60 patients were female, 40 were male. The mean age was 65 years. Altogether a total of 191 bacterial isolates and 25 different bacterial species could be identified.

Results.—The most often detected species were *Staphylococcus aureus* ($n = 60$), *Pseudomonas aeruginosa* ($n = 36$) as well as *Proteus mirabilis* ($n = 17$). In 10 patients (10%) we identified a colonization with methicillin resistant *S. aureus* (MRSA). Merely in 6 patients the taken swabs were sterile. Five years ago a comparable investigation was already carried out in our wound outpatient clinic. At that time we could detect in particular more frequent MRSA (21.5% vs. 10%) and rarely *P. aeruginosa* (24.1% vs. 33.6%).

Conclusion.—The results of our investigation demonstrate the current spectrum of the bacterial colonization in patients with chronic leg ulcers in a university dermatological wound centre in comparison to the last 5 years. In our institution we were able to demonstrate a shift of the detected bacterial species from gram-positive in direction to gram-negative germs. Beside the already known problems with MRSA, in future therapeutic strategies in patients with chronic leg ulcers the increasing amount of gram-negative bacteria and especially of *P. aeruginosa* should considered.

▶ Korber et al provided a useful retrospective study analyzing the current spectrum of microbial colonization of patients with chronic leg ulcers versus comparable data of microbial colonization of chronic leg ulcers from 5 years earlier. The results of the study are both informative and potentially clinically applicable. The study took place in a specialized wound outpatient clinic in the Department of Dermatology at the University of Essen in Germany. The most often detected species was *Staphylococcus aureus*, followed by *Pseudomonas aeruginosa* and *Proteus mirabilis*. Of note was the shift over the last 5 years from gram-positive to gram-negative organisms, including *P aeruginosa* and *P mirabilis*. Interestingly, while methicillin-resistant *S aureus* colonization was identified in 10% of the current patients, its frequency decreased from 5 years ago when it was detected 21.5% of the time. As noted by the article, given this noted shift toward more gram-negative infections, these results should be considered by physicians for targeted future treatment strategies in the care of chronic leg ulcers. Overall, the article is interesting and of practical clinical importance. It is also important to note that controversy exists on treatment of ulcer colonization as opposed to only when infection is observed clinically. Nevertheless, changes in the bacterial ecology of leg ulcers in this setting are noteworthy.

B. D. Michaels, DO
J. Q. Del Rosso, DO

Borrelia in granuloma annulare, morphea and lichen sclerosus: a PCR-based study and review of the literature

Zollinger T, Mertz KD, Schmid M, et al (Kempf und Pfaltz Histologische Diagnostik, Zürich, Switzerland)
J Cutan Pathol 37:571-577, 2010

Background.—Morphea, granuloma annulare (GA) and lichen sclerosus et atrophicans (LSA) have also been suggested to be linked to Borrelia infection. Previous studies based on serologic data or detection of Borrelia by immunohistochemistry and polymerase chain reaction (PCR) reported contradictory results. Thus, we examined skin biopsies of morphea, GA and LSA by PCR to assess the prevalence of Borrelia DNA in an endemic area and to compare our results with data in the literature.

Methods.—Amplification of DNA sequences of *Borrelia burgdorferi sensu lato* by nested PCR from formalin-fixed and paraffin-embedded skin biopsies of morphea, GA and LSA, followed by automated sequencing of amplification products. PCR-based studies on Borrelia species in these disorders published until July 2009 were retrieved by a literature search.

Results.—Borrelia DNA was detected in 3 of 112 skin biopsies (2.7%) including one of 49 morphea biopsies (2.0%), one of 48 GA biopsies (2.1%) and one of 15 LSA biopsies (6.6%). Amplification products belonged to *B. burgdorferi sensu stricto* in two cases available for sequence analysis.

Conclusions.—The results of our and most of other PCR-based studies do not argue for a significant association of *B. burgdorferi sensu lato* with morphea, GA, LSA.

▶ This article weighs in on a rather impassioned controversy surrounding the detection of *Borrelia* species within morphea, granuloma annulare, and lichen sclerosus.

In the past few years, claims have emerged to implicate *Borrelia* species in these otherwise idiopathic and poorly understood diseases. For example, a 2007 article on focus floating microscopy (FFM), which uses immunohistochemical staining and rasterizing in 2 dimensions, purported to be the gold standard in detecting *Borrelia* species in tissue in some of these conditions.[1]

However, in this study from an endemic area, examination of tissue from 115 cases of morphea, 48 cases of granuloma annulare, and 15 cases of lichen sclerosus detected *Borrelia* species DNA by polymerase chain reaction (PCR)-based analysis in only 1 case from each subcategory. Furthermore, in only 2 of the 3 cases was there enough material to verify that *Borrelia burgdorferi sensu stricto* was involved. Lastly, in 1 case where *Borrelia* DNA was detected, treatment with antibiotics was commenced, but there was no improvement in the disease process.

Therefore, the authors of this article proffer that in their minds, this lack of detection and improvement militate against a role for *Borrelia* species with regard to morphea, granuloma annulare, or lichen sclerosus. Of course, this will not stop differing minds from pointing out that it may simply be yet more evidence that PCR is inferior to other techniques such as FFM in detecting *Borrelia*, but as the authors note, this would run contrary to the weight of evidence surrounding use of PCR in a myriad of other infections, such as cutaneous leishmaniasis, where the sensitivity of PCR is superior to all other techniques.[2]

W. A. High, MD, JD, MEng

References

1. Eisendle K, Grabner T, Zelger B. Focus floating microscopy: "gold standard" for cutaneous borreliosis? *Am J Clin Pathol.* 2007;127:213-222.
2. Boggild AK, Ramos AP, Espinosa D, et al. Clinical and demographic stratification of test performance: a pooled analysis of five laboratory diagnostic methods for American cutaneous leishmaniasis. *Am J Trop Med Hyg.* 2010;83:345-350.

Clinical Importance of Purulence in Methicillin-Resistant *Staphylococcus aureus* Skin and Soft Tissue Infections

Crawford SE, David MZ, Glikman D, et al (Univ of Chicago, IL)
J Am Board Fam Med 22:647-654, 2009

Background.—The so-called community-associated methicillin-resistant *Staphylococcus aureus* (MRSA) strains are more frequently susceptible to non−ß-lactam antibiotics (including clindamycin) than health care-associated MRSA strains. We assessed whether predictive clinical characteristics of presumptive MRSA infections can be identified to guide choice of empiric antibiotic therapy.

Methods.—A clinical syndrome was assigned to each inpatient and outpatient at the University of Chicago Medical Center with an MRSA infection in 2004 to 2005. Antimicrobial susceptibilities and molecular characteristics of MRSA isolates were assessed. Patients were stratified by lesion characteristics.

Results.—Of MRSA isolates from 262 patients with purulent skin and soft tissue infections (SSTIs), 231 (88%) were susceptible to clindamycin, 253 (97%) contained staphylococcal chromosomal cassette *mec* (SCC*mec*) IV, and 245 (94%) contained Panton-Valentine leukocidin (*pvl*) genes, characteristics associated with community-associated MRSA strains. The presence of a purulent SSTI had a positive predictive value of 88% for a clindamycin-susceptible MRSA isolate. Among 87 isolates from a nonpurulent SSTI, 44% were susceptible to clindamycin and 34% contained *pvl* genes. In 179 invasive MRSA disease isolates, 33% were clindamycin-susceptible and 26% carried *pvl* genes.

Conclusions.—A purulent MRSA SSTI strongly predicted the presence of a clindamycin-susceptible MRSA isolate. Presence of the *pvl* genes was almost universal among MRSA isolates causing purulent SSTIs; this was less common in nonpurulent SSTIs and other clinical syndromes.

▶ Skin and soft tissue infections (SSTIs) account for most infections caused by community-acquired methicillin-resistant *Staphylococcus aureus* (CA-MRSA) strains. According to researchers, hospital-acquired MRSA (HA-MRSA) isolates are seldom associated with purulent SSTIs. However, HA-MRSA isolates are resistant to multiple antimicrobial drugs, including clindamycin, compared with the common presence of clindamycin-sensitive CA-MRSA isolates. The authors proposed that there may be identifiable clinical features that would distinguish the disease caused by CA-MRSA strains from HA-MRSA strains, which would allow clinicians to choose appropriate initial empiric antibiotic therapy. This analysis included pediatric and adult patients served by the inpatient, outpatient, and emergency department facilities at the University of Chicago Medical Center during 2004 to 2005. Antimicrobial susceptibility and molecular characteristics of MRSA isolates were assessed. For all MRSA isolates, polymerase chain reaction assays for *mecA*, staphylococcal chromosomal cassette *mec* (SCC*mec*) type, *lukF-PV*, and *lukS-PV* were performed. There were 548 MRSA isolates; 362 (66%) contained SCC*mec* type IV and 321 (89%) of these isolates were Panton-Valentine leukocidin (*pvl*) gene positive. SCC*mec* type IV was susceptible to clindamycin. Twenty-three (82%) of these nonabscess purulent MRSA SSTI isolates were susceptible to clindamycin, 24 (86%) contained SCC*mec* type IV, and 22 (79%) were *pvl* positive. Clinical data regarding abscess and nonabscess purulent SSTIs revealed that 88% were caused by MRSA isolates that were susceptible to clindamycin, 97% contained SCC*mec* IV, and 94% were *pvl* positive. It was noteworthy that 97% of the SCC*mec* IV isolates found in patients with purulent SSTIs contained the *pvl* genes compared with only 30 of 44 (68%) isolates that contained SCC*mec* IV obtained from patients with nonpurulent SSTIs ($P < .001$). Of these 91 isolates, 74 (81%) were susceptible to clindamycin, 82 (90%) possessed the *pvl* genes, and 85 (93%) contained SCC*mec* type IV. In contrast, among the 87 isolates from patients with a nonpurulent SSTI, 78 (90%) were identified as HA-MRSA isolates. Of these, 32 (41%) were susceptible to clindamycin, 36 (46%) contained SCC*mec* type IV, and 23 (29%) carried the *pvl* genes. In this study, MRSA SSTIs were significantly more likely to have a clindamycin-susceptible, *pvl*-positive, SCC*mec* type IV isolate compared with patients with nonpurulent SSTIs ($P < .001$). A limitation to this study was that authors only evaluated genes in relation to clindamycin susceptibility. However, these genes may have other functions beside antibiotic susceptibility implications. Also, using a measure such as purulence may be misleading because there are other cutaneous disease processes where purulence may be present without an infection. Although this study may indicate purulence as a clinical indication for CA-MRSA, incision and drainage of abscesses may often be curative without antibiotic therapy, especially for smaller lesions. With multiresistant organisms and patients with drug allergies, this may be a better option. In addition, this study lacked a control group. To add, the authors did not discuss clinical response to medications and only reported MRSA isolate susceptibility to medications. Clinical response to a given antibiotic may also differ, with repeat infections in some cases. Another factor to consider is that purulence may not be visualized by the clinician, such as with respiratory infections or sepsis, and should not be used as an indicator for HA-MRSA or CA-MRSA in these cases. In conclusion, the authors suggest that MRSA isolates that were *pvl* positive frequently caused purulent SSTIs and that this organism type may behave biologically as a virulence factor in CA-MRSA disease.

J. Q. Del Rosso, DO

G. K. Kim, DO

Clinical Management of Rapidly Growing Mycobacterial Cutaneous Infections in Patients after Mesotherapy

Regnier S, Cambau E, Meningaud J-P, et al (Pitié Salpetrière Hosp, Paris, France; Henri Mondor Hosp, Paris, France; et al)
Clin Infect Dis 49:1358-1364, 2009

Background.—Increasing numbers of patients are expressing an interest in mesotherapy as a method of reducing body fat. Cutaneous infections due to rapidly growing mycobacteria are a common complication of such procedures.

Methods.—We followed up patients who had developed cutaneous infections after undergoing mesotherapy during the period October 2006—January 2007.

Results.—Sixteen patients were infected after mesotherapy injections performed by the same physician. All patients presented with painful, erythematous, draining subcutaneous nodules at the injection sites. All patients were treated with surgical drainage. Microbiological examination was performed on specimens that were obtained before and during the surgical procedure. Direct examination of skin smears demonstrated acid-fast bacilli in 25% of the specimens that were obtained before the procedure and 37% of the specimens obtained during the procedure; culture results were positive in 75% of the patients. *Mycobacterium chelonae* was identified in 11 patients, and *Mycobacterium frederiksbergense* was identified in 2 patients. Fourteen patients were treated with antibiotics, 6 received triple therapy as first-line treatment (tigecycline, tobramycin, and clarithromycin), and 8 received dual therapy (clarithromycin and ciprofloxacin). The mean duration of treatment was 14 weeks (range, 1—24 weeks). All of the patients except 1 were fully recovered 2 years after the onset of infection, with the mean time to healing estimated at 6.2 months (range, 1—15 months).

Conclusions.—This series of rapidly growing mycobacterial cutaneous infections highlights the difficulties in treating such infections and suggests that in vitro susceptibility to antibiotics does not accurately predict their clinical efficacy.

▶ Regnier et al report an important consideration that may affect clinicians after medical procedures, specifically after mesotherapy. Although the study that took place in France involved a small sample size (N = 16), the topic is no less significant. The authors report on an outbreak of rapidly growing mycobacterial (RGM) infections following mesotherapy and their relevant findings regarding the clinical management and outcome of these infections. While the study involved RGM infections after mesotherapy, its findings may possibly be applicable to any chronic cutaneous mycobacterial lesion after a medical procedure, as noted by the authors. The importance of this article is in its fostering of awareness of RGM infections and data regarding the difficulty in both diagnosis and treatment of RGM infections. The study identified 2 strains causing cutaneous infections (nodular cutaneous lesions and abscesses): *Mycobacterium chelonae* and *Mycobacterium frederiksbergense*.

What is notable regarding RGMs is that the infections caused by these species are difficult to diagnose and treat. Clinical symptoms are often nonspecific nodules or abscesses, and the time from injection of mesotherapy to the appearance of symptoms may be weeks. The mean time for this study from injection to first signs and symptoms was 9.5 weeks. Compounding this problem is that treatment is difficult even when the mycobacterial species is identified. To date, no optimal treatment is established. In fact, as noted in the article, patients were treated with an antibiotic that showed in vitro susceptibility, but despite treatment, some patients still had persistent disease. Also noted was the lack of efficacy of even double or triple antimycobacterial therapy. Treatment is not only difficult, but the mean duration of therapy was 14 weeks, with the mean time to healing among the sampled patients reported to be 6.2 months. Eventually, all patients except one fully recovered after a 2-year period.

Given the difficulty of RGM infections, the article provides a much-needed suggestion for therapy, indicating that with only a limited number of lesions present, surgical treatment is recommended, and the addition of antibiotic therapy is individualized depending on disease severity. Antimycobacterial antibiotic treatment should still be guided by in vitro results, and patients should be made aware of the difficulty of treatment as well as the risk of scarring. Overall, this article provides a much-needed awareness regarding a difficult cutaneous manifestation that may complicate procedures such as mesotherapy.

B. D. Michaels, DO

J. Q. Del Rosso, DO

Sexually Transmitted Infections and Prostate Cancer among Men in the U.S. Military

Dennis LK, Coughlin JA, McKinnon BC, et al (Univ of Iowa; et al)
Cancer Epidemiol Biomarkers Prev 18:2665-2671, 2009

Studies of self-reported sexually transmitted infections (STI) suggesting an association with prostate cancer may reflect underreporting of such infections among nondiseased subjects. To reduce such bias, we studied archived sera in a cohort of U.S. military personnel known to have high rates of both STIs and prostate cancer. Using a nested case-control design, serum samples from 534 men who served on active duty between September 1, 1993 and September 1, 2003 were examined. Controls were individually matched to cases based on date of serum collection, date of birth, branch of service, military rank, marital status, and race.

Each of the 267 case-control pairs had two serum samples: a recent serum sample, taken ∼1 year before the case's prostate cancer diagnosis, and an earlier serum sample, taken ∼8 years before diagnosis. Each serum specimen was studied for antibodies against human papillomavirus, herpes simplex virus-2 (HSV-2), and *Chlamydia trachomatis*. Logistic regression accounted for matching and potential confounding factors. Study data indicated no association between prostate cancer and serologic evidence of infections just before the reference date. However, a statistically significant association between prostate cancer and serologic evidence of HSV-2 infection was detected in the earlier sample (odds ratio, 1.60; 95% confidence interval, 1.05-2.44). The strength of this association increased when analyses were restricted to sera collected at least 60 months before diagnosis (odds ratio, 2.04; 95% confidence interval, 1.26-3.29; 204 pairs). If this association is causal, then our findings would suggest a long latency period for prostate cancer development after HSV-2 infection.

▶ Despite the fact that 16% of American men will develop prostate cancer, predisposing factors have been poorly defined. One obvious potential factor might be acquisition of 1 or more sexually transmitted diseases (STDs). This study, using a well-chosen case-control—matched subject pool compared with a cohort of men with prostate cancer from the US military, investigated the possible association of STD and neoplasia. The diagnosis of STD was based on objective serological samples, however, rather than on self-reported STD occurrence based upon individual subjects' recollections. The study, as has been true in previous such investigations, failed to show an association of recent STD and prostate cancer. However, because the military stores serum samples for many years, retrospective analysis was also possible. This study did demonstrate a clearly increased risk (roughly 1.5-2.0 odds ratio) of prostate cancer following serologic demonstration of longstanding herpes simplex virus 2 infection (5-7 years). While no direct cause and effect relationship can be inferred, men with a long history of genital herpes might best be served by earlier and more frequent, and certainly more diligent, screening for prostate cancer. The major shortcoming of this study is that it involved only US military personnel. To the degree that those serving in a self-selected volunteer military are not representative of the general male population, this article's conclusions might be less reliable.

T. Rosen, MD

Deep cutaneous fungal infections in immunocompromised children
Marcoux D, Jafarian F, Joncas V, et al (Université de Montréal, Quebec, Canada)
J Am Acad Dermatol 61:857-864, 2009

Background.—Life-threatening infections from ubiquitous fungi are becoming more prevalent in adults and children because of the increased use of immunosuppressive agents and broad-spectrum anti-infective drugs. Extremely low birth weight premature neonates and patients with a disrupted epidermal barrier are also at increased risk. Lethality is high, particularly with delayed diagnosis. As cutaneous lesions are often the first manifestation of such infections, early recognition of suspicious lesions is crucial to decrease associated morbidity and mortality. The clinical features of deep cutaneous fungal infection (DCFI) in immunocompromised children deserve special attention.

Objectives.—This study aimed to characterize our pediatric patients with DCFI, the causative fungi, and the associated risk factors.

Methods.—A medical record review was conducted of pediatric patients with DCFI treated at out institution using data retrieved from the hospital's pathology and microbiology database (1980-2008).

Results.—In all, 26 patients with DCFI were identified (9 girls and 17 boys) ranging in age from 1 day to 18 years (mean age: 8 years), the majority of whom had a hematologic disorder. All patients were immunocompromised, 90% were receiving broad-spectrum antibiotics, and 50% had severe neutropenia (absolute neutrophilic count $\leq 500 \times 10^6$/L). Necrotic ulcers (42%) and papules (34%) represented the most frequent lesion morphology. Fungal species were identified by culture in 20 (87%) of 23 patients tested and were observed histopathologically in 20 of 23 patients tested. *Aspergillus* was identified in 12 (44%) patients and *Candida* in 9 (33%). The other species included *Fusarium* (one), *Exserohilum rostratum* (one), *Alternaria* (one), Zygomycetes (two), and Blatomycetes (one). All but two patients received systemic antifungal therapy; wide surgical excision was performed in 13. Infection resolved in 20 (77%), whereas 6 (23%) died of disseminated infection.

Limitations.—This study was limited by the small number of cases and the retrospective nature of the collected data.

Discussion.—DCFI should rank high in the differential diagnosis of any suspicious skin lesions in immunocompromised children. Early biopsies should be performed for histopathology and microbiological analysis, as lethality is high if appropriate treatment is delayed.

▶ Past studies have suggested that immunocompromised children may be at increased risk for invasive fungal infection (IFI) and deep cutaneous fungal infection (DCFI). This is a study of 26 patients with DCFI at a tertiary care facility describing clinical characteristics, outcomes, and predisposing factors for IFI and DCFI. This retrospective chart review was performed on all patients aged 18 years or younger with DCFI identified through a computerized pathology database and cross-checked with a database of microbiology fungal cultures. Fungal methods, including histopathological descriptions, direct examination, and culture results, were examined. Treatment of the underlying disease at the time of diagnosis of the fungal infection included chemotherapy, other immunosuppressive agents, and corticosteroids, with or without antibiotics, or antibiotics alone. Most children were also neutropenic upon presentation and were already on broad-spectrum systemic antimicrobial agents. Most cases occurred in patients with hematologic disorders (18/26) or in patients who had a disrupted skin barrier. Fungal infections developed within 2 months after the initial diagnosis of the underlying disease in 66% of the cases but developed after a much longer time period (5 years) in 3 of the patients with aspergillosis. Cutaneous lesions were usually presented as a papule and then evolved into a pustule that progressively led to a necrotic ulcer. The most frequently involved anatomic sites were the upper limbs in 77%, followed by the lower limbs, trunk, and then the head and neck region. Multiple sites were involved in 10 cases (38%). Fungal identification results show 12 patients with *Aspergillus* and 9 patients with *Candida* spp, as well as 6 other fungal species. Two organisms were identified in one of the patients. There was systemic fungal involvement in 13 (50%) of 26 patients at the time of DCFI diagnosis, including 6 patients with systemic aspergillosis, 6 patients with systemic candidiasis, and 1 patient with disseminated *Fusarium* spp infection. Twenty (77%) patients recovered from their infections, whereas 6 (23%) died from fungal infections, including 3 from aspergillosis and 3 from candidiasis. All fatal cases had systemic involvement. The authors concluded that secondary DCFI may occur through hematogenous dissemination after initial infection such as impaired skin barrier. However, this study did not examine the exact source of infection from the hospital or from other affected individuals who came into contact with the patient. Future studies examining contamination from intravenous lines, bandages, and medical devices may be of interest so that preventive measures can be taken. To add, at the diagnosis of DCFI, all but 3 cases (90%) were receiving broad-spectrum antibiotics, which may have favored the opportunistic emergence and proliferation of fungal organisms. Almost 80% were on chemotherapeutic agents/immunosuppressive drugs, which may have contributed to the DCFI; however, this study did not include a control group and it may be difficult to make the claim that this cohort of patients is at a higher risk for DCFI as compared with other groups of patients. In conclusion, skin barrier impairment may predispose to primary DCFI, and any skin disease associated with impaired barrier function may allow inoculation of fungi through damaged skin.

J. Q. Del Rosso, DO
G. K. Kim, DO

Emergency Management of Pediatric Skin and Soft Tissue Infections in the Community-associated Methicillin-resistant *Staphylococcus aureus* Era
Mistry RD, Weisz K, Scott HF, et al (Univ of Pennsylvania School of Medicine, Philadelphia)
Acad Emerg Med 17:187-193, 2010

Objectives.—Skin and soft tissue infections (SSTIs) are increasing in incidence, yet there is no consensus regarding management of these infections in the era of community-associated methicillin-resistant *Staphylococcus aureus* (CA-MRSA). This study sought to describe current pediatric emergency physician (PEP) management of commonly presenting skin infections.

Methods.—This was a cross-sectional survey of subscribers to the American Academy of Pediatrics Section on Emergency Medicine (AAP SoEM) list-serv. Enrollment occurred via the list-serv over a 3-month period. Vignettes of equivocal SSTI, cellulitis, and skin abscess were presented to participants, and knowledge, diagnostic, and therapeutic approaches were assessed.

Results.—In total, 366 of 606 (60.3%) list-serv members responded. The mean (± standard deviation [SD]) duration of practice was 13.6 (±7.9) years, and 88.6% practiced in a pediatric emergency department. Most respondents (72.7%) preferred clinical diagnosis alone for equivocal SSTI, as opposed to invasive or imaging modalities. For outpatient cellulitis, PEPs selected clindamycin (30.6%), trimethoprim-sulfa (27.0%), and first-generation cephalosporins (22.7%); methicillin-sensitive *S. aureus* (MSSA) was routinely covered, but many regimens failed to cover CA-MRSA (32.5%) or group A streptococcus (27.0%). For skin abscesses, spontaneous discharge (67.5%) was rated the most important factor in electing to perform a drainage procedure; fever (19.9%) and patient age (13.1%) were the lowest. PEPs elected to prescribe trimethoprim-sulfamethoxazole (TMP-Sx; 50.0%) or clindamycin (32.7%) after drainage; only 5% selected CA-MRSA—inactive agents. All PEPs suspected CA-MRSA as the etiology of skin abscesses, and many attributed sepsis (22.1%) and invasive pneumonia (20.5%) to CA-MRSA, as opposed to MSSA. However, 23.9% remained unaware of local CA-MRSA prevalence for even common infections.

Conclusions.—Practice variation exists among PEPs for management of SSTI. These results can be used to measure changes in SSTI practices as standardized approaches are delineated.

▶ The incidence of pediatric skin and soft tissue infections (SSTIs) has increased rapidly in the past decade. This is a cross-sectional survey with 366 responses from members of the American Academy of Pediatrics Section on Emergency Medicine list-serv. The objective of this study is to describe the current practice for children with SSTI in the era of community-acquired methicillin-resistant *Staphylococcus aureus* (CA-MRSA). Participants were pediatric emergency physicians who were queried about their current approach to SSTIs. All 366 respondents believed that skin abscesses were more likely to be CA-MRSA in origin compared with methicillin-sensitive *S aureus* (MSSA). Respondents used important historical factors when instituting empiric CA-MRSA treatment, including a history of SSTI, documented history of CA-MRSA, and family history of SSTI. Most respondents (72.7%) preferred clinical diagnosis alone for equivocal SSTI, as opposed to invasive or imaging modalities. Also, providers routinely prescribed for coverage of MSSA, but many regimens failed to cover CA-MRSA (32.5%) or group A *Streptococcus* (27.0%). Management strategies for cellulitis varied among survey respondents. With respect to outpatient therapy for cellulitis, clindamycin (35.3%) was the antimicrobial most often selected, followed by trimethoprim-sulfamethoxazole and first-generation cephalosporins. In total, 67.5% of respondents selected treatment regimens that empirically covered CA-MRSA, and all respondents chose therapy adequately covering MSSA. For skin abscesses, spontaneous discharge (67.5%) was rated the most important factor in electing to perform incision and drainage. Because of the nature of this study, patient outcomes and risk factors for *S aureus* infection were not evaluated. Although clinicians prescribed antibiotics, incision and drainage has been shown to be curative without a need for antibiotics in many cases. Also, some lesions may not be infected with *S aureus*, and without appropriate cultures, prophylactic antibiotics may not be necessary. Importantly, it is easy to recommend that there should have been a different approach to treatment after the fact; however, clinical judgment must prevail and needs to be respected. In this study, there is great variation in clinical practice with respect to the treatment of pediatric SSTI.

J. Q. Del Rosso, DO

G. K. Kim, DO

Epidemiology and Susceptibilities of Methicillin-Resistant *Staphylococcus aureus* **in Northeastern Ohio**
Delorme T, Rose S, Senita J, et al (Kent State Univ, Ashtabula, OH; et al)
Am J Clin Pathol 132:668-677, 2009

A retrospective survey was performed on all staphylococcal infections diagnosed by the Ashtabula County Medical Center (Ashtabula, OH) during 2006 and 2007. Of the 1,612 *Staphylococcus aureus* isolates evaluated for their antibiotic resistances, 947 were methicillin-resistant *S aureus* (MRSA). In 2007, MRSA infections reached 589 cases per 100,000 inhabitants, a 77% increase compared with 2006. The increase in MRSA infections was noticeable among youth (6-25 years old), middle-aged people (45-50 years old), and elderly people (86-90 years old). MRSA infections increased among inpatients by 58%, among outpatients by 43%, and among nursing home residents by 183%. More than 66% of MRSA infections were found among healthy people in the community with no apparent risk factors. More than 88.7% of the infections belong to only 9 profiles of antibiotic resistance indiscriminately distributed among inpatients, outpatients, and nursing home residents. This report sheds further light on the rapid spread of MRSA across Northeastern Ohio, stressing the need for better education in preventive measures and infection control at the level of community and health care settings.

▶ This is a good review of the epidemiology surrounding the epidemic of community-acquired methicillin-resistant *Staphylococcus aureus* (CA-MRSA) and many of the factors impacting a local health care environment. Although there are not any clinical pearls from the article to impact management, the recognition of the increasing prevalence among patients and their demographics should spark more awareness among all clinicians. Fig 3 in the original article is especially alarming with the sharp increase in the infection rates among nursing home residents, but the increase among pediatric populations and the multidrug resistance patterns reported here should alert the dermatologist to take more precautions in examining patients and maintaining clinical facilities to slow down the potential for nosocomial spread. The authors also discuss a potential reservoir effect that should be considered in areas of higher incidence of new cases, but their recognition of incomplete and poorly adherent prevention strategies should resonate as the primary source of intervention for controlling further spread of CA-MRSA.

N. Bhatia, MD

Erysipelas: Rare but Important Cause of Malar Rash
O'Connor K, Paauw D (Univ of Washington, Seattle)
Am J Med 123:414-416, 2010

Background.—Malar rash can develop in several local and systemic conditions. Because the morbidity and mortality vary considerably between these conditions, it is important to develop an accurate diagnosis and provide appropriate treatment.

Case Report.—Woman, 45, had a facial rash that began with facial swelling and was accompanied by fever, cervical adenopathy, joint aches, and malaise. She was presumed to have cellulitis and given trimethoprim-sulfamethoxazole (TMP-SMX), but the rash grew worse. The patient had not changed skin care products and had no oral ulcers, chest pain, or hematuria. She had an edematous, erythematous, well-demarcated rash in a malar distribution not accompanied by fever, maxillary or frontal sinus tenderness, or oral lesions. Her white blood cell count was normal, C-reactive protein was high (132 mg/L), and sedimentation rate was 28 mm/h. Antinuclear antibody (ANA) results were negative. Computed tomography revealed bilateral preseptal periorbital soft tissue swelling but no postseptal orbital abscesses. She was hospitalized with a diagnosis of erysipelas and given intravenous (IV) vancomycin to cover for potential methicillin-resistant *Staphylococcus aureus* (MRSA) and IV clindamycin for streptococcal coverage. Her systemic symptoms and rash improved in a few days, and she was discharged taking TMP-SMX for methicillin-sensitive *S aureus* (MSSA) and MRSA coverage as well as dicloxacillin for streptococci.

Differential Diagnosis.—The most common causes of malar rash are erysipelas, cellulitis, systemic lupus erythematosus (SLE), and rosacea.

Erysipelas is a skin infection of the upper dermis and superficial lymphatic system manifest by rapidly expanding, well-demarcated, shiny, erythematous, painful plaque associated with swelling, perifollicular edema, and acute systemic symptoms such as fever, chills, and malaise. Facial rash in a malar or "butterfly" pattern can occur but usually rashes affect the lower extremities. The cause is typically a beta-hemolytic streptococcus.

Cellulitis affects the deeper dermis and subcutaneous fat of the lower extremities and manifests a less well demarcated rash than erysipelas with little or no edema. Systemic symptoms are unlikely. A more indolent course is common if systemic symptoms develop. Bacteria can enter through disruptions in the skin barrier.

SLE is rare, affecting mainly young African American women, but malar rash is a classic finding. Usually the rash is triggered by sun exposure and can be flat or raised, pruritic or painful, but lacks papules and pustules. Both the rash and symptoms of SLE are more indolent than in erysipelas and can occur with periods of relapse and remission. ANA is checked only when two or more organ systems are inexplicably involved and the index of suspicion for SLE is high because the test has a low predictive value.

Malar rash is associated with rosacea more than any other condition. Rosacea is most common in patients with fair skin and involves the forehead, eyelids, cheeks, chin, and nose. Classic findings are nontransient erythema, telangectasias, and papules or pustules with no comedones. The rash is related to periods of flushing triggered by stress, hot drinks, or alcohol. Systemic symptoms are absent.

Conclusions.—Treatment of erysipelas is beta-lactam antibiotics begun immediately on an outpatient basis. With beta-lactam allergy, the patient can be given a broad-spectrum quinolone. Concern about MRSA should prompt the use of combination therapy targeting streptococcus species. For patients already taking these agents, TMP-SMX or doxycycline can be added to treat potential MRSA. If systemic symptoms are present, parenteral therapy may be advisable, including ceftriaxone, cefazolin, or IV vancomycin. Redness and swelling may increase soon after therapy begins but should not extend past the previous line. If the redness progresses while the patient is taking antibiotics, antibiotic resistance should be suspected. Usually patients feel better in 24 to 48 hours, but the rash does not begin to resolve for up to 3 days. On rare occasions complications can develop, leading to recurrence, meningitis, endocarditis, necrotizing fasciitis, or streptococcal toxic shock syndrome. Therefore it is important to distinguish when erysipelas is the cause of malar rash.

▶ This case study highlights the need for a proper history and appropriate laboratory work when confronted with a patient with bilateral erythema of the cheeks. Cultures from lesions of the skin are not frequently helpful, and a high index of suspicion for infection is warranted when a patient presents in such a fashion along with adenopathy and constitutional symptoms, both common in patients with erysipelas. Empiric therapy is indicated to cover for beta-hemolytic streptococcus, and consideration should be given to covering methicillin-sensitive *Staphylococcus aureus* and methicillin-resistant *Staphylococcus aureus*, depending on how ill the patient is and how he/she is progressing.

Clearly, lupus erythematosus (LE) is going to be the primary differential diagnosis in such a patient and is the disease most likely to have systemic or constitutional symptoms. A detailed history regarding previous sun sensitivity and onset of symptoms as well as acute fever and malaise should assist in differentiation of acute systemic LE from erysipelas and should certainly place rosacea much lower on the list. Heat on palpation of affected facial skin likely points to erysipelas. Other entities to consider, but not mentioned in the article, are contact dermatitis, urticaria, and, if unilateral, early onset zoster.

Perhaps as important is a remark made by the authors of this case study and review that in the modern world erysipelas does not most commonly affect the face but the lower extremity. The classic clinical example of the well-demarcated plaque of the cheek is not as common as a similar larger plaque of the shin or calf. Whether this is a result of behavioral patterns and aging population with subsequent lower leg edema issues or a shift in the causative organism is unknown, but cultures of lesions nowadays may show groups B, C, D, or G as well as group A beta-hemolytic streptococcal species.

J. M. Suchniak, MD

Extensive Neonatal Dermatophytoses

Metkar A, Joshi A, Vishalakshi V, et al (Rajiv Gandhi Med College and Chhatrapati Shivaji Maharaj Hosp, Thane, Maharashtra, India)
Pediatr Dermatol 27:189-191, 2010

We report a 25-day-old boy who was referred to our dermatology unit for evaluation of extensive annular erythematous lesions on his body. We initially considered the differential diagnoses of candidiasis and neonatal lupus erythematosus but investigations revealed the case as tinea corporis due to a relatively uncommon causative agent, *Microsporum gypseum*. To the best of our knowledge it is the first case of extensive neonatal dermatophytoses caused by this organism. The possible causes and the role of steroids in producing the clinical picture in our patient are discussed.

▶ This case report from India holds worldwide implications. The geophilic fungus *Microsporum gypseum*, originally believed to be brought to the United States from Brazil, has the potential to infect human and canine alike and is the fifth most common human dermatophyte isolate in Cadiz, Spain.[1] The species can be found from the soils of Brazil to the Tennessee hills.

M.gypseum is a rare cause of dermatophytic infection in neonates but is fast becoming more prevalent because of an increase in immunocompromised patients.[2] The first report of *M.gypseum* infection was in a 40-day-old Japanese child in a study spanning from 1931-1986.[3] Therefore, Metkar et al reported the youngest worldwide. Many reports of immunocompromised patients such as those with human immunodeficiency virus present with tinea capitis, kerion, and tinea corporis. However, this is a case with an unknown cause. Interestingly, a discussion of treatment options can also be raised. The author discusses the use of fluconazole and its general inferiority to griseofulvin. However, Keyvan et al[4] demonstrate that the susceptibility tests for fluconazole are not fully accurate. The medium used to incubate the dermatophyte is not optimal, and therefore, the full clinical effect of fluconazole treatment is not fully represented. This case highlights for the clinician fluconazole as an acceptable alternative, which may be more effective than once thought. This case serves to demonstrate a rare opportunity to standardize treatment of a disease seen worldwide and explores acceptable therapeutic alternatives.

M. McCarty, DO

J. Q. Del Rosso, DO

References

1. García-Martos P, Ruiz-Aragón J, García-Agudo L, Linares M. [Dermatophytoses due to Microsporum gypseum: report of eight cases and literature review]. *Rev Iberoam Micol.* 2004;21:147-149.
2. Pei-Lun S, Hsin-Tsung H. Concentric rings: an unusual presentation of tinea corporis caused by *Microsporum gypseum. Mycoses.* 2006;49:150-151.
3. Hayashi N, Toshitani S. Human infections with *Microsporum gypseum* in Japan. *Mykosen.* 1983;26:337-345.
4. Keyvan P, Bahaedinie L, Rezaei Z, Sodaifi M, Zomorodian K, et al. In vitro activity of six antifungal drugs against clinically important dermatophytes. *Jundishapur Journal of Microbiology.* 2009;2:158-163.

Frequency of detection of methicillin-resistant *Staphylococcus aureus* from rectovaginal swabs in pregnant women
Creech CB, Litzner B, Talbot TR, et al (Vanderbilt Univ Med Ctr, Nashville, TN; Vanderbilt Univ School of Medicine, Nashville, TN)
Am J Infect Control 38:72-74, 2010

Clinical samples from 250 pregnant women undergoing screening for rectovaginal group B streptococcus colonization were evaluated concurrently for the presence of methicillin-resistant *Staphylococcus aureus* (MRSA). Overall, *S aureus* was detected in 21.6% of the women; 53.7% of the isolates were MRSA. Despite a lack of risk factors for MRSA colonization, rectovaginal MRSA was detected in 10.4% of pregnant women in this study.

▶ With the rising prevalence of methicillin-resistant *Staphylococcus aureus* (MRSA), there is a question as to whether an increase in cases of neonatal community-acquired MRSA (CA-MRSA) is associated with horizontal transmission from family members and health care workers. It may also be related to vertical transmission due to staphylococcal rectovaginal colonization from the mother, which is unclear. This retrospective study identified 250 pregnant women (35-37 weeks of gestation) via group B *Streptococcus* (GBS) rectovaginal screening swabs collected in the clinic. Their median age was 28 years, and 47% were white, 32% were black, and 10% were Hispanic. Most women (67%) were multiparous, and 7.6% of women were health care workers. Eight women (3%) had a history of staphylococcal infection by medical chart review. GBS colonization was detected in 66 women. *S aureus* rectovaginal cultures were positive in 55 women: 29 women had cultures positive for methicillin-sensitive *S aureus* (MSSA) and 26 had cultures positive for MRSA. No significant relationship between GBS colonization and either overall *S aureus* detection or MRSA detection was found. The presence of an SCCmec IV cassette was found in 7 women (27% of MRSA carriers). In this cohort of 250 pregnant women, 10.4% had rectovaginal MRSA. The minority of MRSA isolates (27%) had SCCmec cassette found in CA-MRSA strains. Because of the retrospective nature of this study, the outcomes of the neonates were unknown and the potential risk factors for staphylococcal colonization may have been underestimated. Also, the authors did not evaluate whether patients with *S aureus* colonization were also nasal carriers, and cultures were restricted to the rectovaginal area. The study did not include other carriers, such as physicians or health care workers, who may be a source of *S aureus* transmission for neonates. Additionally, although the authors stated that women who were culture positive may possibly increase susceptibility of neonates to infection, it was unknown whether colonization was transient or truly persistent because cultures at delivery were not performed. Additionally, if neonates were at risk for *S aureus* colonization from vertical transmission from the mother, future studies addressing the possible benefit of prophylactic antibiotic therapy would be helpful. Even if neonates had *S aureus* colonization from the mother during birth, it may be transient with no need for treatment. This study concluded that 1 of 9 women had positive rectovaginal culture for *S aureus* with colonization during the third trimester, which may put neonates at risk for colonization. This study is too limited in its scope to allow for a definitive conclusion; additional research in this area is needed.

J. Q. Del Rosso, DO

G. K. Kim, DO

Inpatient treatment patterns, outcomes, and costs of skin and skin structure infections because of *Staphylococcus aureus*
Menzin J, Marton JP, Meyers JL, et al (Boston Health Economics, Inc, Waltham, MA; Pfizer Inc, NY)
Am J Infect Control 38:44-49, 2010

Background.—Staphylococcus aureus (SA) is a common bacterial pathogen in skin and skin structure infections (SSSIs). Limited data exist on hospital treatment patterns and costs for SA-SSSIs.

*Methods.—*This retrospective analysis examined the lengths of stay, treatment patterns, and costs of hospitalized patients with an SA-SSSI diagnosis using a nationally representative inpatient database. Patients were selected if they had an ICD-9-CM diagnosis of an SSSI with SA noted between January 2005 and June 2006, received a study antibiotic (ie, intravenous [IV] vancomycin, IV or oral linezolid, and IV daptomycin), and were not in the intensive care unit before receiving a study antibiotic. Generalized linear models assessed predictors of length of stay and costs. Costs are expressed in 2005 US dollars.

Results.—Thirteen thousand four hundred thirty-three patients met the selection criteria and mean (±SD) age was 48.2 (±18.3) years. Forty percent of patients received a nonstudy antibiotic before receiving their first study antibiotic. Ninety-five percent were prescribed vancomycin as their first study antibiotic. Study antibiotics were administered for an average of 4.3 days, and 8% of patients switched study antibiotics. Nineteen percent of patients receiving IV linezolid stepped down to oral linezolid. Mean (±SD) lengths of hospital stay and costs were 6.1 (±6.0) days and $6830 (±$7100). In-hospital mortality, switching antibiotics, and diagnoses of selected complications or comorbidities were associated with increased lengths of stay and costs. Younger age, location outside the Northeast, and use of oral linezolid were associated with lower lengths of stay and costs.

Conclusion.—The costs of treating inpatient SA-SSSIs are substantial and vary by patient demographics and treatment characteristics.

▶ Two statements made in the first 2 paragraphs of this article should be eye-opening: "...patients hospitalized with SA infections have nearly 5 times the risk of in-hospital death than patients without such infections" and "...patients with SA infections have significantly longer hospital stays (14.3 vs 4.5 days, respectively) and higher direct medical charges than those without SA infections." The parameters for analysis and number of participants (13 433) in the study are also eye-opening, especially for establishing the credibility of the conclusions. However, many of the results that were shown to be predictors of longer hospital stays, such as comorbidities and the need for frequent drug switching, were more obvious than others.

Controlling health care costs and controlling outcomes are rarely predictable; nor are they easily correlated, but the possibility of stratifying a patient's risk of prolonged stay based on data like this is more likely beneficial in retrospective analysis than at a triage door or in the hands of a hospital case manager eager to clear hospital beds or for improving utilization reviews.

In a time when health care costs and efficiency are constantly being scrutinized, studies like this are helpful reminders that sometimes the battles fought for patient health are not just administrative, surgical, or even logical. Given the information provided here, the battles against the enemies we cannot see or predict, namely methicillin-resistant *Staphylococcus aureus* (MRSA), are probably the most difficult. We cannot truly say which patients will have their underlying good health or minor medical problem complicated by MRSA infections or their consequences, even though we can use data like these to better prepare even the least likely patients from superinfection and therefore lengthy and unnecessary complications.

N. Bhatia, MD

Nonrandom Distribution of *Pseudomonas aeruginosa* and *Staphylococcus aureus* in Chronic Wounds

Fazli M, Bjarnsholt T, Kirketerp-Møller K, et al (Univ of Copenhagen, Denmark; Bispebjerg Hosp, Copenhagen, Denmark; et al)

J Clin Microbiol 47:4084-4089, 2009

The spatial organization of *Pseudomonas aeruginosa* and *Staphylococcus aureus* in chronic wounds was investigated in the present study. Wound biopsy specimens were obtained from patients diagnosed as having chronic venous leg ulcers, and bacterial aggregates in these wounds were detected and located by the use of peptide nucleic acid-based fluorescence in situ hybridization and confocal laser scanning microscopy (CLSM). We acquired CLSM images of multiple regions in multiple sections cut from five wounds containing *P. aeruginosa* and five wounds containing *S. aureus* and measured the distance of the bacterial aggregates to the wound surface. The distance of the *P. aeruginosa* aggregates to the wound surface was significantly greater than that of the *S. aureus* aggregates, suggesting that the distribution of the bacteria in the chronic wounds was nonrandom. The results are discussed in relation to our recent finding that swab culturing techniques may underestimate the presence of *P. aeruginosa* in chronic wounds and in relation to the hypothesis that *P. aeruginosa* bacteria located in the deeper regions of chronic wounds may play an important role in keeping the wounds arrested in a stage dominated by inflammatory processes.

▶ Chronic leg wounds and ulcers can be debilitating for patients and are common in both acute hospital and clinic settings. Organisms most commonly isolated in chronic venous leg ulcers are *Staphylococcus aureus* (*S aureus*) (93.5%), *Enterococcus* (71.7%), *Pseudomonas aeruginosa* (*P aeruginosa*) (52.2%), coagulase-negative staphylococci (45.7%), *Proteus* species (41.3%), and anaerobic bacteria (39.1%).[1] This study investigated the distribution of 2 of the more common isolates in chronic wounds: *S aureus* and *P aeruginosa*. Bacterial aggregates were identified with images from peptide nucleic acid—based fluorescence in situ hybridization and confocal laser scanning microscopy. Analysis of 9 patients diagnosed with chronic leg ulcers (4 with *S aureus*, 4 with *P aeruginosa*, and 1 with both) found that *S aureus* frequently colonized wounds superficially compared with *P aeruginosa*, which was found in deeper regions. It is thought that virulence factors produced by *P aeruginosa* destroy polymorphonuclear neutrophils (PMNs) and cause a persistent influx of PMNs in the deeper regions maintaining the wound's inflammatory stage. Clinically, these results are important for the physician in determining appropriate therapy of chronic wounds. Although the prevention and treatment of chronic wounds include a multitude of strategies including dressings, antimicrobial agents, physical therapies, and patient education, these results allow clinicians to obtain more detailed knowledge of the chronic wounds they are treating. Topical antimicrobials and nanocrystalline silver dressings are efficacious for superficial bacteria, such as staphylococci, but ineffective for deeper bacterial aggregates like *P aeruginosa.*

S. Bellew, DO

J. Q. Del Rosso, DO

Reference

1. Gjødsbøl K, Christensen JJ, Karlsmark T, Jørgensen B, Klein BM, Krogfelt KA. Multiple bacterial species reside in chronic wounds: a longitudinal study. *Int Wound J.* 2006;3:225-231.

Primary Skin Abscesses Are Mainly Caused by Panton-Valentine Leukocidin-Positive *Staphylococcus aureus* Strains
del Giudice P, Blanc V, de Rougemont A, et al (Hôpital Bonnet, Fréjus, France; Centre Hospitalier d'Antibes-Juan-les-Pins, France; Université Lyon 1, France)
Dermatology 219:299-302, 2009

Background.—The role of Panton-Valentine leukocidin (PVL) in skin and soft-tissue infections is not clear.

Objective.—Our purpose was to determine the prevalence of PVL gene carriage among *Staphylococcus aureus* strains isolated from primary and secondary skin abscesses.

Methods.—A prospective study was conducted. From July 2003 to June 2008, *S. aureus* isolates from skin abscesses were screened for the PVL genes. The abscesses were considered primary if they occurred on previously healthy skin and secondary in all other cases.

Results.—Fifty-seven patients presenting with *S. aureus* skin abscesses were included in the study. The PVL genes were detected in 40 (70%) of the 57 *S. aureus* isolates. Thirty-eight (92.7%) of the 41 primary skin abscesses were due to PVL-positive strains, compared to only 2 (12.5%) of the 16 secondary skin abscesses (p < 0.001).

Conclusions.—Primary skin abscesses are mainly caused by PVL-positive *S. aureus* strains.

▶ *Staphylococcus aureus* has been established as the causal agent for skin and soft-tissue infections (SSTI). Various toxins have been implicated in the pathogenesis of skin infections. Panton-Valentine leukocidin (PVL) is a toxin that is not entirely elucidated but has been linked to furuncles, abscesses, and necrotizing fasciitis. This is a study to investigate the role of PVL in human SSTI and the prevalence of genes encoding this toxin in *S aureus* strains isolated from primary and secondary skin abscesses. This is a prospective study conducted in a hospital in France during 2003-2008 with *S aureus* isolates from skin abscesses that were screened for PVL genes. There were 57 patients who presented with *S aureus* skin abscess included in the study. The PVL gene was detected in 40 (70%) *S aureus* isolates. There were 41 primary skin abscesses, of which 38 (92.7%) were due to PVL-positive strains, and 16 secondary skin abscesses, of which 2 (12.5%) were due to PVL-positive strains. Of the 57 *S aureus* strains isolated from abscesses, 18 were methicillin-resistant *Staphylococcus aureus* (MRSA) and 39 were methicillin susceptible. PVL genes were more frequently detected from primary abscesses (87.5%) compared with secondary abscesses (13.3%) (*P* < .001). Of the 57 patients, PVL-positive *S aureus* strains caused 70% of the skin abscesses overall. To add, all PVL-positive MRSA strains were community-acquired MRSA. However, the authors did not comment on treatment modalities for PVL-positive strains. Limitations to this study included a small study size and single study site. This study also did not culture other areas of the patients or comment if PVL-positive strains played a role in chronic carriers of *S aureus*. The authors concluded that PVL-positive *S aureus* strains play a role in primary skin abscesses.

J. Q. Del Rosso, DO

G. K. Kim, DO

Onychomycosis Insensitive to Systemic Terbinafine and Azole Treatments Reveals Non-Dermatophyte Moulds as Infectious Agents

Baudraz-Rosselet F, Ruffieux C, Lurati M, et al (Centre Hospitalier Universitaire Vaudois, Lausanne, Switzerland; Private Practice, Fribourg, Switzerland)
Dermatology 220:164-168, 2010

Background.—Dermatophytes are the main cause of onychomycoses, but various non-dermatophyte filamentous fungi are often isolated from abnormal nails.

Objective.—Our aim was the in situ identification of the fungal infectious agent in 8 cases of onychomycoses which could not be cured after systemic terbinafine and itraconazole treatment.

Methods.—Fungal DNA was extracted from nail samples, and infectious fungi were identified by restriction fragment length polymorphism (RFLP) of amplified fungal ribosomal DNA using a previously described PCR/RFLP assay.

Results.—PCR/RFLP identification of fungi in nails allows the identification of the infectious agent: *Fusarium* sp., *Acremonium* sp. and *Aspergillus* sp. were found as a sole infectious agent in 5, 2 and 1 cases, respectively.

Conclusions.—*Fusarium* spp. and other non-dermatophyte filamentous fungi are especially difficult to cure in onychomycoses utilising standard treatment with terbinafine and itraconazole. PCR fungal identification helps demonstrate the presence of moulds in order to prescribe alternative antifungal treatments.

▶ Clinicians are often puzzled when patients with onychomycosis do not respond to standard oral antifungal therapy with terbinafine or itraconazole. This case study of 8 healthy patients with the clinical diagnosis of onychomycosis who were treated with standard oral antifungal therapy (terbinafine and itraconazole) reminds us of the importance of considering other organisms, particularly nondermatophyte molds, as the etiologic organism in their nail disease. Confirmation of the clinical diagnosis of onychomycosis with a potassium hydroxide (KOH) preparation of the subungual nail debris can be helpful, although the positive KOH does not allow the organism to be identified nor does it tell if the organism is viable. The organisms in these 8 cases of nondermatophyte nail disease were identified with polymerase chain reaction (PCR) and restriction fragment length polymorphisms (RFLP) to determine the cause of the nail infection, which in this case were the molds of the genera *Acremonium, Aspergillus,* and *Fusarium.* The author suggests that mixed infections of *Trichophyton* spp (dermatophyte) and a mold may be more common and become apparent after the dermatophyte is treated with terbinafine or itraconazole. PCR/RFLP are not easily performed in the office setting but as a research tool are invaluable for sorting out the complexity of multiple organisms in onychomycosis.

P. Rich, MD

Recent Microbiological Shifts in Perianal Bacterial Dermatitis:
***Staphylococcus aureus* Predominance**
Heath C, Desai N, Silverberg NB (St Luke's-Roosevelt Hosp Ctr, NY)
Pediatr Dermatol 26:696-700, 2009

Traditionally, bacterial infections of the anal skin have been found to be caused by Streptococcus. The aim of this study was to determine the breakdown of bacterial isolates and the current presentation of bacterial diseases involving the perineum. From the chart review of children who had bacterial cultures of the anus from 2005 to 2008 in a pediatric dermatology practice population in New York City, 26 pediatric patients (ages 5 months to 12 yrs) who had the indications of anal erythema or recurrent buttocks dermatitis were identified. Bacterial cultures of 17 patients grew pathogens, that of 14 (82% of identifiably infected patients) grew *Staphylococcus aureus,* in 11 as a solo pathogen (6 MSSA and 5 MRSA in 2 family clusters). Streptococcus was identified in three patients, two on culture and one on latex agglutination test; and two patients were identified as having both group A beta hemolytic Streptococcus and *Staphylococcus aureus* (2 MSSA and 1 MRSA). In patients with *S. aureus* perianally, concurrent small papules and pustules of the buttocks or extension of the erythema to adjacent buttock skin was the primary clinical feature distinguishing this condition from isolated streptococcal disease. Whereas Streptococcal infections of the anus and buttocks occur commonly, *Staphylococcus aureus* has become the leading cause of anal bacterial infection in the setting of skin involvement; therefore, antibacterial therapy for anal and buttock bacterial infections should be tailored accordingly.

▶ Perianal streptococcal infections are recognized as an important problem in the pediatric population, but this report suggests that staphylococci are commonly isolated from perianal skin, especially when erythema is accompanied by papules or pustules. It should be noted that although half of the staphylococcal isolates were methicillin-resistant *Staphylococcus aureus* (MRSA) strains, all but a single patient responded well to a single course of cephalexin. This raises a question of the actual pathogenic role of the staphylococcal organisms. In the setting of impetigo, it has been postulated that the initial invasive organism is a beta-hemolytic *Streptococcus*.[1] Once the skin barrier has been compromised, staphylococci colonize the surface and are easily cultured. A similar situation has been noted with cellulitis, where the invasive tissue pathogen is typically a beta-hemolytic *Streptococcus*, despite isolation of staphylococci from the surface.[2] The impact on therapeutic decisions can be complex. In the setting of cellulitis, some data suggest a better response to beta-lactam drugs than sulfa drugs even when MRSA is isolated from the surface. Sulfa drugs have excellent minimum inhibitory concentrations (MICs) against streptococci but poor in vivo activity, and they are not indicated for the treatment of streptococcal infections. The choice of an antibiotic becomes more complicated when the cellulitis extends directly from an MRSA abscess. For a simple abscess, drainage alone is sufficient, but extensive cellulitis requires coverage with an antibiotic active against MRSA in this setting. When MRSA folliculitis is associated with the cellulitis, an initial trial of a beta-lactam agent may be reasonable. While some clinicians will add a sulfa drug in this setting, it should be noted that this practice has resulted in erythema multiforme in some patients.[3]

So how should we modify practice based on the data presented in this study? I will continue to culture perianal erythema in children, and I will continue to use a beta-lactam drug as the first-line therapy, even when papules or pustules are present. If the patient fails to respond and a resistant strain of *Staphylococcus* is isolated, it would be reasonable to change to an antibiotic to which the isolate is susceptible.

D. M. Elston, MD

References

1. Lee MC, Rios AM, Aten MF, et al. Management and outcome of children with skin and soft tissue abscesses caused by community-acquired methicillin-resistant *Staphylococcus aureus*. *Pediatr Infect Dis J*. 2004;23:123-127.
2. Young DM, Harris HW, Charlebois ED, et al. An epidemic of methicillin-resistant *Staphylococcus aureus* soft tissue infections among medically underserved patients. *Arch Surg*. 2004;139:947-951.
3. Fridkin SK, Hageman JC, Morrison M, et al. Active Bacterial Core Surveillance Program of the Emerging Infections Program Network. Methicillin-resistant *Staphylococcus aureus* disease in three communities. *N Engl J Med*. 2005;352: 1436-1444.

Skin and soft tissue infections caused by community-associated methicillin-resistant *staphylococcus aureus* among children in China

Geng W, Yang Y, Wang C, et al (Beijing Children's Hosp affiliated with the Capital Med Univ, China; Pediatric Hosp of Fudan Univ, Shanghai, China; et al)
Acta Paediatr 99:575-580, 2010

Aim.—To investigate the characteristic of community-associated methicillin-resistant *staphylococcus aureus* (CA-MRSA) skin and soft tissue infections (SSTIs) among children in China.

Methods.—Forty-seven children with CA-MRSA SSTIs were enrolled in this study. Clinical information was collected and analysed. The strains from the children were analysed by multilocus sequence typing (MLST), staphylococcus cassette chromosome mec (SCCmec) typing and spa typing. The Panton-Valentine leukocidin (PVL) gene was also detected.

Results.—The majority of the 47 cases were impetigo (20; 42.6%) and abscesses (14; 29.8%). The rest was cellulites, infected wounds, omphalitis, paronychia and conjunctivitis combined folliculitis. Thirty-two of the isolates (68.1%) were PVL-positive, and the abscesses infected with PVL-positive strains usually required incision and drainage (87.5% vs. 16.7%, p = 0.026). Most of the isolates belonged to ST type 59, which accounted for 46.8%, followed by ST1 (7/47, 14.9%) and ST910 (5/47, 10.6%). The clone of ST59-MRSA-IV with t437 was the most prevalent one. The multi-resistant rate of these strains was 93.6%.

Conclusion.—The most common disease of CA-MRSA SSTIs was impetigo, and PVL-positive abscess was associated with incision and drainage. ST59-MRSA-IV with t437 was the most prevalent clone, and the multiresistant rate was high in Chinese children.

▶ Community-acquired methicillin-resistant *Staphylococcus aureus* (CA-MRSA) is a known cause of skin and soft tissue infections (SSTIs), predominantly among children and younger adults. However, the characteristics of CA-MRSA SSTIs are still being defined. This study provides further clarifying data on the characteristics of CA-MRSA SSTIs among children in China. Although the study sample size was limited to 47 (N = 47) patients, the data are nonetheless informative. It has been previously reported that abscesses and cellulitis were the common SSTIs related to CA-MRSA in Asia. Based on the results of this study, the more prevalent diseases associated with CA-MRSA in this Chinese childhood population were impetigo followed by abscesses. Of the 47 isolates, 32 carried the Panton-Valentine leukocidin (*PVL*) gene, and interestingly, the *PVL*-positive strains usually required incision and drainage in the case of abscesses. The study further elucidated the most common strain of CA-MRSA. In the United States, the most common strain of CA-MRSA is ST8; however, this study found that the most predominant clone of CA-MRSA in Chinese children was ST59-MRSA-IVa with t437. Of clinical importance, the study found that all the strains were sensitive to vancomycin, but they were resistant to 8 non-beta-lactams and had a high multiresistance rate. They specifically noted that 85% of the isolates were resistant to clindamycin, especially the *PVL*-positive isolates, underscoring the importance of *PVL* gene carriage of strains in the choice of treatment method for SSTIs. While the application of this study is limited to the population base of Chinese children, overall, the study is helpful in that it provides important and useful data on SSTIs caused by CA-MRSA.

B. D. Michaels, DO

J. Q. Del Rosso, DO

Subclinical onychomycosis is associated with tinea pedis
Walling HW (Univ of Iowa)
Br J Dermatol 161:746-749, 2009

Background.—Onychomycosis is a common cause of nail dystrophy and may be associated with tinea pedis. The presence of dermatophyte fungi in clinically normal nails is unknown.

Objectives.—To assess the presence of dermatophyte fungi in normal-appearing toenails and to compare the risk of subclinical dermatophytosis in patients without and with concurrent tinea pedis.

Methods.—This is a prospective, University-based study of adults without and with microscopically confirmed tinea pedis. Subjects with dystrophy of any toenail were excluded, as were those ever previously diagnosed as having onychomycosis and those who had used topical anti-fungals in the past year. A great toenail clipping obtained from each subject was submitted for periodic acid-Schiff histology.

Results.—One hundred and one subjects (63 men and 38 women, mean ± SD age 45·4 ± 15·7 years) were included. Overall, septate hyphae (ostensibly dermatophyte) were identified in seven specimens. Of the 66 control subjects, one case (1·5%) of nail dermatophyte was identified. Of the 35 subjects with tinea pedis, six cases (17%) of nail dermatophyte were identified ($P = 0·0066$; odds ratio 13·4, 95% confidence interval 1·6−117). There were no significant differences in age or gender between the experimental and control groups or between the nail dermatophyte-positive and negative cohorts.

Conclusions.—Dermatophyte fungi may be isolated from normal-appearing toenails. The presence of dermatophytes in this situation is strongly associated with the presence of tinea pedis. Subclinical dermatophyte in the nail plate may serve as a reservoir for ongoing local infection.

▶ Onychomycosis is a common disorder of the nail seen in association with dermatophyte infection. However, it may be associated with increasing age, psoriasis, diabetes, malignancy, peripheral arterial disease, and immune dysfunction. This is a prospective university-based study of 101 adults, with and without microscopically confirmed tinea pedis, using clippings of the great toenail for periodic acid-Schiff histology. There were 35 subjects included in the tinea pedis group and 66 patients in the control group. The author sought to assess the presence of dermatophyte in subclinical onychomycosis. All those with nail dystrophy and those with a history of previous topical or oral anti-fungal medication use in the last 12 months were excluded. One of 66 control subjects (1.6%) was identified to have dermatophyte infection. Fungal organisms were detected in 6 of 35 subjects with tinea pedis (17%) with a $P = .0066$. The author concluded that the presence of dermatophyte was associated with the presence of tinea pedis. There was not a significant difference observed between experimental and control groups. There are several limitations to this study. Although the author cites that the great toenail is commonly known to harbor dermatophyte infection, results may differ when clippings of other toenails are examined. Other clinical signs of dermatophyte infection on the body were not mentioned, such as the hands, inguinal area, or fingernails. This information is essential when assessing for chronic carriers of dermatophyte infections. Also, the study did not seek to identify specific fungal species. It is unknown whether patients with dermatophyte organisms were chronic carriers and therefore had subclinical presentations of infections. This also raises the question of whether certain dermatophytes may be commensal organisms and therefore may not cause clinical onychomycosis. On the other hand, dermatophytes may live in the nail plate without causing clinical disease and may reinfect the surrounding structures. This study is significant in that it may have therapeutic implications for chronic carriers in need of nail-directed therapy with oral antifungal agents or long-term nail lacquer application. In conclusion, the author found that dermatophyte fungi may be isolated from clinically normal toenails.

J. Q. Del Rosso, DO

G. K. Kim, DO

Tinea Capitis: Predictive Value of Symptoms and Time to Cure With Griseofulvin Treatment

Lorch Dauk KC, Comrov E, Blumer JL, et al (Rainbow Babies and Children's Hosp, Cleveland, OH)
Clin Pediatr 49:280-286, 2010

Objectives.—To describe (*a*) the predictive value of symptoms for diagnosis of tinea capitis and (*b*) the rate and timing of cure with high-dose griseofulvin treatment.

Methods.—This prospective open-label study enrolled children aged 1 to 12 years with clinical tinea capitis. Participants with a positive dermatophyte culture received oral griseofulvin (20-25 mg/kg/day) and topical selenium sulfide shampoo for 6 weeks.

Main Outcome Measures.—The rate of symptoms of tinea capitis, and rates of mycologic and clinical cure.

Results.—The positive predictive values of any 1, 2, 3, or 4 symptoms for a positive culture were 88%, 82%, 78%, and 77%, respectively. The observed rates of mycologic, clinical, and complete cure were 89%, 66%, and 49%, respectively.

Conclusion.—In a high-risk population it is reasonable to diagnose tinea capitis using one or more cardinal symptoms. Oral griseofulvin at 20 to 25 mg/kg/day with adjunctive shampooing for 6 weeks is moderately successful as treatment.

▶ Tinea capitis is commonly seen in the pediatric setting and characterized with patchy or discrete nonscarring alopecia of the scalp, usually with some inflammation and scaling or scaling without noticeable hair loss with varying degress of inflammation. Tinea capitis may simulate seborrheic dermatitis in children. Although guidelines recommend a single daily dose of 10 to 20 mg/kg/d of microsize oral griseofulvin for 4 to 6 weeks for tinea capitis, it is a well-accepted belief that a higher dosage regimen can be more effective. However, there are few data on high-dose griseofulvin based on well-designed studies. This is a prospective open-label study of children aged 1 to 12 years with clinical tinea capitis using high-dose griseofulvin. Those who participated in this study had a positive dermatophyte culture and received oral griseofulvin (20-25 mg/kg/d) and topical selenium sulfide shampoo twice weekly for 6 weeks. The authors also sought to evaluate the predictive value of symptoms of tinea capitis in a general pediatric population at risk for tinea capitis. Clinical evaluation and dermatophyte culture were performed at enrollment and at weeks 4, 6, and 8. The authors examined rates of mycologic (negative dermatophyte culture), clinical, and complete cure. Symptoms evaluated to establish a predictive value in relation to dermatophyte infection were scaling, alopecia, pruritus, occipital lymphadenopathy, and kerion. The positive predictive values of any 1, 2, 3, and 4 symptoms for a positive culture were 88%, 82%, 78%, and 77%, respectively. There was a significant increase in the rates of culture negativity ($P = .007$) and clinical cure ($P = .02$) from weeks 4 to 6, but after treatment was discontinued, further increases were not statistically significant ($P = .26$ and $P = .11$, respectively). The rate of complete cure increased significantly both from weeks 4 to 6 ($P = .03$) and from weeks 6 to 8 ($P = .03$). One weakness of this study was that 6 (30%) of the 20 children with negative cultures but with the presence of a kerion may have still been infected. Also, this may have represented resistant dermatophyte species, which were not investigated and are overall uncommon. Other weaknesses of this study include high loss of patients (30%-40%) at follow-up and variable patient compliance. Also, the authors concluded that for a high-risk population, it is reasonable for clinicians to make the diagnosis of tinea capitis using 1 or more of the above symptoms. However, clinical signs such as scaling cannot be compared with the presence of a kerion in a child and claiming that scaling alone could give a diagnosis of tinea capitis would seem somewhat incomplete. Laboratory evaluation is suggested to confirm the diagnosis. The authors did not delineate between symptoms that were more clinically supportive of tinea capitis such as a kerion or occipital lymphadenopathy when evaluating the relationship between the presence of symptoms and positive predictive value for dermatophyte infection. To add, when combining oral griseofulvin with topical selenium sulfide, it is difficult to know how much the selenium sulfide shampoo contributed to the resolution of tinea capitis, and it may have been useful to have control groups with shampoo alone. In this study, the authors concluded that high-dose oral griseofulvin with adjunctive shampooing for 6 weeks can be used for tinea capitis.

J. Q. Del Rosso, DO

G. K. Kim, DO

Transmission of Methicillin-Resistant *Staphylococcus aureus* to Household Contacts
Mollema FPN, Richardus JH, Behrendt M, et al (Univ Med Ctr, Rotterdam, the Netherlands; et al)
J Clin Microbiol 48:202-207, 2010

The frequency of and risk factors for methicillin-resistant *Staphylococcus aureus* (MRSA) transmission from a MRSA index person to household contacts were assessed in this prospective study. Between January 2005 and December 2007, 62 newly diagnosed MRSA index persons (46 patients and 16 health care workers) and their 160 household contacts were included in the study analysis. Transmission of MRSA from an index person to household contacts occurred in nearly half of the cases (47%; $n = 29$). These 29 index persons together had 84 household contacts, of which two-thirds (67%; $n = 56$) became MRSA positive. Prolonged exposure time to MRSA at home was a significant risk factor for MRSA transmission to household contacts. In addition, MRSA colonization at least in the throat, younger age, and eczema in index persons were significantly associated with MRSA transmission; the presence of wounds was negatively associated with MRSA transmission. Furthermore, an increased number of household contacts and being the partner of a MRSA index person were household-related risk factors for MRSA acquisition from the index person. No predominant pulsed-field gel electrophoresis (PFGE) type was observed to be transmitted more frequently than other PFGE types. To date, screening household contacts and providing MRSA eradication therapy to those found positive simultaneously with the index person is not included in the "search-and-destroy" policy. We suggest including both in MRSA prevention guidelines, as this may reduce further spread of MRSA.

▶ In the past, carriers of *Staphylococcus aureus* have been a source of transmission of pathogens to their household contacts. This is a prospective study during 2005 to 2007 evaluating the frequency and risk factors for methicillin-resistant *S aureus* (MRSA) from an MRSA index person to household contacts conducted at the University Medical Center Rotterdam, Netherlands. There were 62 newly diagnosed MRSA index persons and their 160 household contacts included in the study analysis. Household contacts were screened for MRSA to determine whether transmission from index persons to household contacts had taken place. Culture samples for MRSA were taken from the throat, anterior nares, and perineum. Other existing skin lesions, wounds, or invasive devices at the present time of MRSA detection were cultured. The index persons had a median of 2 MRSA-colonized sites. Fifty-four of the index persons (87%) were MRSA colonized in the nose, 42 index persons (68%) were MRSA colonized in the throat, and 23 (37%) were colonized in the perinasal area. Transmission of MRSA from an index person to household contacts occurred in 29 of 62 (47%) patients. The attack rate of MRSA transmission in the 84 household contacts was 67%, as 56 household contacts became MRSA positive. Index persons with MRSA transmission to their household contacts were significantly younger than the index persons without transmission (25 vs 45 years, $P = .05$). Index persons who transmitted MRSA to their household contacts had a median of 3 MRSA-colonized sites, and index persons without transmission had a median of 2 MRSA-colonized sites ($P = .15$). Of the index persons, 24 (83%) who transmitted MRSA were at least MRSA colonized in the throat compared with 18 (56%) who did not transmit MRSA ($P = .03$). MRSA throat colonization in combination with 1 or more other MRSA-colonized sites significantly increased the risk of MRSA transmission ($P = .02$). Index persons with eczema had significantly more risk of MRSA transmission than index persons without eczema ($P = .05$). Index persons with transmission had a significantly higher median number of household contacts than index persons without transmission ($P = .007$). The risk of MRSA transmission to household contacts was highest among partners of the index persons ($P = .02$). The hours of contact per day between index persons and household members were not associated with an increased risk of MRSA transmission. However, authors were not able to exclude other contacts besides household members as contacts. A limitation to this study was that the history of previous MRSA carriage or current uses of antibiotics was not discussed. Also, longer follow-up periods are needed because some patients colonized with MRSA may be transient and others may be chronic carriers. To add, this study did not attempt to establish the potential role of the environment in MRSA transmission by collecting environmental specimens in the homes/workplaces of the index person. Several risk factors for MRSA transmission were observed in this study. First, MRSA throat carriage of the index person significantly increased the risk for transmission to household contacts, possibly through coughing, sneezing, or kissing. Second, the risk of transmission from an index person to household contacts depends on MRSA exposure time at home, possibly through crowding and close contacts.

J. Q. Del Rosso, DO
G. K. Kim, DO

Twelve hundred abscesses operatively drained: An antibiotic conundrum?
Zimmerman LH, Tyburski JG, Stoffan A, et al (Wayne State Univ, Detroit, MI)
Surgery 146:794-800, 2009

Background.—The incidence of soft tissue infections from antimicrobial-resistant pathogens is increasing. This study evaluated the epidemiology of operatively drained soft tissue abscesses.

Methods.—This retrospective study evaluated 1,200 consecutive patients from 2002 to 2008 who underwent incision and drainage (I&D) in the main operating room. Patients were excluded for perirectal or hidradenitis infections.

Results.—Of 1,200 consecutive cases with an I&D, 1,005 patients had intraoperative cultures. The 1,817 positive isolates included gram-positive aerobes (1,180 [65%]), gram-negative aerobes (207 [11%]), anaerobes (416 [23%]), and fungi (14 [1%]). The most prevalent organism was Staphylococcus aureus, 30% (536), with 80% (431) being methicillin-resistant S aureus (MRSA). MRSA was the predominant organism in all except the breast abscesses. Anaerobes were identified primarily in the breast in diabetics, and in trunk and extremity abscesses in intravenous drug users. The most frequently prescribed empiric antibiotic was ampicillin/sulbactam (66%). The initial empiric antibiotic did not cover MRSA (82%; $P < .001$), resistant gram-negative aerobes (24%), and anaerobes (26%).

Conclusion.—Gram-positive aerobes plus anaerobes represented approximately 80% of the pathogens in our series, with the anaerobic rates being underestimated. Empiric antibiotics should cover MRSA and anaerobes in patients with superficial abscesses drained operatively.

▶ This article concludes that empiric antibiotics should cover methicillin-resistant *Staphylococcus aureus* (MRSA) and anaerobes when abscesses are drained but does not address whether empiric antibiotic therapy is needed at all. Prior studies have suggested that MRSA abscesses up to 5 cm in diameter respond to drainage alone. Abscesses in intertriginous sites and those that occur in intravenous (IV) drug abusers are more likely to contain anaerobes but may also respond to drainage alone. Even atypical mycobacterial abscesses may respond to drainage alone. In short, the primary treatment for an abscess remains drainage, regardless of the organism involved. The need for antibiotic therapy should be weighed against the risks of adverse effects and development of resistance. Although MRSA was not the predominant organism in breast abscesses in this particular study, it has emerged as an important cause of breast abscesses overall. In labor and delivery units, MRSA breast abscesses have become a major problem, interfering with breast feeding and presenting a risk of necrotizing pneumonitis for the infant.

D. M. Elston, MD

Tinea capitis in early infancy treated with itraconazole: a pilot study

Binder B, Richtig E, Weger W, et al (Med Univ of Graz, Austria)
J Eur Acad Dermatol Venereol 23:1161-1163, 2009

Background.—Tinea capitis is the most common fungal infection of the scalp in childhood, but a very rare disorder in the first year of life.

Objective.—To evaluate the efficacy, tolerability and safety of itraconazole in 7 children aged between 3 and 46 weeks (median: 36 weeks) suffering from tinea capitis caused by *Microsporum canis*.

Methods.—Prospective case note study. In all patients KOH testing and fungal cultivation on Sabouraud dextrose agar were performed.

Results.—7 patients (5 girls and 2 boys) were included in the period between 2001 and 2008. The causative etiologic agent was *Microsporum canis* in all children. The patients received itraconazole 5mg/kg bodyweight daily for 3 to 6 weeks with no clinically side effects being noted. In all patients clinical and mycological cure could be achieved.

Conclusion.—Itraconazole proved to be a safe and effective treatment option for *Microsporum canis* induced tinea capitis in children in their first year of life.

▶ The gold standard for the treatment of tinea capitis has always been systemic treatment with griseofulvin (at least 15 mg/kg/day for *Trichophyton tonsurans* and 20-25 mg/kg/d for *Microsporum canis* in children). This is a prospective study of 7 children aged between 3 and 46 weeks with tinea capitis caused by *M canis* treated with itraconazole. Each child was administered itraconazole capsules or oral suspension in a dosage of 5 mg/kg body weight per day. The parents were instructed to administer either the capsules with the main food of the day or the suspension in the fasting state. In addition to oral antifungal treatment, children applied other antifungal topical agents. Treatment was continued until clinical signs of mycotic infection had disappeared and potassium hydroxide testing as well as fungal culture became negative. Patients were followed up every 2 weeks until completely cured. Laboratory monitoring was not performed in each follow-up visit. The duration of administration of itraconazole was 3 to 6 weeks. There were no significant side effects with systemic and topical treatment. However, adverse events were monitored on a clinical basis. No laboratory values were monitored. The authors did not discuss how they excluded patients with conditions that may preclude the use of itraconazole. Another limitation was the small sample size (N = 7). Tinea capitis is rare in infants in their first year of life, with limited data available on treatment. *M canis* species is a minor cause of tinea capitis in the United States, usually acquired from contact with an affected cat. Oral itraconazole may not be ideal as a first-line treatment for infant patients in the United States but appears to be a viable alternative to griseofulvin if clinically warranted. Also, patients were treated with oral itraconazole and topical antimycotic shampoo and cream (azole agent). Outcome measurements with oral itraconazole alone may be difficult to assess with combination therapy because there were no controls in this study. This may be a reason for the relatively short treatment duration in some of these cases, especially with tinea capitis caused by *M canis*. This pilot study revealed that itraconazole may be a safe and effective alternative for *M canis*—induced tinea capitis in children in the first year of life. Notably, oral terbinafine, which is available in a sprinkle form for use in children, is not very effective for tinea capitis when caused by *M canis*. When using oral itraconazole capsules, the capsules may be opened and the beads sprinkled into applesauce or peanut butter for easier administration to small children. Oral itraconazole solution is better absorbed but may be limited in some children because of diarrhea.

J. Q. Del Rosso, DO
G. K. Kim, DO

Using a Longitudinal Model to Estimate the Effect of Methicillin-resistant *Staphylococcus aureus* Infection on Length of Stay in an Intensive Care Unit
Barnett AG, Batra R, Graves N, et al (Queensland Univ of Technology, Kelvin Grove, Australia)
Am J Epidemiol 170:1186-1194, 2009

Health-care-associated methicillin-resistant *Staphylococcus aureus* (MRSA) infection may cause increased hospital stay, or sometimes death. Quantifying this effect is complicated because the exposure is time dependent: infection may prolong hospital stay, while longer stays increase infection risk. In this paper, the authors overcome these problems by using a multinomial longitudinal model to estimate the daily probability of death and discharge. They then extend the basic model to estimate how the effect of MRSA infection varies over time and to quantify number of excess days in the intensive care unit due to infection. They found that infection decreased the relative risk of discharge (relative risk ratio $= 0.68$, 95% credible interval: 0.54, 0.82). Infection on the first day of admission resulted in a mean extra stay of 0.3 days (95% credible interval: 0.1, 0.5) for a patient with an Acute Physiology and Chronic Health Evaluation II score of 10 and 1.2 days (95% credible interval: 0.5, 2.0) for a patient with a score of 30. The decrease in the relative risk of discharge remained fairly constant with day of MRSA infection but was slightly stronger closer to the start of infection. Results confirm the importance of MRSA infection in increasing stay in an intensive care unit but suggest that previous work may have systematically overestimated the effect size.

▶ Cost considerations and length of stay are becoming national priorities in the health care debate. This article attempted to estimate the true effect of health care-associated methicillin-resistant *Staphylococcus aureus* (MRSA) infections on the length of stay. The challenge, of course, is dissociating this effect from the increased risk of infection strongly associated with longer stays in the hospital. This was a good faith effort, and the data suggest that although health care-associated strains of MRSA do result in longer hospital admissions, the increased length is not as long as has been estimated in prior reports. Of course, health care-associated infections are often associated with sepsis and those who die do not have an increased length of stay, but the authors have made a good faith attempt to capture the true economic impact of health care-associated MRSA infections. The data do not address the effect of infection with community strains, which are now the predominant MRSA strains in some hospitals.

D. M. Elston, MD

Presence of Genes Encoding the Panton-Valentine Leukocidin Exotoxin is not the Primary Determinant of Outcome in Patients with Complicated Skin and Skin Structure Infections Due to Methicillin-Resistant *Staphylococcus aureus*: Results of a Multinational Trial

Bae I-G, Tonthat GT, Stryjewski ME, et al (Duke Univ Med Ctr, Durham, NC; et al)
J Clin Microbiol 47:3952-3957, 2009

The role of Panton-Valentine leukocidin (PVL) in determining the severity and outcome of complicated skin and skin structure infections (cSSSI) caused by methicillin (meticillin)-resistant *Staphylococcus aureus* (MRSA) is controversial. We evaluated potential associations between clinical outcome and PVL status by using MRSA isolates from patients enrolled in two large, multinational phase three clinical trials assessing telavancin for the treatment of cSSSI (the ATLAS program). MRSA isolates from microbiologically evaluable patients were genotyped by pulsed-field gel electrophoresis (PFGE) and PCR for *pvl* and 31 other putative virulence determinants. A single baseline pathogen of MRSA was isolated from 522 microbiologically evaluable patients (25.1%) among 2,079 randomized patients. Of these MRSA isolates, 83.2% (432/519) exhibited the USA300 PFGE genotype and 89.1% (465/522) were *pvl* positive. Patients with *pvl*-positive MRSA were more likely than those with *pvl*-negative MRSA to be young, to be North American, and to present with major abscesses ($P < 0.001$ for each). Patients were significantly more likely to be cured if they were infected with *pvl*-positive MRSA than if they were infected with *pvl*-negative MRSA (91.6% versus 80.7%; $P = 0.015$). This observation remained statistically significant after adjustment for presence of abscess, fever, or leukocytosis; infection size; diabetes; patient age; and study medication received. The *fnbA, cna, sdrC, map-eap, sed, seg, sei, sej*, SCC*mec* type IV, and *agr* group II genes were also associated with clinical response ($P < 0.05$). This contemporary, international study demonstrates that *pvl* was not the primary determinant of outcome in patients with MRSA cSSSI.

▶ Most community-type methicillin-resistant *Staphylococcus aureus* isolates in North America are USA300 genotype and most are Panton-Valentine leukocidin (PVL) positive. It is unclear whether PVL is a primary virulence factor involved in these infections.[1-4] This study suggests that PVL is not the major virulence factor associated with outcome, as most patients studied had better outcomes when the strain was PVL positive. Clearly, more study is necessary to determine the role of individual virulence factors.

D. M. Elston, MD

References

1. Zivkovic A, Sharif O, Stich K, et al. TLR 2 and CD14 mediate innate immunity and lung inflammation to staphylococcal Panton-Valentine leukocidin in vivo. *J Immunol.* 2011;186:1608-1617.
2. Boakes E, Kearns AM, Ganner M, Perry C, Hill RL, Ellington MJ. Distinct bacterio-phages encoding Panton-Valentine leukocidin (PVL) among international methicillin-resistant *Staphylococcus aureus* clones harboring PVL. *J Clin Microbiol.* 2011;49: 684-692.
3. Yeung M, Balma-Mena A, Shear N, et al. Identification of major clonal complexes and toxin producing strains among *Staphylococcus aureus* associated with atopic dermatitis. *Microbes Infect.* 2011;13:189-197.
4. Cataldo MA, Taglietti F, Petrosillo N. Methicillin-resistant *Staphylococcus aureus*: a community health threat. *Postgrad Med.* 2010;122:16-23.

4 Viral Infections (Excluding HIV Infection)

Comparative Study on the Efficacy, Safety, and Acceptability of Imiquimod 5% Cream versus Cryotherapy for Molluscum Contagiosum in Children
Al-Mutairi N, Al-Doukhi A, Al-Farag S, et al (Farwaniya Hosp, Kuwait)
Pediatr Dermatol 27:388-394, 2010

To compare the efficacy, safety and acceptability of imiquimod (IMQ) 5% cream with cryotherapy for the treatment of molluscum contagiosum (MC) in children. Prospective, randomized, comparative, observer blinded study. A total of 74 children, with MC were divided randomly to receive treatment with either IMQ 5% cream (group A) 5 days a week or cryotherapy (group B) once a week until clinical cure or up to a maximum of 16 weeks. All the patients were followed up weekly during active treatment. The patients were followed-up for 6 months after clinical cure to look for recurrence. In the IMQ group (group A), the overall complete cure rate was 91.8% (34 of 37), 22 of the 37 patients cleared by the end of 6 weeks and 12 more patients cleared by the end of 12 weeks, while the remaining three patients (8.1%) did not clear even after 16 weeks. Whereas, in the cryotherapy group, all 37 patients achieved complete cure, 26 of 37 (70.27%) patients cleared after 3 weeks, and the remaining 11 (29.72%) cleared by the end of 6 weeks. No statistically significant difference was found between the overall complete cure rate in both groups at the end of maximum treatment period (16 weeks). Pain, bullae formation, pigmentary changes, and superficial scarring were more significantly common in the cryotherapy group compared with the IMQ group. Imiqimod 5% cream seems to be slow acting but an effective agent for the treatment of MC in children. IMQ appears to be practically painless and more cosmetically accepted treatment when compared with cryotherapy, and may be the preferred treatment of MC in children especially with numerous small lesions. Cryotherapy has the advantage of being rapidly effective, and is less expensive than IMQ and may be the preferred treatment for large solitary or few lesions.

▶ Treatment of molluscum contagiosum is often a challenge to even the most experienced dermatologist. In this study, 74 children (mean age of 8 years) were treated with either cryotherapy once a week or imiquimod 5% cream 5 days a week for up to 16 weeks. The number of lesions varied with a mean of 23.3 in the imiquimod group and 27 in the cryotherapy group. By 16 weeks, both groups showed excellent clearance rates, 100% and 92% respectively. (There was an 8% recurrence rate in the cryotherapy group.) The patients treated with cryotherapy responded much faster than those treated with imiquimod but also experienced more scarring and secondary pigmentary changes. Of note, there are a few important limitations to this study. The authors do not report the time from onset of disease. In a self-limited condition, like molluscum, this is essential information, as the improvement may not be related to treatment. Also, this study was not statistically analyzed. Other studies using imiquimod have been reported. Most are open label and not adequately controlled. One double-blind, placebo controlled pilot study of 23 children with molluscum was published.[1] The results at 12 weeks showed a 33% improvement in the imiquimod-treated group versus 9% in the placebo-treated group. This response rate is much lower than in Al-Mutairi's study, which reported a 92% complete response rate at 12 weeks. Drawing firm conclusions as to the efficacy of imiquimod in particular is difficult.

A. Zaenglein, MD

Reference

1. Theos AU, Cummins R, Silverberg NB, Paller AS. Effectiveness of imiquimod cream 5% for treating childhood molluscum contagiosum in a double-blind, randomized pilot trial. *Cutis.* 2004;74:134-138. 141-142.

Cutaneotropic Human β-/γ-Papillomaviruses are Rarely Shared between Family Members
Gottschling M, Göker M, Köhler A, et al (Univ Hosp of Berlin, Germany; Univ of Tübingen, Germany)
J Invest Dermatol 129:2427-2434, 2009

Several cutaneotropic human papillomavirus (HPV) types seem to be involved in the early onset of cutaneous squamous-cell carcinoma. To test the hypothesis that cutaneotropic HPV infections are facilitated because of close and frequent skin contact (for example, between child and mother), we examined HPV prevalence in hair follicle cells from 134 volunteers (1−89 years of age, median 42 years) from 13 families. We used a high-throughput HPV-typing approach with a sensitive β-/γ-cutaneous PCR method, followed by reverse line blotting, to detect 30 cutaneotropic HPV types. HPV prevalence in all individuals was 42% and increased with age from 5% at $\leq$20 years to 27% at 21−40 years, 53% at 41−60 years, and 76% at >60 years. The effect of life age was significant, independent of couples and family members shown by regression analyses ($P \leq 10^{-8}$). A higher similarity of HPV infection patterns was observed in couples versus two randomly chosen individuals ($P \leq 0.05$). However, the same specific HPV type was rarely found within couples or between children and their parents. Cutaneotropic HPV types are occasionally exchanged between family members during the entire lifetime, but other donors should also be considered in viral transmission.

▶ The role of mucosal-based human papillomavirus (HPV) in the development of both benign and malignant lesions is well established and accepted. Certain cutaneotropic HPV types clearly play a role in the development of benign lesions (eg, warts) and malignant lesions (eg, epidermodysplasia verruciformis). However, the exact role that a myriad of skin-associated HPV types actually play in the development of nonmelanoma skin cancer (NMSC) remains controversial. Understanding if and how these viruses contribute to NMSC would be facilitated by better understanding of how such agents disseminate. This study was designed to detect the β- and γ-HPV viral presence in subjects using sensitive molecular methods on cells derived from the eyebrow follicle. The presence of HPV and the number of different HPV types increased with age. Somewhat surprisingly, the concordance of specifically detected HPV types between children and their mothers was not high but was higher between couples than between randomly selected individuals. The study provides evidence for and against direct skin-to-skin transmission of β- and γ-HPV types. It does not ask, nor help to answer, whether such organisms are merely commensal in nature or etiologic for the development of NMSC. The study also does not address the possibility of variability in cutaneotropic HPV prevalence by geographic area (eg, difference between Europe and the United States). It does suggest that, at least in the population studied, accumulation of cutaneotropic HPV load increases with age. The clinical significance of this finding is uncertain.

T. Rosen, MD

Diversity of human papillomavirus types in periungual squamous cell carcinoma
Kreuter A, Gambichler T, Pfister H, et al (Ruhr-Univ Bochum, Germany; Univ of Cologne, Germany)
Br J Dermatol 161:1262-1269, 2009

Background.—There is accumulating evidence that infections with certain high-risk α-human papillomaviruses (HPVs) are involved in the pathogenesis of digital squamous cell carcinomas (SCCs) and their precursor lesions (SCCs *in situ*).

Objectives.—This study was initiated to search for α- and β-HPV infections in a collective of SCC and SCC *in situ* located on the hands.

Methods.—HPV typing for 36 high-risk and low-risk α-HPV types and 25 β-HPV types was performed in SCCs located at different sites of the hands. Additionally, immunohistochemical staining for p16[INK4a] and Ki67 was performed in 15 samples.

Results.—In total, 25 SCCs/SCCs *in situ* (six periungual lesions, eight lesions from the proximal or lateral part of the finger, and 11 lesions from the dorsal part of the hand) were analysed for the presence of α- and β-HPV types. Only one lesion (an SCC *in situ* positive for HPV11 and HPV31) of the dorsal hand and none of the proximal or lateral part finger lesions were α-HPV positive. In contrast, all six periungual lesions were α-HPV positive, and the majority (83%) of them carried HPV types other than HPV16 (HPV26, HPV33, HPV51, HPV56 and HPV73). β-HPV types were found in only two biopsies. p16^{INK4a} and Ki67 expression was significantly higher in HPV-positive lesions as compared with HPV-negative tumours, and both markers significantly correlated with each other.

Conclusions.—In contrast to other locations of the hands, periungual SCCs are frequently associated with α-HPV infections. Several high-risk HPV types other than HPV16 can induce periungual SCCs. Given the high recurrence rate and high proliferative activity of HPV-associated periungual SCCs, aggressive treatment and close follow-up of these tumours is mandatory.

▶ Certain human papillomavirus (HPV) subtypes have been associated with squamous cell carcinoma (SCC) development. This is a study to analyze 36 high-risk and low-risk α-HPV types and 25 β-HPV types in SCCs located at different sites of the hands. There was a total of 25 SCCs and SCC in situ (6 periungual lesions, 8 lesions from the proximal or lateral part of the finger, and 11 lesions from the dorsal part of the hand) analyzed for α- and β-HPV types. HPV DNA analyses were performed with immunohistochemical staining for p16 and Ki67 in 6 periungual α-HPV lesions and in 9 HPV-negative tumors. The number of p16-expressing cells was significantly higher in the group of HPV-positive tumors (median 87.5%, range 70%-95%) compared with the HPV-negative lesions (median 10%, range 0%-60%; $P = .0004$). Similarly, Ki67 was significantly more expressed in HPV-positive periungual tumors compared with HPV-negative lesions ($P = .0004$). The authors found a significant association of p16 and Ki67 in both HPV-positive ($P = .02$) and HPV-negative ($P = .01$) lesions. β-HPV was found in only 2 biopsies. p16 and Ki67 expression was significantly higher in HPV-positive lesions as compared with HPV-negative tumors. Ki67 may be overexpressed in SCC, and this study found that it was highly expressed in HPV-positive periungual lesions (range 70%-95% of cells). Digital periungual SCC is rare, but there may be evidence that periungual skin is particularly susceptible to HPV acquisition due to microtrauma. However, other factors may also play a significant role in the pathogenesis of periungual SCC, such as exposure to radiation or chemicals, chronic infection, and immune status, which this study did not analyze. Limitations to this study were that other risk factors for SCC development were not discussed and the sample size was small. Also, there were no controls for this study, and HPV subtypes may also be seen in clinically normal lesions.

This study confirmed that most periungual SCCs were associated with α-HPV infections compared with β-HPV.

J. Q. Del Rosso, DO

G. K. Kim, DO

Effectiveness of Pulsed Dye Laser in the Treatment of Recalcitrant Warts in Children
Sethuraman G, Richards KA, Hiremagalore RN, et al (Northwestern Univ, Chicago, IL)
Dermatol Surg 36:58-65, 2010

Background.—To determine the efficacy and safety of the 585-nm pulsed dye laser (PDL) in the treatment of recalcitrant warts in children.

Methods and Material.—Retrospective survey of the medical records of children with recalcitrant warts who were treated with PDL between March 1995 through January 1999 at the Children's Memorial Hospital outpatient subspecialty center, Chicago, Illinois.

Results.—Sixty-one children with recalcitrant warts were treated with PDL; 75% of them had total clearance of warts after an average of 3.1 treatment sessions. Overall success rates were 100% for both perineal and perianal and face-only warts, 93% for hands, 69% for plantar warts, 67% when both face and extremities were involved, and 60% when multiple extremities were involved. Pain and other side effects were minimal. Mild scarring occurred in 2% of patients; 75% of patients remained free of warts after a follow-up period of 24 months or longer.

Conclusion.—PDL therapy is an effective, safe alternative therapy for treatment of recalcitrant warts in children, with few side effects and a low long-term recurrence rate.

▶ Viral warts are a common nuisance seen in the pediatric population. This is a retrospective study surveying medical records of children with recalcitrant warts treated with pulsed dye laser (PDL) to determine the safety and efficacy of 585-nm PDL. There were 61 children with recalcitrant warts treated with PDL; 75% of them had a total clearance of warts after an average of 3.1 treatment sessions. The end result of laser treatment was complete clearance of warts. Warts were considered 100% cleared if there was no recurrence and partially cleared if the patients did not clear completely or had recurrence within the follow-up period. Warts were first pared with a #15 scalpel blade until punctate bleeding, then PDL irradiated all warts, pulsing them multiple times. Patients returned to the laser center for repeat treatment at 2.5 to 4-week intervals until resolution of all warts. A total of 61 children were treated with PDL (age 2-17 years). The overall clearance rate was 75%, with follow-up ranging from 12 to 66 months. The remaining 25% of patients had partial clearance. Body locations such as face and perineum were most likely to clear in 1 treatment (50% and 20%, respectively). Plantar warts cleared in 67% of patients and arm and leg warts in 60% of patients. The side effects of PDL treatments were minimal, with 8% hypopigmentation, 2% hyperpigmentation, and 2% of patients experiencing mild scarring and blistering. The cost of PDL treatment was significant, especially when general anesthesia was needed for younger children. Another weakness in this study was that 1 child developed seizures after general anesthesia. Overall, PDL may not be ideal in terms of cost and safety as first-line treatment in children. It was concluded that PDL is an effective, safe, and well-tolerated procedure for the treatment of extensive recalcitrant warts in the pediatric population; however, limitations need to be recognized. It may be of use to compare PDL with other treatments to evaluate whether PDL results in lower recurrence rates and an increase in response rates. An important limitation was the absence of controls in this study. The authors also suggest that along with photothermolysis, PDL has immumodulating properties, which may be an interest for future study.

J. Q. Del Rosso, DO

G. K. Kim, DO

Herpes Zoster and Exposure to the Varicella Zoster Virus in an Era of Varicella Vaccination
Donahue JG, Kieke BA, Gargiullo PM, et al (Marshfield Clinic Res Foundation, WI; Ctrs for Disease Control and Prevention (CDC), Atlanta, GA; et al)
Am J Public Health 100:1116-1122, 2010

Objectives.—We performed a case–control study to determine if participants with herpes zoster had fewer contacts with persons with varicella or zoster, and with young children, to explore the hypothesis that exposure to persons with varicella zoster virus (VZV) results in "immune boosting."

Methods.—Participants were patients of the multispecialty Marshfield Clinic in Wisconsin. We identified patients aged 40 to 79 years with a new diagnosis of zoster from August 2000 to July 2005. We frequency matched control participants to case participants for age. We confirmed diagnoses by chart review and assessed exposures by interview.

Results.—Interviews were completed by 633 of 902 eligible case participants (70.2%) and 655 of 1149 control participants (57.0%). The number of varicella contacts was not associated with zoster; there was no trend even at the highest exposure level (3 or more contacts). Similarly, there was no association with exposure to persons with zoster or to children, or with workplace exposures.

Conclusions.—Although exposure to VZV in our study was relatively low, the absence of a relationship with zoster reflects the uncertain influence of varicella circulation on zoster epidemiology.

▶ The varicella vaccination program was implemented in the United States in 1995. Since then, there has been speculation as to whether universal vaccination would in turn increase the incidence of herpes zoster because of fewer chances for varicella exposure, which is thought to boost immunity. More specifically, 2 main theories involving the cell-mediated immune response have been described. The first is termed as exogenous boosting whereby the immune response is boosted by exposure to other persons with varicella. The second is endogenous boosting where a subclinical reactivation of latent virus maintains immunity against varicella zoster virus (VZV).[1] This case-control study, 10 years following the start of the vaccination program, showed no relationship between exogenous exposure to VZV and incidence of zoster. Whether a more frequent or intense exposure is required for exogenous boosting is yet to be determined. Limitations of this study include patient recall bias, as results were obtained via telephone interviews and data were dependent on the ability of the participant to accurately remember the number of persons with varicella they came in contact with during the past 10 years before reference date.

S. Bellew, DO

J. Q. Del Rosso, DO

Reference

1. Klein NP, Holmes TH, Sharp MA, et al. Variability and gender differences in memory T cell immunity to varicella-zoster virus in healthy adults. *Vaccine.* 2006;24:5913-5918.

Parental Refusal of Varicella Vaccination and the Associated Risk of Varicella Infection in Children

Glanz JM, McClure DL, Magid DJ, et al (Kaiser Permanente Colorado Inst for Health Res, Denver; et al)

Arch Pediatr Adolesc Med 164:66-70, 2010

Objective.—To quantify both the individual-level and attributable risk of varicella infection requiring medical care in children whose parents refuse varicella immunizations.

Design.—Matched case-control study with conditional logistic regression analysis.

Setting.—Kaiser Permanente of Colorado (KPCO) health plan between 1998 and 2008.

Participants.—Each pediatric physician-diagnosed case of varicella (n = 133) was matched to 4 randomly selected controls (n = 493). Cases were matched by age, sex, and length of enrollment in KPCO.

Main Exposures.—Varicella vaccine refusal.

Outcome Measures.—Varicella infection.

Results.—There were 7 varicella vaccine refusers (5%) among the cases and 3 (0.6%) among the controls. Children of parents who refused varicella immunizations were at a greatly increased risk of varicella infection requiring medical care (odds ratio, 8.6; 95% confidence interval, 2.2-33.3) compared with children of parents who accepted vaccinations (P =.004).

In the entire KPCO pediatric population, 5% of varicella cases were attributed to parental vaccine refusal.

Conclusions.—Children of parents who refuse varicella immunizations are at high risk of varicella infection relative to vaccinated children. These results will be helpful to health care providers and parents when making decisions about immunizing children.

▶ Varicella is an infectious disease caused by the varicella-zoster virus (VZV), a type of human herpes virus spread primarily by aerosol or direct contact. In the United States, the Centers for Disease Control and Prevention recommends the administration of varicella vaccination for all healthy children in 2 doses: 1st dose at age 12 to 15 months and 2nd dose at age 4 to 6 years. The vaccination is currently available singly or in a quadrivalent combination of measles, mumps, rubella, and varicella vaccine. In recent years, growing concern in the media about alleged chronic illness associations with vaccination has led to an increase in the number of parents refusing VZV vaccines for their children. This study investigates the relationship between vaccine refusal and risk of varicella infection. In fact, investigators found a strong association between refusal of VZV vaccine and risk of medically attended childhood varicella disease. However, there were some important limitations to this study as stated by the authors. First, results may not be generalizable, as patients were from a single managed health care plan in Colorado. Second, there were only 10 of 626 patients who refused the vaccine; therefore, the information may not be sufficient to analyze the association between vaccine refusal and varicella infection.

S. Bellew, DO

J. Q. Del Rosso, DO

Risk Factors for Cutaneous Human Papillomavirus Seroreactivity among Patients Undergoing Skin Cancer Screening in Florida
Iannacone MR, Michael KM, Giuliano AR, et al (Moffitt Cancer Ctr, Tampa, FL; German Cancer Res Ctr [Deutsches Krebsforschungszebtrum], Heidelberg, Germany)
J Infect Dis 201:760-769, 2010

Background.—Little is known about the risk factors for cutaneous human papillomavirus (HPV) infection.

Methods.—To investigate factors associated with cutaneous HPV seropositivity, we conducted a cross-sectional study of 411 patients undergoing routine skin cancer screening examinations. Serum antibodies were measured and evaluated for 36 cutaneous HPV types in the genera alpha, beta, gamma, mu, and nu. Associations of demographic and lifestyle factors with cutaneous HPV seropositivity were estimated using odds ratios and 95% confidence intervals calculated using logistic regression.

Results.—The seroprevalence of ≥ 1 cutaneous HPV type was 96% and 90% for men and women, respectively. Seroprevalence was highest for

HPV types 4 (46%), 1 (37%), and 8 (31%) in men and for types 4 (47%), 63 (34%), and 1 (33%) in women. Independent associations of demographic and skin cancer risk factors with genus-specific HPV seropositivity differed by sex. For example, white skin, inability to tan, and lifetime residency in Florida were factors associated with genus-specific HPV seropositivity in men. Heavy smoking, sunscreen use, and green eye color were associated with genus-specific HPV seropositivity in women.

Conclusions.—Seroreactivity to cutaneous HPV types was highly prevalent in our study population. Different risk factors were independently associated with genus-specific cutaneous HPV seropositivity in men and women.

▶ There are limited data on the risk factors associated with cutaneous human papillomavirus (HPV) infection. Accordingly, Iannacone et al sought to elucidate information on risk factors that may be associated with cutaneous HPV seropositivity among patients in Florida undergoing skin cancer screening. Specifically, the study identified the prevalence of HPV seropositivity of the patient population (including ascertaining the common genus and type), but more importantly, sought to distinguish demographic and skin cancer risk factors that may be associated with genus-specific HPV seropositivity by sex. To that end, the study accomplished its objectives; however, as noted by the study itself, further studies with larger sample sizes are needed. Regardless, the conclusions are interesting and provide an important starting framework for further research. Of note, the study found a high prevalence of seroreactivity of cutaneous HPV types in their patient population, noting that 91.2% of the study patients were positive for ≥1 type of cutaneous HPV and 78.8% of the study patients were positive for ≥2 cutaneous HPV types. The most common HPV genus found was genus beta, and the most common HPV type found was type 4. In addition, the study found that the demographic and skin cancer risk factors that were identified to be independently associated with genus-specific cutaneous HPV seropositivity differed ultimately among men and women. Examples included white skin and inability to tan as factors associated with genus-specific cutaneous HPV seropositivity in men, while heavy smoking and sunscreen use were examples of factors associated with genus-specific cutaneous HPV positivity in women. While the goal of the study has been met, additional studies will be needed to expand this base of information and hopefully, provide further clinical relevance.

B. D. Michaels, DO
J. Q. Del Rosso, DO

5 Parasitic Infections, Bites, and Infestations

The Clinical Trials Supporting Benzyl Alcohol Lotion 5% (Ulesfia™): A Safe and Effective Topical Treatment for Head Lice (Pediculosis Humanus Capitis)

Meinking TL, Villar ME, Vicaria M, et al (Global Health Associates of Miami [GHAM], FL; et al)

Pediatr Dermatol 27:19-24, 2010

Benzyl alcohol lotion 5% (BAL 5%) is a non-neurotoxic topical head lice treatment that is safe and effective in children as young as 6 months of age. The safety and efficacy of this pediculicide has been studied in 695 (confirm number) subjects in all phases of clinical development. Scanning electron micrographs (SEM) demonstrated that the active agent appears to stun the breathing spiracles open, enabling the vehicle to penetrate the respiratory mechanism (spiracles), therefore asphyxiating the lice. Initial phase II trials compared this novel product to RID® using identical volumes of treatment (4 oz/application) and yielding, almost, identical efficacy. This outcome pointed to the significant importance of completely saturating the hair with the product in order to achieve maximum treatment success. A second phase II trial, which allowed the use of sufficient product to saturate the hair, resulted in 100% efficacy after both 10 and 30 minute treatments. A third phase II trial verified an effective dose. Phase III trials compared BAL 5% to vehicle placebo for two 10-minute applications. It proved to be safe and effective (p < 0.001) for treatment of head lice and is the first FDA-approved non-neurotoxic lice treatment, now available in the United States as Ulesfia™ lotion.

▶ This is a review of the current phase II and phase III clinical trials done demonstrating the safety and efficacy of benzyl alcohol 5% lotion in the treatment of head lice. Unlike many of the neurotoxic pesticides that are commonly used, benzyl alcohol works as an asphyxiant. It forces the lice spiracles to remain open while the vehicle components fill the louse's respiratory apparatus, effectively asphyxiating it. Three phase II trials determined an optimal concentration of 5% benzyl alcohol with an application time of 10 minutes. In phase III trials, safety and efficacy were determined. Benzyl alcohol 5% lotion was shown to have a 92% success rate at day 8 and a 75% success rate at day 22 (possibly due to reinfestation). The efficacy was equal to the over-the-counter lice treatment, RID. Safety was demonstrated in children as young as 6 months and in pregnant women. Benzyl alcohol 5% lotion should be applied in an adequate volume to saturate the hair and left on for 10 minutes before rinsing. The process should be repeated in 1 week to kill newly hatched nits. This product should prove a useful prescription lice treatment, especially in areas where lice are resistant to standard over-the-counter treatments.

A. Zaenglein, MD

6 Disorders of the Pilosebaceous Apparatus

Trichothiodystrophy and fragile hair: the distinction between diagnostic signs and diagnostic labels in childhood hair disease
Cheng S, Stone J, de Berker D (Bristol Royal Infirmary, UK)
Br J Dermatol 161:1379-1383, 2009

Background.—Hair typically becomes fragile when there are structural abnormalities and/or a reduction in the sulphur-containing amino acids cystine or methionine. This finding in the setting of a neuroectodermal complaint is usually labelled trichothiodystrophy (TTD). The spectrum of features within this diagnostic grouping tests the validity of using sulphur-deficient hair as a central characteristic.

Objectives.—To determine what diagnoses were found within a group of subjects with fragile hair and whether low cystine or methionine were relevant central characteristics.

Methods.—We examined cases referred to us from 12 U.K. centres for hair microscopy over 10 years where hair fragility or clinical characteristics raised the possibility of TTD. All samples underwent amino acid analysis. This was achieved through cation exchange chromatography coupled with spectrophotometric quantification.

Results.—Twenty-five patients (11 male, 14 female) with a mean age of 11 years (0·3—37) were evaluated. Nineteen patients had features of hair damage. Of these, five patients had abnormalities on microscopy only and four patients had microscopic changes and tiger-tail pattern but normal amino acid content. The remaining 10 patients had reduced cystine content, two of whom also had low methionine. All but one had the tiger-tail pattern. Among the wide range of phenotypes there were only three cases matching a diagnosis of TTD.

Conclusions.—Our data suggest that clinically apparent fragile hair in childhood is only rarely associated with a diagnosis of TTD. The tiger-tail change is sensitive but not wholly specific to TTD. We propose that the term trichothiodystrophy be limited in its use to define sulphur-deficient hair rather than as a diagnostic term in a heterogeneous and incoherent multisystem disorder, where sulphur-deficient hair is one feature.

▶ This article challenges the concept that trichothiodystrophy (TTD) is a single condition.[1-5] The authors suggest that when there are 2 or 3 characteristic hair shaft abnormalities together with a partial or complete tiger-tail appearance on polarized light microscopy, the likelihood of a low-sulfur defect (reduced cystine or methionine) is high. They suggest that patients who do not meet all of the above criteria represent a range of complex diseases, including xeroderma pigmentosum group D and argininosuccinate lyase deficiency.

In some patients, the amino acid analysis can be borderline. One subject with a defect in the ornithine carboxylase cycle was identified suggesting a heterogeneous group of disorders with characteristics of TTD. The authors suggest that the term be reserved for those who demonstrate the full complex of findings with low sulfur content.

D. M. Elston, MD

References

1. Lambert WC, Gagna CE, Lambert MW. Trichothiodystrophy: Photosensitive, TTD-P, TTD, Tay syndrome. *Adv Exp Med Biol.* 2010;685:106-110.
2. Wolski SC, Kuper J, Kisker C. The XPD helicase: XPanDing archaeal XPD structures to get a grip on human DNA repair. *Biol Chem.* 2010;391:761-765.
3. Stefanini M, Botta E, Lanzafame M, Orioli D. Trichothiodystrophy: from basic mechanisms to clinical implications. *DNA Repair (Amst).* 2010;9:2-10.
4. Cleaver JE, Lam ET, Revet I. Disorders of nucleotide excision repair: the genetic and molecular basis of heterogeneity. *Nat Rev Genet.* 2009;10:756-768.
5. Morice-Picard F, Cario-André M, Rezvani H, Lacombe D, Sarasin A, Taïeb A. New clinico-genetic classification of trichothiodystrophy. *Am J Med Genet A.* 2009;149A:2020-2030.

Five-year experience in the treatment of alopecia areata with DPC
El-Zawahry BM, Bassiouny DA, Khella A, et al (Cairo Univ, Egypt)
J Eur Acad Dermatol Venereol 24:264-269, 2010

Background.—The effectiveness of Diphencyprone (DPC) in alopecia areata (AA) was demonstrated in several studies with highly variable response rates ranging from 5% to 85%.

Objective.—The response rate and variable factors affecting the prognosis were studied focusing on long-term follow-up with or without maintenance therapy.

Methods.—A total of 135 cases of AA were treated with DPC. Patients were divided into five groups according to the area of scalp affected: Grade 1 AA: 25—49% scalp affection; Grade 2 AA: 50—74% scalp affection; Grade 3 AA: 75—99% scalp affection; alopecia totalis and alopecia universalis. An initial response was defined as appearance of new terminal hair within treated sites. Excellent response was defined as terminal hair covering >75% of the scalp. Relapse meant >25% hair loss. Maintenance therapy meant ongoing therapy once every 1—4 weeks after excellent response. Follow-up was performed to detect any relapse of AA.

Results.—Ninety-seven patients continued therapy for ≥3 months. After an initial 3 month lag, cumulative excellent response was seen in 15 patients (15.4%), 47 patients (48.5%), 51 patients (52.6%) and 55 patients (55.7%) after 6, 12, 18 and 24 months respectively in a mean median time of 12 months. The only patient variable affecting the prognosis was baseline extent of AA. Excellent response was seen in 100%, 77%, 54%, 50% and 41% in Grade 1, Grade 2, Grade 3, AA totalis and AA universalis patients respectively. Side-effects were few and tolerable. Hair fall >25% occurred in 17.9% of patients on maintenance and 57.1% of patients without maintenance therapy (P-value = 0.025).

Conclusion.—Diphencyprone is an effective and safe treatment of extensive AA. A long period of therapy is needed and will increase the percentage of responders especially in alopecia totalis and universalis. Maintenance therapy is recommended to reduce the risk of relapse.

▶ Diphencyprone (DPC), a nonmutagenic chemical substance with a high potential for skin sensitization, has been used to treat alopecia areata (AA) with variable response rates. This is an open-label clinical study of 0.001% diphencyprone (DPC) used in 135 cases of AA, with patients divided into 5 groups according to the area of scalp affected. After initial sensitization with 2.5% DPC, the affected scalp was treated weekly, with the concentration of DPC progressively increased every 4 to 5 weeks. Response was defined based on the presence and extent of new terminal hair within treated sites. Age of onset of disease ranged from 1 to 57 years and included 21 children. Ninety-seven patients continued therapy for > 3 months. The median time needed to achieve excellent response was 12 months. In the group of patients with grade 1 AA (25%-49% scalp area affected), 100% (11/11) of patients achieved excellent response in a median time of 6 months. Of the 27 patients with AA universalis, 3 patients (11%) showed spontaneous regrowth of the eyebrows and eyelashes. In patients with grade 2 AA (50%-74% scalp area affected), 77% (7/9) achieved excellent response in a median time of 12 months. In patients with more extensive grade 3 AA (75%-99% scalp area affected), 54% (15/28) achieved excellent response in a median time of 12 months. In the AA totalis group, 50% (11/22) of patients achieved excellent response in a median of 12 months. In the AA universalis group, 41% (11/27) of patients achieved excellent response in a median of 18 months. One side effect was cervical lymphadenopathy, which occurred in 50% of the cases but was not considered a significant or consequential drug side effect by the authors. Side effects of DPC therapy included localized vitiligo in 2.2% of patients and postinflammatory hyperpigmentation. Forty-six patients were observed from 1 to 48 months. Relapse was noted in 9.5% of patients; however, some patients were lost to follow-up. Hair loss > 25% was noted to be present in 17.9% of patients in the DPC maintenance therapy group as compared with 57.1% not treated with DPC maintenance therapy (P = .025). In this study, a significant benefit of maintenance therapy with DPC in reducing relapses of

AA was found over the follow-up periods reported (*P* = .025). However, the study was not adequately controlled, and many patients with AA can exhibit regrowth of hair spontaneously. The authors concluded that DPC is an effective treatment of extensive AA. However, longer follow-up periods are needed if maintenance therapy is to be recommended, along with a thorough evaluation of the outcomes of cervical lymphadenopathy.

J. Q. Del Rosso, DO

G. K. Kim, DO

---

3 Cases of Dissecting Cellulitis of the Scalp Treated With Adalimumab: Control of Inflammation Within Residual Structural Disease
Navarini AA, Trüeb RM (Univ Hosp of Zürich, Switzerland)
Arch Dermatol 146:517-520, 2010

Background.—Dissecting cellulitis of the scalp (DCS) is a chronic inflammatory disease of scalp hair follicles manifesting as multiple painful nodules and abscesses that interconnect via sinus tracts. The disease tends to run a progressive course that eventually results in scarring alopecia. The condition is thought to represent a follicular occlusion disorder. Sebaceous and keratinous material within dilated pilosebaceous units accumulates until follicles burst, with subsequent neutrophilic inflammatory reaction and abscess formation. Treatment remains unsatisfactory. While oral antibiotics, intralesional corticosteroids, isotretinoin, or dapsone are insufficient, in this case series the inflammation responsible for scarifying tissue destruction was directly targeted by means of the tumor necrosis factor antagonist adalimumab.

Observation.—Clinical signs of inflammation as well as burden of disease measured by a score of 0 to 10 (*P* < .04) was reduced rapidly by adalimumab. Histopathologic characteristics demonstrated marked improvement of inflammation, despite persistence of underlying structural disease. Relapse was observed following discontinuation of adalimumab.

Conclusions.—Adalimumab is effective for treatment of DCS. Relapse on discontinuation of therapy can be expected depending on persisting structural disease. Continuous treatment or combined surgical resection of involved areas could be necessary for definitive resolution of disease.

▶ With the large number of case studies that have examined the efficacy of anti–tumor necrosis factor (TNF) self injectables for the treatment of hidradenitis suppurativa, it stands to reason that, as part of the same follicular occlusion triad, dissecting cellulitis may respond similarly to the same drug class. Use of this drug class is based on the theory that it is the secondary inflammatory process that is responsible for the clinical picture of scarring and tract formation, brought on by an as yet to be determined stimulus creating occlusion of and then destruction of the pilosebaceous unit. This case study found that 3 patients with dissecting cellulitis improved dramatically to the standard psoriasis dosing of adalimumab. However, as appropriately mentioned by the authors, the disease quickly relapsed upon discontinuation of the drug. Moreover, the chronic destructive changes noted pathologically were completely unchanged following 3 months of treatment, and the inflammatory component improved, but in only 2 of the 3 cases. These results in aggregate seem to indicate that, like for psoriasis, the drug diminishes inflammation and allows affected areas to heal but does little to permanently control the disease process.

This case study is clearly limited by the small sample size but provides yet another piece of evidence supporting the need to investigate the TNF inhibitors in earnest for routine treatment of the disfiguring cicatricial inflammatory disease states. The burden of getting insurance companies to cover the cost of the medicine is a very real and significant hurdle that must be overcome, and similar to how these drugs are getting easier to get covered for use in psoriasis and psoriatic arthritis, studies showing such promising results may do the same for the follicular occlusion triad of diseases.

J. M. Suchniak, MD

Alefacept for Severe Alopecia Areata: A Randomized, Double-blind, Placebo-Controlled Study
Strober BE, Menon K, McMichael A, et al (New York Univ School of Medicine; Wake Forest Univ, Winston-Salem, NC; et al)
Arch Dermatol 145:1262-1266, 2009

Objective.—To assess the efficacy of alefacept for the treatment of severe alopecia areata (AA).

Design.—Multicenter, double-blind, randomized, placebo-controlled clinical trial.

Setting.—Academic departments of dermatology in the United States.

Participants.—Forty-five individuals with chronic and severe AA affecting 50% to 95% of the scalp hair and resistant to previous therapies.

Intervention.—Alefacept, a US Food and Drug Administration—approved T-cell biologic inhibitor for the treatment of moderate to severe plaque psoriasis.

Main Outcome Measure.—Improved Severity of Alopecia Tool (SALT) score over 24 weeks.

Results.—Participants receiving alefacept for 12 consecutive weeks demonstrated no statistically significant improvement in AA when compared with a well-matched placebo-receiving group ($P = .70$).

Conclusion.—Alefacept is ineffective for the treatment of severe AA.

▶ Alopecia areata is an autoimmune disease characterized by sharply demarcated areas of variable and unpredictable nonscarring hair loss with a recently identified genetic etiology. The lifetime risk of developing alopecia areata in the general population is approximately 1.7%. Severity of the disease may vary from a few small patches of hair loss to loss of all scalp hair (alopecia totalis) or loss of all scalp and body hair (alopecia universalis). Patients with limited disease are easily treated, usually with intralesional corticosteroids and topical therapy. The spontaneous regrowth rate of limited disease is substantial. In patients with severe disease, including alopecia totalis and alopecia universalis, therapy is more difficult. Treatments such as topical sensitizers, including diphencyprone and squaric acid, are used. Psoralen + ultraviolet A has also been used successfully as have methotrexate and systemic corticosteroids. Patients with severe disease have high relapse rates.

Alefacept is a fusion protein consisting of human lymphocyte function–associated antigen-3 fused to the Fc portion of human immunoglobulin G1. Alefacept binds to CD2 on the surface of naïve T cells, preventing costimulation of those T cells by antigen-presenting cells, thus preventing T-cell activation. Alefacept also induces apoptosis of T lymphocytes that have been implicated in the pathogenesis of alopecia areata. Isolated case reports suggest that Alefacept might be effective in the treatment of alopecia areata.

Forty-five subjects with chronic and severe alopecia areata affecting at least 50% of the scalp participated in this trial. Alefacept was administered weekly for 12 consecutive weeks in the same dose and regimen that it is approved for in psoriasis. A matched control group was treated weekly for 12 consecutive weeks with placebo. At 24 weeks, there were no differences between the active treatment group and the placebo group. While this is a disappointing outcome, the authors suggest that the possibility of future trials of alefacept in combination with other therapies. Based on the results of this trial, there is little reason to pursue alefacept as monotherapy for alopecia areata. However, it is likely that future-targeted biologic therapies may work for this autoimmune disease.

M. Lebwohl, MD

Antimicrobial Property of Lauric Acid Against *Propionibacterium Acnes*: Its Therapeutic Potential for Inflammatory Acne Vulgaris
Nakatsuji T, Kao MC, Fang J-Y, et al (Univ of California, San Diego; Chang Gung Univ, Kweishan, Taoyuan, Taiwan; et al)
J Invest Dermatol 129:2480-2488, 2009

The strong bactericidal properties of lauric acid (C12:0), a middle chain-free fatty acid commonly found in natural products, have been shown in a number of studies. However, it has not been demonstrated whether lauric acid can be used for acne treatment as a natural antibiotic against *Propionibacterium acnes* (*P. acnes*), which promotes follicular inflammation (inflammatory acne). This study evaluated the antimicrobial property of lauric acid against *P. acnes* both *in vitro* and *in vivo*. Incubation of the skin bacteria *P. acnes*, *Staphylococcus aureus* (*S. aureus*), and *Staphylococcus epidermidis* (*S. epidermidis*) with lauric acid yielded minimal inhibitory concentration (MIC) values against the bacterial growth over 15 times lower than those of benzoyl peroxide (BPO). The lower MIC values of lauric acid indicate stronger antimicrobial properties than that of BPO. The detected values of half maximal effective concentration (EC$_{50}$) of lauric acid on *P. acnes*, *S. aureus*, and *S. epidermidis* growth indicate that

P. acnes is the most sensitive to lauric acid among these bacteria. In addition, lauric acid did not induce cytotoxicity to human sebocytes. Notably, both intradermal injection and epicutaneous application of lauric acid effectively decreased the number of *P. acnes* colonized with mouse ears, thereby relieving *P. acnes*-induced ear swelling and granulomatous inflammation. The obtained data highlight the potential of using lauric acid as an alternative treatment for antibiotic therapy of acne vulgaris.

▶ *Propionibacterium acnes* is a gram-positive anaerobic bacterium that has been implicated in the pathogenesis of acne vulgaris. A reduction in *P acnes* colony counts has been correlated with clinical improvement of acne vulgaris in patients with the use of antibiotics, such as the tetracyclines, and antimicrobial agents, such as benzoyl peroxide (BP). Free fatty acids secreted from the sebaceous glands have also been shown to have antibacterial activity against gram-positive bacteria. Lauric acid, a minor free fatty acid found in sebum, has antimicrobial activity and is found commonly in coconut palm and milk. It is unknown whether lauric acid has a significant effect on *P acnes* in in vivo studies. This is a study examining the antibacterial activity of lauric acid in vivo and in vitro against *P acnes*. In vitro models revealed that lauric acid has a much stronger antimicrobial activity at various concentrations compared with BP with a minimal inhibitory concentration that was 15-fold lower. This study also revealed that lauric acid was more active against *P acnes* as compared with *S aureus* and *S epidermidis*. Cytotoxicity of lauric acid was examined using human immortalized sebaceous gland cell lines, and it was found that it did not influence with the viability of sebocytes at high concentrations of $125\mu gml^{-1}$, a level at which *P acnes* was eradicated. Injection of lauric acid showed decreased numbers of *P acnes* colonies in mouse ear models with a decrease in swelling and granulomatous inflammation. Although sebum free fatty acids (FFA) overproduction can induce mild inflammation and assist in bacterial adherence, this is not the case for lauric acid. These results indicate that lauric acid exerts inhibitory effects on the growth of skin bacteria, with activity against *P acnes* at concentrations 15-fold lower than that of BP. To add, lauric acid appears to suppress pathogenicity of *P acnes* in vivo but is harmless to host cells. Limitations of this study were the use of mouse skin, which is thinner than human skin, and also the questionable accuracy of minimal inhibitory concentration (MIC) evaluations for BP. In conclusion, lauric acid appears to exhibit significant antibacterial activity against *P acnes* and is associated with decreased colony counts. Whether or not lauric acid may be a safe and effective alternative treatment for acne vulgaris will require additional studies.

J. Q. Del Rosso, DO
G. Kim, DO

Psychiatric reactions to isotretinoin in patients with bipolar disorder

Schaffer LC, Schaffer CB, Hunter S, et al (Sutter Community Hosps, Sacramento; Univ of California, Davis; Univ of Nevada, Reno)
J Affect Disord 122:306-308, 2010

Background.—Isotretinoin (Accutane®) has been available for the treatment of severe cystic acne for about twenty-five years. There have been several reports of adverse psychiatric reactions to isotretinoin, including depressive symptoms and suicide. However, there have been only three case reports of patients with bipolar disorder (BD) who experienced an untoward psychiatric side effect while receiving isotretinoin treatment. In this study, the psychiatric side effects from isotretinoin were assessed in a larger group of BD patients than has previously been reported.

Methods.—A retrospective chart review of 300 BD outpatients identified ten patients treated with isotretinoin.

Results.—Nine of these ten patients experienced a significant worsening of mood symptoms, and three developed suicidal ideation. Eight experienced a reversal of the relapsed mood symptoms when the isotretinoin was discontinued, whether prematurely or after a full course.

Limitations.—The limitations of this study include small sample size, retrospective data collection, absence of double-blind controlled design, and inability to control for spontaneous mood episodes in patients with BD.

Conclusions.—These results indicate that BD patients treated with isotretinoin for acne are at risk for clinically significant exacerbation of mood symptoms, including suicidal ideation, even with concurrent use of psychiatric medicines for BD. The clinical implications of this study are especially relevant to the treatment of patients with BD because acne usually occurs during adolescence, which is often the age of onset of BD and because a common side effect of lithium (a standard treatment for BD) is acne.

▶ This interesting but small retrospective series appears to show that bipolar patients are at great risk for worsening of depressive symptoms while on isotretinoin. Of 300 bipolar patients, 10 were treated with the drug. Nine of the 10 had worsening of psychiatric symptoms. Wow! Can this be true? I've treated a few bipolar patients with oral isotretinoin and recall no problems arising. Clearly, more information is needed. A prospective study would be helpful but difficult to perform. Dermatologists also need to know more about screening for bipolar disease. Until a larger study is done, it makes sense to use isotretinoin judiciously in known bipolar patients.

G. Webster, MD, PhD

The Effect of Aminolevulinic Acid Photodynamic Therapy on Microcomedones and Macrocomedones

Fabbrocini G, Cacciapuoti S, De Vita V, et al (Univ of Naples Federico II, Italy)
Dermatology 219:322-328, 2009

Background.—Photodynamic therapy (PDT) with aminolevulinic acid (ALA) has been shown to be an effective treatment for acne. However, the effect of ALA PDT on comedo formation has never been objectively evaluated. Cyanoacrylate follicular biopsy (CFB), a noninvasive procedure, has been proposed as the most reliable tool for studying follicular casts.

Objective.—To determine the possible effect of ALA and red light (550—700 nm) on macro- and microcomedones in acne patients.

Patients and Methods.—10 patients with mild-to-moderate facial and/or chest/back acne resistant to conventional therapies received ALA PDT at 2-week intervals in 3 sessions. The severity of acne had been estimated by a system of points, the Global Acne Grading System. The patients underwent PDT utilizing ALA 10% (face) or 15% (back/chest) and red light (15 J/cm^2 each session). CFBs were performed.

Results.—Four weeks after their last PDT session, the patients showed an average global score reduction of 50%. CFBs demonstrated a reduction in the total area, the average area and the density of macrocomedones.

Conclusion.—The results obtained in this study using CFB evaluation demonstrate that ALA PDT exerts an action on the comedogenic phase as well.

▶ This tantalizing article suffers from a common problem in laser and light acne studies; there is no control group. The authors compared before and after microcomedone counts in 10 patients treated with aminolevulinic acid (ALA) + ultraviolet (UV) light and found apparently significant reductions after 3 treatments given 2 weeks apart. But the lack of controls greatly hinders making much of this article. It is possible that UV light + ALA makes counts go down or perhaps only UV light is required—or perhaps it is all artifact and a larger study with controls would show no difference. I would love to see the authors get funding to do that larger study with a controlled methodology.

J. Q. Del Rosso, DO

Dermabrasion for Acne Scars During Treatment with Oral Isotretinoin

Bagatin E, dos Santos Guadanhim LR, Yarak S, et al (Hosp São Paulo, Brazil; Universidade Federal de São Paulo, Brazil)
Dermatol Surg 36:483-489, 2010

Background.—Oral isotretinoin is the criterion standard treatment for severe inflammatory acne associated with scar development. Atypical or exaggerated cicatrization related to oral isotretinoin was reported throughout the 1980s and 1990s. Dermabrasion for atrophic acne scar revision is not recommended 6 to 12 months from the end of oral isotretinoin treatment.

Objective.—To evaluate wound healing after localized dermabrasion in patients receiving oral isotretinoin.

Materials & Methods.—Interventional, prospective study involving seven patients taking oral isotretinoin to treat acne and with atrophic acne scars on the face. Manual dermabrasion was performed on all patients in an area of approximately 1 cm^2, and a 6-month reepithelization follow-up by clinical evaluation was conducted.

Results.—All patients presented normal cicatrization evolution; hypertrophic scarring or keloid as a result of localized abrasion was not observed, and atrophic acne scar revision result was excellent.

Conclusion.—The current recommendation to wait 6 to 12 months after treatment with oral isotretinoin for acne scar revision using dermabrasion should be re-evaluated. Abrasion of a small test area may be a useful predictor of wound healing, enabling earlier acne scar treatment using this procedure.

▶ In an effort to address the concerns regarding increased risk of scarring with dermabrasion performed during or within 6 months to a year following completion of isotretinoin therapy, these authors performed a 1 cm^2 area of manual dermabrasion of atrophic scars on the faces of 7 patients during isotretinoin therapy. Of the 7 patients, only 1 had evidence of hypertrophic scarring from acne. Three patients had dermabrasion on the cheeks; 2 patients received treatment on the forehead; and 1 each on the nose and temple. No evidence of hypertrophic scarring was noted as a result of the procedure. The mean dose of isotretinoin was 25 mg/day. The treatment period was not specified and 1 patient received drug for only 1 month. The authors suggest that additional studies of full facial dermabrasion are needed to reevaluate the recommendation to delay scar revision for 6 to 12 months after the completion of isotretinoin therapy. They recommend manual dermabrasion versus use of the motorized diamond fraise. The small number of patients in this study, the variety of areas treated, the limited exposure of patients to isotretinoin, and the lack of patients predisposed to hypertrophic scarring make it difficult to extrapolate these results to the general population of patients treated with isotretinoin. As a result, these data should be interpreted with caution until more rigorous and definitive studies are performed.

D. Thiboutot, MD

Hydroxychloroquine and lichen planopilaris: Efficacy and introduction of Lichen Planopilaris Activity Index scoring system

Chiang C, Sah D, Cho BK, et al (Dept of Dermatology at Univ of California, San Francisco; Palo Alto Med Foundation, Fremont, CA; Dept of Dermatology at Palo Alto Med Foundation, Mountain View, CA; et al)
J Am Acad Dermatol 62:387-392, 2010

Background.—Lichen planopilaris (LPP) and its variant frontal fibrosing alopecia (FFA) are primary lymphocytic cicatricial alopecias for which there is no evidence-based therapy.

Objective.—We assessed the efficacy of hydroxychloroquine in active LPP and FFA using the LPP Activity Index (LPPAI), a numeric score that allows quantification of the symptoms and signs of the condition for statistical comparison. In addition, we determined with the LPPAI if any improvement (reduction) in the numeric score pretreatment and posttreatment reached statistical significance.

Methods.—This was a retrospective, single-center chart review of 40 adult patients with LPP, FFA, or both who were treated with hydroxychloroquine for up to 12 months from 2004 to 2007 at the University of California, San Francisco Hair Center. Symptoms, signs, activity, and spreading were scored at each visit in the standardized cicatricial alopecia flow chart. A numeric score was assigned to these markers of disease activity and a numeric score was calculated at each visit.

Results.—There was significant reduction (*P* < .001) in the LPPAI at both 6 and 12 months. After 6 months, 69% had improved (reduced) symptoms and signs. At 12 months, 83% had improvement (reduction) in symptoms and signs.

Limitations.—Retrospective analysis and uncontrolled study are limitations.

Conclusions.—Hydroxychloroquine is effective in decreasing symptoms and signs in LPP and FFA as shown by significant reduction in the LPPAI in 69% and 83% of patients after 6 and 12 months of treatment, respectively.

▶ The implementation of the lichen planopilaris activity index (LPPAI) scoring system appears to be a reasonably effective tool for measuring the improvement of patients with lichen planopilaris (LPP). Like psoriasis area and severity index scores, there is subjective variance in the data collection process. However, when used to compare outcomes like in this study, it is effective at establishing a statistical relationship between LPP and hydroxychloroquine therapy. The researchers did downplay their lack of responders (those with 85% improvement of the LPPAI score) by combining the numbers of partial responders and responders and claiming that after 6 months of treatment 69% were full or partial responders. When you look at the table, there were zero responders for LPP and 1 frontal fibrosing alopecia responder at 6 months. At 12 months there were only 14% (4/29) responders for LPP. Moreover, the partial responders could range anywhere from 25% to 85% improvement of the

LPPAI. How many of these partial responders were at the 25% improvement end of the spectrum? It is our opinion that the ranges should be changed in future reports to best represent the actual clinical experience instead of simply presenting the data in an overall fashion, which is hard to translate to the clinical setting.

B. P. Glick, DO, MPH
T. J. Singer, DO
A. Wiener, DO

Inter-observer agreement on acne severity based on facial photographs
Beylot C, Groupe Expert Acné (GEA) (104 Boulevard Wilson, Bordeaux, France; et al)
J Eur Acad Dermatol Venereol 24:196-198, 2010

Background.—The three-grade acne classification (mild, moderate, severe) is widely used to define the licensed indications of acne treatments, and for therapeutic decision-making in clinical practice, but its reproducibility has never been assessed.

Methods.—Ten photographs of facial acne were scored independently by eight experts using the three-grade acne classification. We conducted a descriptive analysis of the results, based on graphical representation of the scores for each photograph.

Results.—Inter-observer agreement on acne severity based on the three-grade acne classification was very poor.

Conclusion.—The classical three-grade acne classification is poorly reproducible. A new rating tool accompanied by a clinical description of each severity level would be extremely useful.

▶ It is well known that there is significant intra- and interobserver variability in grading acne. This is of particular concern in the clinical trial setting. This straightforward study documented the poor interobserver agreement in evaluating photographs of patients with acne using a rating system of mild, moderate, and severe. Challenges in acne grading were noted in evaluating severity based on the amount of the face involved with acne. For example, it was difficult to classify a patient with extensive inflammatory acne on the forehead, yet the remainder of the face was relatively unaffected. As indicated by the authors, these data support the need for an effective acne grading system.

D. Thiboutot, MD

Isotretinoin Is Not Associated With Inflammatory Bowel Disease: A Population-Based Case-Control Study

Bernstein CN, Nugent Z, Longobardi T, et al (Univ of Manitoba IBD Clinical and Res Centre, Canada)
Am J Gastroenterol 104:2774-2778, 2009

Objectives.—There is anecdotal evidence that isotretinoin use is associated with development of colitis. We aimed at determining whether there is an association between isotretinoin use and development of inflammatory bowel disease (IBD).

Methods.—The population-based University of Manitoba IBD Epidemiology Database and a control group matched by age, sex, and geographical residence were linked to the provincial prescription drug registry, a registry that was initiated in 1995. The number of users and duration of isotretinoin use were identified in both IBD cases and controls.

Results.—We found that 1.2% of IBD cases used isotretinoin before IBD diagnosis, which was statistically similar to controls (1.1% users). This was also similar to the number of IBD patients who used isotretinoin after a diagnosis of IBD (1.1%). There was no difference between isotretinoin use before Crohn's disease compared with its use before ulcerative colitis.

Conclusions.—Patients with IBD were no more likely to have used isotretinoin before diagnosis than were sex-, age-, and geography-matched controls. Although there may be anecdotes of isotretinoin causing acute colitis, our data suggest that isotretinoin is not likely to cause chronic IBD.

▶ Isotretinoin has been potentially associated with a variety of side effects such as suicidal ideation and mood alteration. There have also been sporadic reports of inflammatory bowel disease (IBD). This is a population-based case-control study in Manitoba, Canada, from 1995 to 2007 examining the association between isotretinoin use and IBD. A case-control analysis evaluated a cohort of patients with IBD with matched population controls. There were 25 patients (1.2%) who received isotretinoin before their first diagnosis of IBD and 23 patients (1.1%) who used isotretinoin after IBD diagnosis. The mean number of days between the first isotretinoin prescription and initial IBD diagnosis (n = 24) was 1202.4 and the median number of days was 906. For 3 of the 25 patients who had prescriptions before diagnosis and also after diagnosis, their last prescriptions of isotretinoin were 41, 806, and 1107 days after their IBD diagnosis, respectively. The authors felt that the potential link between acne and IBD occurring around the same age may be coincidental. This study showed that there was no greater likelihood for isotretinoin use to be followed by a diagnosis of IBD than for isotretinoin to be used after IBD is diagnosed. There was a median of approximately 3 years between the last drug prescription and the first IBD diagnosis. A limitation to this study was that the authors did not examine whether isotretinoin could cause flaring of pre-existing IBD. The authors also did not comment on any other side effects noted with the use of isotretinoin. In the future, it would be interesting to examine whether specific genotypes for IBD developed disease after isotretinoin use. This study also demonstrated that it is rare for young patients with IBD to have used isotretinoin before their IBD diagnosis (1.2%), which was similar to controls (1.1%). This was also similar to the number of patients with IBD who used isotretinoin after a diagnosis of IBD (1.1%). The authors felt that isotretinoin use in association with true IBD appears to not be likely, and rates are no more elevated in patients using this medication compared to the general population.

J. Q. Del Rosso, DO

G. K. Kim, DO

Practical Guidelines for Evaluation of Loose Anagen Hair Syndrome
Cantatore-Francis JL, Orlow SJ (New York Univ Med Ctr, NY)
Arch Dermatol 145:1123-1128, 2009

Objectives.—To better categorize the epidemiologic profile, clinical features, and disease associations of loose anagen hair syndrome (LAHS) compared with other forms of childhood alopecia.

Design.—Retrospective survey.

Setting.—Academic pediatric dermatology practice.

Patients.—Three hundred seventy-four patients with alopecia referred from July 1, 1997, to June 31, 2007.

Main Outcome Measures.—Epidemiologic data for all forms of alopecia were ascertained, such as sex, age at onset, age at the time of evaluation, and clinical diagnosis. Patients with LAHS were further studied by the recording of family history, disease associations, hair-pull test or biopsy results, hair color, laboratory test result abnormalities, initial treatment, and involvement of eyelashes, eyebrows, and nails.

Results.—Approximately 10% of all children with alopecia had LAHS. The mean age (95% confidence interval) at onset differed between patients with LAHS (2.8 [1.2-4.3] years) vs patients without LAHS (7.1 [6.6-7.7] years) ($P < .001$), with 3 years being the most common age at onset for patients with LAHS. All but 1 of 37 patients with LAHS were female. The most common symptom reported was thin, sparse hair. Family histories were significant for LAHS (n = 1) and for alopecia areata (n = 3). In 32 of 33 patients, trichograms showed typical loose anagen hairs. Two children had underlying genetic syndromes. No associated laboratory test result abnormalities were noted among patients who underwent testing.

Conclusions.—Loose anagen hair syndrome is a common nonscarring alopecia in young girls with a history of sparse or fine hair. Before ordering extensive blood testing in young girls with diffusely thin hair, it is important to perform a hair-pull test, as a trichogram can be instrumental in the confirmation of a diagnosis of LAHS.

▶ Loose anagen hair syndrome (LAHS) is an autosomal dominant disorder with incomplete penetrance. Sporadic cases have also been reported. Clinically, patients are predominantly female children who present with light-colored, thin, sparse, and easily shedding hair without visible areas of hair loss. Some patients may have frizzy, unruly, or unmanageable hair. Subjects had greater than 50% of typical loose anagen hairs on examination of trichogram. In a retrospective review of 374 patients, 37 were found to have LAHS. After further investigation of these young patients, authors present a clinical guideline. Practical guidelines for the diagnosis of LAHS include the following: (1) high index of suspicion for LAHS (younger than 4 years of age; history of sparse, thin hair), (2) female sex or light-colored hair, (3) perform hair-pull test for trichogram before obtaining blood samples, (4) reassure parents that in most instances the condition will improve over time, and (5) treatment of choice is observation. Consider therapy with topical minoxidil in severe cases.

S. Bellew, DO

J. Q. Del Rosso, DO

Refractory Acne and 21-Hydroxylase Deficiency in a Selected Group of Female Patients

Caputo V, Fiorella S, Curiale S, et al (Univ of Palermo, Italy; et al)
Dermatology 220:121-127, 2010

Background.—Excessive androgen production, suspected in women when acne is accompanied by hirsutism and menstrual irregularities, may be due to congenital adrenal hyperplasia. This inherited disorder of cortisol biosynthesis is caused in more than 90—95% of all cases by 21-hydroxylase deficiency (21-OHD). The steroid 21-hydroxylase gene *(CYP21)* has a high degree of variability.

Objective.—This study was conducted to evaluate *CYP21* gene mutations in a selected group of women with papulopustular and comedonal acne refractory to treatment, irregular menses and hirsutism.

Methods.—30 out of 61 women enrolled underwent pelvic ultrasound examination and hormonal screening. In 9 patients with a polycystic ovary and hormonal pattern of adrenal hyperandrogenism a significant elevation of adrenocorticotropic hormone (ACTH) stimulated 17-hydroxyprogesterone was detected. These women positive in the ACTH stimulation test were submitted to *CYP21* gene analysis.

Results.—Genetic testing revealed several different point mutations and demonstrated that a cohort of patients resistant to acne therapy can be carriers or affected by non-classical 21-OHD (late onset).

Conclusion.—Persistent acne can be the unique presenting sign of non-classical 21-OHD. Evaluation of *CYP21* gene mutations may identify female carriers or patients for genetic counselling.

▶ *CYP21* encodes the 21-hydroxylase, which is deficient in 90% to 95% of patients with congenital adrenal hyperplasia (CAH). Sixty-one women with refractory acne, irregular menses, and hirsutism were screened for CAH, and

9 were identified. These women underwent genetic testing to screen for mutations in the *CYP21* gene. Certain point mutations were noted in each of the 9 patients compared that were not present in a control group of 109 subjects. These 9 women were either affected by nonclassical CAH or were carriers. The authors conclude that persistent acne can be the unique presenting sign of nonclassical 21-hydroxylase deficiency and that evaluation of *CYP21* gene mutations may identify female carriers or patients for genetic counseling. Persistent acne in women is known to be a presenting sign of a possible endocrine disorder. Because CAH can be diagnosed with simple testing, such as a serum 17-hydroxyprogesterone level and an adrenocorticotropic hormone stimulation test, the need for genetic testing is unclear. Furthermore, a larger sample would be required to ascertain the relevance of the point mutations found in these patients compared with the general population.

D. Thiboutot, MD

'Relaxers' damage hair: Evidence from amino acid analysis
Khumalo NP, Stone J, Gumedze F, et al (Univ of Cape Town, South Africa; Bristol Royal Infirmary, UK)
J Am Acad Dermatol 62:402-408, 2010

Background.—'Relaxers' are used by more than two thirds of African females to straighten hair, with easy grooming and increased length often cited as reasons. A recent study reported relaxed hair lengths much shorter than expected, suggesting increased fragility; the potential for scalp inflammation and scarring alopecia remains unclear.

Objective.—To investigate the biochemical effects of 'relaxers' on hair.

Methods.—With informed consent, included participants represented 3 groups: natural hair, asymptomatic relaxed hair, and symptomatic (brittle) relaxed hair. Biochemical analysis was performed by using a Biochrom 30 amino acid analyzer. Differences in amino acid levels were assessed using either Wilcoxon rank sum test or matched-pairs signed-rank test.

Results.—There was a decrease in cystine, citrulline, and arginine; however, an increase in glutamine was found in all relaxed compared to natural hair. Cystine levels (milligram per gram amino acid nitrogen) were similar in natural proximal and distal hair: 14 mg/g (range, 4-15 mg/g) versus 14 mg/g (range, 12-15 mg/g); $P = .139$. In asymptomatic relaxed hair, cystine levels were higher in less frequently relaxed samples proximal to scalp: 7.5 mg/g (5.6-12) versus 3.3 mg/g (1.3-9.2); $P = .005$. Cystine levels in distal asymptomatic relaxed and symptomatic relaxed hair were similar to each other and to those in the genetic hair fragility disease trichothiodystrophy.

Limitations.—It was not possible to analyze lye and no-lye 'relaxers' separately.

Conclusions.—'Relaxers' are associated with reduced cystine consistent with fragile damaged hair. A decrease in citrulline and glutamine has been associated with inflammation; prospective studies are needed to investigate whether or how 'relaxers' induce inflammation.

▶ Successful management of ethnic hair diseases means understanding both physiology and daily maintenance issues. The analysis of amino acid metabolism and the breakdown of the different components of the hair shaft provide an excellent review, but I found the correlation to how it impacts the way a patient can benefit from different hairstyles or use of certain products to be very practical. Unless it directly impacts someone close to you, or yourself, it is difficult to truly appreciate how significant alopecia affects a patient's daily life. But when it is augmented by the ethnic predisposition to a hair shaft defect and the progression induced by a necessary agent in maintaining a hairstyle, that frustration definitely escalates. I would read this article again and scrutinize the clinical aspects as closely as the science aspects.

N. Bhatia, MD

Specific dermatologic features of the polycystic ovary syndrome and its association with biochemical markers of the metabolic syndrome and hyperandrogenism
Özdemir S, Özdemir M, Görkemli H, et al (Selçuk Univ, Konya, Turkey)
Acta Obstet Gynecol Scand 89:199-204, 2010

Objective.—To investigate biochemical and metabolic abnormalities in relation with cutaneous features of polycystic ovary syndrome (PCOS).

Design.—Prospective descriptive analysis.

Setting.—University-based tertiary care.

Sample.—One-hundred and fifteen untreated consecutive women diagnosed as having PCOS.

Methods.—Each woman underwent an evaluation of body habitus, acne, hirsutism, seborrhea, androgenic alopecia and acanthosis nigricans. Associations between cutaneous features and hormonal and metabolic parameters were analyzed by means of multivariate logistic regression models.

Main Outcome Measures.—Prevalence of cutaneous features in PCOS and associations among the features and biochemical and metabolic parameters.

Results.—The prevalence of acne, hirsutism, seborrhea, androgenetic alopecia and acanthosis nigricans was 53%, 73.9%, 34.8%, 34.8% and 5.2%, respectively. Acne was not associated with the hormonal, metabolic and anthropometric variables. Hirsutism had positive associations with total testosterone, fasting glucose and total cholesterol, and a negative association with age. Seborrhea was found to be related with free testosterone, fasting glucose and insulin. A negative association was determined among androgenic alopecia and free testosterone, low-density lipoprotein and insulin.

Conclusions.—Acne and androgenic alopecia are not good markers for the hyperandrogenism in PCOS. Hirsutism appears to be strongly related with hyperandrogenism and metabolic abnormalities in PCOS women.

▶ It is clear that acne, hirsutism, androgenetic alopecia, and seborrhea are hormonally related. In this article, the authors examined 115 consecutive women with polycystic ovary syndrome (PCOS) based on the standardized Rotterdam criteria. Patients were evaluated for acne, hirsutism, androgenetic alopecia, seborrhea, and acanthosis nigricans. In addition, hormone levels and other metabolic parameters were examined. The mean age of the patients was 23 years (16-40 years). Acne was defined as the presence of comedones on the face, neck, chest, back, or upper arms. Seborrhea was evaluated based on a question to patients regarding their perception of greasiness of the skin. Androgenetic alopecia and hirsutism were evaluated using standard generally accepted scales. The reported prevalence of acne in the PCOS population ranges from 8% to 34%. This study reports a prevalence of 54% perhaps because of the nonquantitative and relatively nonspecific definition of acne. As in other studies, the authors report increased dehydroepiandrosterone sulfate and free testosterone in those with acne but no association with the other biochemical or metabolic parameters in the multivariate analysis. Seborrhea was more prevalent in the younger women, which is to be expected. It was associated with free testosterone, insulin, and glucose. Hirsutism was strongly correlated with hormones and metabolic parameters. The authors' conclusions in these patients with PCOS support the clinical findings in the general population of female patients in dermatology practices that acne and androgenetic alopecia are not strong markers for hyperandrogenism. That is not to discount, however, the need for a hormonal evaluation in women with a constellation of findings suggestive of hyperandrogenism. In addition, this study points to the need for standardized evaluation criteria for acne and seborrhea.

D. Thiboutot, MD

Adapalene—benzoyl peroxide, a unique fixed-dose combination topical gel for the treatment of acne vulgaris: a transatlantic, randomized, double-blind, controlled study in 1670 patients
Gollnick HPM, for the Adapalene—BPO Study Group (Otto-von-Guericke Universität Magdeburg, Germany; et al)
Br J Dermatol 161:1180-1189, 2009

Background.—Combination therapy utilizing agents with complementary mechanisms of action is recommended by acne guidelines to help simultaneously target multiple pathogenic factors. A unique, topical, fixed-dose combination gel with adapalene 0·1% and benzoyl peroxide (BPO) 2·5% has recently been developed for the once-daily treatment of acne.

Objectives.—To evaluate the efficacy and safety of adapalene 0·1%—BPO 2·5% fixed-dose combination gel (adapalene—BPO) relative to

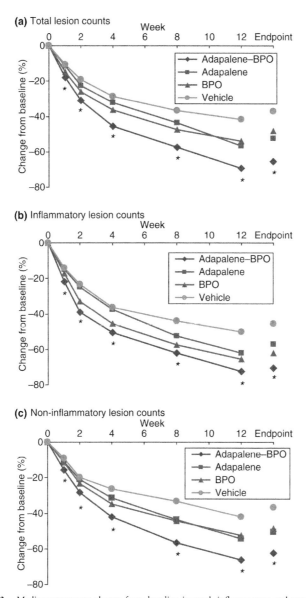

FIGURE 3.—Median percentage change from baseline in total, inflammatory and noninflammatory lesions (intent-to-treat population). (a) Total. *Differences between adapalene—benzoyl peroxide (BPO) and other treatment groups were all statistically significant (at least $P < 0.05$). (b) Inflammatory. *Differences between adapalene—BPO and other treatment groups were all statistically significant (at least $P < 0.05$) (c) Noninflammatory. *Differences between adapalene—BPO and other treatment groups were all statistically significant (at least $P < 0.05$), with the exception of week 1 vs. BPO ($P = 0.08$). (Reprinted from Gollnick HPM, for the Adapalene—BPO Study Group. Adapalene—benzoyl peroxide, a unique fixed-dose combination topical gel for the treatment of acne vulgaris: a transatlantic, randomized, double-blind, controlled study in 1670 patients. *Br J Dermatol.* 2009;161:1180-1189.)

adapalene 0·1% monotherapy (adapalene), BPO 2·5% monotherapy (BPO), and the gel vehicle (vehicle) in a large population for the treatment of acne vulgaris.

Methods.—In total, 1670 subjects were randomized in a double-blind controlled trial to receive adapalene—BPO, adapalene, BPO or vehicle for 12 weeks (1 : 1 : 1 : 1 randomization). Evaluations included success rate (subjects 'clear' or 'almost clear'), percentage change in lesion count from baseline, cutaneous tolerability and adverse events.

Results.—Adapalene—BPO was significantly more effective than corresponding monotherapies, with significant differences in percentage lesion count change observed as early as 1 week. Cutaneous tolerability profile was similar to adapalene. Adverse events were more frequent with the combination therapy (mainly due to an increase in mild-to-moderate dry skin), occurred early in the study, and were transient.

Conclusions.—Adapalene—BPO provides significantly greater and synergistic efficacy and a faster onset of action with an acceptable safety profile in the treatment of acne vulgaris when compared with the corresponding vehicle and the adapalene and BPO monotherapies (Fig 3).

▶ This is an interesting article that shows what is described as the synergistic activity of adapalene + benzoyl peroxide in reducing acne lesions. In Fig 3, the data for all lesions, inflammatory and noninflammatory lesions, are presented separately. The synergism seems to reside mainly in the reduction of comedones. To me, this is an unexpected and useful finding. Traditionally, comedones have been viewed as retinoid territory, but in this study that involves antibiotics in acne, it has been found that comedones are also reduced by drugs with anti—*Propionibacterium acnes* or anti-inflammatory activity. This study makes it quite clear that maximal comedones reduction is achieved with retinoid + anti—*P acnes* therapy, a lesson worth remembering the next time a patient with stubborn comedonal acne is in your office.

G. Webster, MD, PhD

Depressive symptoms and suicidal ideation during isotretinoin treatment: a 12-week follow-up study of male Finnish military conscripts
Rehn LMH, Meririnne E, Höök-Nikanne J, et al (Helsinki City Health Ctr, Finland; Centre for Military Medicine, Lahti, Finland; Lohja Hosp, Finland; et al)
J Eur Acad Dermatol Venereol 23:1294-1297, 2009

Objective.—To investigate the putative association between isotretinoin treatment and depressive symptoms or suicidal ideation among Finnish male military conscripts.

Methods.—Consecutive acne patients were enrolled into an uncontrolled, prospective 12-week follow-up study conducted at the Central Military Hospital, Helsinki, Finland. Of the 135 patients prescribed isotretinoin, 126 (93.3%) completed the follow-up. Depression and suicidal ideation were investigated with the Beck Depression Inventory (BDI) at baseline, weeks 4—6, and weeks 10—12.

Results.—BDI mean score was low at baseline and declined further significantly ($p < 0.001$) during the follow-up from 3.0 (SD 3.948) to 1.8 (SD 3.783) among patients on isotretinoin. Moreover, the proportion of patients with clinically significant depressive symptoms (BDI $\geq$ 10) declined non-significantly from 7.1 % to 3.2 %. Suicidal ideation was reported by 17 (13.5 %) patients at baseline and 9 (7.1%) patients at the end of the follow-up (NS). During the follow-up, one non-depressed patient attempted suicide while intoxicated by alcohol.

Conclusion.—On group level, isotretinoin seems not to be typically associated with treatment-emergent depression or suicidal ideation among young men. However, the possibility that individual patients may be susceptible for mood effects of isotretinoin as a rare idiosyncratic reaction can not be excluded.

▶ It's nice to have another article that finds no association between isotretinoin and mental issues, but the sample size is small. I doubt that one could expect to have a problem turn up in a group of this size because even if the association of isotretinoin and depression is real, it is an extremely uncommon one.

G. Webster, MD, PhD

Diet and acne
Bowe WP, Joshi SS, Shalita AR (State Univ of New York Downstate Med Ctr, Brooklyn; Northwestern Univ Feinberg School of Medicine, Chicago, IL)
J Am Acad Dermatol 63:124-141, 2010

Historically, the relationship between diet and acne has been highly controversial. Before the 1960s, certain foods were thought to exacerbate acne. However, subsequent studies dispelled these alleged associations as myth for almost half a century. Several studies during the last decade have prompted dermatologists to revisit the potential link between diet and acne. This article critically reviews the literature and discusses how dermatologists might address diet when counseling patients with acne. Dermatologists can no longer dismiss the association between diet and acne. Compelling evidence exists that high glycemic load diets may exacerbate acne. Dairy ingestion appears to be weakly associated with acne, and the roles of omega-3 fatty acids, antioxidants, zinc, vitamin A, and dietary fiber remain to be elucidated. This study was limited by the lack of randomized controlled trials in the literature. We hope that this review will encourage others to explore the effects of diet on acne.

▶ A dietary effect in acne has been claimed for generations. Invariably, food that is liked by teens or food that is greasy is blamed for causing zits. In most cases, this had the effect of blaming the kid for the disease and acne became another focus for rebellion. Some recent articles suggest that milk or more likely carbohydrates in general can worsen acne. Clearly, there appears to be something to this, but still there is not a coherent story that can reliably be given to patients. Until the value of diet in acne therapy is more clear, I'm going to focus on what I know will work.

G. Webster, MD, PhD

Infliximab therapy for patients with moderate to severe hidradenitis suppurativa: A randomized, double-blind, placebo-controlled crossover trial
Grant A, Gonzalez T, Montgomery MO, et al (Florida Academic Dermatology Ctrs, Miami; Centocor Inc, Horsham, PA)
J Am Acad Dermatol 62:205-217, 2010

Background.—Biologic therapies with anti—tumor necrosis factor agents are promising treatments for hidradenitis suppurativa (HS).

Objective.—We assessed the efficacy and safety of infliximab (IFX) for the treatment of moderate to severe HS.

Methods.—A prospective double-blind treatment phase of 8 weeks where patients received IFX or placebo was followed by an open-label phase where patients taking placebo were given the opportunity to cross over to IFX, and an observational phase. Primary treatment efficacy was based on HS Severity Index. Secondary end points included Dermatology Life Quality Index, visual analog scale, and Physician Global Assessment scores. Inflammatory markers erythrocyte sedimentation rate and C-reactive protein were also assessed.

Results.—More patients in the IFX than in the placebo group showed a 50% or greater decrease from baseline HS Severity Index score. In addition, statistically and clinically significant improvement from baseline was observed at week 8 in Dermatology Life Quality Index score, visual analog scale score, erythrocyte sedimentation rate, and C-reactive protein compared with placebo. Patients in the placebo group treated with IFX after week 8 (crossover) responded similarly to the original IFX group. Many patients withdrew during the observational phase to continue anti—tumor necrosis factor-alfa therapy. No unexpected serious adverse events were observed.

Limitations.—Results are representative of a single center, patients were treated by a single physician, some patients did not return after their last infusion, and the HS Severity Index requires validation.

Conclusions.—This clinical study represents the first formal assessment of IFX for treatment of moderate to severe HS. IFX was well tolerated, no unexpected safety issues were identified, and improvements in pain intensity, disease severity, and quality of life were demonstrated with concomitant reduction in clinical markers of inflammation.

▶ Hidradenitis suppurativa (HS) is a chronic debilitating inflammatory disease involving the intertriginous areas of the body where apocrine glands are abundant. HS is frustrating for the patient and the clinician, as existing treatment modalities have shown to be of limited value. These include general measures (weight loss, smoking cessation, and loose clothing), medical treatments (antibiotics, hormone therapy, retinoids, and corticosteroids), radiotherapy, carbon dioxide laser treatments, and surgical management; biologic therapies have emerged as a new treatment option for HS.[1] This is the first formal investigation of the safety and efficacy of infliximab (IFX) in treatment of moderate to severe HS. Thirty-eight patients were randomly assigned to either placebo or IFX treatment at 5 mg/kg administered intravenously. IFX is a chimeric IgG1 (kappa) monoclonal antibody against tumor necrosis factor-α. It is Food and Drug Administration approved for the treatment of rheumatoid arthritis, Crohn disease, ankylosing spondylitis, psoriatic arthritis, plaque psoriasis, and ulcerative colitis. Results indicate that IFX was well tolerated by patients with improvement of pain, disease severity, and quality of life. Concomitantly, there was reduction in clinical inflammatory markers. As stated by authors, limitations of the study include a single-center investigation, evaluation by a single physician, and most patients not returning following last infusion. IFX and other biologics may be a viable option for patients with HS; however, further investigations are needed in a multicenter trial.

S. Bellew, DO

J. Q. Del Rosso, DO

Reference

1. Slade DEM, Powell BW, Mortimer PS. Hidradenitis suppurativa: pathogenesis and management. *Br J Plast Surg.* 2003;56:451-461.

Photodynamic therapy of acne vulgaris using 5-aminolevulinic acid 0.5% liposomal spray and intense pulsed light in combination with topical keratolytic agents

de Leeuw J, van der Beek N, Bjerring P, et al (Outpatient clinic for dermatology and laser treatment, Hilversum, The Netherlands; Swansea Univ, Wales, UK; et al)
J Eur Acad Dermatol Venereol 24:460-469, 2010

Background.—Increasing antibiotic resistance of *Propionibacterium acnes* and growing awareness on the side effects of topical and systemic drugs in the treatment of acne vulgaris by physicians and patients have paved the way for a search into new efficacious and safe treatment modalities such as photodynamic therapy (PDT). Although the efficacy of PDT using 20% 5-aminolevulinic acid (ALA) cream has been established, phototoxic side effects limit its use. The 5-ALA concentration can be lowered by a factor of 40 by changing the vehicle of 5-ALA from a moisturizing cream to liposome encapsulation.

Objectives.—Assessment of the efficacy and the safety of PDT using 5-ALA 0.5% in liposomal spray and intense pulsed light (IPL) in combination with topical peeling agents (Li-PDT-PC) in acne vulgaris.

Materials and Methods.—32 patients suffering from acne participated in this randomized, prospective, single blind study. All patients were treated with Li-PDT-PC. During the study nine patients were additionally treated with topical or systemic antibiotics (Li-PDT-PC-AT). These patients were removed from the study although their results were recorded.

Results.—After a mean period of 7.8 months and a mean number of 5.7 treatments the mean total number of lesions dropped from 34.6 lesions to 11.0 lesions, resulting in a mean improvement of 68.2%. Side effects were minimal. Additionally, an intention to treat analysis was conducted.

Conclusion.—Photodynamic therapy of acne vulgaris using 5-ALA 0.5% liposomal spray and IPL in combination with topical peeling agents is safe and efficacious, even in patients with acne recalcitrant to standard therapy.

▶ In 2000 a benchmark study demonstrated that 20% aminolevulinic acid (ALA) photodynamic therapy (PDT) using high-dose red light to treat nodulocystic acne produced sustained clearances equivalent to isotretinoin therapy.[1] Efficacy was attributed to the destruction of the sebaceous gland and was confirmed by histology. However, the epidermal side effects of crusting, burning, scabbing, and prolonged hyperpigmentation caused by high-dose red light ALA-PDT created an engineering challenge in treating acne: how to impact the sebaceous gland without causing significant epidermal side effects. A novel ALA formulation used in this study (0.5% ALA in a liposomal vehicle) combined with a keratolytic agent and coupled with an intense pulsed light as the activating light source provides us with several interesting observations. Inflammatory and noninflammatory lesions could be significantly reduced, while cutaneous side effects were minimized. What was not addressed by the study and remains to be determined is the length of sustained clearance following this therapy. The numerous in-office treatments (mean 5.7 months over 7.8 months) and less-than-complete clearance (68%) in treated patients without long-term clearance data will give physicians cause for consideration before adopting this as a mainstream or an alternative acne therapy.

G. Martin, MD

Reference

1. Hongcharu W, Taylor CR, Chang Y, Aghassi D, Suthamjariya K, Anderson RR. Topical ALA-photodynamic therapy for the treatment of acne vulgaris. *J Invest Dermatol.* 2000;115:183-192.

Effect of Smooth Pulsed Light at 400 to 700 and 870 to 1,200 nm for Acne Vulgaris in Asian Skin

Kawana S, Tachihara R, Kato T, et al (Nippon Med School, Tokyo, Japan)
Dermatol Surg 36:52-57, 2010

Background.—Intense pulsed light (IPL) treatment is effective for acne in Caucasians, but no significant improvements have been observed in studies on Asian skin.

Objective.—To evaluate the efficacy and safety of IPL on acne vulgaris in Asian skin.

Methods.—Twenty-five Japanese patients, mainly of skin phototypes III or IV and moderate to severe acne, were treated five times with IPL at wavelengths of 400 to 700 nm and 870 to 1,200 nm. Results were evaluated in terms of changes in numbers of noninflammatory comedones and inflammatory papules, pustules, and cysts and acne grade before and after treatment.

Results.—After the first exposure, numbers of noninflammatory and inflammatory acne lesions decreased to 36.6% and 43.0%, respectively, of their pretreatment values. After five treatments, they decreased to 12.9% and 11.7%, respectively, of their pretreatment values. Acne grade improved significantly over the course of the study. Transient erythema, with or without burning or stinging, was noted in 20 (80%) patients, but no major adverse reactions were observed.

Conclusion.—IPL with dominant wavelengths of 400 to 700 nm had a satisfactory effect on acne vulgaris in Asians.

▶ Most articles reporting success in the treatment of acne with laser or light suffer from 2 critical flaws: different dosages of light are given to each patient and/or other acne medicines are continued during the phototherapy. This article commits neither of these sins but still is imperfect. Lesion counts done from photos are highly unreliable and insensitive (and the photos shown in the article are not in good focus). Moreover, the results are expressed as percent improvement with no raw lesion counts presented. This can be misleading. A patient with 4 zits who has 2 go away has the same percentage of improvement as a one with starting count of 50 that went to 25. Also milder acne is more prone to spontaneous improvement. Having said all that, this is still one of the better articles in the field of "lasers and lights for acne" and is probably true. Two big questions remain with the treatment. The mechanism of action of light in acne is still unknown. I suspect that the primary action is anti-inflammatory rather than anti-P acnes, but definitive studies are lacking. The other more pressing question is how cost effective is light compared with say benzoyl peroxide (BP)? BP is a drug with no major safety concerns and is cheap. Light is safe but decidedly not cheap. Which patients would benefit from light and which should stay on standard medications? Well-done studies, and more of them, are needed.

G. Webster, MD, PhD

7 Photobiology

A 20-year analysis of previous and emerging allergens that elicit photoallergic contact dermatitis
Victor FC, Cohen DE, Soter NA (New York Univ School of Medicine)
J Am Acad Dermatol 62:605-610, 2010

Background.—Retrospective chart reviews are periodically needed to update allergen series to detect changes in photoallergic contact dermatitis (PACD) over time.

Objective.—We sought to evaluate photopatch test results during a 13-year period and extend the observations to 20 years.

Methods.—A retrospective chart review was conducted in patients who were photopatch tested.

Results.—In all, 76 patients were evaluated. A total of 69 positive photopatch and 45 positive patch test reactions were detected in 30 and 23 patients, respectively. The frequencies of the positive photopatch test reactions were sunscreens 23.2%, antimicrobial agents 23.2%, medications 20.3%, fragrances 13%, plants and plant derivatives 11.6%, and pesticides 8.7%. Of the positive photopatch reactions to antimicrobial agents, 60% were caused by Fentichlor.

Limitations.—This study was a retrospective chart analysis, and the number of patients was small.

Conclusions.—Sunscreens and antimicrobial agents were the most frequent allergens eliciting PACD, and there was a decrease in PACD caused by fragrances. The number of reactions to medications increased. This study also demonstrated that pesticides can be a cause of PACD. The detection of reactions to Fentichlor was unexpected and, although they have been attributed in some studies to cross-reactions to sulfanilamides and bithionol, such a robust association was not observed in this study. This study extends our experience of the changes in the allergens that elicit PACD to 20 years.

▶ The thorough evaluation of suspected photoallergic contact dermatitis is often hampered by a lack of availability of testing centers, the complexity of the test performance, and the inconvenience of many visits within a 1-week period. Consequently, the infrequent nature of this disorder in the differential diagnosis of eczematous dermatitis results in a relative dearth of literature on the prevalence of antigens that are responsible for the disease. This is compounded by regional variations in the reactivity of some allergens based on the usage of personal hygiene products and through natural variation in airborne plant allergens. The use of longitudinal studies in the field of contact allergy allows for the detection of trends in human reactivity that may mimic certain exposure patterns. Because photoallergic dermatitis also requires the cofactor of ultraviolet light, the genesis of the disorder is more difficult to detect. As observed in some other studies, the reactivity to fragranced products has decreased somewhat, while those to sunscreens remains more robust. Even if elaborate photopatch testing is not readily available, reasonable recommendations may be able to be dispatched to patients based on the population studies done regionally.

D. E. Cohen, MD, MPH

Contact and photocontact sensitization in chronic actinic dermatitis: a changing picture
Chew A-L, Bashir SJ, Hawk JLM, et al (St Thomas' Hosp, London, UK; King's College Hosp, Denmark Hill, London, UK; et al)
Contact Dermatitis 62:42-46, 2010

Background.—Patients with chronic actinic dermatitis (CAD) frequently have positive patch or photopatch tests. In our previous study (period 1987—1992), the most prominent contact allergen was the sesquiterpene lactone mix (36% of patients with CAD).

Objective.—To assess whether contact allergy profiles in CAD patients between 2000 and 2005 have changed in respect to our previous data (1987—1992).

Patients and Methods.—Fifty CAD patient records from 2000 to 2005 for patch and photopatch testing were retrospectively analysed and data were compared with that from 86 patients seen between 1987 and 1992.

Results.—Thirty-two (64%) and 64 (74%) patients had positive patch or photopatch tests in 2000—2005 and 1987—1992, respectively. The allergen profile has altered. A decline in sesquiterpene lactone mix positive reactions was noted: 29 (36%) patients were positive in 1987—1992 and 10 (20%) patients in 2000—2005, but this was not significant ($P = 0.08$). Reactions to non-fragrance consumer allergens (i.e. p-phenylenediamine and preservatives) had risen from 7 reactions (1987—1992) to 21 reactions in 13 individuals (2000—2005) ($P < 0.001$). Of these allergens, p-phenylenediamine was the most common (12%; $P = 0.004$).

Conclusions.—A significant rise in positive patch tests to non-fragrance consumer allergens, particularly p-phenylenediamine, was seen in CAD patients in 2000—2005. We speculate this alteration of allergen profile may be partly due to changes in exposure patterns.

▶ Chronic actinic dermatitis is a relatively rare disorder characterized by a photo-distributed eruption occurring in patients with documented reduced minimum erythema doses to ultraviolet (UV) A, UVB, or visible light. These patients frequently have positive patch and photopatch test reactions to several classes of chemicals. Their clinical relevance has been challenging to determine and consequently connect to the genesis of the eruption. This study from England exemplifies the necessity to continue to monitor the prevalence of reactions to patch test and photopatch test chemicals because the emergence of trends is likely to mirror exposure patterns in patients over time. The reduction, if the airborne sesquiterpene lactone reactivity with an increase in p-phenylenediamine, suggests that exposure patterns at home and work may influence these reactions. As our patients use different products either from our clinical recommendations or through marketing means, their reactivity may be reflected in population trends in reactivity.[1] Further study to survey these trends is necessary to determine whether they are actual in chronic actinic dermatitis or a phenomenon of earlier detection and evaluation.

D. E. Cohen, MD, MPH

Reference

1. Victor FC, Cohen DE, Soter NA. A 20-year analysis of previous and emerging allergens that elicit photoallergic contact dermatitis. *J Am Acad Dermatol.* 2010;62:605-610.

The relation between the amount of sunscreen applied and the sun protection factor in Asian skin
Kim SM, Oh BH, Lee YW, et al (Konkuk Univ School of Medicine, Seoul, Korea)
J Am Acad Dermatol 62:218-222, 2010

Background.—The measurement of the sun protection factor (SPF) is the usual method in the examination of the effectiveness of sunscreen. The declared SPF is based on the use of a sunscreen layer of 2 mg/cm^2. However, only around a quarter (0.5 mg/cm^2) of this amount is generally used in real life. Theoretical calculations have suggested that the effectiveness of SPF is related to sunscreen quantity in an exponential way but this was not confirmed in Asian skin.

Objectives.—This study was performed to investigate the change in SPF values when less than the recommended amount of sunscreen was applied.

Methods.—A board divided into 10 areas measuring 7×4 cm was placed on the back of 15 healthy volunteers. Low- and high-SPF standard reference sunscreens, and two types of sunscreen (SPF 30 and 35) were each applied on 4 areas, 0.5, 1.0, 1.5, and 2.0 mg/cm^2, respectively, and were left to dry for 20 minutes. The irradiation was conducted at a distance of 50 cm using a template (1×1 cm) placed directly on the skin with 10 windows allowing ultraviolet (UV) radiation to pass through with a dose increment of 20%. Erythema was evaluated 20 to 24 hours after exposure to UV radiation.

Results.—Sunscreen showed its expected SPF value when 2.0 mg/cm^2 was applied. The SPF values of the different amounts were significantly different from each other and decreased when less was applied ($P < .05$).

The relation between the amount of sunscreen applied and the SPF provided was most likely to follow exponential growth.

Limitations.—Spectral differences between our solar simulator and the UV sources of commercial laboratories are likely to be important. In addition, differences in sunscreen application techniques may have influenced the ultimate SPF values.

Conclusions.—This study concludes that to get the expected SPF value, it is important to apply the UV protective sunscreen precisely in the amount of 2.0 mg/cm^2 on Asian skin as recommended by the Food and Drug Administration. In addition, it was difficult to predict the SPF values when the usual amount of 0.5 mg/cm^2 was applied.

▶ Sunscreen has been encouraged by clinicians to prevent malignant and premalignant skin lesions. An amount of 2 mg/cm^2 needs to be applied for the claimed sun protective factor (SPF) according to the Federal Drug Administration. However, in real life, an average of 0.5 mg/cm^2 is usually applied. In the past, dermatologists believed that the amount of sunscreen applied was linear in relation to SPF protection, and there may be data to suggest otherwise. This is a study of 15 healthy Korean volunteers using 2 types of sunscreen (SPF 30, 35), applying them in an area of 0.5, 1.0, 1.5, 1.5, and 2.0 mg/cm^2, and examining the outcome. All patients had Fitzpatrick skin types III and IV. Sunscreen A (SPF 30) contained titanium dioxide and octocrylene and sunscreen B (SPF 35) contained octyl methoxycinnamate and were applied 20 minutes before irradiation to a solar simulator. Minimal erythema dose (MED) was determined as the lowest of 10 ultraviolet doses at which faint erythema was observed. The SPF decreased when less was applied ($P < .05$). When 2.0 mg/cm^2 of sunscreen was applied, the mean SPF values of sunscreen A and B were 82.1% and 92.9%, respectively. The authors found that the amount of sunscreen applied and the SPF was nonlinear but rather exponentially related. Limitations to this study were that it was conducted only on Asians with a Fitzpatrick skin type III/IV, and results may vary with other skin types with varying MED. Also, the study was conducted on the back of patients, and results may vary on other locations of the body. To add, artificial sunlight may also yield different results as compared with natural sunlight. This study may suggest that patients may need more explicit instructions on correct sunscreening application. Clinicians may also need to suggest higher SPF, anticipating that patients may not be applying sunscreen correctly. However, this study does not address the effect of reapplication and if reapplication may then also have an exponential benefit or demonstrate additive SPF. In conclusion, this study illustrates that SPF and the amount applied should not be considered linear but rather exponential.

J. Q. Del Rosso, DO
G. K. Kim, DO

Topical aminolaevulinic acid- and aminolaevulinic acid methyl ester-based photodynamic therapy with red and violet light: influence of wavelength on pain and erythema

Mikolajewska P, Iani V, Juzeniene A, et al (Rikshospitalet-Radiumhospitalet Medical Center, Montebello, Oslo, Norway)
Br J Dermatol 161:1173-1179, 2009

Background.—Photodynamic therapy (PDT) is based on the combination of an exogenously administered precursor of photosensitizer [protoporphyrin IX (PpIX)] synthesis and exposure to light. Choosing the optimal wavelength is important. Red light penetrates deeper into tissue, while violet light is more efficient in activating PpIX but does not penetrate so deeply.

Objectives.—We studied PpIX formation and the PDT effect after application to human skin of creams containing aminolaevulinic acid (ALA) and aminolaevulinic acid methyl ester (MAL). The aim of the study was to investigate whether the wavelength of the light used has an influence on pain sensations during topical PDT with the different prodrugs.

Methods.—Methods ALA cream (10%) and MAL cream (10%) were topically applied on the skin of 10 healthy volunteers. After 24 h the application site was exposed to 8 mW cm^{-2} violet laser or to 100 mW cm^{-2} red laser light. The erythema index was monitored up to 24 h after light exposure. For the first time the pain during topical ALA- and MAL-PDT was assessed by measuring the time taken for pain to occur. Also, for the first time, the intensities of the light sources were calibrated so as to have the same relative quantum efficiency.

Results.—The pain sensation during ALA-PDT with red light came 22 s sooner than during ALA-PDT with violet light, which is statistically significant ($P < 0.05$). Moreover, ALA-PDT with red light gave stronger and more persistent erythema than ALA-PDT with violet light. ALA induced about three times more PpIX than MAL. No statistically significant differences were found for erythema, or for the time for pain to occur, in the case of MAL-PDT with red vs. violet light.

Conclusions.—Topical ALA-PDT with violet light allows longer exposure times before pain is induced and gives less erythema as compared with topical ALA-PDT with red light.

▶ Pain during photodynamic therapy (PDT) limits its use in many patients. Presumably, the sensory nerves would be beneath the level of actinic keratosis pathology and thus a regimen/light source could be developed that makes this therapy more tolerable. If pain is to be minimized with the use of PDT for deeper processes such as nodular basal cell carcinoma or acne vulgaris, it would seem to require a targeted therapy rather than modulating light dosages with a nonspecific photoactive drug.

G. Webster, MD, PhD

Treatment of Angiofibromas of Tuberous Sclerosis with 5-Aminolevulinic Acid Blue Light Photodynamic Therapy Followed by Immediate Pulsed Dye Laser
Weinberger CH, Endrizzi B, Hook KP, et al (Univ of Minnesota, Minneapolis)
Dermatol Surg 35:1849-1851, 2009

Angiofibromas of tuberous sclerosis are often disfiguring, proliferative, and symptomatic. We sought to develop a treatment that would fulfill several criteria. First, discomfort should be minimal, alleviating the need for general anesthesia. Second, wound care should be simple. Third, improved appearance and symptoms are critical. Finally, because recurrence occurs even with aggressive treatments, the treatment must be repeatable. Here we report a novel treatment meeting these objectives.

▶ This study presents some interesting data on the use of topical aminolevulinic acid photodynamic therapy to treat angiofibromas of tuberous sclerosis. There was some response in some patients that deserves further study in a randomized controlled manner. Hopefully, the optimization of the treatment parameters will occur in these future studies.

E. A. Tanghetti, MD

8 Collagen Vascular and Related Disorders

A rare case of frontal linear scleroderma (*en coup de sabre*) with intra-oral and dental involvement
Pace C, Ward SE, Pace A (Charles Clifford Dental Hosp/Royal Hallamshire Hosp, Sheffield, UK; Rotherham Community Centre, UK)
Br Dent J 208:249-250, 2010

En coup de sabre is a linear scleroderma that presents on the frontal or frontoparietal scalp. This case describes a 36-year-old female who presented with a history of *en coup de sabre* with subsequent oral and dental involvement which to the authors' knowledge has never been reported previously. The clinical presentation, pathology and laboratory findings together with a brief discussion of the management of this case are discussed.

▶ Linear scleroderma describes a localized area of excessive collagen deposition usually without the involvement of systemic organs as seen in systemic sclerosis. It can in some cases also affect underlying structures, producing bony defects, visual disturbances, and dental abnormalities. This is a single-case report of a 36-year-old female presenting with a hypopigmented atrophic linear plaque approximately 6-cm wide on the right side of the forehead, extending to the frontal scalp with associated alopecia. Intraoral examination revealed extension with involvement of the upper right central incisor together with gingival recession. The patient underwent a number of surgical procedures including excision of the lesion on the forehead followed by tissue expansion of the scalp. For correction of the incisor, tooth extraction with a prosthesis replacement was completed. The patient also had a computerized tomogram (CT) of the head that was normal with no underlying cerebral lesions or bone loss. The incidence of dental abnormalities is sporadic, and progressive hemifacial atrophy (Parry-Romberg Syndrome) has also been associated with localized scleroderma with the relationship between the 2 disease entities being controversial. Although this was a single-case report, it reiterates a point that patients who present with linear scleroderma deserve a thorough examination that includes an oral exam. This report also demonstrated the importance of a CT of the head to rule out other cerebral abnormalities that may accompany linear scleroderma. In addition, patients can present with new symptoms after the disease has been quiescent for many years and should be monitored for any new neurological changes, a caveat not discussed in this article. Another important aspect of the disease that was demonstrated in this case report was the importance of surgical repair and reconstructive surgery being best performed after the disease has essentially burned out, which may take several months to years depending on the individual. Although this was a single-case report, it re-emphasized many clinically relevant aspects of linear scleroderma and important monitoring suggestions to aid the clinician.

J. Q. Del Rosso, DO

G. K. Kim, DO

Scar classification in cutaneous lupus erythematosus: morphological description
Al-Refu K, Goodfield M (Mutah Univ, Karak, Jordan)
Br J Dermatol 161:1052-1058, 2009

Background.—Scarring represents the single most debilitating aspect of discoid lupus erythematosus (DLE) in patients with cutaneous lesions alone. Despite this, there have been no studies which have attempted to classify the types of scars seen in this chronic disease.

Objectives.—The aim was to classify the types of scars based on morphological description.

Patients and Methods.—Forty-five patients with histologically confirmed DLE were included in the study. In the assessment of the types of scars, the scars were scored initially according to their anatomical localization. Each anatomical area was assessed for the types of scars which occurred in these areas.

Results.—Scars in patients with DLE were initially classified morphologically into six types according to the site of the scar and then each type was classified into subtypes according to the morphology of the scar. Scars were seen in the majority of the patients and scarring affected mostly areas including the scalp, other hairy areas such as the eyebrows, nonhairy areas, mucosa, fatty layers of the skin and the nails. This study demonstrated that scars may not only produce textural changes but may also produce pigmentary changes. It is possible that other types of scars may yet occur in DLE but have not so far been detected.

Conclusions.—Early classification and identification of the types of scars in these patients may change management towards more aggressive therapy in those with continued disease activity, and it is possible that different types of scarring require different therapies.

▶ Chronic cutaneous lupus erythematosus is characterized by lesions of discoid lupus erythematosus (DLE) that can be localized or generalized. The authors reason that early classification of scar types in patients with DLE might affect management and even go further to suggest that different types of scarring require different therapies.

Forty-five patients with DLE were studied. Twenty-six had generalized disease, and 19 had localized disease. Thirteen of the patients fulfilled American Rheumatism Association criteria for the diagnosis of systemic lupus erythematosus, and 44 of 45 had scarring. Scars were classified according to site and then morphology. The 6 possible sites were scalp, other hairy areas, nonhairy areas, mucosa, fatty layers of the skin, and nails. Scars were further evaluated as to whether they produced textural changes and/or pigmentary changes. The authors observed that multiple scars were most common with only 6.6% of patients having a single lesion, 20% having a few lesions, and 71% having multiple scarred lesions. The scalp was the most common site of involvement affecting 50% of patients. All of the patients with scarring of the scalp had scars elsewhere as well. Atrophic scars were the most common type, occurring in 55% of patients and pigmentary changes, including hypopigmented or hyperpigmented patches, occurred in 47% of patients. Poikiloderma-like changes, cribriform scarring, pitting acneiform scars, hypertrophic scars, and anetoderma were described. Lupus profundus resulting in loss of cutaneous tissue and significant deformity occurred in 8.8% of patients. There were 4 cases of nail involvement, including subungual hyperkeratosis, longitudinal striae, discoloration, and nail crumbling. Mucosal scarring occurred in 11% of patients and included nasal, oral, and perineal lesions.

Albrecht et al[1] previously developed the Cutaneous Lupus Erythematosus Disease Area and Severity Index to measure the severity of skin changes in this disorder. Their score includes an activity scale measuring erythema, scaling and hypertrophy, and mucous membrane disease and a damage scale that measures hyperpigmentation, atrophy, and scarring alopecia. The authors of this article make a bold attempt to further classify the scars that occur in cutaneous lupus erythematosus. Unfortunately, the scars are too varied, occurring in multiple sites and have very variable clinical presentations. The authors did point out some clinically useful information, including the presence of multiple scars, the frequency of scalp involvement, and the wide variations found in the scars of chronic cutaneous lupus erythematosus. Unfortunately, we are still without a simple classification system for this disorder.

M. Lebwohl, MD

Reference

1. Albrecht J, Taylor L, Berlin JA, et al. The CLASI (Cutaneous Lupus Erythematosus Disease Area and Severity Index): an outcome instrument for cutaneous lupus erythematosus. *J Invest Dermatol.* 2005;125:889-894.

Histopathology and immunohistochemistry of depigmented lesions in lupus erythematosus

França AFEC, de Souza EM (Univ of Campinas [UNICAMP], SP, Brazil)
J Cutan Pathol 37:559-564, 2010

Background.—Depigmented lesions (DL) have been described in areas previously damaged by inflammation in lupus erythematosus (LE). In the absence of typical lesions, distinction with other achromic diseases might be challenging. We studied the histological features and the behavior of melanocytes in these lesions.

Methods.—Tissue sections of 12 patients with lupus and DL were stained with hematoxylin-eosin, periodic acid-Schiff and Fontana-Masson. Melanocytes were counted by immunohistochemistry methods using Melan A and HMB-45. Ten biopsies of normal skin were used as controls.

Results.—The most common histological findings were: cellular infiltration (75%); hyperkeratosis (66.7%); thickening of basement membrane (66.7%); thinning and flattening of the epidermis (58.3%) and degenerative changes in collagen fibers (50%). Epidermal melanin and melanocytes were found in 41.7%. The melanocyte counts by HMB-45 and Melan A were significantly lower than in normal skin.

Conclusions.—The DL still fulfill histological criteria for lupus. In the absence of a precise histological diagnosis, thickening of basement membrane, hyperkeratosis, cellular infiltration, epidermal atrophy and elastosis are the most common features. Loss of melanocytes and the dermal fibrosis suggests that DL in cutaneous LE behave as post-inflammatory scars.

▶ In this study, the histopathologic features of depigmented lesions in lupus erythematosus (LE) were evaluated. Clinically, the depigmented lesions of LE may be indistinguishable from other dermatoses, such as vitiligo. The authors evaluated biopsy specimens from 12 patients with LE with depigmented lesions. Thickened basement membrane was noted in 66% of cases. Other common findings were hyperkeratosis, epidermal atrophy, loss of rete ridges, and the presence of inflammatory infiltrates. Evaluation of melanocytes revealed decreased number of melanocytes but no loss of melanocyte activity. Overall, the findings suggested scarring. Although the number of cases is small, the data suggest that histopathologic features of depigmented lesions in LE may help to distinguish these from other clinical entities with depigmented lesions.

S. M. Purcell, DO

Immune-mediated skin lesions in patients treated with anti-tumour necrosis factor alpha inhibitors

Exarchou SA, Voulgari PV, Markatseli TE, et al (Univ of Ioannina, Greece)
Scand J Rheumatol 38:328-331, 2009

Objective.—To describe immune-mediated skin lesion (IMSL) development in patients during anti-tumour necrosis factor (TNF) therapy.

Methods.—Two hundred and fifty-two patients with rheumatoid arthritis (RA) and 183 with spondyloarthropathies (SpA) treated with anti-TNF inhibitors were analysed to identify IMSLs.

Results.—Of the 252 patients with RA (146 treated with infliximab, 72 with adalimumab, and 34 with etanercept), 32 developed IMSLs. Eleven patients developed psoriatic skin lesions, 10 presented with granuloma annulare (GA), five had skin vasculitis, two alopecia areata, two discoid lupus erythematosus, one lichenoid eruption (lichen planus), and one vitiligo. Of the 183 patients with SpA (138 treated with infliximab, 37 with etanercept, and eight with adalimumab), 10 cases with IMSLs were identified. All were treated with infliximab. More specifically, six patients with ankylosing spondylitis (AS) developed psoriatic skin lesions, one developed GA, one lichen planus, and one alopecia areata. In addition, one patient with psoriatic arthritis (PsA) developed skin vasculitis. The occurrence of these IMSLs ranged from 3 to 36 months with a median of 20 months. Of all the patients with IMSL development, two with psoriatic skin lesions, two with GA, and one with vasculitis stopped anti-TNF therapy because of the extent and severity of the skin lesions.

Conclusions.—Our results on patients treated with TNF antagonists strongly support a link between TNF inhibition and IMSL development. Although these clinical complications are rare, clinicians should be aware of their occurrence and should recognize them.

▶ Antitumor necrosis factor alpha (anti-TNF-α) has been used in several inflammatory conditions, such as rheumatoid arthritis (RA), ankylosing spondylitis (AS), psoriatic arthritis (PsA), cutaneous psoriasis, and Crohn disease. This is a cohort of 252 patients with RA and 183 patients with AS treated with anti-TNF inhibitors analyzed for immune-mediated skin lesions (IMSLs). In this study, 32 patients (12.7%) developed IMSLs. There were 11 patients who developed psoriatic skin lesions, 10 granuloma annulare (GA), 5 cutaneous vasculitis, 2 alopecia areata, 2 discoid lupus erythematosus, 1 lichen planus, and 1 vitiligo. Of the 93 patients with AS, 9 developed IMSLs (6 psoriatic skin lesions, 1 GA, 1 lichen planus, and 1 alopecia areata), whereas only 1 patient with PsA developed vasculitis. The occurrence of these IMSLs ranged between 3 to 36 months with a median of 20 months of TNF therapy. All patients with IMSLs were treated with local corticosteroid therapy with good results. There was no difference in outcome comparing different anti-TNF-α therapies. However, proving that the drug alone was the precipitating agent with a median of 20 months may not be substantial evidence. Patients may either have a predisposition to developing IMSLs, may have been taking other drugs not identified as possible causative factors, or have other unidentified precipitating agents to IMSLs other than anti-TNF therapy. Also, no auto-immune workup or screen was conducted for these patients, such as the 2 patients who developed discoid lupus erythematosus. Although the authors concluded that there may be a strong association between anti-TNF therapy and IMSL development, it may be that patients have a genetic predisposition to developing IMSL, or it may accompany their pre-existing disease. In the future, age and sex-matched controls are needed to examine whether anti-TNF therapy is the true culprit in causing or promoting IMSLs.

J. Q. Del Rosso, DO

G. K. Kim, DO

Interstitial Lung Disease in Classic and Skin-Predominant Dermatomyositis: A Retrospective Study With Screening Recommendations

Morganroth PA, Kreider ME, Okawa J, et al (Philadelphia VA Med Ctr, PA; Univ of Pennsylvania, Philadelphia)
Arch Dermatol 146:729-738, 2010

Objectives.—(1) To determine the prevalence of interstitial lung disease (ILD) and isolated low diffusing capacity for carbon monoxide (DLCO) in a large cohort of outpatients with dermatomyositis. (2) To compare the pulmonary abnormalities of patients with classic dermatomyositis and those with skin-predominant dermatomyositis.

Design.—Retrospective cohort study.

Setting.—University hospital outpatient dermatology referral center.

Patients.—Medical records of 91 outpatients with adult-onset dermatomyositis seen between May 26, 2006, and May 25, 2009, were reviewed.

Main Outcome Measures.—Presence of ILD on thin-slice chest computed tomographic (CT) scans and DLCO.

Results.—Of the 71 patients with dermatomyositis who had CT or DLCO data, 16 of 17 (23%; 95% confidence interval [CI], 13%-33%) had ILD as defined by CT results. All patients with ILD had a reduced DLCO, and the ILD prevalence was not different between patients with skin-predominant dermatomyositis (10 of 35 [29%]) and those with classic dermatomyositis (6 of 36 [17%]) ($P = .27$). Eighteen of 71 patients with dermatomyositis (25%; 95% CI, 15%-36%) (7 of 35 [20%] with skin-predominant dermatomyositis; 11 of 36 [31%] with classic dermatomyositis; $P = .41$) had a low DLCO in the absence of CT findings showing ILD. The prevalence of malignant disease was higher in patients with classic dermatomyositis than in those with skin-predominant dermatomyositis ($P = .02$), and no patients with skin-predominant dermatomyositis had internal malignant disease.

Conclusions.—Radiologic ILD and isolated DLCO reductions, which may signify early ILD or pulmonary hypertension, are common in dermatology outpatients with both classic and skin-predominant dermatomyositis.

Because DLCO testing is both inexpensive and sensitive for pulmonary disease, it may be appropriate to screen all patients with dermatomyositis with serial DLCO measurements and base further testing on DLCO results.

▶ Interstitial lung disease (ILD) has been known to be associated with certain autoimmune diseases, such as dermatomyositis (DM). This is a retrospective study to determine the prevalence of ILD by evaluating diffusion capacity for carbon monoxide (DLCO) and CT scans in a large cohort of patients in a tertiary care center. Patients were classified as classic DM (CDM) or predominant skin DM (SDM). Pulmonary function tests (PFTs) with DLCO values without corrected hemoglobin were recorded. CT scans of the chest were also recorded to help confirm the diagnosis of ILD. There were 7 patients who had overlap with other connective tissue diseases. Authors found that 13% (6 of 47) of patients had higher rates of internal malignant disease in patients with CDM compared with none in patients with SDM. Sixteen of 71 (23%) patients were considered to have ILD based on CT results. There was no statistically significant difference ($P = .27$) between the prevalence of ILD in patients with SDM and those with CDM. Patients with at least 1 normal lung test and no abnormal test results were considered to have no evidence of ILD. Eighteen of 71 patients fell into the middle category with lung diffusion abnormality of uncertain clinical significance. The mean duration of follow-up was 25 months, which was a limitation of the study because patients may have developed lung disease later on in life. Eleven of 12 patients were treated with high-dose glucocorticoids and 10 of 12 patients were treated with immunosuppressants. Of the patients with at least 6 months of follow-up, 8 of 11 (73%) experienced improvement from the lowest DLCO compared with the last date of PFT follow-up. This study demonstrated that ILD prevalence is significant in patients with DM and is deserving of attention. Twenty-three percent of patients with DM with at least 1 CT or DLCO measurement had ILD as defined by CT imaging. However, 2 patients with ILD had a recent history of methotrexate use, which is also a drug known to cause ILD but generally occurs after chronic administration. In these cases, ILD secondary to DM or methotrexate-induced ILD was indistinguishable. Also, each patient's baseline PFT values were unknown before they were diagnosed with DM, and the presence of pre-existing lung disease, such as pulmonary hypertension and low DLCO from anemia or smoking, was not explored in this study. There were also no controls, no mention of current medications, and smokers were not excluded, which may have affected the results. However, authors recommended that patients with DM should be screened for respiratory symptoms, which is a valid point. Patients should also have a baseline PFTs with a pulmonary specialist if they are symptomatic, and a high-resolution CT scan may also help confirm ILD. Also, DLCO testing is relatively inexpensive and sensitive for pulmonary disease and can be used to screen patients with DM serially for ILD. Larger randomized controlled studies need to be done to evaluate if patients with DM and other connective tissue disease are at a higher risk of pulmonary disease than originally believed.

J. Q. Del Rosso, DO
G. K. Kim, DO

Lupus erythematosus tumidus is a separate subtype of cutaneous lupus erythematosus

Schmitt V, Meuth AM, Amler S, et al (Univ of Münster, Germany; et al)
Br J Dermatol 162:64-73, 2010

Background.—Lupus erythematosus tumidus (LET) is a rare disease which was first described in 1909 but has not always been considered as a separate entity of cutaneous lupus erythematosus (CLE) in the international literature.

Objectives.—To compare characteristic features of different subtypes of CLE and to analyse whether LET can be distinguished as a separate entity in the classification system of the disease.

Methods.—The study involved 44 patients with CLE, including 24 patients with LET, 12 with discoid lupus erythematosus (DLE) and eight with subacute CLE (SCLE), from two centres in Germany. A core set questionnaire and an SPSS database were designed to enable a consistent statistical analysis.

Results.—Location of skin lesions did not differ significantly between the CLE subtypes; however, the activity score was significantly lower in LET than in DLE $(P < 0·01)$, and the damage score was significantly lower in LET than in SCLE $(P < 0·01)$ and DLE $(P < 0·01)$. Photosensitivity and antinuclear antibodies were confirmed to be different in LET compared with SCLE and DLE but without statistical significance. Moreover, histological analysis of skin biopsy specimens showed that abundant mucin deposition is significantly more present in LET compared with SCLE $(P < 0·01)$ and DLE $(P < 0·01)$ while prominent interface dermatitis and alteration of hair follicles were absent in LET.

Conclusions.—Several significant differences were found between LET and other subtypes of CLE with regard to clinical, histological and laboratory parameters. These data strongly indicate that LET should be defined as a separate entity in the classification of CLE.

▶ There are recent data to suggest that lupus erythematosus tumidus (LET) should be recognized with clinical, photobiological, histological, immunohistochemical, and serological features separate from other subtypes of cutaneous lupus erythematosus (CLE). This study sought to characterize features of different subtypes of CLE compared with LET, with 44 patients with CLE, 24 with LET, and 12 with discoid lupus erythematosus (DLE). Researchers diagnosed and classified subtypes according to histological and clinical examination, photoprovocation (UVA/UVB), and serological markers of patients. Also, disease severity was measured in each patient with a damage score calculated by the Cutaneous Lupus Erythematosus Disease Area and Severity Index. The damage and activity was also calculated using the "Activity and Damage of Disease" calculation. The onset of disease in patients with LET was significantly lower, 38.5 years old compared with 42.9 years old (CLE, $P = .026$). Twenty-three (96%) of the patients (LET) had lesions in sun-exposed areas at the time of data collection, with only 1 (4%) of the patients having skin lesions on the back, which was considered a non–sun-exposed area. However, it was unknown if sun exposure in these areas were controlled for. Photosensitivity was most frequently reported in those with LET, with 17 (71%) patients compared with 5 (62%) with subacute CLE (SCLE) and 7 (58%) with DLE. The mean standard deviation time between UV exposure and appearance of characteristic skin lesions was 7.3 (9.5 days) in patients with LET. Skin lesions were induced by UVA irradiation in 7 (41%) of the 17 patients with LET, in 4 (80%) of the 5 patients with SCLE, and in 3 (38%) of the 8 patients with DLE. Histological confirmation revealed that alteration of hair follicles was not present with LET compared with DLE ($P = .034$). To add, vacuolar degeneration at the dermoepidermal junction was abundant with SCLE and DLE compared with LET ($P < .001$). Mucin deposition was frequently seen more in patients with LET than in those with DLE and SCLE ($P < 0.001$). Overall, patients with LET displayed a lower activity of the disease than those with DLE ($P = .003$) but similar level of activity compared with those with SCLE. Scarring alopecia was not present in any of the patients with LET compared with those with SCLE ($P < .001$ and $P = .011$, respectively). Spontaneous resolution of skin lesion without topical and systemic treatment was observed most frequently in 10 (42%) of 24 patients with LET, in only 1 (12%) patient with SCLE, and in 3 (25%) patients with DLE. Laboratory examination revealed that there was less anti–double-stranded DNA positivity in LET compared with DLE ($P = .034$). Anti-Ro/SSA and Anti-Lo/SSB were less frequent in LET compared with SCLE ($P = .009$ and $P = .039$, respectively). The limitation to this study was that it was performed in a single institution with limited follow-up period. Although there were differences observed in serological markers, it was unknown if these were patient's baseline serological markers or done at the time of the study, as serological markers may change with time and disease activity. In conclusion, LET has many distinctive features compared with subtypes of CLE and should be considered a separate entity in the classification of CLE.

J. Q. Del Rosso, DO

G. K. Kim, DO

Rituximab in diffuse cutaneous systemic sclerosis: an open-label clinical and histopathological study
Smith V, Van Praet JT, Vandooren B, et al (Ghent Univ Hosp, Belgium)
Ann Rheum Dis 69:193-197, 2010

Objectives.—The safety and potential efficacy of rituximab was examined in diffuse cutaneous systemic sclerosis (dc-SSc).

Methods.—A 24 week open-label study in which eight patients with dc-SSc received an infusion of 1000 mg rituximab administered at baseline and day 15, together with 100 mg methylprednisolone at each infusion. Assessment included CD19+ peripheral blood lymphocyte number, skin sclerosis score, indices of internal organ functioning, the health assessment questionnaire disability index, the 36-item Short Form health survey and histopathological evaluation of the skin.

Results.—Ritixumab induced effective B-cell depletion in all patients (<5 CD19+ cells/μl blood). There was a significant change in skin score at week 24 (p<0.001). Also, significant improvements were measured in the dermal hyalinised collagen content (p = 0.014) and dermal myofibroblast numbers (p = 0.011). Two serious adverse events occurred, which were thought to be unrelated to the rituximab treatment.

Conclusions.—Rituximab appears to be well tolerated and may have potential efficacy for skin disease in dc-SSc. This study is registered with ClinicalTrials.gov, number NCT00379431.

▶ Diffuse cutaneous systemic sclerosis (dcSS) is a clinically heterogeneous disease in which excessive collagen deposition causes skin and internal organ changes. The rationale for using rituximab was based on its potential efficacy to deplete B cells. This effect was found in all 8 patients and resulted in decreased fibrosis, which correlates to previous findings in animal models. The direct effect of this drug on the disease pathophysiology is crucial since the excessive collagen deposition and fibrosis can be immunomodulated and prevented. The results offered by the authors are fundamental and propose rituximab as a promising therapy for dcSS. Rituximab appeared to decrease the hyalinized collagen score and myofibroblast positivity, which leads to the idea that the drug has more effect on the skin. It did not appear to result in a significant beneficial effect on the internal organs. As the authors recognized, double-blind, placebo-controlled studies with longer follow-up are needed and warranted to evaluate the potential efficacy of rituximab on internal organs as well as to further support it as a first-line therapeutic option for dcSS.

B. Berman, MD, PhD

Successful Immunosuppressive Treatment of Dermatomyositis: A Nailfold Capillaroscopy Survey
Riccieri V, Vasile M, Macri V, et al (Sapienza Univ of Rome, Italy)
J Rheumatol 37:443-445, 2010

Background.—Patients with dermatomyositis (DM) often have vascular involvement. Nailfold capillaroscopy (NC) can be done to evaluate the condition, which can be severe in DM. NC abnormalities are more common with skin involvement in untreated DM, but also correlate with disease activity in inflammatory myopathies. An association was noted between NC findings, disease activity, and treatment response.

Case Report.—Man, 40, had arthromyalgias, asthenia, fatigue, and muscle weakness mainly affecting the lower limbs. Both hands, face, and neck had erythematous-desquamative lesions, and Raynaud's phenomenon was evident. His erythrocyte sedimentation rate was 54/hr, C-reactive protein was 48 mg/l, creatine kinase was 530 U/l, lactate dehydrogenase was 485 U/l, and the anti-Jo-1 test was positive. Electromyography revealed myositic impairment with increased junctional activity as well as polyphasic potentials in the upper and lower limbs. Perivascular lymphomononuclear infiltrates with degenerative zones and necrosis were noted on muscle biopsy.

Treatment was conducted in the hospital because of progressive dyspnea. The patient was given 40 mg daily of 6-methylprednisolone (6-MP). On pulmonary high-resolution computed tomography, he had severe interstitial lung disease (ILD), particularly affecting the perihilar and basal levels, and bilateral pleural effusion. His forced vital capacity was 55% and diffusion capacity for carbon monoxide was 36%; he also had respiratory alkalosis. NC was performed to evaluate Raynaud's phenomenon and demonstrated abnormal morphology, with capillary loops demonstrating a marked architectural derangement, frequent ramified and bizarre configurations, and megacapillaries. Neoangiogenesis alternated with avascular areas, and many microhemorrhages were seen.

For the next 6 months the patient was given 750 mg/month intravenous cyclophosphamide plus 80 mg/day 6-MP that was gradually tapered to 8 mg/day. Assessment at that point demonstrated improvements in cutaneous lesions, strength, dyspnea status, and muscle weakness. Mild basal interstitial involvement, seen as dyspnea with extended effort and restrictive lung impairment, remained. The patient's acute-phase reactant and serum muscle enzyme levels had normalized. A repeat NC done by the same clinician under the same conditions as the first one demonstrated marked improvement. The number, morphology, and distribution of the capillary loops and neovascularized zones were normal, and there were no microhemorrhages or giant capillaries. The patient was started on an immunosuppressive maintenance regimen of azathioprine 50 mg twice a day.

Conclusions.—This patient with DM had severe NC results that improved dramatically with treatment. NC testing could add useful information for the diagnosis, follow-up, and assessment of responses to treatment in patients with DM.

▶ This is a case report of a 40-year-old male presenting with arthromyalgias and muscle weakness diagnosed with dermatomyositis (DM). Authors evaluated the patient's symptoms, laboratory findings, and nailfold capillaroscopy (NC) before and after immunosuppressive treatment. In DM, there may be vascular involvement, which can be visualized with capillaroscopy. Some investigators have reported that capillaroscopy findings can be related to disease activity or response to treatment. The patient was started on 40 mg of 6-methylprednisonlone (6MP) and continued on 6-month therapy with 750 mg/month of cyclophosphamide started with 80 mg/day 6MP. NC was repeated on the same section of the nail fold and revealed marked improvement with normalization in the number, morphology, and distribution of capillary loops and neovascularized zones and absence of microhemorrhages and giant capillaries. An immunosuppressive maintenance regimen was started with azathioprine 50 mg twice a day. This case showed improvement with NC findings correlating with improved clinical and laboratory outcomes after immunosuppressive therapy. Limitations to this study included a single-case report, and more randomized prospective studies will be needed in the future to evaluate NC improvement correlating with disease activity. Also improvement in NC is a visual evaluation and a more precise way to evaluate vascular improvement may be with biopsies of nail folds. Authors suggest that NC may be a useful diagnostic tool for assessing clinical response in patients with DM.

J. Q. Del Rosso, DO

G. K. Kim, DO

The Localized Scleroderma Skin Severity Index and Physician Global Assessment of Disease Activity: A Work in Progress Toward Development of Localized Scleroderma Outcome Measures
Arkachaisri T, for the Localized Scleroderma Clinical and Ultrasound Study Group (LOCUS) (Univ of Pittsburgh School of Medicine, PA; et al)
J Rheumatol 36:2819-2829, 2009

Objective.—To develop and evaluate a Localized Scleroderma (LS) Skin Severity Index (LoSSI) and global assessments' clinimetric property and effect on quality of life (QOL).

Methods.—A 3-phase study was conducted. The first phase involved 15 patients with LS and 14 examiners who assessed LoSSI [surface area (SA), erythema (ER), skin thickness (ST), and new lesion/extension (N/E)] twice for inter/intrarater reliability. Patient global assessment of disease severity (PtGA-S) and Children's Dermatology Life Quality Index (CDLQI) were collected for intrarater reliability evaluation. The second phase was aimed to develop clinical determinants for physician global assessment of disease activity (PhysGA-A) and to assess its content validity. The third phase involved 2 examiners assessing LoSSI and PhysGA-A on 27 patients. Effect of training on improving reliability/validity and sensitivity to change of the LoSSI and PhysGA-A was determined.

Results.—Interrater reliability was excellent for ER [intraclass correlation coefficient (ICC) 0.71], ST (ICC 0.70), LoSSI (ICC 0.80), and PhysGA-A (ICC 0.90) but poor for SA (ICC 0.35); thus, LoSSI was modified to mLoSSI. Examiners' experience did not affect the scores, but training/practice improved reliability. Intrarater reliability was excellent for ER, ST, and LoSSI (Spearman's rho = 0.71–0.89) and moderate for

SA. PtGA-S and CDLQI showed good intrarater agreement (ICC 0.63 and 0.80). mLoSSI correlated moderately with PhysGA-A and PtGA-S. Both mLoSSI and PhysGA-A were sensitive to change following therapy.

Conclusion.—mLoSSI and PhysGA-A are reliable and valid tools for assessing LS disease severity and show high sensitivity to detect change over time. These tools are feasible for use in routine clinical practice. They should be considered for inclusion in a core set of LS outcome measures for clinical trials.

▶ This article provides an excellent tool that should be considered for objective measurement of localized scleroderma (LS), providing a high sensitivity to detect changes over time. The use of this index system is adaptable to clinical practice, and its incorporation should be considered by clinicians caring for patients with LS.

B. P. Glick, DO, MPH

B Cell-Targeted Therapies for Systemic Lupus Erythematosus: An Update on Clinical Trial Data
Looney RJ (Univ of Rochester School of Medicine and Dentistry, NY)
Drugs 70:529-540, 2010

In the past year there has been remarkable activity and some important success in the development of B cell-targeted therapies for the treatment of systemic lupus erythematosus (SLE). The most promising studies were BLISS-52 and BLISS-76, large phase III studies that demonstrated measurable efficacy for belimumab, a monoclonal antibody against B cell-activating factor (BAFF). The moderate-sized phase IIIII trials EXPLORER and LUNAR that tested rituximab, an anti-CD20 monoclonal antibody, for treatment of non-renal and renal lupus, disappointed many investigators with anecdotal success in refractory patients. These rituximab trials were intended to detect a large clinical effect in patients with very active disease and this was not found. Nevertheless, arguments can be made for additional studies in targeted populations or with a change in design to detect smaller or longer-term effects. Epratuzumab, a monoclonal antibody against the B cell surface antigen CD22, and atacicept, a chimeric molecule formed by a receptor for BAFF and a proliferation-inducing ligand (APRIL) with immunoglobulin (Ig)-G, have both been promising in initial small trials and now larger clinical trials are underway. Thus, recent clinical trial data show that B cell-targeting therapies are beginning to fulfil their promise as treatments for SLE and there are good reasons to hope for further progress in the near future.

▶ B cells (B lymphocytes) have been shown to play a role in the pathogenesis of autoimmune diseases. As a result, there are a number of clinical trials that have evaluated the use of B-cell-targeted therapies as treatment for conditions such as systemic lupus erythematosus (SLE). To that end, this article provides a well-written update on the latest larger clinical trials on B-cell-targeted therapies for SLE and identifies the outcomes of the available clinical data. The 4 main B-cell-targeted therapies reviewed in the treatment of SLE were rituximab, belimumab, epratuzumab, and atacicept. The most successful trials have been associated with belimumab, a fully human monoclonal antibody against B-cell-activating factor. Although there are 5 trials to date studying belimumab for SLE, 2 larger phase III trials (Belimumab International SLE Study [BLISS]-52 and BLISS-76) have shown notable clinical efficacy in the treatment of SLE, and according to this article, the results represent a significant breakthrough in new drug development for SLE. In addition, belimumab was noted to be well tolerated, and there were no described safety issues, but questions regarding the magnitude of belimumab's benefits remain. However, given this initial promising data, belimumab may well be the first new drug approved for SLE in over 40 years, which would certainly be much anticipated. One of the first B-cell-targeted therapies in clinical use (for treatment other than SLE) is rituximab. Unfortunately, while rituximab has shown clinical trial success in other disease entities, such as rheumatoid arthritis, 2 moderate-sized high-quality studies (Exploratory Phase II/III SLE Evaluation of Rituximab and LUpus Nephritis Assessment with Rituximab) have not proven rituximab to be beneficial in the treatment of SLE. The other 2 therapies, epratuzumab and atacicept, have undergone smaller trial studies and fortunately, have shown initial promising results. Both therapies are now undergoing larger trials.

Ultimately, this article provides an insightful synopsis on the state of B-cell-targeted therapy. At least initially, the data appear to be promising, but there is certainly additional studies needed on B-cell-targeted therapies for SLE. However, given the recent success of belimumab in clinical studies, there is at least hope for the expectation that additional promising therapies will be available for the treatment of SLE in the near future.

B. D. Michaels, DO

J. Q. Del Rosso, DO

A randomized controlled trial of R-salbutamol for topical treatment of discoid lupus erythematosus
Jemec GBE, Ullman S, Goodfield M, et al (Univ of Copenhagen, Roskilde, Denmark; Bispebjerg Hosp, Copenhagen NV, Denmark; Leeds General Infirmary, UK; et al)
Br J Dermatol 161:1365-1370, 2009

Background.—In a recent open pilot trial, R-salbutamol sulphate, a well-known molecule with anti-inflammatory effects, was tested successfully on patients with therapy-resistant discoid lupus erythematosus (DLE).

Objectives.—To compare the efficacy and safety of R-salbutamol cream 0·5% vs. placebo on DLE lesions in a multicentre, double-blinded, randomized, placebo-controlled phase II trial.

Methods.—Thirty-seven patients with at least one newly developed DLE lesion were randomized — 19 to the R-salbutamol cream 0·5% and 18 to placebo — and treated twice daily for 8 weeks. Efficacy was evaluated through scores of erythema, scaling/hypertrophy and induration as well as pain and itching; general improvement scored by the investigator and global improvement scored by patients' assessment were also evaluated.

Results.—The mean area under the curve of improvement for scaling/hypertrophy, pain, itching and global patient assessment was significantly better for the actively treated patients as compared with placebo (scaling/hypertrophy, $P = 0·0262$; pain, $P = 0·0238$; itching, $P = 0·0135$; global patient assessment, $P = 0·045$). Moreover, the percentage of patients without induration was significantly higher in the active group compared with the placebo group ($P = 0·013$), and a statistically significantly greater decrease in the size of the lesional area was also seen in the overall analysis of the R-salbutamol-treated patients ($P = 0·0197$). No serious adverse events were reported.

Conclusions.—Application of R-salbutamol cream 0·5% was safe and well tolerated. Statistically significant effects were seen on scaling/hypertrophy, induration, pain and itching as well as patient global assessment, suggesting that R-salbutamol could be a promising new topical therapy alternative for DLE.

▶ Discoid lupus erythematosus (DLE) often begins with erythematous papules or plaques with scaling. Lesions can progress to thicker plaques with pigmentary changes and can eventually lead to atrophy and scarring when left untreated. Successful treatment can be challenging. This randomized, double-blinded, placebo-controlled, phase II study further investigates the efficacy of topical R-salbutamol 0·5% cream in the treatment of therapy-resistant DLE. R-salbutamol is a β_2-receptor agonist and appears to have an anti-inflammatory effect, which may be beneficial in the treatment of inflammatory dermatoses such as DLE. It was found that R-salbutamol was efficacious with statistically significant improvement in scaling/hypertrophy, induration, pain, and itching and also based on patient global assessment scores as compared with placebo. The topical therapy was safe and generally well tolerated with the most common side effect being headaches, back pain, and nasopharyngitis. Limitations of the study include small number of patients ($N = 37$) and short duration of therapy (8 weeks). R-salbutamol may be a valid alternative in treating refractory DLE. Further studies need to be performed utilizing a larger group of patients with a longer treatment duration to further evaluate efficacy and safety, including long-term results.

S. Bellew, DO
J. Q. Del Rosso, DO

Treatment of Pediatric Localized Scleroderma: Results of a Survey of North American Pediatric Rheumatologists

Li SC, Feldman BM, Higgins GC, et al (Hackensack Univ Med Ctr, NJ)
J Rheumatol 37:175-181, 2010

Objective.—We surveyed pediatric rheumatologists (PR) in North America to learn how they treat pediatric localized scleroderma (LS), a disease associated with significant morbidity for the growing child.

Methods.—A Web based survey was sent to the 195 PR members of the pediatric rheumatology research alliance CARRA (Childhood Arthritis and Rheumatology Research Alliance). Members were asked which medications they use to treat LS and which factors modify their treatment strategies. Clinical vignettes were provided to learn the specific treatment regimens used.

Results.—A total of 158 PR from over 70 clinical centers in the United States and Canada participated in the survey, representing 81% of the CARRA membership. These PR saw over 650 patients with LS in the prior year. Nearly all respondents treated LS with methotrexate (MTX) and corticosteroids; most of them intensify treatment for lesions located on the face or near a joint, and about half intensify treatment for recent disease onset (< 6 months). Most PR reserve topical medications for limited treatment situations. Clinical vignettes showed that PR use a broad range of treatment doses and durations for MTX and corticosteroids.

Conclusion.—Most PR in North America treat localized scleroderma with a combination of MTX and corticosteroids. However, there is no consensus on specific treatment regimens. There is a need for controlled treatment trials to better determine optimal therapy for this potentially disabling disease.

▶ Localized scleroderma (LS) may cause significant morbidity and disability in the pediatric patient. This is a web-based survey sent to the 195 pediatric rheumatology (PR) clinics in North America to evaluate treatment protocols among pediatric rheumatologists there, including multiple-choice questions, open-ended options, and clinical vignettes. There were a total of 158 PR clinics that took the survey, representing 81% of the Child Arthritis and Rheumatology Research Alliance pediatric rheumatology membership. The respondents reported treating a total of 1041 patients with LS in the previous year, with 757 who received systemic medications during the previous year. PR clinics were asked if they thought all patients with a specific LS subtype should be treated with systemic medication at some point during their disease course. Most respondents used topical medications (78/121, 64.5%), while other PR clinics used them in conjunction with systemic therapy (38/121, 31.4%). The most common topical treatment was corticosteroids (47/78, 60.3%) and calcipotriene (33/78, 42.3%). Most respondents treated lesions on the face or limb joints more aggressively. PR clinics stopped treatment according to the clinical appearance of remission (erythema, new lesions, and shrinkage). This study illustrated the difference in approach for PR as compared with adult rheumatologists and dermatologists who frequently use topical treatments and phototherapy. PR clinics feel that topical medications have limited role and reserve them for use in conjunction with systemic treatment or for small minimally active lesions. The clinical vignette response revealed that there was no clear consensus on dosing regimens. PR clinics were also asked to detail their treatment of the same clinical vignette to evaluate treatment protocols. All respondents answered that they would use methotrexate (MTX), with most using the subcutaneous route. There was more than a 3-fold range in MTX dose and more than a 16-fold spread in MTX treatment duration for the first vignette patient. Respondents also showed an even greater variation for corticosteroid treatment, with more than a 30-fold range in total treatment amount and more than a 100-fold difference in total treatment duration. Treatment was determined based on signs of activity and specific patient features. LS subtypes were not a major factor in determining treatment; instead, treatment was based on activity and presence of new lesions. A limitation to this study was that the ages of pediatric patients were not discussed and may be a factor in the treatment with MTX. Also, side effects and adverse events were not discussed. To add, this was a survey, and recall bias may have affected results. More controlled trials determining optimal treatment options for LS are needed in the pediatric population.

J. Q. Del Rosso, DO
G. K. Kim, DO

9 Blistering Disorders

A population-based study of acute medical conditions associated with bullous pemphigoid
Langan SM, Hubbard R, Fleming K, et al (Univ of Nottingham, UK)
Br J Dermatol 161:1149-1152, 2009

Background.—Bullous pemphigoid is associated with poorly understood dramatically increased early mortality rates.

Objectives.—To assess the incidence of acute events predisposing to early mortality.

Methods.—Computerized medical records from the Health Improvement Network, a large population-based U.K. general practice database, were used to conduct a cohort analysis. Outcome measures were incidence rates of myocardial infarction, pulmonary embolism, pneumonia and sepsis compared with a matched control population.

Results.—People with bullous pemphigoid were three times as likely to develop pneumonia, adjusted rate ratio 2·94 [95% confidence interval (CI) 2·01−4·31] or pulmonary embolism, adjusted rate ratio 3·12 (95% CI 1·37−7·12) compared with matched controls. No statistically significant increase was seen for myocardial infarction, adjusted rate ratio 1·24 (95% CI 0·66−2·33), or sepsis, adjusted rate ratio 2·02 (95% CI 0·78−5·21).

Conclusions.—The risk of pulmonary embolism and pneumonia is increased following a diagnosis of bullous pemphigoid. It may be possible to reduce associated mortality through considering prophylaxis with either antithromboembolic measures or antibiotic therapy and vaccination.

▶ In the past, bullous pemphigoid (BP) has been associated with an increase in mortality compared with the general population. This randomized, age and sex-matched, large, population-based cohort study between 1996-2006 evaluated incidence rates of myocardial infarction, pulmonary embolism, pneumonia, and sepsis following a diagnosis of BP. Included were 868 patients with BP with a median age of 80 years. Patients with BP had an incidence rate of 21/1000 person-years for pneumonia and were almost 3 times as likely as matched controls to develop pneumonia. There was a similar 3-fold relative increase (3.12) with pulmonary embolism compared with matched controls. However, the incidence of sepsis and myocardial infarction was similar to matched controls. These findings were consistent with past reports to suggest that patients with BP had higher association with bronchopneumonia and pulmonary embolism. The authors suggest that this may be due to patients

231

with BP being frequently exposed to high doses of corticosteroids after a diagnosis of BP is made. However, this study did not evaluate current or past usage of corticosteroid in the study population. This study does not give a definitive explanation as to why patients with BP have higher incidences of pneumonia and pulmonary embolisms. In the future, a hypercoagulation workup would be helpful to study in order to evaluate if patients with BP have an inherent risk for a thromboembolic event. Also, it would be helpful to identify if patients with BP develop atypical pneumonia as seen with immunocompromised patients or a pattern of pneumonia similar to that seen in the general population. It is also suggested that patients with BP may need to be vaccinated against potential pneumonias, and these findings may also suggest that at least some patients with BP be placed on anticoagulation therapy. However, the risks associated with anticoagulation may not be ideal for patients with BP, especially with a mean age of 80 years. Future studies are needed to evaluate the risk and benefits of anticoagulation therapy and vaccination in this population of patients.

J. Q. Del Rosso, DO

G. K. Kim, DO

Anti–Bullous Pemphigoid 180 and 230 Antibodies in a Sample of Unaffected Subjects
Wieland CN, Comfere NI, Gibson LE, et al (Mayo Clinic, Rochester, MN)
Arch Dermatol 146:21-25, 2010

Objective.—To evaluate the prevalence of autoantibodies against 2 hemidesmosomal proteins typically found in patients with bullous pemphigoid (BP), BP antigen II (BP180) and BP antigen I (BP230), in persons without BP.

Design.—Cross-sectional study.

Setting.—Academic medical center.

Patients.—An age- and sex-stratified, random, population-based sample of local county patients seen during 2007: 20 men and 20 women per decade of age (from age 20 to 89 years) and 57 patients (33 women and 24 men) aged 90 to 99 years.

Intervention.—Stored serum samples were retrieved for analysis by enzyme-linked immunosorbent assay and indirect immunofluorescence.

Main Outcome Measure.—Presence of circulating autoantibodies to BP180 and BP230.

Results.—Of the 337 study patients, 25 (7.4%) were positive for 1 or both autoantibodies; these 25 samples all tested negative with indirect immunofluorescence. Autoantibody levels did not vary by age or sex.

Conclusions.—Bullous pemphigoid has a higher incidence in the elderly population, but the prevalence of antibodies to BP180 and BP230 did not increase significantly with age or vary by sex in this population-based sample. Other exogenous factors may affect the development of these autoantibodies in a population without clinically evident immunobullous disease, including limitations inherent to the test (false-positive rate).

▶ The pathogenesis of bullous pemphigoid (BP) has been characterized by circulating autoantibodies against basement membrane zone proteins. Patients with BP have been known to have BP180 and BP230, which may follow pathogenicity of autoantibodies and disease activity. However, little is known about BP antigen prevalence in the general population. The main objective of the authors was to determine the prevalence of autoantibodies, specifically BP180 and BP230, in the general population of patients without immunobullous disease. Of the 337 patients without known bullous disease, 25 (7.4%) had a positive result by enzyme-linked immunosorbent assay (ELISA) for autoantibodies against BP180 only (n = 11), BP230 only (n = 11), or both (n = 3). Autoantibodies did not appear to vary significantly with age or sex. However, variation between ethnicities was not commented on. The incidence rates of positive ELISA were 7.3% and 7.6% among patients < 60 years of age and > 60 years of age, respectively. To rule out other autoimmune disease possibilities or undetected BP, all 25 ELISA-positive serum samples were tested with indirect immunofluorescence. Although other studies have shown that BP autoantibodies are higher in the elderly population, this study did not reveal this. None of the 25 patients with positive ELISA had evidence of clinical BP; however, it is unknown whether these patients developed BP later on in life because of limited follow-up. Authors speculated that there may be other secondary triggers to BP that may not be revealed. Limitations to this study were that other unknown autoantibodies may exist besides BP180 and BP230. This study was also limited because it was a single-center study, and larger cohort studies comparing the general population with patients with BP would shed additional light on this fascinating subject in dermatology.

J. Q. Del Rosso, DO
G. K. Kim, DO

Bacteremia in Stevens-Johnson Syndrome and Toxic Epidermal Necrolysis: Epidemiology, Risk Factors, and Predictive Value of Skin Cultures
de Prost N, Ingen-Housz-Oro S, anh Duong T, et al (Université Paris XII, Créteil, France)
Medicine 89:28-36, 2010

Toxic epidermal necrolysis (TEN) is a rare drug-related life-threatening acute condition. Sepsis is the main cause of mortality. Skin colonization on top of impaired barrier function promotes bloodstream infections (BSI). We conducted this study to describe the epidemiology, identify early predictors of BSI, and assess the predictive value for bacteremia of routine skin surface cultures.

We retrospectively analyzed the charts of all patients with Stevens-Johnson syndrome (SJS) and TEN hospitalized over an 11-year period.

Blood cultures and skin isolates were recovered from the microbiology laboratory database. Early predictors of BSI were identified using a Cox model. Sensitivity, specificity, and negative and positive predictive values of skin cultures for the etiology of BSI were assessed.

The study included 179 patients, classified as having SJS (n = 54; 30.2%), SJS/TEN overlap (n = 59; 33.0%), and TEN (n = 66; 36.9%). Forty-eight episodes of BSI occurred, yielding a rate of 15.5/1000 patient days. Inhospital mortality was 13.4% (24/179). Overall, 70 pathogens were recovered, mainly *Staphylococcus aureus* (n = 23/70; 32.8%), *Pseudomonas aeruginosa* (n = 15/70; 21.4%), and Enterobacteriaceae organisms (n = 17/70; 24.3%). Variables associated with BSI in multivariate analysis included age >40 years (hazard ratio [HR], 2.5; 95% confidence interval [CI], 1.35−4.63), white blood cell count >10,000/mm^3 (HR, 1.9; 95% CI, 0.96−3.61), and percentage of detached body surface area ≥30% (HR, 2.5; 95% CI, 1.13−5.47). Skin cultures had an excellent negative predictive value for bacteremia due to S aureus (especially methicillin-resistant strains) and P aeruginosa, but not for those due to Enterobacteriaceae organisms. In contrast, the positive predictive value was low for all pathogens studied. To our knowledge, this is the largest study describing the epidemiology and risk factors of BSI in patients with SJS/TEN. The body surface area involved is the main predictor of BSI. Excellent negative predictive values of skin cultures for S *aureus* and P *aeruginosa* bacteremia should help clinicians consider targeted empirical antibiotic choices when appropriate.

▶ Toxic epidermal necrolysis (TEN) is a life-threatening dermatosis. TEN differentiates from Steven-Johnson syndrome (SJS) based on the extent of the detached skin relative to the body surface area (BSA). This is a retrospective cohort study reviewing the medical records of 179 patients hospitalized for TEN/SJS and examining the epidemiology and early predictors of bloodstream infection (BSI). Treatment course and affected BSA and other variables such as age, sex, medical history, and other medical conditions were noted. The severity of TEN/SJS was assessed from the SCORTEN grading system and from generic scores of organ dysfunction. Aerobic and anaerobic samples were taken on admission from peripheral vascular access sites or from central lines. Blood cultures were also taken upon clinical suspicion of sepsis. BSI was defined as 1 blood culture yielding a recognized pathogen from a single sample or an organism of the normal skin flora isolated from more than 1 culture within a 48-hour period. In 92 patients (51.4%), the percentage of detached BSA increased during hospitalization. The overall in-hospital mortality was 13.4% (24/179). Forty-eight episodes of BSI occurred in 48 patients (26.8%) over 3095 patient days, yielding a rate of BSI of 15.5/1000 patient days. Twenty-four patients (13.4%) had a polymicrobial episode with 2 to 3 pathogens recovered within the same blood sample. Overall, 70 pathogens were recovered, mainly *Staphylococcus aureus* (23/70), *Pseudomonas aeruginosa* (15/70), and Enterobacteriaceae organisms (17/70). In-hospital mortality associated with these pathogens was 5/23 (21.7%) for S aureus, (3/15) for P aeruginosa, and 4/17 for Enterobacteriaceae organisms. The median time that elapsed between the first symptom of the disease and BSI was 11 days and between the hospital admission and BSI was 5 days. The results of this study showed that 48/179 patients had an episode of BSI, with the main pathogens being *S aureus, P aeruginosa,* and Enterobacteriaceae organisms. The overall median length of stay in hospital was 22 days in patients in whom bacteremia occurred and 12 days in the others ($P < .0001$). There was no association between the BSI and treatment with intravenous immunoglobulin G ($P = .88$) or cyclo-sporine ($P = .39$). Age > 40 years, diabetes, serum urea > 10 mM, white blood cell count > 10 000, and percentage of detached BSA > 30% yielded a *P* value of < 0.10. Limitations to this study included that it was a retrospective study and from a single institution. To add, the authors were not able to analyze the predictive factors of BSI for each pathogen group. Also, when patients do develop BSI from TEN/SJS, it is recommended for clinicians to first choose an appropriate broad-spectrum antibiotic. In this study, the authors concluded that BSA was the main predictor of BSI, and skin cultures had an excellent negative predictive value for bacteremia due to *S aureus* and *P aeruginosa* and not for those due to Enterobacteriaceae organisms.

J. Q. Del Rosso, DO
G. K. Kim, DO

Common Wound Colonizers in Patients with Epidermolysis Bullosa
Brandling-Bennett HA, Morel KD (Columbia Univ, NY)
Pediatr Dermatol 27:25-28, 2010

One of the major morbidities of patients with epidermolysis bullosa is the tendency to develop chronic wounds, which predisposes them to multiple complications including life-threatening infections, failure to thrive, and squamous cell carcinomas. Chronic wounds frequently become colonized with bacteria, and we sought to identify the most common microorganisms isolated on cultures from patients with epidermolysis bullosa. We conducted a retrospective review of positive wound, nasal, and blood cultures, including bacterial, fungal and viral, in 30 patients with epidermolysis bullosa. *Staphylococcus* sp., *Streptococcus* sp., diptheroids, *Pseudomonas aeruginosa,* and *Candida* sp. were the most commonly isolated microorganisms in wound cultures from our epidermolysis bullosa patients. Two patients had viral cultures that grew herpes simplex virus type-1. Bacterial colonization of chronic wounds can lead to infections and may also impact wound healing. Results from this study provide data on which to base empiric antibiotic choice in patients with epidermolysis bullosa when needed and may be useful in planning strategies for decolonization and improved wound healing in this population.

▶ In this retrospective chart review, the authors catalog the results of 203 positive wound (192), nasal (3), and blood (8) cultures obtained from 30 patients with various subtypes of epidermolysis bullosa (EB) over a 10-year period in an effort to help to guide empiric antibiotic selection. Patients were selected by author recall and search of the electronic medical record for EB. *Staphylococcus* sp, *Streptococcus* sp, diphtheroids, and *Pseudomonas aeruginosa* were the most frequently recovered bacteria from wound cultures. Nearly half of cultures grew more than 1 type of bacteria, and 20% of cultures grew 3 or more bacteria. The authors note that growth of 4 or more bacteria from chronic leg ulcers in patients without EB has been associated with delayed wound healing. However, additional study is necessary to determine the implications of these findings on patients with EB. Two patients had positive herpes simplex virus type 1 cultures, underscoring the importance of considering herpetic infection in these patients who are prone to developing noninfectious blisters.

The study has several limitations, including no distinction between cultures obtained because of concern for infection and those taken for surveillance purposes. Culture methods were not standardized, and no data on treatment or outcomes were obtained. Nevertheless, results provide some guidance for clinicians considering empiric treatment for infected wounds in patients with EB.

D. Dasher, MD

Pulsed intravenous cyclophosphamide and methylprednisolone therapy in refractory pemphigus
Saha M, Powell A-M, Bhogal B, et al (St Thomas' Hosp, London, UK)
Br J Dermatol 162:790-797, 2010

Background.—Pemphigus is a rare autoimmune blistering disorder. The mainstay of current treatment is high-dose oral corticosteroid therapy in combination with a steroid-sparing agent. Adjuvant therapy is important for disease control and to reduce the iatrogenic effects of oral prednisolone. Pulsed therapy with intravenous methylprednisolone and cyclophosphamide (PPC) has been shown to be an effective treatment but there are currently few data on its use in patients who have failed to respond to conventional immunosuppression.

Objectives.—To report the clinical and immunological responses of 21 patients with pemphigus refractory to prednisolone and azathioprine or mycophenolate mofetil treated in our department with a standard protocol of monthly PPC.

Methods.—Patients with pemphigus were identified who had undergone PPC therapy during the period between 1997 and 2006. Initial clinical severity and response to treatment was assessed. In addition, change in intercellular antibody titres and desmoglein 1 and 3 antibodies to PPC therapy was also recorded.

Results.—Of the 21 patients treated, seven had an excellent response, two a good response, five a moderate response, six a minimal response and one patient had no clinical response. Four patients achieved complete clinical remission and the number of pulses for these patients varied between 11 and 22. We observed significant reductions in indirect immunofluorescence titres for normal human skin substrate ($P = 0 \cdot 0078$) and antidesmoglein 1 and 3 autoantibody levels ($P = 0 \cdot 007$ and $P = 0 \cdot 0085$, respectively) from pre-PPC therapy to 1 year after the last pulse. All patients were able to reduce their prednisolone dose from a pre-pulsing median dose of 40—10 mg at the last pulse with a median dose reduction of 66% ($P < 0 \cdot 001$). The most common adverse effect was transient lymphopenia (12 patients); nonlife-threatening sepsis (seven patients) and premature ovarian failure (two patients) also occurred.

Conclusions.—PPC can be an effective treatment for refractory pemphigus but its adverse effects should be considered prior to therapy and closely monitored in patients on treatment.

▶ The combination of pulsed cyclophosphamide and steroid therapy for pemphigus is fairly well written about in the world literature, but most studies include patients with all grades of severity and presentation. This study looks at only those patients who have already failed the steroid-sparing modalities of mycophenolate mofetil and azathioprine and treats them with monthly 3-day pulses of methylprednisolone and a 1 day per month pulse of cyclophosphamide, with daily oral cyclophosphamide in between. Only 4 of 21 patients obtained a complete remission, but overall, the data were fairly impressive on this refractory subset of patients with pemphigus, as 9 patients (43%) had a 1- or 2-grade improvement in oral and/or skin disease and only 1 patient had no clinical response. Furthermore, all study patients were able to diminish their precyclophosphamide oral steroid dependence by nearly 40%, at a minimum, and in some cases by over 80%, and kept them low 1 year post pulsed therapy. The clinical responses were mirrored by the significant drop in antibodies to desmoglein (Dsg)-1 and Dsg-3. The rates of complete clinical remission in this study were much lower when compared with other studies, but this was most certainly because of the sample of more recalcitrant patients who were selected. At the same time, some of the more feared side effects of this drug were not seen in this study either, such as hemorrhagic cystitis or bladder cancer. The authors attribute this to the relatively lower doses used (50 mg daily) versus weight-based daily dosing at 2 to 2.5 mg/kg/d or complete immunoablative therapy as has been attempted for oncologic regimens. Nonetheless, it must be kept in mind that cyclophosphamide treatment carries with it not only a risk of transitional cell carcinoma of the bladder but also severe infections, gross hematuria, non-Hodgkin lymphoma, leukemia, and squamous cell skin cancers. Perhaps even more traumatic is the possibility of premature gonadal failure as was seen in 3 patients in this study. While the goal of diminishing the exposure to steroids in patients with pemphigus is worthwhile, this is yet another study that reinforces the fact that cyclophosphamide can have its own very serious complications and that monthly pulsing with lower daily oral doses may be an improvement but still must be administered with meticulous monitoring of side effects and careful counseling regarding fertility planning.

J. M. Suchniak, MD

Stevens-Johnson syndrome and toxic epidermal necrolysis in Asian children

Koh MJ-A, Tay Y-K (Changi General Hosp, Singapore)

J Am Acad Dermatol 62:54-60, 2010

Background.—Stevens-Johnson syndrome (SJS) and toxic epidermal necrolysis (TEN) are rare but severe drug reactions. There have been few reviews of SJS and TEN in children.

Objectives.—To evaluate the clinical profile and treatment outcomes of 15 pediatric patients with SJS or TEN.

Methods.—We retrospectively reviewed the case notes of all patients diagnosed with SJS or TEN admitted to a tertiary care pediatric hospital from 2001 to 2006.

Results.—We identified 13 cases of SJS, 1 case of SJS/TEN overlap and 1 case of TEN. Four patients were treated with intravenous immunoglobulin (IVIg), 5 patients were treated with systemic corticosteroids, and 6 patients were treated with supportive therapy only. The time to cessation of progression of disease was not significantly different in these 3 groups of patients. The duration of hospital stay was longer for patients treated with IVIG compared with those treated with systemic corticosteroids or supportive therapy. The only death was the patient with TEN treated with IVIG.

Limitations.—This was a retrospective study with a very small number of patients.

Conclusion.—The use of intravenous immunoglobulins or systemic corticosteroids did not improve the outcome of SJS and TEN.

▶ Stevens Johnson syndrome (SJS) and toxic epidermal necrolysis (TEN) have been known to occur in children in association with infection and drugs. Treatment options, especially with corticosteroids, remain controversial. This is a retrospective study with 15 Asian patients with patient's clinical characteristics, causes, treatment regimens, complications, and treatment outcomes. In this study, drugs such as anticonvulsants and beta-lactam antibiotics were the most common cause of SJS. The mean onset of symptoms was 9 days (range 2-18 days). The most common skin manifestations were an exanthematous eruption and atypical target lesions. All patients had at least 2 mucosal surface sites of involvement with eye involvement in 11 cases. However, there was no mention of an ophthalmological evaluation, but patients were treated with ophthalmologic agents. Three patients had positive mycoplasma serology, and herpes simplex virus isolated from mouth erosions was negative in 9 patients tested. Other viral studies, including Epstein-Barr virus serology and immunofluorescence, for respiratory viruses were performed. Only 3 patients had skin biopsies to confirm the diagnosis, which was a limitation to this study. Four patients were treated with intravenous immunoglobulin, 5 treated with systemic corticosteroids, and 6 patients treated with supportive therapy only. The time of cessation of progression of disease was not significant in all these 3 groups. Other limitations were that all patients were Asian, with the majority being of Chinese descent, and a small study size. This study also found that anticonvulsants were the most common cause of disease, with other studies revealing that HLA-B*1502 is associated with carbamazepine-induced SJS in Chinese patients, which this study did not evaluate. Another limitation was that although some patients had positive mycoplasma serology, this may not necessarily be the inciting agent, and it may be difficult to prove a definitive causal relationship. Also researchers did not disclose if patients were on other drugs during their hospital stay, as patients may have taken multiple drugs before their hospital stay, and provocation tests were not performed to confirm the offending drug. To add, cessation of progression of rash and blistering was made on a clinical basis to evaluate if treatment outcomes differed from one another, and one investigator's end point may have differed from another. In conclusion, this study found that intravenous immunoglobulin or systemic corticosteroids did not improve the outcome of SJS and TEN in Asian patients.

J. Q. Del Rosso, DO

G. K. Kim, DO

Elevation of serum prolactin levels in patients with pemphigus vulgaris: A novel finding with practical implications

Fallahzadeh MK, Lashkarizadeh H, Kamali-Sarvestani E, et al (Shiraz Univ of Med Sciences, Iran)
J Am Acad Dermatol 62:1071-1072, 2010

Background.—Receptors for the cytokine prolactin are found throughout immune cells. This hormone has an antiapoptotic effect on B cells, enhances autoantibody production, upregulates tumor necrosis factor-alpha production, and increases interleukin-2 secretion and its proliferative effects on lymphocytes. The severity of some autoimmune diseases has been linked to serum prolactin levels. An investigation was undertaken to determine the serum prolactin levels of patients with pemphigus vulgaris (PV) and if these levels correlate with the extent of cutaneous involvement.

Methods.—Twenty-four PV patients and 24 healthy controls were matched for age and gender. Participants had a 30-minute period of absolute rest before morning samples were obtained. Enzyme-linked immunosorbent assay was used to determine serum prolactin levels, with differences between the two groups analyzed using the parametric Mann-Whitney U test. The correlation between percentage of body surface involvement and prolactin levels was assessed using the Pearson test.

Results.—Patients' mean serum prolactin levels were significantly higher than controls' levels (21.66 and 11.38 ng/mL, respectively). Hyperprolactinemia was found in six women with PV but none of the controls. Serum prolactin levels correlated positively with the extent of body surface area involved, but site of involvement, whether mucosal or cutaneous, did not show an association with prolactin levels.

Conclusions.—Patients with PV had elevated prolactin levels compared to healthy individuals. Patients with severe pemphigus should be evaluated for prolactin levels.

▶ The scientific understanding of how prolactin extends the life of B cell lymphocytes allowing increased production of autoantibodies is not entirely clear.[1,2] Elevations in prolactin have a wide range of disease associations including celiac disease, antiphospholipid antibody syndrome (APS), systemic lupus erythematosus (SLE), rheumatoid arthritis (RA), Sjögren syndrome (SS), type I diabetes, Addison disease, multiple sclerosis, autoimmune thyroid disease, and uveitis.[1] Therefore, linking levels of prolactin to pemphigus vulgaris (PV) remains an illusive task. This study attempts to screen a PV population in order to prove a clinical validity to monitor prolactin. However, the study did not exclude patients with primary thyroid disease, type I diabetes, RA, SLE, APS, or SS. The attempt of the authors to demonstrate that monitoring prolactin levels may be a clinically relevant tool appears to be difficult to conclude at this time. However, development of a serum screen for cytokine-specific prolactin activity may hold clinicotherapeutic relevance, for instance, stratifying PV cases that may respond to bromocriptine therapy, in the future.

M. McCarty, DO
J. Q. Del Rosso, DO

References

1. Praprotnik S, Agmon-Levin N, Porat-Katz BS, et al. Prolactin's role in the pathogenesis of the antiphospholipid syndrome. *Lupus.* 2010;19:1515-1519.
2. Fojtíková M, Cerná M, Pavelka K. [A review of the effects of prolactin hormone and cytokine on the development and pathogenesis of autoimmune diseases]. *Vnitr Lek.* 2010;56:402-413.

10 Drug Actions, Reactions, and Interactions

Cetuximab-induced cutaneous toxicity

Tomková H, Kohoutek M, Zábojníková M, et al (T Bata's Regional Hosp, Zlín, Czech Republic)

J Eur Acad Dermatol Venereol 24:692-696, 2010

Background.—Epidermal growth factor receptor inhibitors are recently utilized by oncologists in advanced cases of certain malignancies. However, these agents are associated with numerous cutaneous adverse reactions.

Objective.—To systematically review the cutaneous toxicity of cetuximab-treated patients.

Methods.—An analysis of a series of 24 patients (20 men and 4 women) treated with cetuximab (12 patients with head and neck cancer and 12 patients with colorectal cancer) was performed with respect to relevant clinical characteristics.

Results.—A total of 22 patients (91.7%) developed pustular or maculopapular follicular eruption, often referred to as acneiform rash. One patient (4.2%) developed paronychia in the course of cetuximab therapy. All patients with head and neck cancer had a combination treatment with radiotherapy and experienced radiation dermatitis accompanied by skin xerosis. Anaphylactic reaction was observed in three patients (12.5%).

Conclusions.—The most frequent cutaneous side effect reported in this series was acneiform eruption. The authors observed that all women with acneiform rash had only limited facial involvement, whereas all but one man experienced more widespread lesions of the face, the back and the chest. We found no association between the extent and severity of cutaneous eruptions (grade 1 vs. grade 2) and patients' response to therapy.

▶ Epidermal growth factor receptor (EGFR) inhibitors are increasingly being used to treat malignancies, including head and neck and colorectal cancers. Dermatologists should be aware of cutaneous side effects associated with these medications, as they occur frequently. This article focuses on side effects seen in patients on cetuximab. The most common side effect reported was acneiform rash. I would like to point out that the term acneiform is not truly accurate based on histologic evaluation and also clinical presentation in many cases. The eruption presents as erythematous papules and pustules, which may be associated with pruritus. Although the cutaneous eruption may sometimes resemble acne vulgaris clinically, an important distinction is that it is not associated with comedones or cystic lesions, and it does not resemble acne vulgaris pathologically.[1] Also, in many cases, the lesions tend to be predominantly monomorphic or demonstrate greater confluence of lesions, both of which are not characteristic of acne vulgaris. There is no alteration of the sebaceous glands in patients treated with EGFR inhibitors, which is in contrast with findings in acne patients.

S. Bhambri, DO

Reference

1. Bhambri S, Del Rosso JQ, Michaels B. Epidermal growth factor receptor inhibitors and associated cutaneous drug eruptions: mechanisms, recognition, and management. *Cosmet Dermatol.* 2008;21:45-51.

Cutaneous adverse effects in patients treated with the multitargeted kinase inhibitors sorafenib and sunitinib
Lee WJ, Lee JL, Chang SE, et al (Univ of Ulsan College of Medicine, Songpagu, Seoul, Korea)
Br J Dermatol 161:1045-1051, 2009

Background.—The multitargeted kinase inhibitors sorafenib and sunitinib have improved treatment of solid tumours including renal cell carcinoma and hepatocellular carcinoma by offering better clinical responses. However, sorafenib and sunitinib are commonly associated with cutaneous toxicity.

Objectives.—We conducted this study to make a clinical assessment of the cutaneous toxicities induced by the oral multitargeted kinase inhibitors sorafenib and sunitinib.

Methods.—Retrospectively, we reviewed medical records of patients receiving multitargeted kinase inhibitors, including 109 patients on sorafenib for the treatment of renal cell carcinoma or hepatocellular carcinoma and 119 patients receiving sunitinib for treatment of renal cell carcinoma or a gastrointestinal stromal tumour. Clinical data on cutaneous toxicities were collated. We describe the incidences and intensities of toxicities, and analyse the data statistically.

Results.—The most common cutaneous toxicity was hand-and-foot skin reaction (HFSR). Other cutaneous toxicities included alopecia, stomatitis, skin discoloration (hair or face), subungual splinter haemorrhage, facial swelling, facial erythema and xerosis. HFSR and severe stomatitis required therapy modifications to relieve symptoms, but other cutaneous toxicities did not affect treatment course. HFSR was observed in 48% of patients treated with sorafenib and 36% of those treated with sunitinib. Median time to onset was 18·4 days in patients receiving sorafenib and 32·4 days in those receiving sunitinib. HFSR and stomatitis were early symptoms compared with other cutaneous toxicities. Patients with severe HFSR were likely to develop the symptoms at early phases of therapy. A significant correlation between the severity of HFSR and development of alopecia and stomatitis was found.

Conclusions.—Multitargeted kinase inhibitors are associated with a significant risk of various cutaneous adverse events. HFSR is the commonest and most serious cutaneous toxicity in patients treated with these drugs.

▶ The goal of this study was to look at the cutaneous side effects encountered in patients on oral multitargeted kinase inhibitors sorafenib and sunitinib. The multitargeted kinase inhibitors are increasingly being used in patients with solid tumors, including renal cell carcinoma and hepatocellular carcinoma. A total of 228 patients (109 patients on sorafenib and 119 patients on sunitinib) were part of the study. Hand-and-foot skin reaction (HFSR) was the most common cutaneous reaction seen in 48% (52) of the patients in the sorafenib group followed by alopecia and stomatitis. The most common cutaneous reaction in the sunitinib group was HSFR followed by stomatitis and facial swelling. This article was well written and was thorough. Because these medications are routinely being used, dermatologists should be aware of cutaneous effects that may be encountered.

S. Bhambri, DO

Cutaneous Adverse Reactions to Psychotropic Drugs: Data From a Multicenter Surveillance Program

Lange-Asschenfeldt C, Grohmann R, Lange-Asschenfeldt B, et al (Heinrich-Heine Univ, Düsseldorf, Germany; Ludwig-Maximilians Univ, Munich, Germany; Charité Univ Hosp, Berlin, Germany)
J Clin Psychiatry 70:1258-1265, 2009

Objective.—Cutaneous adverse drug reactions (CADRs) in psychiatric pharmacotherapy are common, potentially harmful, and among the most frequent types of adverse events. To date, most of the data regarding CADRs to psychotropic medications are anecdotal, and systematic studies are lacking, particularly with respect to modern "second-generation" drugs.

Method.—Data were drawn from a database of 208,401 psychiatric inpatients monitored by the multicenter drug safety surveillance project Drug Safety in Psychiatry (Arzneimittelsicherheit in der Psychiatrie [AMSP]) during the years 1993—2005. The project surveys clinically relevant adverse reactions to all marketed psychotropic drugs.

Results.—Two hundred fourteen cases of clinically relevant CADRs with a "probable" or "definite" attribution to a single psychotropic compound were identified (0.1%), of which 7 were life threatening

(3.3% of CADR cases). Eruptions occurred irrespective of age and mainly in women. The gender effect was significant only for mood-stabilizing antiepileptic drugs (AEDs; P =.001). Substances with the highest and statistically significant CADR risk were AEDs (P <.0001), particularly lamotrigine and carbamazepine. For the most part, the incidence in antidepressants did not differ from the mean CADR rate of the monitored drugs in this survey (0.103%). However, CADRs were seen significantly less often with modern antidepressants (such as selective serotonin reuptake inhibitors and dual-mechanism or other second-generation antidepressants) than with classical tricyclic and tetracyclic antidepressants (P =.048). Conventional and atypical antipsychotics alike had the lowest rates of dermatologic side effects.

Conclusions.—Although serious complications are rare, clinicians should be aware of CADRs, particularly with AED mood stabilizers. Modern second-generation drugs appear to be associated with a rather low CADR risk.

▶ Cutaneous adverse drug reactions (CADRs) are frequently encountered adverse events to medications, ranging from urticaria to Stevens-Johnson syndrome. This is an open-ended study database of 208 401 psychiatric inpatients monitored by the multicenter drug safety surveillance project during the years 1993-2005, providing an overview of all cases with respect to age, sex, and diagnosis. Clinically relevant CADRs were attributed to 49 of 172 psychotropic drugs used during the observation period and were documented in 214 cases. With an incidence of 0.23%, mood stabilizers accounted for the highest CADR rate as a drug group, with high statistical significance compared with the mean CADR rate ($P < .0001$). Within this group, lamotrigine (0.62%) and carbamazepine (0.32%) had the highest rates, followed by oxcarbazepine (0.21%) and valproate (0.06%). Lithium carbonate had a lower rate of cutaneous adverse effects (0.01%). Antidepressants were the second most frequent psychotropic drug group to cause clinically relevant drug eruptions (0.054%). Papular eruptions comprised 78.9% of reactions, and urticaria and vesicular manifestations occurred at a rate of 9.6% and 6.3%, respectively. The median clinical latency for these subtypes was 9, 5, and 4 days, respectively. The most common symptom was pruritus (50.0%), followed by edema (12.0%) and exudative lesions (1.4%). Concurrent conjunctivitis occurred in 1.0%, fever in 5.8%, and dyspnea in 1.9%. In the majority of cases, the trunk was affected (65.1%), and large body areas were covered. In 11 cases (5.1%), transfer to a medical monitoring or intensive care unit became necessary. Drug treatment involved antihistamines applied topically or systemically in 106 cases and corticosteroids in 75 cases. The highest rate of CADRs occurred during the winter months (35.9%). This study reports findings associated with 172 drugs under surveillance, with only 49 drugs identified as offending agents and with only 7 having a CADR incidence above the mean. This study suggests that the majority of drug eruptions were caused by only a limited number of psychotropic drugs, with the highest rate being mood stabilizers. One weakness of this study was that spontaneous reporting may be incomplete, with some elements of bias. In conclusion, this study provided valuable information in comparing CADR frequencies with psychotropic drugs and emphasized the importance of patient education.

J. Q. Del Rosso, DO

G. K. Kim, DO

Dermatologic Infections in Cancer Patients Treated With Epidermal Growth Factor Receptor Inhibitor Therapy
Eilers RE Jr, Gandhi M, Patel JD, et al (Northwestern Univ Feinberg School of Medicine, Chicago, IL; et al)
J Natl Cancer Inst 102:47-53, 2010

Background.—Patients treated with epidermal growth factor receptor inhibitors (EGFRIs) frequently experience dermatologic toxic effects. Whereas the impact of these effects on quality of life and EGFRI dosing has been described, their impact on physical health has not been ascertained. We examined the prevalence of infections that complicate dermatologic toxic effects of EGFRIs.

Methods.—We used retrospective chart review methods to analyze 221 patients who were treated in the Skin and Eye Reactions to Inhibitors of EGFR and Kinases clinic, a referral clinic for dermatologic toxic effects of cancer therapies. We reviewed results of bacterial cultures, histopathologic assessment of biopsy samples, and immunohistochemical staining of skin specimens for viral pathogens that were recorded in the patients' medical records. Associations between patient demographic and treatment characteristics and the development of infections were examined using the Fisher exact test. All statistical tests were two-sided.

Results.—Eighty-four (38%) of the 221 patients showed evidence of infection at sites of dermatologic toxic effect. Fifty (22.6%) of the 221 patients had cultures positive for *Staphylococcus aureus*, and 12 (5.4%) of the 221 patients cultured positive for methicillin-resistant *S aureus*. Less frequent infections included herpes simplex (3.2%), herpes zoster (1.8%), and dermatophytes (10.4%). The seborrheic region was the most prevalent site of infection, and patients with leukopenia had higher risk for infection than patients who did not have leukopenia ($P = .005$). Demographic factors and associated treatments were not associated with the occurrence of a dermatologic infection ($P \geq .05$).

Conclusions.—Patients with dermatologic toxic effects following treatment with EGFRIs have a high prevalence of cutaneous infections. Most notably, bacterial infections developed at sites previously affected by dermatologic toxic effects, with leukopenic patients being at greater risk.

▶ Epidermal growth factor receptor (EGFR) regulates cellular processes such as cell proliferation, differentiation, and survival. EGFR dysregulations in certain malignancies have been observed in lung, gastrointestinal, and head and neck cancers and are associated with poor prognosis, with increased resistance to chemotherapy and radiotherapy. This is a retrospective chart review of patients receiving EGFR inhibitors (EGFRI), with examination of the dermatologic toxic effects of these drugs and how they can predispose to secondary infection in patients on EGFRI therapy. The authors did a review of bacterial, viral, and fungal cultures and stains as well as histochemical findings from skin biopsies. In this study, EGFRI therapy was used currently with ongoing treatment with radiation and/or previous oncologic treatment with chemotherapy, topical corticosteroids, and antibiotics for prophylaxis of skin eruptions. The results were clinical and demographic characteristics of 221 EGFRI-treated patients with and without dermatologic infections. Of the 221 patients investigated in this study, 189 (86%) patients received topical corticosteroid treatment (86.9%) and 116 patients were without infection (84.7%). Nineteen uninfected patients (13.9%) and 7 infected patients (8.3%) were treated with prophylactic topical corticosteroids. There was no association between prophylactic topical corticosteroid use and incidence of infections. Of 221 patients included in this study, 33 patients were referred to the clinic before initiation of EGFRI therapy and were treated prophylactically with topical corticosteroids (12%), oral tetracycline antibiotics (15%), or both (14%). Among the 221 EGFRI-treated patients, bacterial infection was the most common subtype affecting 64 patients (29%). Bacteria were the sole cause of infection in 52 patients (23.5%), and 12 patients (5.4%) had polymicrobial infections with bacteria and/or viral and/or dermatophyte infection. *Staphylococcus aureus* was the most common bacterial pathogen observed in 50 (22.6%) of the 221 patients who received EGRFI therapy. Twelve (5.4%) of the 221 EGFRI-treated patients were infected with methicillin-resistant *S aureus* (MRSA) and 8 of these 12 MRSA infections were caused by tetracycline-resistant strains. The majority of infections were polymicrobial and localized to the seborrheic region. Fungal infection occurred in 23 patients (10.4%), whereas viral infection occurred in 13 patients (5.9%), and the most common viral infections were with herpes simplex virus and herpes zoster, occurring in 7 (3.2%) and 4 (1.8%) patients, respectively. Twenty-two (10.0%) of the 221 EGFRI-treated patients had *S aureus* colonization in the nasopharyngeal region in addition to a cutaneous bacterial, dermatophyte, or viral dermatologic infection. Five patients (2.2%) without a dermatologic infection had nasopharyngeal cultures positive for *S aureus*, of which 2 (0.9%) had MRSA colonization. Leukopenia was statistically significantly associated with the presence of a dermatologic infection ($P < .001$). A total of 20 (50%) of the 40 leukopenic patients compared with 25 (24.3%) of the 103 nonleukopenic patients had a dermatologic infection ($P = .005$). There was no association between any other clinical or demographic variable and the type of dermatologic infection ($P > 0.05$). The compromised barrier function of skin or alterations in the cutaneous immune system in patients with dermatologic toxic effects of EGFRIs may contribute to the high prevalence of infection. However, biopsies of the skin were not done to evaluate whether those on EGFRI therapy had a compromised stratum corneum as compared with those who were not on EGFRI therapy. Also, other skin conditions, such as atopic dermatitis and psoriasis, and pre-existing skin disease may contribute to increased rates of infection; however, these potential factors were not addressed in this study. Another weakness of this study was that there were no controls.

J. Q. Del Rosso, DO

G. K. Kim, DO

Epicutaneous patch testing in drug hypersensitivity syndrome (DRESS)
Santiago F, Gonçalo M, Vieira R, et al (Coimbra Univ Hosp, Portugal, et al)
Contact Dermatitis 62:47-53, 2010

Background.—In some patterns of cutaneous adverse drug reactions, and depending on the culprit drug, patch testing has been helpful in confirming its cause. Its value in Drug Rash with Eosinophilia and Systemic Symptoms (DRESS) has not been established in a large cohort of patients.

Objective.—The aim of the present study is to evaluate the safety and usefulness of patch testing in DRESS.

Patients/Methods.—Between January 1998 and December 2008, we studied 56 patients with DRESS induced by antiepileptic agents in 33 patients (59%), allopurinol in 19 (34%) and sulfasalazine, cotrimoxazole, tenoxicam, and amoxicillin in 1 patient each (7%).

Results.—A positive patch test reaction was observed in 18 patients (32.1%), of which 17 were with antiepileptics and 1 with tenoxicam. In the antiepileptic group, carbamazepine alone was responsible for 13 of 17 positive reactions (76.5%). Patch tests with allopurinol and its metabolite were negative in all cases attributed to this drug.

Conclusions.—In this study, patch testing was a safe and useful method in confirming the culprit drug in DRESS induced by antiepileptic drugs, whereas it had no value in DRESS induced by allopurinol. The pathogenesis of DRESS is not yet entirely clarified, but positive patch tests suggest a drug-dependent delayed hypersensitivity mechanism.

▶ Drug rash with eosinophilia and systemic symptoms (DRESS) is a severe life-threatening drug hypersensitivity dermatoses involving the skin and viscera. Common drugs causing DRESS include antiepileptics, dapsone, allopurinol, minocycline, and antiretroviral drugs, such as nevirapine and abacavir. Over time, the list of offending drugs continues to expand.[1] Three to 8 weeks following ingestion of the culprit drug, patients may present with fever, diffuse erythematous exanthematous skin eruption, eosinophilia, lymphocyte activation, and multivisceral involvement.[1] Fatality rate has been reported to be around 10% to 40%. The objective of this study is to evaluate the safety and application of patch testing in DRESS where rechallenges are contraindicated. Investigators studied 56 patients with DRESS from 1998 to 2008 in the Dermatology Department of Coimbra University Hospital in Portugal. Results indicate that patch testing is relatively safe where serious adverse reaction is unlikely to occur even at higher concentrations (20% petrolatum). Patch-test positivity was high (18 patients) in the antiepileptics, especially carbamazepine. In summary, clinicians may use patch testing as a safe method of identifying the culprit drug in patients with DRESS, particularly if antiepileptics are suspected. As the authors mentioned, it is important to note that patch testing should be delayed at least 4 to 6 weeks after resolution of skin symptoms, so that there is normal skin to test on, and iatrogenic immunosuppression does not reduce skin reactivity.

S. Bellew, DO

J. Q. Del Rosso, DO

Reference

1. Wolf R, Orion E, Marcos B, Matz H. Life-threatening acute adverse cutaneous drug reactions. *Clin Dermatol.* 2005;23:171-181.

High Prevalence of Potential Drug-Drug Interactions for Psoriasis Patients Prescribed Methotrexate or Cyclosporine for Psoriasis: Associated Clinical and Economic Outcomes in Real-World Practice

Saurat J-H, Guérin A, Yu AP, et al (Hôpital Cantonal Universitaire de Genève, Geneva, Switzerland; Analysis Group, Inc, Boston, MA; et al)
Dermatology 220:128-137, 2010

Background.—Methotrexate (MTX) and cyclosporine (CYC) may adversely interact with common medications in patients with psoriasis.

Objective.—Our purpose was to investigate the prevalence and outcomes of MTX/CYC polypharmacy.

Methods.—We evaluated rates of events that may be associated with drug-related toxicity, health care resource utilization and costs for patients with psoriasis in the Ingenix® Impact National Managed Care Database (1999–2007) who were exposed or not exposed to potential drug-drug interactions.

Results.—Among 4,583 (57.6%) exposed and 3,372 (42.4%) nonexposed patients, nonsteroidal anti-inflammatory drugs and antibiotics were the most common drugs with potential interactions. The exposed patients had significantly greater risks of developing renal [adjusted odds ratio (OR): 2.58; p = 0.0145], gastrointestinal (OR: 1.36; p = 0.0197) and pulmonary events (OR: 1.20; p = 0.0470), and significantly greater health care resource utilization (e.g. OR for inpatient and emergency department visits: 1.47; p < 0.0001) and costs (adjusted incremental cost: USD 1,722; p < 0.0001).

Conclusions.—MTX/CYC polypharmacy is prevalent in patients with psoriasis and associated with significant risks.

▶ Saurat et al offer an interesting article with clinical impact for physicians who prescribe methotrexate (MTX) and cyclosporine (CYC) for psoriasis. Specifically, the article looked at the prevalence of polypharmacy associated with MTX and CYC use and provides information on the most common drugs that are prescribed among clinicians, have potential drug interactions when administered along with MTX and CYC, and further, provide the most commonly associated health risks. The article reviewed a large national managed care database and remarkably found that over half of patients taking MTX or CYC also have been prescribed medications with potential interactions. The most commonly prescribed medications with the potential for interaction were nonsteroidal anti-inflammatory drugs and antibiotics, specifically, sulfonamides. In addition, it was also found that patients who were exposed to these interactions did indeed experience a greater risk of adverse events associated with pulmonary, renal, and gastrointestinal events. This in turn resulted in greater health care costs to the patient. Ultimately, this article is important from the perspective of providing awareness to dermatologists about the importance of exercising caution when prescribing both MTX and CYC in the treatment of this common chronic skin disease, especially if either medication is routinely used as a treatment option for patients. Given the significant reported prevalence of interactions, the dermatologist is reminded that a high level of awareness is both necessary and essential before any medication is prescribed because of possible drug-drug interactions that are clinically significant. To this end, the article achieves its objective and is a clinically relevant and beneficial article for all dermatologists.

B. D. Michaels, DO

J. Q. Del Rosso, DO

Investigation of papulopustular eruptions caused by cetuximab treatment shows altered differentiation markers and increases in inflammatory cytokines
Han SS, Lee M, Park GH, et al (Asan Med Ctr, Seoul, Korea; et al)
Br J Dermatol 162:371-379, 2010

Background.—Epidermal growth factor receptor (EGFR) critically regulates tumour cell division, survival and metastasis. Agents that inhibit EGFR have been used in the treatment of advanced-stage malignancies, but cause variable cutaneous side-effects, most often papulopustular eruptions and xerosis.

Objectives.—We assayed expression of inflammatory cytokines [interleukin (IL)-1α, tumour necrosis factor (TNF)-α, interferon (IFN)-γ, human leucocyte antigen (HLA)-DR and intercellular adhesion molecule (ICAM)-1], differentiation markers (filaggrin, involucrin and loricrin) and phosphorylated EGFRs (pEGFRs) in papulopustular eruptions to determine the association between these markers and the eruptions caused by cetuximab.

Patients/Methods.—Twelve papulopustular lesion biopsies were selected from patients with colon cancer who had received cetuximab treatment. Immunohistochemistry and immunofluorescence with a confocal laser scanning microscopy were performed.

Results.—Filaggrin expression decreased and expression of involucrin, various inflammatory markers (IL-1α, TNF-α, ICAM-1 and HLA-DR) increased and the expression of pEGFR was markedly downregulated in papulopustular eruptions. In perilesions, decreased pEGFR expression was noted in hair follicles compared with interfollicular epidermis. The increase of IL-1α and TNF-α was observed in perilesions as in the lesions.

Conclusions.—The early inflammatory events (IL-1α and TNF-α expression) seen, and the lack of pEGFR in perilesional follicles, indicate that inflammatory events induced by EGFR inhibition may initiate papulopustular eruptions along with the altered differentiations. The decrease of filaggrin may contribute to the pathogenesis of the xerosis caused by cetuximab.

▶ Cetuximab and other epidermal growth factor inhibitors developed for the treatment of certain malignancies have a well-recognized side effect of inducing a sterile dose-related papulopustular eruption of the face and trunk, frequently in the first 2 weeks after initiating treatment. The difficulty for clinicians is in determining the best therapy to treat and possibly prevent such eruptions. Understanding how these eruptions occur may help us in that endeavor. By using immunohistochemical techniques, the authors in this study show that keratinocyte markers, such as involucrin and filaggrin, are expressed in abnormal amounts or at irregular times in follicular lesions of those patients treated with cetuximab. They propose that the drug, by inhibiting epidermal growth factor receptor, alters the natural process of differentiation and proliferation of keratinocytes leading to inflammation, xerotic skin, and ruptured follicles.

Importantly, the details of the study help to elucidate the histology observed in these lesions and the inflammatory factors involved in the process of developing them. What is clear from this study is that this process appears to be pathogenically distinct from that of acne vulgaris, in as much as histologically; there is no mention of sebaceous gland hypertrophy or comedone formation. Additionally, cultures of lesions have generally been shown to be sterile, at least initially. Furthermore, several inflammatory modulators, such as interleukin-1 alpha, tumor necrosis factor alpha, and intercellular adhesion molecule 1, are specifically upregulated in lesional skin but not as a result of *Propionibacterium acnes* stimulation, rather likely as a direct result of downregulation of epidermal growth factor receptor. It, therefore, appears that while this process can appear clinically similar to acne, it is not likely going to respond to similar therapeutic maneuvers. Retinoids, therefore, would not be expected to be helpful in this disease state and may in fact only contribute to irritation and dryness. Based on the results of this study, it is conceivable to hypothesize that therapies such as topical steroids or calcineurin inhibitors would be of benefit. Similarly, oral tetracycline class antibiotics would also be first-line choices for more severe grades of the disease owing to their anti-inflammatory properties, as would some topical antibiotics, such as topical clindamycin or erythromycin.

Such investigational work is essential to our understanding of not only how these drugs may distort the normal order of keratinocyte differentiation leading to dermatologic side effects but may also begin to shed light on how aberrant keratinocyte maturation may influence other disease states, such as psoriasis and pemphigus.

J. M. Suchniak, MD

Management of cutaneous side-effects of cetuximab therapy in patients with metastatic colorectal cancer
Ocvirk J, Cencelj S (Inst of Oncology, Ljubljana, Slovenia; Regulatory and Med Dept, Ljubljana, Slovenia)
J Eur Acad Dermatol Venereol 24:453-459, 2010

Background.—Cetuximab is a chimeric human-murine monoclonal antibody against the epidermal growth factor receptor (EGFR). It has shown activities against multiple malignancies in clinical trials. EGFR-inhibitors (EGFRI) often cause skin toxicity, most frequently acneiform eruption. Xerosis, eczema, fissures, teleangiectases, nail changes and paronychia can be seen in some cases, rarely hyperpigmentation.

Materials and Methods.—We reviewed local practice of skin toxicity management during treatment with cetuximab. From November 2005 to January 2007, 31 patients with metastatic colorectal cancer were treated with cetuximab in combination with chemotherapy. They all suffered from acne-like rash. They were followed up for at least 3 months, once per week. Skin toxicity was evaluated according to NCI CTCAE, v3.0.

Results.—Of 31 patients, six had grade three rash, 16 patients Grade 2 and nine patients Grade 1 acne like rash. Less frequently, pruritus, dry skin, desquamation, hair modification, conjunctivitis, telangiectases, paronychia or fissures were observed. After the first documented cutaneous toxicity, topical use of emollients was started. For Grade 2 rash, we used emollients and topical antibiotics. Therapy with cetuximab was discontinued at Grade 3 until skin reactions resolved. Skin reactions at Grade 3 were generally manageable with emollients, topical and systemic antibiotics. No Grade 4 skin reactions were observed.

Conclusion.—During the treatment with EGFRI, it is necessary to recognize and manage adverse reactions promptly to assure better patient quality of life and allowing continuation of therapy without dose reduction or drug discontinuation.

▶ Since their approval, epidermal growth factor inhibitors have been on dermatologists' radar owing to their near universal and often debilitating cutaneous side effects on the patients who receive them. Cetuximab acts by inhibiting and subsequently downregulating the epidermal growth factor receptor and, by extension, the proliferative cytokines that promote tumor development. However, epidermal and follicular cells also express this receptor, and unintended side effects of the drug are commonplace. This study describes the therapeutic approaches of 1 clinic to the most common cutaneous side effects in

31 patients. Their approach to the most common of these, acneiform eruptions, is to judge the severity of the outbreak, then begin applying emollients, followed by topical clindamycin, and, if needed, oral clindamycin. Interestingly, the authors eschewed the use of topical steroids, a treatment that some in the United States find helpful, especially in symptomatic patients. The next most common side effects, xerosis and fissures, were seen in about half the patients, and conservative measures with emollients were recommended. Pyogenic granulomas of the nailbeds were treated with topical antibiotics, with limited success, and conjunctivitis was ameliorated with topical neomycin/dexamethasone.

This study reminds us that these cutaneous side effects are exceedingly common in this patient population and that prompt intervention is necessary to avoid interruption or complete cessation of therapy. At the same time, the study also underscores the reality that many of the side effects are very difficult to treat and that if necessary, cessation of therapy may be the best option to limit morbidity. Overall, the standard tenets of skin care apply in these patients: proper bathing with mild cleansers, frequent emollition, and local wound care as needed. The more frequent acneiform eruption should be treated with topical and oral systemic antibiotics. We must also keep in mind that the need for innovative and esoteric approaches may at times be necessary to achieve the desired outcome.

J. M. Suchniak, MD

The Safety and Efficacy of Pimecrolimus, 1%, Cream for the Treatment of Netherton Syndrome: Results From an Exploratory Study
Yan AC, Honig PJ, Ming ME, et al (Univ of Pennsylvania School of Medicine, Philadelphia; Hosp of the Univ of Pennsylvania, Philadelphia)
Arch Dermatol 146:57-62, 2010

Background.—Impaired skin integrity in patients with Netherton syndrome (NS) results in significant systemic absorption of topically applied medications. Some have advocated the administration of pimecrolimus, 1%, topical cream for the treatment of patients with NS. Insufficient data exist with regard to its safety, systemic absorption, and efficacy.

Observations.—An exploratory study was conducted involving 3 children with NS who received twice-daily application of pimecrolimus, 1%, cream over 18 months. There were no notable abnormalities in hematologic or chemistry profiles. Blood levels of pimecrolimus ranged from 0.625 to 7.08 ng/mL, with peak levels reached during the first month in all 3 patients. Dramatic reductions were observed in the Netherton Area and Severity Assessment, Eczema Area and Severity Index, Investigator Global Evaluation of Disease, and pruritus scores compared with baseline levels.

Conclusions.—Use of pimecrolimus, 1%, cream was well tolerated and demonstrated marked improvements in nearly all of the parameters evaluated. Patients treated with pimecrolimus responded rapidly, within the first month of treatment, and improvement persisted throughout the study period. In adult patients receiving oral pimecrolimus, blood levels as high as 54 ng/mL for 3 months have not shown clinically significant immunosuppression. Absorption of pimecrolimus, 1%, cream was detectable, but levels were much lower than expected even when applied to 50% of total body surface area. Larger studies are warranted to determine the safety and efficacy of pimecrolimus, 1%, cream in the treatment of NS. *Trial Registration.*—clinicaltrials.gov Identifier: NCT00208026.

► Netherton syndrome is classically comprised of the triad of trichorrhexis invaginata, ichthyosis linearis circumflexa, and atopic diathesis. It is caused by a genetic defect in *SPINK5* gene. Controlling the chronic pruritus and eczematous skin rashes can be very difficult. Management and limiting use of corticosteroids were made even more difficult when reports of significant cutaneous absorption of tacrolimus surfaced.[1] In this report of 3 patients with Netherton syndrome, the use of pimecrolimus 1% cream was closely monitored with laboratory testing, including complete blood cell counts, hepatic function testing, electrolytes, blood urea nitrogen, glucose monitoring, and serum pimecrolimus levels. Clinical improvement was also determined by Netherton Area and Severity Assessment, Eczema Area and Severity Index, Investigator's Global Evaluation of Disease, and Children's Dermatology Quality of Life Index. Significant clinical improvement was noted fairly quickly with the use of pimecrolimus 1% cream twice daily as needed. Over the course of treatment, cutaneous absorption of pimecrolimus was documented, with levels highest during the first month. These elevations were considered mild, and no evidence of immunosuppression was noted either clinically or evidenced by changes in laboratory values. While not every dermatologist treats patients with Netherton syndrome, this study highlights the need to determine safe use of topical medications in patients with impaired barrier function. Safety should not be assumed when using medications for off-label use.

A. Zaenglein, MD

Reference

1. Allen A, Siegfried E, Silverman R, et al. Significant absorption of topical tacrolimus in 3 patients with Netherton syndrome. *Arch Dermatol.* 2001;137:747-750.

Phenytoin-induced acute generalized exanthemous pustulosis
Aziz N, Toerge S, Nigra T (Riverside Regional Med Ctr, Newport News, VA; Washington Hosp Ctr, DC)
J Am Acad Dermatol 62:718-719, 2010

Background.—The most common antiepileptic drugs that have been associated with the development of acute generalized exanthemous pustulosis (AGEP) are carbamazepine and phenobarbital. A case in which phenytoin was implicated occurred in an African American man whose seizure disorder was related to a traumatic head injury.

Case Report.—Man, 57, came to the emergency department
(ED) complaining of multiple pustular lesions that had begun on
his face and spread to his trunk and upper extremities. Five days
earlier he had come to the same ED in status epilepticus, for
which he was given 1 g phenytoin and increased doses of the lora-
zepam and levetiracetam he was taking for his seizures. The seizure
resolved and he was discharged after 2 days on increased doses of
levetiracetam and valproic acid. Physical examination revealed
a febrile patient with nonfollicular round pustules 1 to 3 mm in
size covering his face. Erythematous plaques studded with pustules
were seen over the chest, back, and upper extremities. Severe
edema of the right eye and irregular macular erythema with diffuse
edema of the right hand were also noted. Laboratory investigation
found leukocytosis with increased band neutrophil levels and hypo-
calcemia. A lesional punch biopsy with hematoxylin-eosin stain
demonstrated neutrophilic spongiosis in some epidermal areas
and patchy intraepidermal neutrophilic infiltrates with slight aggregation in the upper epidermis consistent with pustules. Edema and
sparse perivascular lymphoid infiltrates were noted in the superficial dermis, consistent with a diagnosis of AGEP. The patient was
started immediately on a regimen of 20 mg prednisone four times
daily for 4 days and improved within 48 hours. Most pustules
had ruptured after the fourth day of therapy, leaving exfoliated
areas. On the sixth day the patient was discharged with a prednisone taper prescription.

Conclusions.—This is the first case to demonstrate phenytoin as the
cause of AGEP. It was considered the likely cause since it was the only
new drug the patient received. Although not previously one of the antiepileptics associated with this diagnosis, phenytoin should be added to the
suspect list. AGEP is fortunately largely self-limited, with most patients
having a full recovery.

▶ Acute generalized exanthematous pustulosis (AGEP) is characterized by
a sudden onset of sterile nonfollicular pustules on an erythematous base usually
accompanied by leukocytosis, fever, and elevated blood neutrophilia. Histologic examination reveals spongiform intraepidermal neutrophilic pustules,
papillary edema, and perivascular lymphoid infiltrates. Drugs are often the
offending agent in most cases, and the current report illustrates a patient with
phenytoin-induced AGEP. In review of literature, there are 2 additional reports
that support this finding.[1,2] More commonly, drugs that were found to have
a higher association with AGEP include pristinamycin, aminopenicillins, quino-
lones, hydroxychloroquine, sulfonamides, terbinafine, and diltiazem.[1] Interestingly, a study of 36 Korean patients found that herbal medications, lacquers,
and radiocontrast media were the main causative agents.[3] In evaluating patients
with pustular dermatoses, an extensive medical history along with recent medications used is imperative for diagnosis and treatment. The interval between

administration of offending drug and the onset of skin findings vary from 2 days to 2 to 3 weeks.[1] Fortunately, the overall prognosis is good for most patients, and discontinuation of causative drug will often resolve clinical signs and symptoms. Additionally, systemic corticosteroids may be used according to disease severity.

S. Bellew, DO

J. Q. Del Rosso, DO

References

1. Sidoroff A, Dunant A, Viboud C, et al. Risk factors for acute generalized exanthematous pustulosis (AGEP) — results of a multinational case-control study (EuroSCAR). *Br J Dermatol.* 2007;157:989-996.
2. Lee HY, Chou D, Pang SM, Thirumoorthy T. Acute generalized exanthematous pustulosis: analysis of cases managed in a tertiary hospital in Singapore. *Int J Dermatol.* 2010;49:507-512.
3. Choi MJ, Kim HS, Park HJ, et al. Clinicopathologic manifestations of 36 Korean patients with acute generalized exanthematous pustulosis: a case series and review of the literature. *Ann Dermatol.* 2010;22:163-169.

Role of minor determinants of amoxicillin in the diagnosis of immediate allergic reactions to amoxicillin

Torres MJ, Ariza A, Fernández J, et al (Carlos Haya Hosp, Malaga, Spain; F-IMABIS-Carlos Haya Hosp, Malaga, Spain; UMH, Elche, Spain; et al)
Allergy 65:590-596, 2010

Background.—Skin testing of subjects with immediate hypersensitivity to amoxicillin is performed using major and minor determinants of benzylpenicillin plus amoxicillin. However, sensitivity is not optimal, and other determinants need to be considered. We assessed the sensitivity of stable, well-characterized minor determinants of amoxicillin in subjects with immediate allergic reactions to amoxicillin to improve skin test sensitivity.

Methods.—Amoxicillin, amoxicilloic acid, and diketopiperazine were prepared and characterized by reverse-phase HPLC, tested *in vivo* by skin testing and *in vitro* by basophil activation test and RAST inhibition assay.

Results.—Patients with immediate hypersensitivity to amoxicillin were selected: Group A ($n = 32$), skin test positive just to amoxicillin; Group B ($n = 19$), skin test positive to benzylpenicillin determinants; Group C ($n = 10$), skin test negative and amoxicillin drug provocation test positive. In Group A, 27 subjects (81.8%) were skin test positive to amoxicillin, ten (30.3%) to amoxicilloic acid, two (6.1%) to diketopiperacine, and six (18.2%) negative. In Group B, nine (50%) were positive to amoxicillin, eight (42.1%) to amoxicilloic acid, none to diketopiperacine, and nine (50%) negative. In Group C, skin tests were negative. BAT was positive to amoxicillin in 26 patients (50.9%), to amoxicilloic acid in 15 (29.1%), and diketopiperazine in four (7.8%). RAST inhibition studies showed

> 50% inhibition in all sera, with the highest concentration of amoxicillin and amoxicilloic acid.

Conclusions.—The combination of minor determinants of amoxicillin, amoxicilloic acid, and diketopiperazine seems to be of no greater value than the use of amoxicillin alone. Further efforts are needed to find new structures to improve sensitivity in the diagnosis of immediate hypersensitivity to betalactams.

▶ Improved sensitivity of the present diagnostic skin testing for immediate hypersensitivity allergic reactions to amoxicillin is needed. As it stands now, the sensitivity of the existing combination of skin testing determinants is less than optimal. Testing is currently being performed using the major and minor determinants of benzylpenicillin plus amoxicillin for allergies to betalactams, including amoxicillin. In hopes of finding increased sensitivity for skin testing, the goal of this study was to analyze whether there would be increased skin test sensitivity using other minor skin determinants, specifically amoxicillin, amoxicilloic acid, and diketopiperazine. While the objective of this study was certainly met, their findings unfortunately revealed that the used combination of minor determinants would not improve the diagnosis and be of no greater value than the use of amoxicillin. Ultimately, this study is certainly a step in the right direction, but the finding of new structures for testing will be needed if there is an expectation of improving skin test sensitivity for those individuals with an immediate allergic hypersensitivity to amoxicillin.

B. D. Michaels, DO
J. Q. Del Rosso, DO

11 Drug Development and Promotion

A randomized, controlled comparative study of the wrinkle reduction benefits of a cosmetic niacinamide/peptide/retinyl propionate product regimen vs. a prescription 0·02% tretinoin product regimen
Fu JJJ, Hillebrand GG, Raleigh P, et al (Private Practice, Mason, OH; The Procter and Gamble Company, Cincinnati, OH; et al)
Br J Dermatol 162:647-654, 2010

Background.—Tretinoin is considered the benchmark prescription topical therapy for improving fine facial wrinkles, but skin tolerance issues can affect patient compliance. In contrast, cosmetic antiwrinkle products are well tolerated but are generally presumed to be less efficacious than tretinoin.

Objectives.—To compare the efficacy of a cosmetic moisturizer regimen vs. a prescription regimen with 0·02% tretinoin for improving the appearance of facial wrinkles.

Methods.—An 8-week, randomized, parallel-group study was conducted in 196 women with moderate to moderately severe periorbital wrinkles. Following 2 weeks washout, subjects on the cosmetic regimen ($n = 99$) used a sun protection factor (SPF) 30 moisturizing lotion containing 5% niacinamide, peptides and antioxidants, a moisturizing cream containing niacinamide and peptides, and a targeted wrinkle product containing niacinamide, peptides and 0·3% retinyl propionate. Subjects on the prescription regimen ($n = 97$) used 0·02% tretinoin plus moisturizing SPF 30 sunscreen. Subject cohorts ($n = 25$) continued treatment for an additional 16 weeks. Changes in facial wrinkling were assessed by both expert grading and image analysis of digital images of subjects' faces and by self-assessment questionnaire. Product tolerance was assessed via clinical erythema and dryness grading, subject self-assessment, and determinations of skin barrier integrity (transepidermal water loss) and stratum corneum protein changes.

Results.—The cosmetic regimen significantly improved wrinkle appearance after 8 weeks relative to tretinoin, with comparable benefits after 24 weeks. The cosmetic regimen was significantly better tolerated than tretinoin through 8 weeks by all measures.

Conclusions.—An appropriately designed cosmetic regimen can improve facial wrinkle appearance comparably with the benchmark prescription treatment, with improved tolerability.

▶ This study by Fu et al is a groundbreaking study for the cosmeceutical industry. It is the first study to compare the effectiveness of an over-the-counter (OTC) cosmetic product to a prescription retinoid in a large, double blinded, well-designed, and objective study.

The reviewers are impressed with the authors for using about 100 subjects per group for up to 24 weeks and the use of 3 different methods to evaluate product efficacy (self assessment by the subject, expert graders via photographs, and objective computer analysis via VISIA CR imaging technology). However, a split face trial would have made these study results even stronger, and it would have been more complete for the authors to have included their inclusion/exclusion criteria for selecting patients for the trial.

The niacinamide/peptide/retinyl propionate (NPP) formulas contain 3 of the strongest OTC ingredients for antiaging: an OTC retinoid, 2 polypeptides, and niacinamide. Niacinamide in the literature is shown to be a potent antioxidant, decreases hyperpigmentation, increases skin barrier function, increases ceramide synthesis, and decreases wrinkles. Polypeptides stimulate collagen synthesis. Retinoids increase collagen production, decrease hyperpigmentation, and decrease surface roughness. However, the use of retinyl propionate as the retinoid of choice in the NPP formulas was surprising. The most studied OTC retinoids are as far from skin permeation and metabolism as retinoic acid is to retinol and retinaldehyde.

One of the main signs and symptoms of aging is decreased barrier function evidenced by increased transepidermal water loss (TEWL). Despite both tretinoin and NPP having similar clinical antiaging effects at 24 weeks, in our opinion the NPP products may be a the better overall antiaging regimen given its ability to increase skin barrier function and decrease TEWL. This antiaging effect in the NPP formula is likely due to the niacinamide.

Also, the subjects using tretinoin even at a low percentage struggled with irritation, dryness, and erythema throughout the 24 weeks of the study. Many believe that irritation and inflammation as evidenced by the erythema, dryness, and increased TEWL may actually cancel out some of the antiaging effects of tretinoin.

Overall, this is an excellent study proving the effectiveness of these antiaging OTC formulas and the possible role for cosmeceuticals for patients that cannot tolerate prescription retinoids.

J. Levin, DO
J. Q. Del Rosso, DO

Hydrosoluble medicated nail lacquers: *in vitro* drug permeation and corresponding antimycotic activity

Monti D, Saccomani L, Chetoni P, et al (Univ of Pisa, Italy; et al)
Br J Dermatol 162:311-317, 2010

Background.—Two nail lacquers, containing ciclopirox (CPX) or amorolfine (MRF), based on water-insoluble polymers are currently considered mainstays of topical treatment of onychomycosis. The present study aimed at evaluating the antimycotic activity of a new water-soluble nail lacquer containing CPX (CPX/sol), easily removable by washing with water and applicable to periungual skin.

Objectives.—To compare transungual permeation of CPX with that of MRF in the same hydroxypropyl chitosan-based nail lacquer (MRF/sol) and with a nonwater-soluble reference (Loceryl®; Galderma International, La Défense, France), and to evaluate the antimycotic activity of CPX/sol and Loceryl® against the most common fungal strains that cause onychomycosis.

Methods.—*In vitro* drug permeation experiments with CPX/sol, MRF/sol and Loceryl® were carried out through bovine hoof slices. Experimental permeates from CPX/sol and Loceryl® underwent *in vitro* susceptibility testing against clinical isolates of dermatophytes, moulds and yeast.

Results.—MRF transungual flux from MRF/sol lacquer was significantly higher when compared with Loceryl®. CPX was able to permeate hoof membranes more easily compared with MRF. CPX and MRF concentrations in the subungual fluids collected after application of CPX/sol or Loceryl® were sufficient to inhibit fungal growth, with the exception of *Candida parapsilosis*. Smaller amounts of fluid containing CPX were required for complete inhibition of fungal growth. Efficacy index values were significantly higher for CPX/sol.

Conclusions.—Application of the CPX/sol nail lacquer allows rapid nail penetration of CPX, providing CPX levels sufficient to inhibit fungal growth for a prolonged period of time (30 h) after application of lacquer dose. CPX/sol nail lacquer appeared superior to the market reference Loceryl® in terms of both vehicle (hydroxypropyl chitosan) and active ingredient (CPX) as witnessed by its higher efficacy on all nail pathogens.

▶ Dermatologists desperately want an effective topical antifungal drug to treat onychomycosis, and there is a lot of research in this area involving novel vehicles, drugs, and devices. This article presents a new water-soluble nail lacquer containing ciclopirox (CPX). The lacquer is easily removed without acetone-based removers. The nail plate prevents drug from acting on the nail bed where the fungus resides, so products that facilitate penetration of the nail plate have promise. The application of the CPX/water-soluble and water-based nail lacquer allows rapid nail penetration of CPX, providing CPX levels sufficient to inhibit fungal growth for up to 30 hours after the application of a lacquer dose. This study is an in vitro permeation study in bovine hooves, testing the new preparation against common fungal strains that cause onychomycosis. While this is novel and interesting, it may have little relevance to human onychomycosis, and in vivo studies in human nails would be more compelling.

P. Rich, MD

Predicting Migraine Responsiveness to Botulinum Toxin Type A Injections
Kim CC, Bogart MM, Wee SA, et al (Harvard Med School, Boston, MA)
Arch Dermatol 146:159-163, 2010

Background.—Botulinum toxin type A (BTX) is used prophylactically to reduce the frequency of migraine headaches, with inconsistent responses reported in the literature. The purpose of our study was to determine whether BTX injections at doses used for upper-face cosmetic purposes, which differ from doses typically used by headache specialists, could prevent imploding and ocular but not exploding migraines.

Observations.—Study participants were recruited among patients who had received or were planning to receive BTX injections for upper-face cosmetic purposes but also reported having migraines. Among the 18 patients who completed the study, most with imploding and ocular migraines experienced a significant reduction in their headache frequency, whereas those with exploding migraines generally did not.

Conclusions.—Our study supports the hypothesis that patients with imploding and ocular migraines are more responsive to BTX than those with exploding migraines. Injections of BTX at doses appropriate for cosmetic purposes may be sufficient to prevent migraine attacks.

▶ Botox (BTX) treatment for migraine headaches shows inconsistent efficacy data. The authors of this study suppose that the inconsistent success rate in BTX for the treatment of migraines may be because of the fact that BTX may only effectively treat a certain subset of migraine headache types. The objective of this study is to determine if BTX may have a higher success rate in treating imploding, exploding, or ocular migraines.

This study had several limitations related to study design, which included the small number of participants of the study, the inclusion criteria for patients accepted into the study, the lack of a placebo injection, the subjective classification of the migraine headache type, and the potential for recall bias when reporting the effect of the BTX treatments.

Regarding the number of participants in this study, it is hard to characterize a reliable trend when less than 50 subjects are analyzed.

The inclusion criteria of this study allowed for patients who had already had BTX of the upper face/glabella area to be included into the study. Patients that have had BTX in these areas for cosmetic reasons may have partial coincidental treatment of their migraine headaches before starting the study, therefore, not establishing an accurate baseline prior to the study resulting in an inaccurate measure of change after the migraine-specific BTX treatment.

Because migraine headaches are debilitating but not life threatening, it would have been an excellent study design to include a placebo control group with patients receiving saline injections to see if patients obtained relief of their headaches from the placebo effect of injection.

Pain is often very difficult for patients to characterize or localize. Therefore, we can assume that the subjective self-assessment of the patient's migraine headache type may be difficult and vary from person to person. In addition, the authors never addressed the possibility of patients having multiple overlapping symptoms of exploding, imploding, and ocular migraines that may lead to the improper patient characterization of headache type and hence incorrect analyses of the results.

The study also never mentioned whether the patients were required to keep a headache diary throughout the 3-month treatment window. This may result in a recall bias at the end of the 3-month treatment period, and patients may overstate or underreport the actual number of migraine headaches they had over the time period.

The reviewers also believe that there may be a major flaw with the theory in general that BTX may treat imploding with better efficacy than exploding headaches. Given the mechanism of action of BTX, perhaps it may best to treat migraine headaches that are triggered by muscular tension. In other words, BTX works by relaxing the muscles, so it seems likely that BTX may actually decrease migraines that stem from muscle tension or strain instead of factors like food, sunlight, and/or dehydration.

In general, it is commonly known that pharmacologic prophylactic migraine therapy only works for a small subset of patients with chronic migraines. It would have been interesting for the authors to report previously reported success rate of pharmacologic prophylactic migraine therapy so that we could compare it to success rate of BTX for the treatment of migraine patients.

J. Levin, DO

J. Q. Del Rosso, DO

Reduction in the appearance of facial hyperpigmentation after use of moisturizers with a combination of topical niacinamide and *N*-acetyl glucosamine: results of a randomized, double-blind, vehicle-controlled trial

Kimball AB, Kaczvinsky JR, Li J, et al (Harvard Med School, Boston, MA; The Procter & Gamble Company, Cincinnati, OH; et al)
Br J Dermatol 162:435-441, 2010

Background.—Topical niacinamide and N-acetyl glucosamine (NAG) each individually inhibit epidermal pigmentation in cell culture. In small clinical studies, niacinamide-containing and NAG-containing formulations reduced the appearance of hyperpigmentation.

Objectives.—To assess the effect of a combination of niacinamide and NAG in a topical moisturizing formulation on irregular facial pigmentation, including specific detection of changes in colour features associated with melanin.

Methods.—This was a 10-week, double-blind, vehicle-controlled, full-face, parallel-group clinical study conducted in women aged 40–60 years. After a 2-week washout period, subjects used a daily regimen of either a morning sun protection factor (SPF) 15 sunscreen moisturizing lotion and evening moisturizing cream each containing 4% niacinamide + 2% NAG (test formulation; $n = 101$) or the SPF 15 lotion and cream vehicles (vehicle control; $n = 101$). Product-induced changes in apparent pigmentation were assessed by capturing digital photographic images of the women after 0, 4, 6 and 8 weeks of product use and evaluating the images by algorithm-based computer image analysis for coloured spot area fraction, by expert visual grading, and by chromophore-specific image analysis based on noncontact SIAscopy™ for melanin spot area fraction and melanin chromophore evenness.

Results.—By all four measures, the niacinamide + NAG formulation regimen was significantly ($P < 0.05$) more effective than the vehicle control formulation regimen in reducing the detectable area of facial spots and the appearance of pigmentation.

Conclusions.—A formulation containing the combination of niacinamide + NAG reduced the appearance of irregular pigmentation including hypermelaninization, providing an effect beyond that achieved with SPF 15 sunscreen.

▶ This is an excellently designed and executed study looking at the effectiveness of niacinamide 4% combined with *N*-acetyl glucosamine (NAG) 2% for reducing facial hyperpigmentation associated with photoaging. The product combination is excellent in theory because of the dual mechanism of action for preventing pigmentation. Simply stated, niacinamide prevents pigment transfer from melanocytes to keratinocytes, and NAG reduces the pigment production by slowing down the enzyme tyrosinase. This combination product has the potential to be a great over the counter product for treating patients with hyperpigmentation.

The reviewers were extremely impressed with the number of patients in this study, the methods implemented to measure patient compliance, the objective measurements of pigmentation and spot size, the photography methods, the division of treatment group versus placebo to equalize age and pigmentation level between the groups, and the use of a wash-out period.

However, we do question why only 4% niacinamide was used in this formula (as most of the clinical studies on niacinamide is based on a 5% formula), why the study was only conducted for 8 weeks instead of 12 or 24 weeks, the use of only a 2-week wash out period, and it was not mentioned whether patients were excluded based on previous cosmetic procedures, such as laser treatments, peels, or hydroquinone use. We also believe that a split face trial would have allowed even greater comparison of the tested product versus placebo.

Even with the above limitations, overall, this is one of the best cosmeceutical studies that we the reviewers have seen to date. Given the significant results of this study, this product is an excellent treatment option for patients with hyperpigmentation. However, a comparison to the effectiveness of other treatment products of its kind like vitamin C, hydroquinone, soy proteases, and retinoids should be made to determine whether this product offers superior results for patients with hyperpigmentation secondary to photoaging.

J. Levin, DO
J. Q. Del Rosso, DO

12 Miscellaneous Topics in Clinical Dermatology

A double-blind, randomized study to assess the effectiveness of different moisturizers in preventing dermatitis induced by hand washing to simulate healthcare use

Williams C, Wilkinson SM, Mcshane P, et al (Univ of Leeds, UK)

Br J Dermatol 162:1088-1092, 2010

Background.—Healthcare-associated infection is an important worldwide problem that could be reduced by better hand hygiene practice. However, irritant contact dermatitis of the hands as a result of repeated hand washing is a potential complication that may be preventable by the regular use of an emollient.

Objectives.—To assess the effect of moisturizer application after repeated hand washing (15 times daily) vs. soap alone.

Methods.—In a double-blind, randomized study, the effect of five different moisturizers on skin barrier function was determined by assessment after repeated hand washing over a 2-week period in healthy adult volunteers. Assessments of transepidermal water loss (TEWL), epidermal hydration and a visual assessment using the Hand Eczema Severity Index (HECSI) were made at days 0, 7 and 14.

Results.—In total, 132 patients were enrolled into the study. A statistically significant worsening of the clinical condition of the skin as measured by HECSI was seen from baseline to day 14 ($P = 0.003$) in those subjects repeatedly washing their hands with soap without subsequent application of moisturizer. No change was seen in the groups using moisturizer. Subclinical assessment of epidermal hydration as a measure of skin barrier function showed significant increases from baseline to day 14 after the use of three of the five moisturizing products ($P = 0.041$, 0.001 and 0.009). Three of the five moisturizers tested led to a statistically significant decrease in TEWL at day 7 of repeated hand washing. This effect was sustained for one moisturizing product at day 14 of hand washing ($P = 0.044$).

Conclusions.—These results support the view that the regular application of moisturizers to normal skin offers a protective effect against repeated exposure to irritants, with no evidence of a reduction in barrier efficiency allowing the easier permeation of irritant substances into the skin as has been suggested by other studies. Regular use of emollient in the healthcare environment may prevent the development of dermatitis.

▶ Health care–associated infection is an important public health concern that can be largely remedied by better hand hygiene practice. However, the detrimental effects of frequent hand washing, including dryness, irritation, and skin barrier dysfunctions cause a decrease in compliance by health care workers. This double-blinded randomized study (N = 132) looked at whether routine use of emollients following hand washing would provide better protection against the repeated assaults by skin irritants. Subjects were followed for a 2-week period. Measurements were made of transepidermal water loss (TEWL) using a Delfin VapoMeter, epidermal hydration measured via a Corneometer CM825, and product tolerability was assessed using a clinical grading system of hand dermatitis with the Hand Eczema Severity Index. Results support the protective effects of regular moisturization against repeated exposure to irritants. In fact, 3 of the 5 moisturizers used increased epidermal hydration and 1 led to significant reduction in TEWL. The type of emollients used in the study is an important factor when evaluating this type of data, as previous investigations have shown a significant difference in the mechanisms of action between nonphysiologic, physiologic, and incomplete physiologic lipid applications.[1] These studies showed that physiologic lipid mixtures (ie, ceramides and cholesterol sulfate) facilitate the barrier recovery mechanism, whereas nonphysiologic ointments (ie, petrolatum) remain localized and restricted to the stratum corneum in an occlusive fashion, and incomplete mixtures actually delay the repair process.[2]

S. Bellew, DO

J. Q. Del Rosso, DO

References

1. Mao-Qiang M, Feingold KR, Elias PM. Influence of exogenous lipids on permeability barrier recovery in acetone-treated murine skin. *Arch Dermatol.* 1993; 129:728-738.
2. Mao-Qiang M, Brown BE, Wu-Pong S, Feingold KR, Elias PM. Exogenous nonphysiologic vs physiologic lipids. Divergent mechanisms for correction of permeability barrier dysfunction. *Arch Dermatol.* 1995;131:809-816.

A global survey of the role of ultraviolet radiation and hormonal influences in the development of melasma
Ortonne JP, Arellano I, Berneburg M, et al (Univ of Nice-Sophia Antipolis, France; Hosp General de México, Mexico City; Eberhard-Karls Univ, Tubingen, Germany; et al)
J Eur Acad Dermatol Venereol 23:1254-1262, 2009

Background.—It has been generally believed that the four main causes of melasma are pregnancy, hormonal contraception, family history and sun exposure; however, there are few published comprehensive studies that confirm these assertions. The Pigmentary Disorders Academy – an international group of experts in pigmentary disorders — designed and conducted a global survey of women to investigate the effect of these factors on onset and chronicity of melasma and the course of the disease in order to gain a better understanding of the causative factors associated with this disorder, with a particular focus on hormonal factors and UV exposure in females.

Methods.—A 40-item largely self-administered questionnaire was completed by 324 women being treated for melasma in nine clinics worldwide.

Results.—The mean age at onset of melasma was 34 years, and 48% of subjects questioned had a family history of melasma (97% in a first-degree relative). Subjects with family history of melasma tended to have darker skin (90% types III—VI) compared to those without (77% types III—VI). The most common time of onset was after pregnancy (42%), often years after the last pregnancy, with 29% appearing pre-pregnancy and 26% during pregnancy. Onset was related to darker skin type post-pregnancy ($P = 0.002$). Risk of onset during pregnancy was associated with having spent more time outdoors (an extra 10 h per week spent working outside increases the odds of onset of melasma during pregnancy by approximately 27%) and an increased maternal age at pregnancy (increased by approximately 8% for each year of age at first pregnancy; $P = 0.02$). The odds of melasma occurring for the first time during a pregnancy were also increased with multiple pregnancies (twice the odds if 2 vs. 1 pregnancies, three times higher if 3 or more vs. 1 pregnancy). Of the women, 25% who had used hormonal contraception claimed that melasma appeared for the first time after its use, the rate being higher for those without vs. with a family history.

Conclusions.—The results suggest that, whilst accepted causes do affect onset of melasma, a combination of these factors often triggers this disorder. These factors may provide further insights into how physicians can manage individual melasma cases, support recommendation of preventative measures and even anticipate treatment results and recurrence.

▶ The authors introduce the formation of the first Pigmentary Disorders Academy—an international group of experts in disorders of pigmentation. In their article, a 40-question global survey of 324 women with melasma was initiated to investigate the relationship between and the effects of 4 factors, that is, pregnancy, hormonal contraception, family history, and sun exposure on this common form of dyschromia and to use the data to determine the course and chronicity of melasma.

The article is of high quality and is well organized, supplying data that are properly stratified. Appropriate parameters defining melasma and its apparent etiologies were analyzed and underwent careful logistic regression. Additionally, the authors substratify the data by using recursive partitioning to identify further those subjects who fell into more distinct groups.

The article provides interesting, informative, and useful data that has clinical relevance and may have some impact on the clinicians approach to the management of melasma (eg, 48% of subjects with a positive family history of melasma—97% first-degree relatives—29% of subjects with melasma following contraceptive use—match data from previous studies).

The limitations of this study/survey include its lack of investigation of the prevalence of melasma within subgroups, as all survey subjects were known diagnosed melasma patients. The authors acknowledge further that hormonal contraception and the timing of its use relative to pregnancy in some subjects was not recorded, which may have an impact as to which triggering factor, if either, may have been responsible for the development of melasma in a particular study subject. Furthermore, there is a lack of randomization and controls with this type of study and survey results, which may affect the interpretation of the data. The authors, therefore, acknowledge the need for additional randomized investigations.

B. P. Glick, DO, MPH

Over-the-counter scar products for postsurgical patients: Disparities between online advertised benefits and evidence regarding efficacy
Morganroth P, Wilmot AC, Miller C (Univ of Pennsylvania, Philadelphia)
J Am Acad Dermatol 61:e31-e47, 2009

Surgical patients frequently read about over-the-counter (OTC) scar products online and ask physicians for advice about product use. We summarized the characteristics of the 20 best-selling scar products on the Web site drugstore.com and reviewed the medical literature for data supporting the efficacy of OTC scar products used on fresh postsurgical wounds. Products had an average price of $16.25 (range $9.49-$59.99) and an average of 9.2 ingredients (range 1-29). Silicone, vitamin E, and onion extract were common ingredients. Although weak evidence indicates that silicone gel dressings may improve postsurgical scar appearance, published evidence does not support postoperative use of most scar products. However, many products have multiple ingredients, and few clinical trials assess the ingredient combinations of specific products. The practical information about OTC scar products and published efficacy data found in this review may help physicians to counsel patients about postsurgical product use and counter unrealistic expectations gained from online advertisements.

▶ This is a study identifying 20 best-selling over-the-counter (OTC) scar products on the web site drugstore.com and characterizing the products according to price, advertised benefits, ingredients, vehicles, directions for use, regulation, and efficacy data. Inclusion criteria were prospective controlled clinical trials involving application of silicone gel dressings or topical agents containing onion extract, vitamin E, or sunscreen, or topical corticosteroids to fresh postsurgical wounds. Studies of mature scars, evolving scars exhibiting hypertrophic or keloid changes, and burn wounds were excluded. The 10 most common ingredients were silicone, vitamin E, water, methylparaben, glycerin, onion extract, carbomer, polyethylene glycol, vitamin A, and vitamin C. Many products had specific warnings against application near the eyes, mucous membranes, or infected wounds. Only 4 of the 20 products from drugstore.com differentiated between active and inactive ingredients. The authors found that despite laboratory data, clinical data did not support the benefits of onion extract for improvement of postoperative scar appearance. Vitamin E and its derivatives were the second most common ingredients in the OTC scar products. Silicone was the most common ingredient in the OTC products. Studies revealed that the force of occlusion was at least as important or possibly more important than silicone itself in modulating fibroblast activity and improving scar appearance. There were also 2 products that contained copper peptide complexes, which may increase extracellular matrix accumulation observed in copper peptides in rat models. Only 9 clinical trials met the inclusion criteria, with most of the trials evaluating a single ingredient as compared with the OTC product with multiple active and inactive ingredients. There is a need for more and better randomized clinical trials evaluating the specific combinations of ingredients. To add, concentration in each OTC scar medication may vary, and because these OTC products are not regulated by the Food and Drug Administration, any given product may have insufficient concentration for efficacy. This study illustrated a notable disparity between the online advertised benefits of many OTC products and existing data to support their efficacy.

J. Q. Del Rosso, DO

G. K. Kim, DO

Acitretin for Severe Lichen Sclerosus of Male Genitalia: A Randomized, Placebo Controlled Study
Ioannides D, Lazaridou E, Apalla Z, et al (Aristotle Univ Med School, Thessaloniki, Greece; et al)
J Urol 183:1395-1399, 2010

Purpose.—Genital lichen sclerosus is a chronic inflammatory and fibro-sclerotic disease associated with substantial morbidity. Acitretin has been reported to be of benefit in many dermatological indications including lichen sclerosus. We evaluated the efficacy and tolerability of acitretin for biopsy confirmed, severe lichen sclerosus of the male genitalia.

Materials and Methods.—A randomized, double-blind, placebo controlled study was performed in which 52 male patients with severe, long-standing lichen sclerosus were randomized in a 2:1 ratio to receive daily acitretin (35 mg) or placebo for 20 consecutive weeks. Followup lasted for 36 weeks from baseline. The primary end point was complete response of active lichen sclerosus as well as improvement of patient quality of life. Secondary end points were partial response and recurrence rates after treatment discontinuation.

Results.—A total of 49 patients completed the study and were eligible for statistical analysis. Complete response was achieved by 36.4% (12 of 33) of the acitretin group vs 6.3% (1 of 16) of the controls, while 36.4% (12 of 33) vs 12.5% (2 of 16) achieved partial resolution, respectively. Mean total clinical score of the acitretin group was significantly lower than that of the controls at week 20 [t (47) = −4.146, p = 0.00 < 0.5], which was also accompanied by a significant improvement in mean Dermatology Life Quality Index score [t (32) = 6,441, p = 0.000 < 0.05]. Acitretin was well tolerated and only minimal transient side effects were recorded.

Conclusions.—Acitretin is safe and effective for the management of severe, long-standing lichen sclerosus of the male genitalia. Study limitations included bias during clinical evaluation considering the expected side effects of acitretin.

▶ Although less commonly found in males, lichen sclerosus can be both physically disfiguring as well as emotionally traumatic, given the location and the potential to affect sexual relationships. Penile lichen sclerosus is a recognized cause of phimosis in uncircumcised males. The evidence provided in the article for improvement with a 20-week course of acitretin is encouraging, knowing that more than two-thirds of the study group achieved either complete or partial resolution of the lesional surface area, although most patients experienced the highest benefits well into the course, which per the author suggests that a longer treatment protocol might serve patients better. Moreover, the improvement scores in relation to the side effect profile that was experienced for that course duration were significant, given the potential morbidity of the disease and known correlation to malignancy, which was encouraging. The main side effects of systemic retinoids such as cheilitis, xerosis, and pruritus, otherwise known as the nuisance effects, were much more common than the more dose-limiting effects of alopecia, hyperlipidemia, and headache. This study, despite the low numbers of patients treated in each group, gives light to another use of systemic retinoids, which are often underused in many dermatoses, given risks of lack of efficacy and limiting side effects. There is an excellent explanation at the end of the discussion section regarding the applied mechanisms of retinoids to this class of dermatoses, which should be reviewed by the reader.

N. Bhatia, MD

Addiction to Indoor Tanning: Relation to Anxiety, Depression, and Substance Use
Mosher CE, Danoff-Burg S (Memorial Sloan-Kettering Cancer Ctr, NY; Univ at Albany, NY)
Arch Dermatol 146:412-417, 2010

Objective.—To assess the prevalence of addiction to indoor tanning among college students and its association with substance use and symptoms of anxiety and depression.

Design.—Two written measures, the CAGE (Cut down, Annoyed, Guilty, Eye-opener) Questionnaire, used to screen for alcoholism, and the *Diagnostic and Statistical Manual of Mental Disorders (Fourth Edition, Text Revision) (DSM-IV-TR)* criteria for substance-related disorders, were modified to evaluate study participants for addiction to indoor tanning. Standardized self-report measures of anxiety, depression, and substance use also were administered.

Setting.—A large university (approximately 18 000 students) in the northeastern United States.

Participants.—A total of 421 college students were recruited from September through December 2006.

Main Outcome Measures.—Self-reported addiction to indoor tanning, substance use, and symptoms of anxiety and depression.

Results.—Among 229 study participants who had used indoor tanning facilities, 90 (39.3%) met *DSM-IV-TR* criteria and 70 (30.6%) met CAGE criteria for addiction to indoor tanning. Students who met *DSM-IV-TR* and CAGE criteria for addiction to indoor tanning reported greater symptoms of anxiety and greater use of alcohol, marijuana, and other substances than those who did not meet these criteria. Depressive symptoms did not significantly vary by indoor tanning addiction status.

Conclusion.—Findings suggest that interventions to reduce skin cancer risk should address the addictive qualities of indoor tanning for a minority of individuals and the relationship of this behavior to other addictions and affective disturbance.

▶ This study reinforces the relationships found in several other studies on addiction of indoor tanning. The authors also found an increased rate of anxiety and substance abuse in those who were considered addicted to indoor tanning. With 421 total participants, it more than meets statistical relevance for sample size. The modified (Cut down, Annoyed, Guilty, Eye opener) Questionnaire and modified (*Diagnostic and Statistical Manual of Mental Disorder,* Fourth Edition) criteria for substance-related disorders were effective tools for measuring this behavior. Previous research supports an actual physical release of endorphins after ultraviolet exposure.[1] This phenomenon could help explain the correlation between addictive indoor tanning and substance abuse.

This research is clinically relevant for our patients who may present with excessive photodamage or early skin cancers. The authors suggest that correction of the underlying mood disorder may be a necessary step to reduce the skin cancer risk in such individuals. Though probably not the conventional thought process of most dermatologists, certainly this option should be considered for select patients.

B. P. Glick, DO, MPH

Reference

1. van Steensel MA. UV addiction: a form of opiate dependency. *Arch Dermatol.* 2009;145:211.

Aggressive Fibromatosis in Children and Adolescents: The Italian Experience

Meazza C, Bisogno G, Gronchi A, et al (Natl Cancer Inst, Milano, Italy; Padova Univ Hosp, Italy; et al)
Cancer 116:233-240, 2010

Background.—Aggressive fibromatosis (AF) is a rare tumor of intermediate malignancy that has a strong potential for local invasiveness and recurrence. To date, there are no general recommendations for the clinical management of pediatric AF.

Methods.—The authors retrospectively analyzed 94 patients aged ≤21 years, including 23 patients who underwent complete surgery (Group I), 42 patients who underwent incomplete surgery with microscopic residual tumor (Group II), and 29 patients who underwent either biopsy or macroscopically incomplete surgery (Group III).

Results.—The 5-year event-free survival (EFS) and overall survival rates were 44% and 99%, respectively. Local recurrences developed in 22% of patients in Group I, in 76% of patients in Group II, and in 76% of patients in Group III. Two of 7 patients with abdominal disease died of tumor progression, whereas none of the patients with extra-abdominal AF died of their disease. Systemic treatment was given to 15 patients as first-line treatment and to 34 patients at the time they developed recurrent disease: The response rate was 47% in the former patients and 50% in the latter patients. Objective responses were observed in 11 of 19 patients who received combined methotrexate plus vinblastine/vinorelbine, in 7 of 15 patients who received alkylating-agent chemotherapy, and in 4 of 11 patients who received other therapies (tamoxifen, sulindac, interferon alfa).

Conclusions.—The current analysis suggested that the clinical course of AF in children may resemble that of AF in adults. Local recurrences did not affect the chance of responding to systemic therapy or the survival rate. The completeness of initial resection was the main factor that influenced EFS, whereas disease control after marginal resection was much the same as that achieved after intralesional surgery/biopsy. Good responses to systemic treatments, and particularly to low-dose chemotherapy, were observed as reported previously in adults.

▶ Aggressive fibromatosis, or desmoid tumor, is a very rare musculoaponeurotic tumor. It occurs more commonly in childhood with a peak occurrence at 8 years of age (0-19 years). A second peak occurs in females at around 40 years of age. Aggressive fibromatosis is associated with Gardner syndrome, familial adenomatous polyposis, and familial infiltrative fibromatosis, or hereditary desmoids tumors, all due to defects in the *APC* gene. Primary treatment, universally, consists of surgical excision. Unfortunately, obtaining clear margins is not possible in many cases with local invasion and recurrence being common. Needless to say, prognosis is directly correlated to the ability to obtain clear margins. In those with incomplete resection or recurrence, a multimodal customized approach is recommended. Various chemotherapy regimens and radiation therapy are second-line treatments. In general, pediatric cases of desmoid tumor are more likely to recur and to be less responsive to radiation therapy. In this study, the cases of 94 patients younger than 21 years were reviewed. Five-year event-free survival and overall survival rates were 44% and 99%, respectively. Intrabdominal tumors and patients with Gardner syndrome had more aggressive disease. (The 2 patients who died of disease in this series had Gardner syndrome.) The authors concluded that the pediatric course and response rates were similar to adult cases. Radiation therapy was less effective in this series of pediatric patients than in reported adult cases. However, other published studies suggest that radiation can be a useful adjunctive therapy and effective in pediatric patients.[1]

A. Zaenglein, MD

Reference

1. Jabbari S, Andolino D, Weinberg V, et al. Successful treatment of high risk and recurrent pediatric desmoids using radiation as a component of multimodality therapy. *Int J Radiat Oncol Biol Phys.* 2009;75:177-182.

Chemical Matricectomy with 10% Sodium Hydroxide for the Treatment of Ingrown Toenails in People with Diabetes

Tatlican S, Eren C, Yamangokturk B, et al (Diskapi Yildirim Beyazit Education and Res Hosp, Ankara, Turkey; et al)
Dermatol Surg 36:219-222, 2010

Background.—Treatment of ingrown toenails using chemical matricectomy in patients with diabetes has been difficult, because delayed wound healing, wound infections, and digital ischemia can interfere with the procedure. Chemical matricectomy with 10% sodium hydroxide is an effective treatment for ingrown toenails in a normal population.

Objectives.—Investigation of the effectiveness and safety of chemical matricectomy with 10% sodium hydroxide solution for ingrown toenails in patients with diabetes.

Material and Methods.—Thirty patients with diabetes with 40 ingrown toenails and 30 patients without diabetes with 41 ingrown toenails were enrolled in the study. After partial avulsion of the affected edge, germinal matrix was treated for 1 minute with 10% sodium hydroxide. Patients were observed on alternate days until complete healing was achieved and followed for up to 24 months for recurrence.

Results.—Assessment of the treatment in both groups for complete healing, postoperative pain, tissue damage, drainage, infections, and rate of recurrences revealed no statistically significant difference.

Conclusions.—The partial avulsion of the affected edge and the treatment of the germinal matrix for 1 minute with 10% sodium hydroxide

TABLE 2.—Postoperative Complications, Complete Healing Time, and Recurrences

Variable	With Diabetes	Without Diabetes	P-Value
Duration of pain, days, mean ± SD	1.7 ± 1.5	1.6 ± 1.5	.79
Duration of drainage, days, mean ± SD	9.3 ± 4.1	9.1 ± 4.8	.85
Duration of tissue damage, days, mean ± SD	5.6 ± 2.8	5.6 ± 2.8	.88
Complete healing time, days, mean ± SD	10.5 ± 3.6	10.3 ± 4.4	.79
Infections, n (%)	0 (0.0)	0 (0.0)	
Recurrences, n (%)	1 (2.5)	1 (2.4)	>.99

SD = standard deviation.

preceded by matrix curettage is an effective and safe treatment modality for ingrown toenails in people with diabetes (Table 2).

▶ Ingrown toenail treatment in patients with diabetes can be challenging because of the potential for poor wound healing, infection, and ischemic changes in the diabetic foot. This study shows that chemical matricectomy of ingrown toenails with 10% sodium hydroxide (NaOH) applied to the nail matrix for 1 minute after partial nail avulsion was as safe and effective in patients with diabetes (n = 30) as in nondiabetic (n = 30) patients with ingrown toenails. The patients were followed for complications and recurrences of ingrown toenails for 24 months after the toenail partial matricectomy with NaOH. There was no statistical difference in healing rate, pain, drainage, infection, or recurrence rates between the diabetic and nondiabetic groups (see Table 2) in this study.

P. Rich, MD

Control of negative emotions and its implication for illness perception among psoriasis and vitiligo patients

Kossakowska MM, Cieścińska C, Jaszewska J, et al (Warsaw School of Social Sciences and Humanities Faculty in Sopot, Poland; Nicolaus Copernicus Univ in Torun, Poland; New Line Learning Academy, Maidstone, Kent, UK)
J Eur Acad Dermatol Venereol 24:429-433, 2010

Background.—The purpose of the study was to determine the intensity of control over negative emotions of anger, depressed mood, and anxiety in certain skin diseases such as psoriasis and vitiligo, and to define the predictors of this emotional control in terms of the illness perception in the following context: duration of illness, age at onset, subjective knowledge of the causes of illness, subjective sense of control over the disease.

Methods.—The study included 60 patients with psoriasis (n = 30) and vitiligo (n = 30) as well as healthy persons (n = 60) matched to the experimental group in terms of gender, age, and level of education. Control of negative emotions was examined by means of Watson and Greer's Courtauld Emotional Control Scale (Polish adaptation by Juczynski) and the illness perception by means of Kossakowska's Chronic Patients Questionnaire.

Results.—The research concludes that psoriasis patients control negative emotions more intensively than healthy people. Vitiligo patients on the other hand do not differ in the control of negative emotions compared with healthy subjects. There are no significant predictors of negative emotional control in vitiligo. In psoriasis gender and age are the main contributors to negative emotional control and anger control is predicted by the age at onset as well.

Conclusion.—The specificity of the skin disease affects maladaptive negative emotional control and the suggestion is to use psychological treatment in hospitalised psoriasis in particular.

▶ Many dermatological diseases are associated with negative emotions because of the psychological or social aspect of the disease. This study attempted to determine the intensity of control over negative emotions of anger, depressed mood, and anxiety in certain skin diseases such as psoriasis and vitiligo. The conclusions suggest that psoriatic patients dealt with negative emotions more intensively. This could be because of the disease itself or the fact that all patients were hospitalized for their treatment. Factors that made negative emotions more prevalent were age of onset of their disease, older patients more frequently negatively affected than younger patients. Perhaps the perception of unsatisfactory life at an older age plays a part in these negative emotions. There was no difference in the vitiligo group versus control as far as negative emotions displayed. A plausible explanation may be that these patients are in general healthy, and they adapt well to their skin condition compared with those in the placebo group.

J. L. Smith, MD

Cutaneous Manifestations in Renal Transplant Recipients of Santiago, Chile

Sandoval M, Ortiz M, Díaz C, et al (Pontificia Universidad Católica de Chile, San Joaquín, Santiago)
Transplant Proc 41:3752-3754, 2009

Introduction.—Renal transplant recipients have a heightened risk of developing various cutaneous manifestations, such as skin infections, skin cancer, and secondary effects of immunosuppressive drugs. These manifestations differ depending on the evaluated population. The objective of this study was to describe the prevalence of cutaneous manifestations among renal transplant recipients in Chile between 1979 and 2008.

Methods.—Patients were recruited and then evaluated using a standardized questionnaire. Dermatologic physical examination was performed in every patient describing skin lesions, immunosuppressive drug effects, and malignant diseases. All suspicious lesions were biopsied for analysis. Every patient was queried for the development of skin cancer after his or her transplantation.

Results.—A total of 91 patients were enrolled; ages 10–67 years. Sixty percent of the patients presented with an infection at the initial evaluation. The most common infection was onychomycosis (58%) and verruca vulgaris (25%). In this study 58% of patients developed cutaneous side effects of immunosuppressive drugs. Among the evaluated patients, 16% showed premalignant or malignant manifestations on physical examination. The most frequent manifestations were actinic keratosis (17%), basal cell carcinoma (1%), and squamous cell carcinoma (1%). On a retrospective analysis, 12% of patients developed skin cancer after transplantation, 66% squamous cell carcinoma and 34% basal cell carcinoma, with a ratio of 1.9 to 1.

Discussion.—Cutaneous manifestations in renal transplant recipients are generally secondary to immunosuppression. These patients show a greater risk of having human papilloma virus (HPV) infections and nonmelanoma skin cancer. Periodic dermatologic evaluation of these patients should be performed to detect early lesions and modify risk factors.

▶ Sandoval et al compile further convincing data reiterating the importance of consistently evaluating patients with renal transplant for skin manifestations. Although this study evaluated only a portion of the patients (N = 91) who underwent renal transplantation from 1970-2008 in the focused patient population base in Central Chile, the data nonetheless serve as an important reminder of the increased prevalence of skin manifestations in patients who undergo renal transplants. Notable findings in the study included the prevalence of fungal infections (over 50% of patients), the increased side effects of immunosuppressive medications, the greater risk of contracting human papillomavirus, and the frequency of premalignant and malignant skin lesions that may develop in patients with renal transplants. Of the 91 patients evaluated (with an average age of 46.6 years), 16 had premalignant or malignant lesions on physical exam, and 11 patients on retrospective analysis were noted to have developed skin cancer after transplantation. Unfortunately, the answer to the question as to how many of these patients would have developed precancerous and even cancerous lesions without renal transplant for comparison would not have been possible to obtain. Further data comparing skin manifestations of nonrenal transplant patients and renal transplant patients (of approximately the same median age and study years) at this institution would provide additional support for their objective. Nonetheless, the authors achieved their goal and provided enough evidence to support the position that a long-term dermatologic evaluation plan is important to implement for patients with renal transplant to help detect skin lesions early.

B. D. Michaels, DO
J. Q. Del Rosso, DO

Topical Calcipotriol for Preventive Treatment of Hypertrophic Scars: A Randomized, Double-Blind, Placebo-Controlled Trial

van der Veer WM, Jacobs XE, Waardenburg IE, et al (VU Univ Med Ctr, Amsterdam, the Netherlands; Univ Med Ctr Groningen, the Netherlands)
Arch Dermatol 145:1269-1275, 2009

Objectives.—To evaluate the efficacy of topical application of calcipotriol to healing wounds in preventing or reducing hypertrophic scar formation and to investigate the biochemical properties of the epidermis associated with hypertrophic scar formation.

Design.—Randomized, double-blind, placebo-controlled trial using the reduction mammoplasty wound-healing model.

Setting.—University Medical Center Groningen.

Patients.—Thirty women who underwent bilateral reduction mammoplasty.

Interventions.—For 3 months, scar segments were treated with either topical calcipotriol or placebo.

Main Outcome Measures.—Three weeks, 3 months, and 12 months postoperatively, the scars were evaluated and punch biopsy samples were collected for immunohistochemical analysis.

Results.—No significant difference in the prevalence of hypertrophic scars was observed between the placebo- and calcipotriol-treated scars. Only scars with activated keratinocytes 3 weeks postoperatively became hypertrophic ($P = .001$).

Conclusions.—Topical application of calcipotriol during the first 3 months of wound healing does not affect the incidence of hypertrophic scar formation. We observed a strong association between keratinocyte activation and hypertrophic scar formation.

Trial Registration.—trialregister.nl Identifier: NTR1486.

▶ As calcipotriol has been shown to promote the terminal differentiation of keratinocytes and diminish keratinocyte proliferation in patients with psoriasis, it makes sense that it may have a similar effect during scar formation. The results of this study suggest that topical calcipotriol histopathologically had the opposite desired effect on healing wounds, showing increased keratinocyte proliferation. However, no difference, as compared with the group applying the placebo vehicle, was seen clinically concerning the prevention or stimulation of hypertrophic scars. This study is well designed using intraindividual comparison of groups using placebo vehicle alone and topical calcipotriol, including clinical and histologic evaluations of wound healing. Given the results of this study, we clearly do not fully understand the mechanisms involved in the keratinocyte proliferation in wound healing versus psoriasis. The authors of the study astutely suggest that psoriasis may have defective proliferative keratinocytes that are affected differently by calcipotriol as compared with normal keratinocytes during wound healing. Another thought may be that activated keratinocytes in wound healing may somehow be resistant to any inhibitory signals that would normally diminish keratinocyte proliferation until a certain level of wound healing is attained. In either case, further research is needed to clarify the role of calcipotriol in wound healing.

J. Levin, DO

Early high-dose immunosuppression in Henoch–Schönlein nephrotic syndrome may improve outcome
Andersen RF, Rubak S, Jespersen B, et al (Aarhus Univ Hosp, Skejby, Denmark)
Scand J Urol Nephrol 43:409-415, 2009

Objective.—Renal involvement in Henoch–Schönlein purpura (HSP) constitutes a risk of end-stage renal disease (ESRD), especially in patients presenting with nephrotic syndrome.

Patients and Methods.—The clinical courses of six patients (mean age 13.2 years; four boys and two girls) admitted from 2000 to 2007 with HSP and nephrotic syndrome were reviewed. Average follow-up was 44 months (28−59). Treatment protocols included oral prednisolone and in non-responders cyclosporin A, cyclophosphamide, mycophenolate mofetil or tacrolimus. Five patients were treated immediately after presentation of nephrotic syndrome/nephrotic range proteinuria (median 277 mg/m²/h). The last patient was treated locally with low-dose prednisolone (0.2−0.9 mg/kg/day) and 3 months of low-dose cyclophosphamide (1 mg/kg/day).

Results.—All five patients treated promptly with high-dose immunosuppressant had normal estimated glomerular filtration rate (eGFR) (median 159 ml/min/1.73 m²) at follow-up. One obtained complete remission, two had positive dipstick proteinuria and two needed angiotensin-converting enzyme inhibitors to stay normotensive. The patient receiving low-dose immunosuppression at onset progressed to ESRD 44 months later. At initial presentation eGFR, blood pressure, renal biopsy grading, proteinuric range and plasma albumin were similar in all patients.

Conclusion.—Follow-up data from the patients suggest that an early aggressive immunosuppressive approach improves long-term renal outcome in HSP patients with nephrotic syndrome.

▶ Henoch-Schönlein purpura (HSP) is the most common primary vasculitis in children involving the skin, joints, gastrointestinal tract, and kidneys. Studies have shown a positive correlation with increased risk of progression to end-stage renal disease (ESRD). This is a retrospective study of 6 patients from 2000 to 2007 with HSP and nephrotic syndrome, with a follow-up period of 44 months. This is a report of the prevalence of severe renal complications in HSP and the clinical course and long-term outcome in 6 patients. HSP was defined as palpable purpura and at least one of the following symptoms: diffuse abdominal pain, arthritis or arthralgias, renal involvement, hematuria and/or proteinuria, and biopsy-proven immunoglobulin A deposition. HSP and nephrotic syndrome range proteinuria were defined as proteinuria

> 40 mg/m^2/h. Renal biopsy was performed in all patients and graded according to the International Study of Kidney Disease in Children grade I-IV. The 6 patients had a mean age of 13.2 years at HSP presentation. Mild renal involvement was present in all patients at the time of HSP diagnosis. Median duration from time of HSP diagnosis to appearance of nephrotic range proteinuria was 17 days (7-90 days). Nephrotic range proteinuria, median 277 mg/m^2/h, was seen in all 6 patients, and manifest nephrotic syndrome was seen in 5 patients with median plasma albumin of 18.1 g/L. The protocol was oral prednisolone 60 mg/m^2/dfor 6 weeks followed by 6 weeks with alternate-day prednisolone 40 mg/m^2 and then a slowly tapering dose of alternate-day prednisolone (5-10 mg) for several months. Nonresponders were treated with cyclophosphamide, mycophenolate mofetil, or tacrolimus. Renal biopsy was performed within 7 to 84 days after the development of nephritic range proteinuria. Five patients were treated after presentation of nephrotic syndrome (median 277 mg/m^2/h). The last patient was treated with low-dose prednisolone (0.2-0.9 mg/kg/d) and 3 months of low-dose cyclophosphamide (1 mg/kg/d). The 5 patients receiving early high-dose immunosuppression according to the study protocol had preserved kidney function at follow-up, while the patient receiving low doses of immunosuppressant therapy progressed to ESRD during follow-up. A limitation to this study was the small study size, understandable because of the relative rarity of HSP. Also, all patients were treated with angiotensin-converting enzyme inhibitors, and the contribution of this nonimmunosuppressant is unclear and needs further investigation. This study also did not discuss any complications, such as infection, with any of these patients or any changes with baseline laboratory test results. When considering immunosuppressant therapy in children, other more conservative approaches may need to be considered. This study did not evaluate the etiology of HSP and also baseline renal biopsies were not performed; therefore, pre-existing renal disease or a predisposition to developing HSP was also unknown. This study also did not discuss whether cutaneous findings or any other associated clinical features of HSP responded better to high-dose immunosuppressants. Although severe glomerulonephritis with nephrotic syndrome is an uncommon complication of HSP, this study suggests that early intervention with high-dose prednisolone may prevent patients from progressing to ESRD.

J. Q. Del Rosso, DO

G. K. Kim, DO

Sun-Protection Behaviors Among African Americans

Pichon LC, Corral I, Landrine H, et al (Univ of Michigan, Ann Arbor; American Cancer Society, Atlanta, GA; et al)
Am J Prev Med 38:288-295, 2010

Background.—Data suggest that the prevalence of sun-protection behaviors is low (44%) among African Americans; the samples in such studies, however, tended to be small or nonrepresentative.

Purpose.—This article aims to examine the prevalence and correlates of sun-protection behaviors among a large, random, statewide sample of African-American adults living in California to ascertain behavioral patterns and highlight directions for targeted interventions.

Methods.—From September 2006 through May 2008, an anonymous health survey collected data on sunscreen, sunglasses, and wide-brim hat use among a random sample of 2187 African-American adults, and assessed demographic, regional, skin type, and other potential correlates of these behaviors. The analysis was conducted in 2009.

Results.—Only 31% engaged in at least one sun-protection behavior; of the three behaviors, sunscreen use was the least prevalent, with 63% never using sunscreen. Multivariate logistic regressions revealed that gender, SES, and skin type were significant predictors of sun-protection behaviors.

Conclusions.—Tailored interventions to increase sun-protection behaviors among African Americans (men in particular) are needed.

▶ Melanoma is predominantly an ultraviolet light—induced skin cancer more commonly associated with light-skinned Caucasians than with individuals of darker skin. However, when affected, these minority populations, including African Americans (AAs) are more likely to present with a more advanced stage of skin cancer and have a poorer prognosis. Subsequently, authors analyzed data to investigate sun-protection behaviors in a randomly selected AA population in the state of California. The study found low levels of sun-protection behaviors among AAs, including low prevalence of sunscreen use and less than 10% reporting regular use of wide-brim hats. In addition, men and low-socioeconomic status groups were less likely to wear sunglasses on a regular basis. It is important to remember that there is significant diversity in skin color amongst AAs and that this variation is a strong predictor of sun-protective behaviors. Clearly, skin cancer prevention education is needed in minority populations. Given the poor survival rates in AAs with skin cancer and its propensity for unusual locations, clinicians should maintain a high index of suspicion in this minority population.

S. Bellew, DO

J. Q. Del Rosso, DO

Pulsed High-Dose Corticosteroids Combined With Low-Dose Methotrexate Treatment in Patients With Refractory Generalized Extragenital Lichen Sclerosus
Kreuter A, Tigges C, Gaifullina R, et al (Ruhr-Univ Bochum, Germany)
Arch Dermatol 145:1303-1308, 2009

Background.—Lichen sclerosus (LS) is a rare, chronic inflammatory skin disease that predominantly affects the anogenital area. A few patients exhibit widespread extragenital disease that may lead to blister formation and superficial erosions. We evaluated the efficacy of pulsed high-dose corticosteroids combined with low-dose methotrexate treatment in patients with refractory generalized LS that had failed to respond to standard topical corticosteroid therapy.

Observation.—Seven patients were included in this retrospective study, all of whom were treated with pulsed high-dose corticosteroids combined with low-dose methotrexate for at least 6 months. The outcome measure was an individual, nonvalidated clinical score. Overall, a significant decrease in the clinical score was observed, from a median score of 8 (range, 5 to 24) before treatment to 2 (range, 1 to 4) after treatment. Adverse effects observed during therapy were moderate and disappeared after the end of treatment. During the follow-up period of at least 3 months (mean, 4.7 [range, 3-8] months), none of the patients experienced a relapse of extragenital LS.

Conclusions.—Patients with severe extragenital LS benefit from pulsed high-dose corticosteroids combined with low-dose methotrexate therapy. This combination therapy should be considered in generalized disease, especially disease that is refractory to conventional treatment.

▶ This article provides reassuring evidence of an effective treatment option for refractory lichen sclerosus. Long-term results from a larger cohort of subjects are needed to assess long-term treatment response and sequelae.

B. P. Glick, DO, MPH

A. Wiener, DO

Gadolinium deposition in nephrogenic systemic fibrosis: An examination of tissue using synchrotron x-ray fluorescence spectroscopy
High WA, Ranville JF, Brown M, et al (Univ of Colorado Health Sciences Ctr, Denver; Colorado School of Mines, Golden; et al)
J Am Acad Dermatol 62:38-44, 2010

Background.—Nephrogenic systemic fibrosis is a fibrosing disorder associated with gadolinium (Gd)-based contrast agents dosed during renal insufficiency.

Objective.—In two patients, Gd deposition in tissue affected by nephrogenic systemic fibrosis was quantified using inductively coupled plasma mass spectrometry. The presence of Gd was confirmed and mapped using synchrotron x-ray fluorescence spectroscopy.

Results.—Affected skin and soft tissue from the lower extremity demonstrated 89 and 209 ppm (μg/g, dry weight, formalin fixed) in cases 1 and 2, respectively. In case 2, the same skin and soft tissue was retested after paraffin embedding, with the fat content removed by xylene washes, and this resulted in a measured value of 189 ppm (μg/g, dry weight, paraffin embedded). Synchrotron x-ray fluorescence spectroscopy confirmed Gd in the affected tissue of both cases, and provided high-sensitivity and high-resolution spatial mapping of Gd deposition. A gradient of Gd deposition in tissue correlated with fibrosis and cellularity. Gd deposited in periadnexal locations within the skin, including hair and eccrine ducts, where it colocalized to areas of high calcium and zinc content.

Limitations.—Because of the difficulty in obtaining synchrotron x-ray fluorescence spectroscopy scans, tissue from only two patients were mapped. A single control with kidney disease and gadolinium-based contrast agent exposure did not contain Gd.

Conclusions.—Gd content on a gravimetric basis was impacted by processing that removed fat and altered the dry weight of the specimens. Gradients of Gd deposition in tissue corresponded to fibrosis and cellularity. Adnexal deposition of Gd correlated with areas of high calcium and zinc content.

▶ It is difficult to provide objective commentary on ones' own article, but that is why the editor of this book delegated it to me. Perhaps the greatest importance in this piece is 2-fold: (1) it provides yet another technology that has affirmed the presence of gadolinium deposition in the tissue of patients diagnosed with nephrogenic systemic fibrosis (NSF) and (2) it highlights, also via another technology, that there is a gradient of deposition within the tissue.

It is interesting to note that when my research group, which includes me, Dr Shawn Cowper of Yale University, and engineering professionals from the Colorado School of Mines, became the first to identify gadolinium in the tissue of patients with NSF, our article was submitted first to a well-regarded general medicine publication. After considerable time of nearly 6 weeks, and multiple editorial meetings, that publication was declined with the explanation that all consultants to that editorial board were of the opinion that gadolinium would be unlikely to deposit in tissue given the thermodynamic considerations of the chelating agents, in sum, that it was effectively an impossibility.

Now, after confirmation of this finding by many other research groups, using a variety of biochemical techniques, while the means and conditions of deposition remain rather cryptic, it is readily apparent that for reasons poorly understood gadolinium is deposited within the tissue. It will be interesting to observe, in the years to come, what effect this might have on the development and approval of additional metal-based radiological contrast agents and whether dermatologic expertise and interests will be more fully represented during toxicological evaluations.

W. A. High, MD, JD, MEng

Growth rate of human fingernails and toenails in healthy American young adults

Yaemsiri S, Hou N, Slining MM, et al (Univ of North Carolina at Chapel Hill)
J Eur Acad Dermatol Venereol 24:420-423, 2010

Background.—Human nail clippings are increasingly used in epidemiological studies as biomarkers for assessing diet and environmental exposure to trace elements or other chemical compounds. However, little is known about the growth rate of human nails.

Objective.—To estimate the average growth rate of fingernails and toenails and examine factors that may influence nail growth rate.

Methods.—Twenty-two healthy American young adults marked their nails close to the proximal nail fold with a provided nail file following a standardized protocol, and recorded the date and the distance from the proximal nail fold to the mark. One to three months later, participants recorded the date and distance from the proximal nail fold to the mark again. Nail growth rate was calculated based on recorded distance and time between the two measurements.

Results.—Average fingernail growth rate was faster than that of toenails (3.47 vs. 1.62 mm/month, $P < 0.01$). There was no significant difference between right and left fingernail/toenail growth rates. The little fingernail grew slower than other fingernails ($P < 0.01$); the great toenail grew faster than other toenails ($P < 0.01$). Younger age, male gender, and onychophagia were associated with faster nail growth rate; however, the differences were not statistically significant.

Conclusion.—Nail growth rates have increased compared with previous estimates conducted decades ago. Toenail clippings may reflect a long exposure time frame given the relatively slow growth rate.

▶ Fingernail analysis is useful for determining environmental exposure to elements such as arsenic and drugs such as nicotine. While blood and urine are useful to measure recent exposures to drugs and chemicals, the nail clippings provide a convenient record of exposure for time periods of up to a year. By knowing the rate of growth of the nail, the approximate time of exposure to an element or drug can be determined from distal nail clippings. In this study, nail growth rate of 22 healthy young adults was calculated by making a shallow notch on the nails with a file at the cuticle and then measuring the distance that the notch grew out from the cuticle at various time points so that the growth rate could be determined. One hundred ninety fingernails and 188 toenails were measured. The data showed that the rate of fingernails was greater than toenails, and there was no difference in the left and right digit nail growth in fingers or toes. The great toenail grew faster than other toenails, and the little fingernail grew slower than other fingernails. The average rate of fingernail growth was 3.47 mm/month, twice as fast as toenails, which grew at an average rate of 1.62 mm/month. The average rate of growth of all nails was greater than that calculated in the last large studies, which were all performed prior to the 1980s.

There were several limitations with this study. Each individual subjects notched and measured the growth of their own nails rather than having an investigator measure all of the nails for consistency. Previous nail growth studies showed that nail growth rate varies greatly by age, but that was not confirmed in this study because all of the subjects were young adults, and children or elderly were not included in the study population.

P. Rich, MD

Haematological deficiencies in patients with recurrent aphthosis

Compilato D, Carroccio A, Calvino F, et al (Univ Hosp of Palermo, Italy; Univ Hosp of Palermo and Hosp of Sciacca, Italy)
J Eur Acad Dermatol Venereol 24:667-673, 2010

Background.—Recurrent aphthosis is a common oral ulcerative condition consisting also of a subset of similar ulcers, properly named 'aphthous-like' ulcers (ALU), linked to systemic diseases and among these, to iron, folic acid and vitamin B_{12} deficiencies.

Objectives.—The main objectives of this study were: (i) to evaluate the association between recurrent aphthosis and the most common predisposing factors; (ii) to assess the frequency of ALU in recurrent aphthosis; (iii) to verify the efficacy of a replacement therapy in all ALU patients.

Methods.—Thirty-two adults with recurrent aphthosis and 29 otherwise healthy controls were consecutively recruited, interviewed and subjected to haematological investigations.

Results.—Family history of recurrent aphthosis was significantly associated ($P < 0.01$). The overall frequency of haematinic deficiencies was 56.2% in recurrent aphthosis patients vs. 7% in controls ($P < 0.0001$). All ALU patients with a negative family history showed a complete remission of the ulcerative episodes after replacement therapy, while those with a positive family history only had a reduction in frequency and severity. In the logistic regression model, only family history was associated with recurrent aphthosis ($P = 0.0137$).

Conclusion.—The strong association with familiarity, the unexpected higher frequency of ALU (compared with the idiopathic variant) and the good response to replacement therapy means that familiarity should always be investigated. Furthermore, routine haematological screening and tests for serum iron, folic acid and vitamin B_{12} deficiencies should be assessed in all patients with recurrent aphthosis to treat any nutritional deficiency and to prevent more important related systemic manifestations.

▶ The objective of this article is to look at patients with recurrent aphthosis ulcers and to indicate common etiologies that have been well documented. Replacement controls all did well, and family histories improved but not dramatically. This article had a small patient population but is important for the dermatologist.

Based on a study of 32 adults with recurrent aphthosis and 29 otherwise healthy controls, the definition of recurrent aphthosis is a chronic ulcerative condition with a properly named aphthous-like ulcer (ALU) linked to systemic disease in iron, folic acid, and vitamin B_{12} deficiencies. A determination of a family history of recurrent aphthosis was significantly associated. The overall incidence of etiologic deficiencies was 56.2% in the patients with the recurrent aphthosis and 7% in the controls. All ALU patients with a negative family history showed a complete remission after replacement therapy. Those with a positive family history showed only a reduction in frequency and severity. The article did not mention links to trauma, citrus, and other exogenous factors other than smoking. This article suggests recommendations for hematological screenings and tests for serum iron, folic acid, and vitamin B_{12} deficiencies in patients with recurrent aphthosis to both treat and prevent related systemic manifestations.

L. Cleaver, DO

Hypoglycemia in Children Taking Propranolol for the Treatment of Infantile Hemangioma

Holland KE, Frieden IJ, Frommelt PC, et al (Med College of Wisconsin, Milwaukee; Univ of California, San Francisco; et al)
Arch Dermatol 146:775-778, 2010

Background.—Propranolol hydrochloride has been prescribed for decades in the pediatric population for a variety of disorders, but its effectiveness in the treatment of infantile hemangiomas (IHs) was only recently discovered. Since then, the use of propranolol for IHs has exploded because it is viewed as a safer alternative to traditional therapy.

Observations.—We report the cases of 3 patients who developed symptomatic hypoglycemia during treatment with propranolol for their IHs and review the literature to identify other reports of propranolol-associated hypoglycemia in children to highlight this rare adverse effect.

Conclusions.—Although propranolol has a long history of safe and effective use in infants and children, understanding and recognition of deleterious adverse effects is critical for physicians and caregivers. This is especially important when new medical indications evolve as physicians who may not be as familiar with propranolol and its adverse effects begin to recommend it as therapy.

▶ More than any other medication in recent years, propranolol has changed how pediatric dermatologists practice medicine. With the alternatives being long-term oral corticosteroids, vincristine, and interferon, the use of propranolol in the treatment of infantile hemangioma has been eagerly embraced, and in many cases, the results are quite dramatic. Propranolol is by no means a new medication, it has been used in neonates with various cardiac and noncardiac conditions for many years, and its side effects are well established. How to safely use this medication in infantile hemangioma is the subject of much debate.[1] This report details the cases of 3 children who experienced symptomatic hypoglycemia while on propranolol in treatment of infantile hemangioma. Their ages varied, from 5 weeks to 18 months. Each child was found to be cold and lethargic or unresponsive by their caregiver. While propranolol-associated hypoglycemia is more common in the neonatal period, it can occur in older children as well, as evidenced by these reports and others. The authors reviewed available data on hypoglycemia related to propranolol use in an effort to identify risk factors for drug-associated hypoglycemia. They advise making parents and caregivers aware of signs of hypoglycemia (which can be difficult to assess in infants), evaluating carefully for concomitant hypoglycemic states or medications that can cause hypoglycemia, and holding doses of propranolol when there is decreased food intake or associated illness. It is important that any clinician who is considering the use of propranolol in the treatment of infantile hemangioma be aware of the potential side effects and carefully weighs the risks and benefits before using this medication.

A. Zaenglein, MD

Reference

1. Frieden IJ, Drolet BA. Propranolol for infantile hemangiomas: promise, peril, pathogenesis. *Pediatr Dermatol.* 2009;26:642-644.

Lip and oral mucosal lesions in 100 renal transplant recipients
Güleç AT, Haberal M (Baskent Univ Faculty of Medicine, Ankara, Turkey)
J Am Acad Dermatol 62:96-101, 2010

Background.—Renal transplant recipients (RTRs) appear to be more susceptible to the development of oral mucosal disease and lip cancer as a result of graft-preserving immunosuppressive therapy. However, reports regarding these pathologies other than lip cancer are scarce and not studied in a detailed manner in this patient population.

Objective.—The aim of this study was to determine the prevalence rates and clinical features of lip lesions and oral mucosal lesions (OMLs) in RTRs.

Methods.—In all, 100 consecutive RTRs (21 female and 79 male) and 79 healthy age- and sex-matched control subjects (23 female and 56 male) were screened for all pathologic and pseudopathologic lip lesions and OMLs, with special interest on precancerous and cancerous lesions. Information about possible associated risk factors such as smoking and alcohol consumption was also obtained. Dermatologic investigation included clinical observation and direct microscopic examination, culture, and histopathological evaluation when indicated.

Results.—One or more lip lesions, OMLs, or both were noted in every participant of both groups. Fordyce spots on the lips was the most common lesion in the patient group (73%), followed by diffuse gingival enlargement (39%), fissured tongue (35%), and oral candidiasis (26%). The last 3 disorders were significantly more common in RTRs, whereas the frequency of Fordyce spots in patients and control subjects was similar. No actinic cheilitis, lip cancer, or oral malignancy was observed.

Limitations.—This was a relatively small sample size for evaluating precancerous and cancerous lip lesions and OMLs, as they are less frequently observed than benign lesions.

Conclusions.—Some of the benign OMLs (oral candidiasis and diffuse gingival enlargement) are increased in RTRs mainly as a result of the immunosuppressive therapy or drug side effects. Precancerous or cancerous lesions were not observed on the lips or the oral mucosa of our RTRs.

This finding is in direct contrast with those of previous studies, yet this can be related to the limited sample size of this study regarding these lesions.

▶ Renal transplant recipients (RTRs) are more susceptible to developing oral disease and lip cancer due to their immunosuppressive state. This is a study of 100 RTRs and 79 age- and sex-matched randomized controls that were screened for pathologic and nonpathological oral lip lesions. One or more lip lesions, oral mucosal lip lesions, or both were seen in every participant of both the RTRs and controls. The mean number of lesions within the 2 groups were similar (P > .05). Fordyce spots on the lips were the most common in the RTR group (73%), followed by diffuse gingival enlargement (39%), fissured tongue (35%), and oral candidiasis (26%). Fordyce spots were also common in the control subjects. Furthermore, 21 (60%) patients with fissured tongue had intraoral candidiasis, whereas 2 (5.7%) with fissured tongue had geographic tongue. Smoking was significantly associated with gingival hyperpigmentation in control subjects (P = .018). Analysis showed no significant effect of age, sex, or duration of immunosuppression on the rates of lip lesions or oral mucosal lesions in RTRs. However, longer duration of immunosuppression with cyclosporine (CsA) had a significant effect on the rate of diffuse gingival enlargement (P = .002). No association between oral findings in RTRs and primary renal disease was found. Diffuse gingival enlargement was the second most common disorder found in RTRs and there were also no significant CsA dose differences in these patients. In addition, there were no precancerous lesions either on the lips or oral mucosa of RTRs. However, with an increase in squamous cell carcinoma in transplant patients, the authors did not biopsy all lesions or specify which lesions were biopsied. Limitations were small sample size and that all patients were RTRs. There may be a higher incidence of both cancerous and precancerous lesions in other transplant patients, who may require a greater degree of immunosuppression. In conclusion, benign oral mucosal lesions were increased in RTRs possibly due to impaired immune surveillance or side effects of drugs. With an increased risk of cancerous lesions in this group of patients, a routine lip/oral examination is an important part of the overall dermatologic examination.

J. Q. Del Rosso, DO
G. K. Kim, DO

Malignancies associated with dermatomyositis and polymyositis in Taiwan: a nationwide population-based study
Huang YL, Chen YJ, Lin MW, et al (Natl Yang-Ming Univ, Taipei, Taiwan; et al)
Br J Dermatol 161:854-860, 2009

Background.—Previous studies showed that idiopathic inflammatory myopathies (IIM) carried an increased risk of cancers. However, no large-scale study of IIM has been conducted in the Chinese population.

Objectives.—We sought to delineate the association of IIM and various cancer types from a nationwide database in Taiwan.

Methods.—We analysed the published national data from records of National Health Insurance claims. Cases of dermatomyositis (DM) and polymyositis (PM) from 2000 to 2005 and cancers registered in the catastrophic illness profile from 1997 to 2006 were collected. A nationally representative cohort of 1 000 000 enrollees was included for comparison.

Results.—In total, 136 patients (12·8%) among 1059 cases of DM and 46 persons (7·0%) among 661 cases of PM carried internal malignancies. Patients with DM tended to have cancers of nasopharynx, lung and breast. On the other hand, patients with PM tended to have breast, uterine cervix and lung cancers. Compared with the general population, DM gave a 10-fold increased risk for cancers, in which a 66-fold increased risk for nasopharyngeal carcinoma and a 31-fold increased risk for lung cancer were the two most significant. For patients with PM, a 6-fold increased risk for cancer was observed. Juvenile DM had a 16-fold increased risk for haematopoietic or lymphoid malignancy. Two thirds of comorbid malignancies were detected shortly after the diagnoses of IIM, within a mean of 1—2 years. Overall, younger patients with IIM carried the highest risk for malignancies, especially those in their twenties and thirties.

Conclusions.—This is the first large-scale study to report the associated malignancies and the cancer risk of IIM in Taiwan.

▶ Cancers have a known association with idiopathic inflammatory myopathies (IIMs). However, the association of IIMs with various cancer types has never been delineated within the Chinese population. Huang et al sought to review a large nationwide Taiwanese database to analyze the associated cancers with IIMs in this population. To this end, the study itself is certainly informative. The authors analyzed a large cohort of patients from a large database in Taiwan and discovered, among other notable findings, that dermatomyositis (DM) had a 10-fold increase and polymyositis (PM) had a 6-fold increase for cancers DM-associated cancers included nasopharyngeal, lung, and breast cancers. PM-associated cancers included breast, uterine, cervix, and lung cancers. Juvenile DM had a 16-fold increase for hematopoietic or lymphoid malignancy. It was also interesting to note that younger patients (especially those aged 20-30 years) with IIM carried the highest risk for malignancies.

The study itself did have some limitations. First, the patients included in the study recruited from the database records were based on a definite diagnosis, fulfilling strict criteria for both DM and PM. Thus, it is possible that not all patients with DM or PM would have been included during the period studied, thus possibly, but unlikely, affecting the percentage of associated cancers with DM and PM. In addition, this study was based on a database from Taiwan, and thus, the findings of the study can only be applied to the Taiwanese population. Regardless, this study provides needed additional data on the types of cancer and their prevalence in patients with DM and PM in the Taiwanese population, and as a result, the study accomplished its objective.

B. D. Michaels, DO
J. Q. Del Rosso, DO

Measurement of skin texture through polarization imaging

Bargo PR, Kollias N (Johnson & Johnson Consumer Products Company, Skillman, NJ)
Br J Dermatol 162:724-731, 2010

Background.—Determination of skin surface texture is of particular importance in the field of dermatology as such measurements can be used for skin diagnostics and evaluation of therapeutic or cosmetic treatments. Profilometry of skin replicas, three-dimensional imaging and computer vision have been successfully used to measure and document skin texture. Nevertheless, the development of a simpler and faster technique may prove to be advantageous in a clinical setting.

Objectives.—We propose the use of polarization imaging with high angles of incidence as a simple alternative to measure/document skin texture/roughness.

Methods.—A system based on digital photography and polarization optics was developed to acquire and compute texture images. Optimization of the system configuration was conducted to enhance the contrast for measuring skin roughness. The method was validated against roughness standards and tested in clinical studies. Measurements were made in subjects aged from 9 to 70 years and image analysis was used to evaluate texture.

Results.—The developed texture scale was shown to correlate closely to the results from clinical assessment and from roughness standards. Frequency domain analysis showed a significantly different power spectrum for the texture images of young subjects when compared with older subjects. The evaluation of texture as a function of age showed that facial skin roughness increased linearly from teenage to 40 years followed by a plateau thereafter.

Conclusions.—The system proved to be a useful clinical tool for assessing skin texture. The age-related results may indicate that some skin texture features are formed before the age of 40 years.

▶ This article describes the usefulness of skin texture measurements using polarization imaging. The use of a goniometric arm to take photos at 150 intervals was well thought out and executed. They had a total of 130 patients, with ages ranging from 9 to 70 years, a good population spread. The patients applied 4 different cosmetic products designed to decrease the appearance of textural age-related changes.

Limitations of this study include patient population, limited to healthy females with Fitzpatrick skin types I to III, and excluding males. There was a brief mention that further articles would be published to include male patients and those with darker skin types. There was no mention if the expert evaluator was a physician, an aesthetician, a nurse, or a random person off the street. Also, the scales used to rate the textural changes were very subjective, relying on the expert to be able to determine the difference between very slight improvement and slight improvement without any blinding to the rater.

They evaluated periorbital improvement in a 1 cm^2 area. It would have been better to compare one side with the other or take a bigger area like 25 cm^2 or the entire cheek. There was no mention as to whether the patients had prior cosmetic procedures or had been using prescribed or nonprescribed wrinkle creams that could alter the results.

In summary, this article does a good job at describing the use of skin texture analysis and has a good study design to test this with a polarizing imaging system, but the overall study design has a lot of limitations.

A. Torres, MD, JD

Nail changes in kidney transplant recipients
Abdelaziz AM, Mahmoud KM, Elsawy EM, et al (Mansoura Univ, Egypt)
Nephrol Dial Transplant 25:274-277, 2010

Background.—Nail changes are common complications of end-stage renal disease, and reports of nail changes in kidney transplant recipients (KTR) are rare. Few reports have documented a higher prevalence of ony-chomycosis in KTR compared with controls, while others found no signif-icant differences. In this study, we investigated the prevalence and nature of nail changes in a large series of KTR.

Methods.—Three hundred and two KTR (216 males and 86 females) were included in this study, and the mean transplant duration was 6.57 years (range 1.5 month–23 years). They were screened for the pres-ence of nail changes. Nail clippings were collected when indicated and cultures were performed for patients with suspected onychomycosis. The patients were compared with 302 age- and sex-matched healthy controls (220 males and 82 females).

Results.—One hundred and twenty-one KTR (40.1%) had nail changes compared with 104 (34.4%) in controls. Onychomycosis, Muehrcke's nail and leuconychia were significantly more common in KTR [23 (7.6%), 13.3 (4.3%), 11 (3.6%), respectively] compared with controls [7 (2.3%), 1 (0.3%), 2 (0.66%), $P = 0.002$, 0.001 and 0.02, respectively]. However, the most frequent nail change among KTR and controls was absent lunula, 90 (29.8%) and 80 (26.5%), respectively $P = 0.36$. Longitudinal ridging was also a frequent nail pathology among KTR and controls, 21 (6.9%) and 19 (6.3%), respectively, $P = 0.74$.

Conclusion.—KTR have higher prevalence rates of onychomycosis, Muehrcke's nail and leuconychia than the healthy population. On the other hand, absent lunula could be a normal variation among Egyptian people.

▶ Nails are often a marker of renal disease, but few studies have looked specif-ically at kidney transplant recipients (KTRs) for the prevalence of nail changes. In this study, 302 KTR and 302 age/sex-matched controls were examined for the presence of nail changes. Those with clinical features of onychomycosis (OM) had distal nail clippings taken for culture. In the KTR group, 121 patients (40.1%) had nail findings compared with 104 (34.4%) of normal controls. The most common nail findings were OM, Muehrcke lines, and leukonychia. Of the patients who had nail changes consistent with OM, 8.6% of patients with KTR versus 2.6% of controls had positive fungal cultures. In the KTR group, roughly 65% of the cultures grew dermatophtytes, and of the remaining, 35% were equally divided into yeast and molds. It is not clear how much the immunosuppression plays a role in the rate of nail infections in the transplant patients because there are no good studies looking at the prevalence of OM in other immunosuppressed populations.

P. Rich, MD

Narrowband ultraviolet B course improves vitamin D balance in women in winter
Vähävihu K, Ylianttila L, Kautiainen H, et al (Päijät-Häme Central Hosp, Lahti, Finland; Non Ionizing Radiation Laboratory, Helsinki, Finland; ORTON Foundation, Helsinki, Finland; et al)
Br J Dermatol 162:848-853, 2010

Background.—Vitamin D insufficiency is common in winter in the Nordic countries.

Objectives.—To examine whether a short course of narrowband ultraviolet B (NB-UVB) improves vitamin D balance.

Methods.—Fifty-six healthy, white women (mean age 41 years) volunteered and 53 completed the study. NB-UVB exposures were given on seven consecutive days either on the whole body ($n = 19$), on the head and arms ($n = 9$) or on the abdomen ($n = 14$). Similarly, seven solar simulator exposures were given on the face and arms ($n = 11$). The cumulative UVB dose was 13 standard erythema doses in all regimens. Serum calcidiol (25-hydroxyvitamin D) concentration was measured by radioimmunoassay before and after the NB-UVB exposures. Follow-up samples were taken from the whole-body NB-UVB group at 2 months.

Results.—At onset 41 women (77%) had vitamin D insufficiency (calcidiol < 50 nmol L^{-1}) and six (11%) had vitamin D deficiency (calcidiol < 25 nmol L^{-1}). Calcidiol concentration increased significantly, by a mean of 11·4 nmol L^{-1} when NB-UVB was given on the whole body, by 11·0 nmol L^{-1} when given on the head and arms and by 4·0 nmol L^{-1} when given on the abdomen. Solar simulator exposures given on the face and arms increased calcidiol by 3·8 nmol L^{-1}. After 2 months serum calcidiol was still higher than initially in the group who received NB-UVB exposures on the whole body.

Conclusion.—NB-UVB exposures given on seven consecutive days on different skin areas of healthy women significantly improved serum calcidiol concentration. A short low-dose NB-UVB course can improve vitamin D balance in winter.

▶ Vitamin D synthesis, metabolism, toxicity, supplementation guidelines, and perceived health benefits have been at the forefront of virtually all medical disciplines over the past year. This study originating from Finland measured vitamin D levels on professional health care women (nurses or physicians) in the winter before, during, and after exposure to narrowband ultraviolet B (UVB) light for 7 consecutive days. As expected, vitamin D levels increased in all 4 groups:

1. Narrowband UVB to whole body—vitamin D increase 11.4 nmol/L.
2. Narrowband UVB to head/arms—vitamin D increase 11.0 nmol/L.
3. Narrowband UVB to abdomen—vitamin D increase 4.0 nmol/L.
4. Solar simulator (broadband UVB) to head/arms—vitamin D increase 3.8 nmol/L.

The expected increase in vitamin D is because of the close proximity of the wavelength for maximum vitamin D synthesis ($\sim$297 nm) and narrowband UVB wavelength (311-313 nm). Of interest is that vitamin D synthesis from head/arms (which is approximately one-fourth bovine serum albumin) than whole body was about the same. One explanation might be that the sun-exposed areas of the head and arms has a more advanced processing and synthesis of vitamin D than non—sun-exposed skin. Also of interest is that vitamin D levels persisted above baseline 2 months after exposure.

J. L. Smith, MD

Neonatal and Early Infantile Cutaneous Langerhans Cell Histiocytosis: Comparison of Self-regressive and Non—Self-regressive Forms
Battistella M, Fraitag S, Teillac DH, et al (Assistance Publique-Hôpitaux de Paris, France; et al)
Arch Dermatol 146:149-156, 2010

Objectives.—To describe clinical and immunohistochemical findings in patients with cutaneous Langerhans cell histiocytosis (LCH) beginning in the first 3 months of life and to define predictors of disease evolution.

Design.—Observational retrospective survey from July 15, 1989, to April 30, 2007.

Setting.—Referral center in pediatric dermatology.

Patients.—Thirty-one patients with a diagnosis of cutaneous LCH in the first 3 months of life and no previous visceral LCH.

Main Outcome Measures.—Cutaneous lesion characteristics, regulatory T-lymphocyte density, and E-cadherin expression were assessed. Data were compared between the patient groups with selfregressive vs non—self-regressive forms of cutaneous LCH. Pathologic analysis was performed blinded to patient group.

Results.—Self-regressive cutaneous LCH was found in 21 patients and non-self-regressive cutaneous LCH in 10 patients. Monolesional forms, necrotic lesions, hypopigmented macules at presentation, and distal topography of limb lesions were seen only in patients with self-regressive cutaneous LCH. Regulatory T-lymphocyte density correlated with interleukin 10 expression in lesions ($r=0.77$, $P=.003$) but was not predictive of disease evolution. E-cadherin expression by Langerhans cells was found in 7 patients with disease limited to the skin whether self-regressive or not. One patient with secondary disseminated disease showed loss of E-cadherin expression in Langerhans cells.

Conclusions.—Some morphologic traits of skin lesions can orient the diagnosis to a self-regressive form of cutaneous LCH. Regulatory T-lymphocyte density does not seem to be predictive of disease evolution. E-cadherin expression seems to be an indicator of limited skin disease but not of disease regression. Additional immunohistochemical study is required to confirm these data.

▶ Conclusive criteria distinguishing self-regressive forms of Langerhans cell histiocytosis (SR-LCH) from non–self-regressive forms of LCH (NSR-LCH) in neonatal patients continue to be lacking. Accordingly, Battistella et al sought to describe whether there were any decisive clinical features (such as cutaneous lesion characteristics) or immunohistochemical findings (such as T-lymphocyte density and E-cadherin expression) in patients with cutaneous LCH in the first 3 months of life and to define what, if any, predictive variables are there for disease evolution in patients with neonatal and early infantile self-regressive and non–self-regressive forms of LCH.

The findings of the study were interesting. As noted by the article, this is the first study to demonstrate that there are some morphologic traits that point toward a diagnosis of SR-LCH, including necrosis, a solitary lesion, and involvement of the extremities. Other notable findings included that there was no histopathological difference between SR-LCH and NSR-LCH and that T-regulatory lymphocytes density did not seem to be predictive of disease evolution. The study did note that E-cadherin expression may be an indicator of good prognosis and limited disease in skin lesional Langerhans cells. The study included only 31 patients and admittedly prospective validation of these conclusions would be helpful, especially with a larger number of patients. Overall, the study was helpful in providing much needed additional evidence in the continued efforts to elucidate both SR-LCH and NSR-LCH.

B. D. Michaels, DO
J. Q. Del Rosso, DO

Pediatric Mastocytosis Is a Clonal Disease Associated with D^{816}V and Other Activating c-*KIT* Mutations
Bodemer C, Hermine O, Palmérini F, et al (Hôpital Necker, Paris, France; Centre de Référence des Mastocytoses, Paris, France; et al)
J Invest Dermatol 130:804-815, 2010

Adult mastocytosis is an incurable clonal disease associated with c-*KIT* mutations, mostly in exon 17 (D^{816}V). In contrast, pediatric mastocytosis often spontaneously regresses and is considered a reactive disease. Previous studies on childhood mastocytosis assessed only a few patients and focused primarily on codon 816 mutations, with various results. In this study, we analyzed the entire c-*KIT* sequence from cutaneous biopsies of 50 children with mastocytosis (ages 0−16 years). A mutation of codon 816 (exon 17) was found in 42% of cases, and mutations outside exon 17 were observed in 44%. Unexpectedly, half of the mutations were located in the fifth Ig loop of c-KIT's extracellular domain, which is encoded by exons 8 and 9. All mutations identified in this study were somatic and caused a constitutive activation of c-KIT. There was no clear phenotype−genotype correlation, no clear relationship between the mutations and familial versus spontaneous disease, and no significant change in the relative expression of the c-KIT GNNK+ and GNNK isoforms. These findings strongly support the idea that, although pediatric mastocytosis can spontaneously regress, it is a clonal disease most commonly associated with activating mutations in c-KIT.

▶ This article gives us new insight into our understanding of pediatric mastocytosis. Previously, it was believed that pediatric mastocytosis was reactive and as such was differentiated from adult disease by the absence of c-*KIT*-activating mutations.[1-2] This is not only the largest sample size of pediatric patients evaluated to date but in these patients, the entire c-*KIT* gene was sequenced for mutational analysis.

All of the identified mutations caused constitutive activation of c-*KIT*. The D816V mutation most commonly associated with adult mastocytosis was found in 36% of patients. Evaluation of genomic DNA in 13 patients showed the absence of c-*KIT* mutations in all patients suggesting mutations to be primarily somatic. There was no clear phenotype-genotype correlation nor any specific mutation associated with familial versus spontaneous disease. However, familial childhood-onset mastocytosis was found to occur both with and without c-*KIT* mutations. In addition, it was noted that children with onset of mastocytosis between 3 and 16 years of age lacked 816 codon mutations.

The data in this study support the conclusion that pediatric mastocytosis is a clonal disease causing c-*KIT*-activating mutations.[3] However, this leads us to question how and why pediatric and adult mastocytosis differ in their behavior and their association with systemic disease and malignancy. It is not clear how spontaneous resolution of pediatric mastocytosis occurs and whether uncovering a common mutation or factor might help us in the treatment of this condition. As in adult mastocytosis, KIT targeting might also be a consideration in treating systemic disease in children. It is also promising that all identified extracellular and juxtamembrane intracellular domain mutations were found to be sensitive to imatinib. The results from this study may help spur further research and have the potential to impact our evaluation and treatment of pediatric disease.

S. Fallon Friedlander, MD

References

1. Ben-Amitai D, Metzker A, Cohen HA. Pediatric cutaneous mastocytosis: a review of 180 patients. *Isr Med Assoc J.* 2005;7:320-322.
2. Kiszewski AE, Durán-Mckinster C, Orozco-Covarrubias L, Gutiérrez-Castrellón P, Ruiz-Maldonado R. Cutaneous mastocytosis in children: a clinical analysis of 71 cases. *J Eur Acad Dermatol Venereol.* 2004;18:285-290.
3. Yanagihori H, Oyama N, Nakamura K, Kaneko F. c-kit Mutations in patients with childhood-onset mastocytosis and genotype-phenotype correlation. *J Mol Diagn.* 2005;7:252-257.

Prevalence and distribution of solitary oral pigmented lesions: a prospective study
De Giorgi V, Sestini S, Bruscino N, et al (Univ of Florence, Italy)
J Eur Acad Dermatol Venereol 23:1320-1323, 2009

Solitary pigmented lesions are uncommon in the oral mucosa. A review of the literature reveals no information regarding the relative frequency of these lesions. The purpose of this study is to determine the relative prevalence of solitary oral pigmented lesions in a selected population of patients. This study includes 265 consecutive patients who accessed the dermatology out-patients' surgery of the Department of Dermatology, University of Florence between March 2006 and July 2007. The sample we studied presented 5.7% of oral pigmented lesions; the most frequent being vascular lesions. Despite the various methods used, the differential diagnosis for these particular lesions is not always easy. There is some difficulty in distinguishing between a benign pigmented lesion and a growing melanoma which, though rare (1% of all oral malignancies), is a serious and often fatal disease. Therefore, biopsy with histological exam represents the diagnostic gold standard.

▶ A complete oral cavity examination is often not part of a practitioner's routine skin examination. This report provides useful information on the types of solitary pigmented lesions one may encounter with a complete intraoral examination.

The histology of the oral mucosa is varied and is sprinkled with ducts as well as glandular and neural structures. One in 10 million patients develops an intraoral melanoma. Most of the pigmented lesions we encounter in our intraoral examinations will be one of the many benign lesions discussed in this article.

A limitation of this prospective study would be the small number of individuals included. It would be interesting to know the ethnic mix of this cohort since some studies have reported increased numbers of oral pigmented lesions in darker skin types (Fitzpatrick III-VI), Hispanics, and black populations.

Contrary to some other studies, this study did not show a connection with increased number of cutaneous nevi and the presence of intraoral nevi.

R. I. Ceilley, MD

A. K. Bean, MD

Recurrent erythema multiforme: Clinical characteristics, etiologic associations, and treatment in a series of 48 patients at Mayo Clinic, 2000 to 2007
Wetter DA, Davis MDP (Mayo Clinic, Rochester, MN)
J Am Acad Dermatol 62:45-53, 2010

Background.—Recurrent erythema multiforme (EM) is a condition of substantial morbidity. Our efforts toward the etiologic attribution and treatment of recurrent EM have been less fruitful than those previously described.

Objective.—We sought to further characterize clinical characteristics, etiologic associations, and treatment of recurrent EM.

Methods.—We conducted a retrospective review of patients with recurrent EM seen between 2000 and 2007.

Results.—Of 48 patients (mean age at disease onset, 36.4 years), 28 (58%) were female (mean duration of recurrent EM, 6 years). Thirty (63%) patients had oral involvement. Herpes simplex virus caused recurrent EM in 11 (23%) patients, and the cause remained unknown in 28 (58%). In all, 37 (77%) patients received systemic corticosteroids, 33 (69%) received continuous antiviral treatment, and 23 (48%) used immunosuppressive or anti-inflammatory agents. Sixteen of 33 patients receiving continuous antiviral treatment had either partial or complete disease suppression. Patients had varied responses to immunosuppressants, with mycophenolate mofetil providing partial or complete response in 6 of 8 patients. Features of recalcitrant cases included clinicians' inability to identify a specific cause, lack of improvement with continuous antiviral therapy, severe oral involvement, extensive corticosteroid therapy, and immunosuppressive therapy (two or more agents).

Limitation.—This study is retrospective.

Conclusions.—More than half of patients in this study did not have an identifiable cause for recurrent EM, and herpes simplex virus was found less frequently than reported in previous studies. Response to systemic treatments, including continuous antivirals and immunosuppressants, was varied and oftentimes suboptimal.

▶ Wetter and Davis performed a retrospective analysis of patients with recurrent erythema multiforme (EM), seeking to further clarify the clinical characteristics, etiologic associations, and treatment options. The results of their study were not necessarily reassuring to practitioners from a treatment standpoint but regardless, were both interesting and insightful. Although their study comprises a total of 48 patients in a tertiary referral center and, thus, admittedly not necessarily representative of the general population, the findings of the study helped to emphasize the complexity of this disease. Noteworthy findings included that in over half the patients, an identifiable cause was not established. Additionally, herpes simplex virus was found as the cause of disease in only 11 of the 48 patients, certainly less than that had been reported in previous studies. From a treatment standpoint, systemic medications, including continuous antiviral therapy and immunosuppressants, proved to be suboptimal often. As the authors emphasize, treatment of recurrent EM can be prolonged and challenging. For example, after corticosteroid treatment to control the disease, many times the disease flared when therapy was tapered or discontinued. This is not to suggest that treatment with either corticosteroids, antivirals, or immunosuppressants was never effective. In 33 patients treated with antivirals, 12 showed complete response, and of the 23 treated with immunosuppressants, 11 showed complete response. Thus, although these treatments can be effective in some cases, no one treatment regimen was proven to be optimal in most cases.

Ultimately, this article does a great job of calling to light the problematic nature of this disease to the general practitioner, from the difficulty in identifying an underlying cause to the difficulty in treatment options, all the while underlying the need for future research on this disease entity, especially for the patients suffering with this enigmatic disease.

B. D. Michaels, DO

J. Q. Del Rosso, DO

School-Based Condom Education and Its Relations With Diagnoses of and Testing for Sexually Transmitted Infections Among Men in the United States
Dodge B, Reece M, Herbenick D (Indiana Univ, Bloomington)
Am J Public Health 99:2180-2182, 2009

An intense social and political debate continues in the United States regarding sexuality education. Included in the debate are those who favor comprehensive approaches, those who favor abstinence-only approaches, and those who favor no sexuality education. In this study, we showed that men who received school-based condom education were less likely to have been diagnosed with sexually transmitted infections (STIs) and were more likely to ever have been tested for sexually transmitted infections than were men without such education. School-based condom education is associated with less, rather than more, STI risk.

▶ This is an interesting attempt to demonstrate that high-school—based sexually transmitted disease (STD) education, including, and specifically, condom-use education, will reduce the risk of subsequent development of STDs. While the desired outcome was indeed demonstrated (with the exception of chlamydial infection), the study itself is replete with serious shortcomings that diminish its impact. The most glaring deficiency is that minorities were grossly underrepresented in the study subject pool. This is the exact group at highest risk for STD acquisition. Moreover, all data collected depended upon the subjects' recollection of events some decade earlier. The quality of STD (and condom use) education could not be assessed. Thus, the study results are suggestive, but hardly conclusive, that high-school sex education may help to reduce subsequent risky behavior and STD acquisition. Despite these reservations, the study does provide additional evidence that STD education is better than simply ignoring the issue altogether in terms of subsequent medical consequences.

T. Rosen, MD

Seborrhoeic keratoses in patients with internal malignancies: a case–control study with prospective accrual of patients
Fink A, Filz D, Krajnik G, et al (Wilhelminenspital, Vienna, Austria; et al)
J Eur Acad Dermatol Venereol 23:1316-1319, 2009

Background.—The association between the eruption of numerous seborrhoeic keratoses as a result of an underlying malignancy is controversially discussed. The aim of this case–control study with prospective accrual of patients was to determine whether a direct association exists between the number seborrhoeic keratoses and internal malignancies.

Methods.—The numbers and sites of seborrhoeic keratoses were counted in 150 oncological patients and 150 matched controls. Additionally, the presence or absence of pruritus, acanthosis nigricans, and the sudden appearance of seborrhoeic keratoses were assessed.

Results.—Seborrhoeic keratoses did not differ significantly between patients with internal malignancies and controls. Only two patients fulfilled the criteria of the Leser-Trélat sign, defined as the eruption of numerous seborrhoeic keratoses as a cutaneous marker of an underlying internal malignancy.

Conclusion.—No association was found between seborrhoeic keratoses and cancer. Furthermore, our data did not provide support to the validity of the Leser-Trélat sign in patients with internal malignancies.

▶ Ah, the elusive sign of Leser-Trélat, harder to identify than the Loch Ness Monster or Bigfoot, yet everyone familiar with it wants to make the diagnosis when a patient unfortunately diagnosed with a systemic malignancy has multiple seborrheic keratoses (SKs). And yet for decades, we have had nothing but scrutiny that this link truly exists,[1] although the link to malignant acanthosis nigricans and its correlation as a paraneoplastic syndrome can be supported.[2] The truth of the elusive diagnosis, which the authors remind us is "the eruption of numerous seborrhoeic keratoses as a cutaneous marker of an underlying internal malignancy" is that many of the patients we consider for it are elderly, who also have a higher incidence of SKs and typically do not remember when they first showed up. In this article, those concepts are revisited because the abrupt onset of the SKs was only seen in 2 of the 150 patients. The other important part of the study was how the authors randomized the subjects, all with visceral cancers, into the 4 groups divided by quantity of SKs. This took out any bias of age, type of malignancy, and onset of lesions, which are the common screening criteria in the clinic. Finally, the 2 patients identified as having met the criteria for the diagnosis did not have any signs of acanthosis nigricans.

Although traditional teaching has perpetuated the notion that the sign of Leser-Trélat is linked to abrupt onset of SKs, perhaps articles and studies that continue to refute the linkage should also be part of that teaching.

N. Bhatia, MD

References

1. Rampen HJ, Schwengle LE. The sign of Leser-Trélat: does it exist? *J Am Acad Dermatol.* 1989;21:50-55.
2. Schwartz RA. Sign of Leser-Trélat. *J Am Acad Dermatol.* 1996;35:88-95.

Significant upregulation of antimicrobial peptides and proteins in lichen sclerosus

Gambichler T, Skrygan M, Tigges C, et al (Ruhr-Univ Bochum, Germany; et al)
Br J Dermatol 161:1136-1142, 2009

Background.—Lichen sclerosus (LS) is a chronic inflammatory T cell-driven sclerotic skin condition in which skin barrier disruption frequently occurs. Inflamed and injured epithelia are a particularly rich source of antimicrobial peptides and proteins (AMPs).

Objectives.—We aimed to investigate for the first time the expression pattern of AMPs in lesions of LS as compared with healthy skin.

Methods.—Twenty-four women with LS as well as 10 healthy women were included in the study. In order to assess the expression of human β-defensin (hBD)-1, hBD-2, hBD-3, psoriasin (S100A7), the cathelicidin LL-37 and RNase 7, real-time reverse transcriptase—polymerase chain reaction and immunohistochemistry were performed on skin specimens obtained from lesional and healthy skin of the genital region, respectively.

Results.—Median hBD-2 mRNA levels observed in LS were significantly higher than in controls ($0 \cdot 15$ vs. $0 \cdot 008$; $P = 0 \cdot 0037$). Moreover, psoriasin ($98 \cdot 2$ vs. $28 \cdot 1$; $P = 0 \cdot 0052$) mRNA expression was significantly higher in LS lesions as compared with controls. Significant differences in mRNA expression of hBD-2 and psoriasin were also confirmed by immunohistochemistry. For hBD-1, hBD-3, LL-37 and RNase 7, levels did not differ significantly or were significant only at the gene level but not protein level.

Conclusions.—We have demonstrated that hBD-2 and psoriasin expression levels in lesional skin of patients with LS are significantly increased when compared with healthy controls. Whether this observation simply reflects an innate defence response caused by an increased risk of local infection, or whether our data indicate a pathogenetic role of AMPs in LS, will be addressed in future studies.

▶ The abnormal expression of antimicrobial peptides (AMPs) shows a linkage to a wide variety of dermatoses, such as rosacea and psoriasis. The authors bring lichen sclerosus (LS) into that category with this demonstration of defensins, specifically human β-defensin-2 (inducible epidermal keratinocyte AMP from interleukin-1 stimulation) and psoriasin (S-100 epidermal protein). There were no significant increases in constitutive AMPs such as LL-37 and other defensins, which means in LS, there is still host immunity against infections. Superinfections are not commonly observed, according to the article based on these findings similar to psoriasis, compared with atopic dermatitis, yet both conditions are associated with disruptions in epidermal barrier integrity. In the clinical setting, these conditions are often treated with high-potency steroids and immunomodulators, yet antibiotics are often unnecessary. This emphasizes the important point that the authors introduce in the abstract: that it is unclear and difficult to demonstrate "whether this observation simply reflects an innate defence response" or "a pathogenetic role of AMPs in LS." More important for the clinician is the understanding of treating the entire disease process and exploring where retinoids, vitamin D analogs, and other nonsteroid alternatives might impact the disease process, namely the abnormal AMP expression, than just the disease symptoms by simply using steroids alone.[1-3]

N. Bhatia, MD

References

1. Schauber J, Gallo RL. The vitamin D pathway: a new target for control of the skin's immune response? *Exp Dermatol.* 2008;17:633-639.
2. Dombrowski Y, Peric M, Koglin S, Ruzicka T, Schauber J. Control of cutaneous antimicrobial peptides by vitamin D3. *Arch Dermatol Res.* 2010;302:401-408.
3. Peric M, Koglin S, Dombrowski Y, et al. Vitamin D analogs differentially control antimicrobial peptide/"alarmin" expression in psoriasis. *PLoS One.* 2009;4:e6340.

Studying Regression of Seborrheic Keratosis in Lichenoid Keratosis with Sequential Dermoscopy Imaging
Zaballos P, Salsench E, Serrano P, et al (Hosp de Sant Pau i Santa Tecla, Tarragona, Spain; et al)
Dermatology 220:103-109, 2010

Background.—Lichenoid keratosis (LK) is a well-described entity that has been proposed to represent a regressive response to a pre-existent epidermal lesion.

Aims.—To evaluate the natural evolution of a series of cases showing the intermediate stage of the regression of seborrheic keratosis in LK using sequential dermoscopy imaging over time.

Material and Methods.—A series of lesions with dermoscopic areas of seborrheic keratosis and LK in the same tumor were consecutively collected for over 3 years at the Dermatology Department of the Hospital de Sant Pau i Santa Tecla, Tarragona, Spain. Sequential dermoscopic images of each case were collected quarterly for 1 year. At the end of the follow-up, all the lesions were biopsied.

Results.—A total of 22 cases were collected. At the end of the follow-up, the LK part increased in all the lesions. In 11 cases (50%), the seborrheic keratosis part disappeared completely, and in another 5 cases (22.7%), seborrheic keratosis comprised only 10% of the remaining area.

Conclusions.—These dermoscopic study findings support the proposal that LK represents a regressive response to a pre-existent epidermal lesion, in this case seborrheic keratosis.

▶ This is a fascinating article outlining the evolution of seborrheic keratoses to lichenoid keratoses. The authors use sequential dermoscopic images to elucidate the evolution of lichenoid keratoses. The premise is that lichenoid keratoses result from an immunologic reaction to a pre-existing lesion with resultant inflammation that ultimately destroys the original lesion. In this article, the authors use previously described dermoscopic findings to follow 22 patients every 3 months for 1 year. Initially, all patients had areas of seborrheic keratosis and lichenoid keratosis defined by dermoscopy. At the end of the year, 50% of the cases showed complete disappearance of the seborrheic keratosis and another 22% showed 90% disappearance of the seborrheic keratosis. This article offers compelling evidence that lichenoid keratoses are indeed the result of inflammatory regression of seborrheic keratoses.

S. M. Purcell, DO

The 5-D itch scale: a new measure of pruritus
Elman S, Hynan LS, Gabriel V, et al (Univ of Texas Southwestern Med Ctr, Dallas)
Br J Dermatol 162:587-593, 2010

Background.—Itching is a subjective and multidimensional experience which is difficult to quantify. Most methodologies to assess itching suffer from being unidimensional, for example only measuring intensity without impact on quality of life, or only measuring scratching activity. None has actually been demonstrated to be able to detect change over time, which is essential to using them as an outcome measure of response to an intervention. The 5-D itch scale was developed as a brief but multidimensional questionnaire designed to be useful as an outcome measure in clinical trials. The five dimensions are degree, duration, direction, disability and distribution.

Objectives.—To study the 5-D with respect to validity, reliability and response to change.

Methods.—The 5-D was administered to 234 individuals with chronic pruritus due to liver disease ($n = 63$), kidney disease ($n = 36$), dermatological disorders ($n = 56$), HIV/AIDS ($n = 28$) and burn injuries ($n = 51$). The 5-D was administered at baseline and after a 6-week follow-up period. A subset of 50 untreated patients was retested after 3 days to assess test—retest reliability.

Results.—The 5-D score correlated strongly with a visual analogue score: $r = 0.727$ at baseline ($P < 0.0001$), $r = 0.868$ at the 3-day repeat ($P < 0.0001$), and $r = 0.892$ at the 6-week follow-up ($P < 0.0001$). There was no change in mean 5-D score between day 1 and day 3 in untreated individuals (intraclass correlation coefficient $= 0.96$, $P < 0.0001$). The 5-D did, however, detect significant changes in pruritus over the 6-week follow-up period ($P < 0.0001$). Subanalysis of the different patient groups revealed similar response patterns and scores, with the exception of lower total scores for the burn victims due to lower scores on the distribution domain because they itched only at the site of their burn.

Conclusions.—The 5-D, therefore, is a reliable, multidimensional measure of itching that has been validated in patients with chronic pruritus to be able to detect changes over time. The 5-D should be useful as an outcome measure in clinical trials.

▶ The authors have developed a new tool for measuring itch. The 5-domains (5-D) itch scale is a single-page simple questionnaire, which is easy to administer, complete, and score. The questionnaire measures itching in 5 domains: duration, degree, direction, disability, and distribution.

The article analyzes the validity of the 5-D questionnaire comparing it with the standard visual analog scale and determined that the new tool was both reliable and valid. As opposed to the visual analog scale, the questionnaire is straightforward and easy to understand and does not require abstract thinking by the taker. The 5-D questionnaire appears to be a simple and reasonable tool for itch assessment that would be useful in clinical research and clinical practice.

S. M. Purcell, DO

The effects of topical isoflavones on postmenopausal skin: Double-blind and randomized clinical trial of efficacy
Moraes AB, Haidar MA, Soares Júnior JM, et al (UNIFESP, Brazil; et al)
Eur J Obstet Gynecol Reprod Biol 146:188-192, 2009

Objective.—The aim of this study was to evaluate the effects of estrogen and isoflavones on postmenopausal skin morphological parameters.

Study Design.—A randomized, double-blind, estrogen-controlled trial was performed on postmenopausal women treated in the Gynecology Department of the Federal University of São Paulo. This study was designed to analyze the effects of topical administration of estradiol and isoflavones on facial skin for 24 weeks. The participants were divided into two groups: G1—17-betaestradiol 0.01% ($n = 18$) and G2—isoflavones 40% (genistein 4%, $n = 18$). Skin biopsies were performed on each patient before and after the treatment. The skin samples were processed for histological analysis, stained with haematoxylin and eosin, and examined using light microscopy.

Results.—After 24 weeks of treatment, the estradiol group had a significant increase in skin parameters analyzed compared to the isoflavone group and to the baseline measurements: epidermal thickness (a 75% increase in the estrogen group and 20% in the isoflavone group), number of dermal papillae (a rise of 125% with estrogen, no significant gain with isoflavones), fibroblasts (a 123% accretion with estradiol, no significant gain with isoflavones), and vessels (a 77% increase with estrogen and 36% with isoflavones).

Conclusion.—Our data suggest that estrogens may have a stronger effect on histomorphometrical parameters than isoflavones.

▶ Soy isoflavones are phytoestrogens and therefore by definition exhibit only a weak estrogenic effect. In part this may be because of the necessary conversion of soy to its free isoflavone form to exert estrogenic activity. If the objective of this study was to compare topical estrogen with the topical estrogenic effects of soy isoflavones, then the article is just in essence reproving the already established information. The unique aspect of this study is the histologic comparisons of the effects of topical estradiol with the effects of soy isoflavones. The results of this study clearly demonstrate that soy isoflavones only minimally affect epidermal thickness and cutaneous vessel formation, while topical estrogens significantly affect epidermal thickness, number of dermal papillae, fibroblasts, and vessel formation. Why estrogens and phytoestrogens have different histological effects on the skin is unclear. Perhaps an additional study with more participants, a higher dose of isoflavones, and intraindividual comparisons may have demonstrated that phytoestrogens may produce similar changes in histology in all 4 categories but to a lesser extent, as expected from a weak estrogen. This is of course speculative at best. Assuming that the results of this study hold strong and phytoestrogens do not increase new vessel formation in the skin, this may not be such a bad thing. As seen in patients with cirrhosis who have too much circulating estrogen, they classically develop numerous spider angiomas and palmer erythema due to the increased vessel formation. These are the 2 undesired effects of estrogens that may potentially occur with topical application and may be avoided by using soy isoflavones instead of topical estrogens. Additional studies are needed.

J. Levin, DO

The impact of obesity on skin disease and epidermal permeability barrier status

Guida B, Nino M, Perrino NR, et al (Univ Federico II, Naples, Italy)
J Eur Acad Dermatol Venereol 24:191-195, 2010

Background.—Obese subjects frequently show skin diseases. However, less attention has been paid to the impact of obesity on skin disorders until now.

Objective.—The purposes of this study are: to highlight the incidence of some dermatoses in obese subjects and to study the water barrier function of the obese skin using transepidermal water loss (TEWL).

Methods.—Sixty obese subjects and 20 normal weight volunteers were recruited. Obese group was further divided into three body mass index (BMI) classes: class I (BMI 30—34.9 kg/m²), class II (BMI 35—39.9 kg/m²) and class III (BMI 40 g/m²). All subjects attended dermatological examination for skin diseases. To assess barrier function, TEWL measurements were performed on the volar surface of the forearm using a tewameter.

Results.—The results of this study showed that: (i) obese subjects show a higher incidence of some dermatoses compared with normal-weight controls; in addition the dermatoses are more, frequent as BMI increases; (ii) the rate of TEWL is lower in obese subjects, than in the normal-weight subjects, particularly in patients with intra-abdominal obesity.

Conclusion.—Specific dermatoses as skin tags, striae distensae and plantar hyperkeratosis, could be considered as a cutaneous stigma of severe obesity. The low permeability of the skin to evaporative water loss is observed in obese subjects compared with normal weight control. Although the physiological mechanisms are still unknown, this finding has not been previously described and we believe that this may constitute a new field in the research on obesity.

▶ Previous studies have recognized that an increase in adipose tissue causes changes in skin physiology in relation to an increase in sweat gland activity, dry skin, high transepidermal water loss (TEWL), altered collagen structure and function, and impaired wound healing. This is a study examining differences in skin lesions and TEWL of 60 obese subjects separated into body mass index (BMI) class I, II, and III compared with 20 normal-weight patients. Plantar hyperkeratosis was not observed in subjects of BMI class I but was found in 29% of BMI class II and 80% of BMI class III. Pseudoacanthosis nigricans was observed in 60% of subjects in BMI class III. Striae distensae was observed more frequently in obese subjects in up to 80% in BMI class III and predominant more in women as compared with men (76% and 33%, respectively). However, this observation may have been seen because women go through more dramatic weight changes such as pregnancy and may not be a marker for obesity, which was not discussed in this article. Skin tags were found in 83% of subjects of BMI class I compared with 86% in class II and 100% in class III. The authors noted that all obese subjects showed clinical signs of hyperandrogenism; however, no androgenic laboratory studies were conducted to confirm these findings. Sebaceous gland hypertrophy and seborrheic dermatitis were not found frequently in obese subjects. A significant lower TEWL rate ($P < .05$) was observed in subjects with abdominal obesity compared with those without abdominal obesity. Findings suggest that TEWL at the forearm site was significantly lower ($P < .05$) in obese subjects compared with those in the control group. However, taking TEWL measurements at only the volar surface of the arms may not be sufficient data to assess total TEWL in a patient. To add, those on current topical treatment that may affect TEWL were not excluded or identified. Another limitation to this study was that controls were not matched for age and sex, and statistical significance with dermatoses in obese subjects was not discussed. Also, patient's current medical conditions were not discussed that could have explained such clinical observations as hyperandrogenism in obese patients. However, those who were treated with insulin, oral glucose, or lipid-lowering agents were excluded. In conclusion, the authors found that obese patients may have a predisposition to develop dermatoses such as skin tags, striae distensae, and plantar hyperkeratosis as compared with normal-weight individuals.

J. Q. Del Rosso, DO

G. K. Kim, DO

Trends of skin diseases in organ-transplant recipients transplanted between 1966 and 2006: a cohort study with follow-up between 1994 and 2006

Wisgerhof HC, Edelbroek JRJ, de Fijter JW, et al (Leiden Univ Med Centre, the Netherlands)
Br J Dermatol 162:390-396, 2010

Background.—Skin diseases are frequently observed in organ-transplant recipients (OTRs).

Objectives.—To count the registered skin diseases in all 2136 OTRs who had been transplanted in a single centre between 1966 and 2006 and to calculate their relative contribution in relation to the number of years after transplantation.

Methods.—All registered skin diseases which were entered into a computerized system between 1994 and 2006 at the Leiden University Medical Centre were counted and their relative contributions were calculated.

Results.—Between 1994 and 2006, 2408 skin diseases were registered in 801 of 1768 OTRs who were at risk during this specific time period. The most commonly recorded diagnoses were skin infections ($24 \cdot 0\%$) followed by benign skin tumours ($23 \cdot 3\%$) and malignant skin lesions ($18 \cdot 2\%$). The relative contributions of infectious and inflammatory disorders decreased with time after transplantation, whereas the contribution of squamous cell carcinomas strongly increased with time.

Conclusions.—This study gives a systematic overview of the high burden of skin diseases in OTRs. The relative distributions of skin diseases importantly changed with time after transplantation, with squamous cell carcinoma contributing most to the increasing burden of skin diseases with increasing time after transplantation.

▶ Skin disorders are frequently seen in organ-transplant recipients (OTRs). The aim of this study was to estimate the frequency of registered skin diseases diagnosed in a single center between 1994 and 2006. The authors also sought to calculate the relative contributions of the different skin diseases in relation to the number of years after transplantation. There were 2136 patients who received a kidney transplantation (n = 1910) or a pancreas and kidney transplantation (n = 226) between 1994 and 2006. The 2408 registered skin diseases were equally distributed among skin tumors (1274) and other skin diseases (1134). The diagnoses of skin tumors tended to concentrate in fewer patients (456 patients) than other skin diseases (591 patients). Skin diseases other than tumors were diagnosed almost 10 years earlier compared with skin tumors at a median of 5.2 and 14.8 years after transplantation, respectively. The most frequent diagnoses were skin infections (21.3%) consisting of viral, bacterial, parasitic, fungal, and yeast infections. Herpes simplex and yeast infections occurred relatively early at a median of 2.0 and 2.2 years after transplantation. Inflammatory skin conditions were also regularly observed in OTRs (11% of the patients at risk), of which eczematous dermatitis, acne, and drug-related rashes were the most frequently registered skin diseases. Skin tumors were seen in 44% of the benign tumors (19.2% of the patients at risk), 21.6% of the premalignant tumors (10.4% of the patients at risk), and 34.4% of the malignant tumors (10.5% of the patients at risk). The median time from transplantation to the registration of the benign tumors was 9.9 years. The median time from transplantation to premalignant and malignant tumors was much longer, 16.5 and 17.8 years, respectively. The most frequently diagnosed benign skin tumors were human papillomavirus (HPV)-related warts (verrucae). The median time period after transplantation to the diagnoses of common warts was 11.1 years, actinic keratoses (15.2 years), basal cell carcinomas (15.9 years), and squamous cell carcinomas was (19.5 years). There were no age- or sex-matched controls, which was a limitation to this study. In addition, the authors were unable to exclude patient visitation to other hospitals or clinics for treatment of other skin diseases that may have been missed in this study. The study confirmed earlier publications that skin infections occur early after transplantation and that skin cancers increase exponentially after transplantation. This study also revealed that patients may also have vascular problems as shown in 7.8% of this study population.

J. Q. Del Rosso, DO
G. K. Kim, DO

Truncal Pruritus of Unknown Origin May Be a Symptom of Diabetic Polyneuropathy

Yamaoka H, Sasaki H, Yamasaki H, et al (Wakayama Med Univ, Japan)
Diabetes Care 33:150-155, 2010

Objective.—Our goal was to ascertain the prevalence of pruritus in diabetic and nondiabetic subjects and the relevance of symptoms, signs, and nerve functions of diabetic polyneuropathy (DPN) of pruritus.

Research Design and Methods.—A large-scale survey of 2,656 diabetic outpatients and 499 nondiabetic subjects was performed. In diabetic subjects, the relationship between pruritus and age, sex, diabetic duration, A1C, Achilles tendon reflex (ATR), and abnormal sensation in legs was evaluated. In 105 diabetic subjects, nerve conduction studies, quantitative vibratory threshold (QVT), heart rate variability, and a fall of systolic blood pressure at a head-up tilt test (ΔBP) were performed, and the relationships between pruritus and nerve functions were evaluated.

Results.—Although the prevalence of truncal pruritus of unknown origin (TPUO) in diabetic subjects was significantly higher than that in age-matched nondiabetic subjects (11.3 vs. 2.9%, $P = 0.0001$), the prevalence of other pruritus was not different between the two groups. Multiple logistic regression analysis revealed that abnormal sensation and ATR areflexia were independent risk factors for TPUO in age, sex, duration of diabetes, and A1C. ΔBP in diabetic subjects with TPUO was significantly impaired compared with that in those without TPUO. Larger ΔBP was identified as a significant risk factor of TPUO independent of other nerve dysfunctions by multiple logistic regression analysis.

Conclusions.—TPUO is significantly more frequent in diabetic than in nondiabetic individuals. TPUO is significantly associated with symptoms and signs of DPN, including impaired blood pressure response in a head-up tilt test. TPUO, therefore, might be a newly recognized symptom of DPN.

▶ This is a good-quality large-scale survey of 2656 diabetic outpatients and 499 nondiabetic subjects. The objective of the study was to ascertain the prevalence of pruritus in diabetic and nondiabetic subjects and the relevance of such symptoms, signs, and nerve functions in patients with diabetic polyneuropathy. The authors were only able to identify a correlation of truncal pruritus of unknown origin (TPUO) in patients with diabetes. They also noticed a correlation with change in blood pressure in patients with diabetes with TPUO versus those without TPUO. Their conclusion that TPUO may be a symptom of diabetic polyneuropathy is interesting. However, their suggested possible etiologic mechanisms of sympathetic nerve dysfunction leading to xerosis or direct damage to sensory c-fibers do not explain the predilection of TPUO for the trunk.

Their sample size is relatively adequate. However, the geographic distribution is very limited and must be considered as a possible confounding variable in this study. Although there is some clinical relevance to having another symptom to help assess peripheral neuropathy in patients with diabetes, the diagnosis of TPUO creates somewhat a challenge of its own. Nonetheless, it does present alternative treatments for TPUO if it is neuropathically induced. Further studies are needed to assess for geographic variance as well as clinical and histopathological correlation before definitive clinical relevance can be determined.

B. P. Glick, DO, MPH

A. Wiener, DO

T. J. Singer, DO

Visual and Pathologic Analyses of Keloid Growth Patterns
Akaishi S, Ogawa R, Hyakusoku H (Nippon Med School Hosp, Tokyo, Japan)
Ann Plast Surg 64:80-82, 2010

Keloids grow and spread not only vertically but also horizontally, although hypertrophic scars do not grow beyond the boundaries of the original injury. Clinically, we have encountered keloids with regular and irregular (untypical) shapes. As the characteristics of the irregular growth patterns of keloids have not been studied yet, we analyzed the irregular growth of keloids both visually and pathologically.

A total of 220 keloid specimens, each from a different patient, were surgically removed and used in this study. Through visual analysis, the preoperative shapes of these 220 keloids were classified into those with a regular shape (R group) and those with an irregular shape (IR group). Moreover, we distinguished between cases that had received keloidectomy previously and those that had not. We also determined whether the keloids were recurrent keloids or not. In both the R and IR groups, keloid specimens were studied histologically to examine for infection.

In the R group, there were 156 cases (70.9%; 55 males and 101 females with a mean age of 33.68 years). Three patients (1.9%) had infection and 2 patients (1.3%) had undergone keloidectomy previously. In the IR group, there were 64 cases (29.1%; 24 males and 40 females with a mean age of 45.27 years). Thirty patients (46.9%) had infection and 24 patients (37.5%) had undergone keloidectomy previously. Statistically, the rates of infection and keloidectomy were significantly different between the R group and the IR group.

Severe infection or operative history may be the cause of irregularly shaped keloids. Thus, in the absence of significant infection or a surgical history, the shape of keloids may be determined uniquely by skin tension.

▶ This study offers an interesting analysis about growth patterns of keloids with obvious therapeutic and planning implications and, although all keloids received postoperative radiation therapy, it underscores the importance of treating keloids with a combination of modalities to avoid recurrences usually ranging between 45% and 100% when treated with resection alone. In addition, the study shows how infections, well-known disruptors of the normal healing process, can also interfere and modify later stages of this process, resulting in scarring. Statistically significant results such as the influence of infections and prior keloid resection in the development of irregular keloids, compared with those keloids with regular shapes and minimal association with infections or prior resection, constitute important findings that prompt further investigation, including for example, systemic and/or local antibiotic therapy for the control of fibroblast proliferation, excessive collagen synthesis, and dermal remodeling, with possible implications in other fibroproliferative disorders of the skin; an old concept that has been in debate for many years. Additional interesting observations were obtained with the computer analysis of keloid growth pattern including higher skin tension in the edges of the keloid than in the center, keloid expansion in the direction of the skin being pulled, and the stiffness of the skin at the circumference of a keloid correlating directly with the degree of skin tension at the circumference.

B. Berman, MD, PhD

DERMATOLOGIC SURGERY AND CUTANEOUS ONCOLOGY

13 Nonmelanoma Skin Cancer

A basal-cell-like compartment in head and neck squamous cell carcinomas represents the invasive front of the tumor and is expressing MMP-9
Sterz CM, Kulle C, Dakic B, et al (Univ Hosp Giessen and Marburg, Germany; et al)
Oral Oncol 46:116-122, 2010

Head and neck squamous cell carcinomas (HNSCCs) are the most frequent malignancies of the upper aerodigestive tract. The cancer stem cell (CSC) hypothesis concludes that CSCs constitute the dangerous tumor cell population due to their ability of self-renewal and being associated with relapse of tumor disease, invasiveness and resistance to chemo (radio)therapy. The aim of this study was to look for CSC candidates and expression of MMP-9 that previously was implicated in HNSCC invasiveness.

Immunohistochemical, immunofluorescence and Western blot analysis were performed on HNSCC tumor specimens using antibodies specific for MMP-9, CD44, ALDH1 and CK14. Gelatinolytic activity was assessed by zymography. Pearson correlation analysis was used for statistical comparison.

Immunohistochemical analysis found CD44 and MMP-9 to co-localize in tumor cells at the invasive front. Western blot analysis demonstrated a significant correlation ($p = 0.0047$) between CD44 and MMP-9 in the tested tissues. In addition gelatinolytic activity of HNSCC tissues was found to significantly correlate ($p = 0.0010$) with MMP-9 expression. The CD44$^+$ invasive front of the tumor was also positive for ALDH1 and CK14, all of them being typically expressed by cells in the basal cell layer of normal stratified squamous epithelia that also harbors the epithelial stem cells.

The observations point to a role of a MMP-9 positive basal-cell-like cell layer in the process of HNSCC invasiveness. This compartment likely contains CSCs since it is expressing the putative CSC markers CD44, ALDH1 and CK14. This cell layer therefore should be considered a major therapeutic target in the treatment of head and neck cancer.

▶ This interesting study reinforces the possibility that cancer stem cells (CSCs) are present within basal-cell-like tumor cells of head and neck squamous cell carcinomas, providing a possible target for tumor invasion inhibition. Previous studies have associated CSCs with tumor perpetuity, tumor invasion, metastatic capability, resistance to treatment, and tumor relapse; all signs of aggressive biological behavior. The authors showed that this small subset of cells (ie, CSCs) are located within epidermal basal cells, which are part of the invasive front of the tumor (CD44+, ALDH1+, CK14+, and matrix metalloproteinase [MMP]-9+), contrary to normal basal cells that share positivity to those markers except to MMP-9. Gelatinase B (MMP-9)-positive cells were found to be co-localized with CSCs CD44+. This co-expression and particular distribution of MMP-9 and CD44+ cells limited to the invasive front of the tumor may be related to and may explain one of the molecular mechanisms of tumor invasion. MMP-9 inhibition has proven in the past to inhibit prostate cancer invasiveness. Further studies are needed to elucidate the clinical value of MMP-9 inhibition for the treatment and/or prevention of tumor invasion.

B. Berman, MD, PhD

A Randomized Trial of Tailored Skin Cancer Prevention Messages for Adults: Project SCAPE
Glanz K, Schoenfeld ER, Steffen A (Univ of Pennsylvania, Philadelphia; Stony Brook Univ, NY; Univ of Hawaii, Honolulu)
Am J Public Health 100:735-741, 2010

Objectives.—We evaluated the impact of a mailed, tailored intervention on skin cancer prevention and skin self-examination behaviors of adults at moderate and high risk for skin cancer.

Methods.—Adults at moderate and high risk for skin cancer were recruited in primary health care settings in Honolulu, HI, and Long Island, NY. After completing a baseline survey, participants were randomized to 2 groups. The treatment group received tailored materials, including personalized risk feedback, and the control group received general educational materials. Multivariate analyses compared sun protection and skin self-examination between groups, controlling for location, risk level, gender, and age.

Results.—A total of 596 adults completed the trial. The tailored materials had a significant effect on overall sun-protection habits, the use of hats, the use of sunglasses, and the recency of skin self-examination. Some effects were moderated by location and risk level.

Conclusions.—Tailored communications including personalized risk feedback can improve sun-protection behaviors and skin self-examination among adults at increased risk for skin cancer. These convenient, low-cost interventions can be implemented in a variety of settinas and should be tested further to assess their long-term effectiveness.

▶ The objective of this study is to evaluate the impact of mail-tailored educational intervention on skin cancer and self-examination behaviors of adults in moderate-risk and high-risk patients with skin cancer. This is a comparative study between patients recruited in the primary care setting in Honolulu, Hawaii and in Long Island, New York; the patients were with moderate to high risk for skin cancer. This was obtained via the Brief Skin Cancer Risk Assessment Tool Survey Instrument, which has been successfully used in other studies to indicate those patients who are found to be of higher risk of skin cancer and have good reproducibility. A group of 596 adults completed the trial, and 1 group received tailored educational materials that had specific messages regarding overall sun protection habits, the use of hats, the use of sunglasses, and the recency of skin self-examinations. The other group was assessed on these categories without the tailored informational brochures that were mailed. The information showed an improvement over all parameters. The major parameters were looking at the exposure of sun between 10 AM and 4 PM, and the habits were measured with 6 protective behaviors, wearing a long sleeve shirt, sunglasses, staying in the shade, using sunscreen, limiting time in the midday, and wearing a hat. The sunscreen usage survey diary was kept along with telephone interviews. The reaction to interventions were assessed with 1 through 5, with 1 being not at all to 5 being very on these 6 features. Three approaches were used in a multivarying analysis. Treatment efforts included sun protection habit index, individual habits, sunscreen application index, sun exposure, and number of sunburns. The original study was performed over 2 summers, and 238 people completed a risk analysis. A total of 137 people were eligible after 724 completed a baseline survey and were randomized. The study completion rate was 82.3% for 596 patients. Participants were equally divided across both groups. They include analysis for college education and household incomes. There was no significant difference between treatment and control groups and gender, education, ethnicity, age, percent risk, high risk, or mean baseline sun habits scores for all participants. Sole differences were noted between the Honolulu and the Long Island participants, specifically for men and people with lower income who were more likely to have had a sunburn in the previous 3 months.

As expected, the outcomes indicate that both from multiple analysis with telephone interviews and with diary that the targeted use of patient education materials in a high-risk or moderate-risk patient population does improve their compliance with preventive measures. This study was a good study to assess this because it had a relatively large size, 564 patients, and because it had multiple geographic locations and measured prevention exposure behaviors. The weakness of the study was the lack of the ability of the targeted educational materials and that there may be a possibility that this relatively well-educated and affluent group may do well, but a less educated group may not work so well. The percent change and behavioral change from baseline was significant in the treatment group both from multiple modalities, the average sun protection habits, any sun protection, and the use of sunscreen, wearing a shirt, wearing a hat, and staying in the shade. Factors that had poor correlation with the treatment group were the sun exposure totals, sun exposure on weekend, and sun exposure on weekdays.

L. Cleaver, DO

A study of mitochondrial DNA D-loop mutations and p53 status in nonmelanoma skin cancer
Prior SL, Griffiths AP, Lewis PD (Swansea Univ, UK; Morriston Hosp, Swansea, UK)
Br J Dermatol 161:1067-1071, 2009

Background.—Mitochondrial DNA (mtDNA) displacement-loop (D-loop) mutations have previously demonstrated potential as smoking-induced biomarkers in oral squamous cell carcinoma (SCC). Additionally, they have been observed in SCC and basal cell carcinoma of nonmelanoma skin cancer (NMSC). However, they have not been examined in the SCC precursor lesions, Bowen disease or actinic keratosis.

Objectives.—Here, we present a novel study of mtDNA D-loop mutations in these two precursors, a rare keratoacanthoma and NMSC (all tumours not related to smoking).

Methods.—We used a polymerase chain reaction and direct sequencing approach. Furthermore, as the tumour suppressor protein p53 has been reported as having a novel role in maintaining mitochondrial genetic stability, we assessed p53 status using immunohistochemistry, evaluating potential association with the presence of mtDNA mutations.

Results.—Of 36 tumours, nine (25%) exhibited mutations in the D-loop. In total, 13 base substitutions were observed across all patients: seven (53·8%) were A : T to G : C; two (15·4%) were G : C to T : A; two (15·4%) were G : C to A : T and two (15·4%) were G : C to C : G. Four of the 13 (30·8%) base substitutions were observed at nucleotide 146. We observed abnormal p53 accumulation in over half of the samples analysed (55·5%), suggesting it to be a major part of the carcinogenic process of NMSC; however; there was no association between p53 positivity and the presence of mtDNA mutations (P = 0·47).

Conclusions.—It is unlikely that alteration in p53 status is a contributing factor to mtDNA mutagenesis.

▶ P53 is a tumor suppressor gene, which when mutated is known to be involved in the pathogenesis of human cancers. Whether these mutations occur early or late in malignant transformation is debated. In this study, Prior et al found that mutations in p53 were present in precancerous lesions as well: 4/4 actinic keratosis (AK) lesions and 4/5 Bowen's disease (BD) lesions. Importantly, these results provide evidence that p53 mutations occur early in malignant transformation and may be used in the future as a marker for early detection of cancer.

In addition, it is believed that p53 may play a role in stabilizing mitochondrial DNA, and therefore, mutations in p53 may have a relationship to mutations in mitochondrial DNA. Prior et al found mutations in the D-loop of mitochondrial DNA in 9/36 lesions studied (including basal cell carcinoma, squamous cell carcinoma, and BD), but only 3 were also positive for p53 mutations. This is inconsistent with the previous findings of Achanta et al,[1] and therefore, supports the need for larger future studies to determine whether there is a relationship between mitochondrial DNA mutations and p53 mutations.

B. Berman, MD, PhD

Reference

1. Achanta G, Sasaki R, Feng L, et al. Novel role of p53 in maintaining mitochondrial genetic stability through interaction with DNA Pol gamma. *EMBO J.* 2005;24:3482-3492.

Agreement on the Clinical Diagnosis and Management of Cutaneous Squamous Neoplasms
Terushkin V, Braga JC, Dusza SW, et al (Memorial Sloan-Kettering Cancer Ctr, NY; et al)
Dermatol Surg 36:1514-1520, 2010

Background.—Diagnostic accuracy and preferred therapeutic strategies for actinic keratoses (AKs) and squamous cell carcinoma (SCC) have significant public health implications.

Objective.—To evaluate clinical–pathologic agreement on the diagnosis of AKs and early SCCs and to characterize the effect of diagnosis on therapeutic decisions.

Methods & Materials.—Nine dermatologists and two dermatopathologists reviewed an image-based dataset of AKs and early SCCs. Clinical–pathologic agreement, inter- and intraobserver reliability for clinical diagnosis, and frequencies of therapies according to pathologic diagnosis were assessed.

Results.—Clinical-pathologic ($\kappa = 0.10$) agreement was poor, whereas interobserver ($\kappa = 0.24$) and intraobserver ($\kappa = 0.28$) agreements were fair. Participants were more likely to treat AKs with cryotherapy (64.2%) and to manage SCCs with surgery (72.8%). Therapeutic choice rarely changed after participants were shown histological photomicrographs. Participating clinicians treated most lesions histologically diagnosed as SCC in situ arising within AK using surgery, whereas pathologists selected cryotherapy or curettage and electrodesiccation for these lesions.

Conclusion.—We found poor clinical–pathologic agreement and reproducibility for clinically distinguishing between AK and early SCC even between skin cancer specialists from a single academic group practice. Nomenclature used in the pathologic diagnosis of AK and SCC affects clinicians' therapeutic decisions. The authors have indicated no significant interest with commercial supporters.

▶ Controversy exists in the classification of cutaneous squamous cell neoplasms. From actinic keratosis (AK) to invasive squamous cell carcinoma (SCC), distinctive diagnostic lines can be blurred. One study found that 1 in 25 clinically diagnosed AK lesions were actually early SCC.[1] Some believe that AKs are SCCs in their earliest phase.[2-4] In general, clinicians will agree that most AK can be treated with nonsurgical means, whereas invasive SCC is typically treated with surgery. In fact, results of this study indicate that most evaluators recommended cryotherapy for treatment of AKs and excision, including Mohs surgery, for SCCs depending on the location, size, tumor features, and other factors. In addition, there was poor clinical-pathologic agreement among participants. The use of only photographs may be a contributing factor, as some lesions are better appreciated by tactile means. Additional limitations include small number of participants (9 dermatologists and 2 dermatopathologists) and evaluators that were from a single academic institution. Guidelines on diagnosis and treatment of lesions that fall between the 2 extremes are currently lacking in consensus. Therefore, it is extremely important to work in conjunction with the clinician's dermatopathologist in providing optimal therapy for patients.

S. Bellew, DO

J. Q. Del Rosso, DO

References

1. Ehrig T, Cockerell C, Piacquadio D, Dromgoole S. Actinic keratoses and the incidence of occult squamous cell carcinoma: a clinical-histopathologic correlation. *Dermatol Surg.* 2006;32:1261-1265.
2. Röwert-Huber J, Patel MJ, Forschner T, et al. Actinic keratosis is an early in situ squamous cell carcinoma: a proposal for reclassification. *Br J Dermatol.* 2007; 156:8-12.
3. Lober BA, Lober CW. Actinic keratosis is squamous cell carcinoma. *South Med J.* 2000;93:650-655.
4. Kessler GM, Ackerman AB. Nomenclature for very superficial squamous cell carcinoma of the skin and of the cervix: a critique in historical perspective. *Am J Dermatopathol.* 2006;28:537-545.

Basal cell carcinoma with perineural invasion: reexcision perineural invasion?
Bechert CJ, Stern JB (Univ of Texas Med Branch, Galveston; Natl Cancer Inst, Bethesda, MD)
J Cutan Pathol 37:376-379, 2010

Background.—Perineural invasion (PI) in basal cell and squamous cell carcinomas, especially of the head and neck, has been reported to indicate an increased morbidity. Reexcision perineural invasion (RPI), a benign mimic of tumoral perineural invasion, may present a difficult histologic differential diagnosis.

Methods.—We surveyed the medical literature for PI occurring in basal cell carcinomas to investigate the degree to which the reported cases occurred in reexcision specimens vs. primary biopsy specimens.

Results.—We found large retrospective studies of 14,120 basal cell carcinomas evaluated for PI in which 310 cases of PI were identified (2.2%), and 20 sporadic case reports of basal cell carcinomas with PI. Of 310 cases of

basal cell carcinoma with PI, 196 (63%) were in reexcision specimens. Of 20 sporadic reports, 17 (85%) were in reexcision specimens.
Conclusion.—The high percentage of PI occurring in reexcision specimens vs. primary excisions may indicate that many of the reported cases of basal cell carcinomas with PI are actually examples of RPI.

▶ Perineural invasion (PI) in basal cell carcinoma (BCC) is rare. Re-excision PI (RPI) is presence of benign perineural epithelial cells in previously biopsied areas. In this article, the authors surveyed the literature and hypothesized that majority of the PI reported were in fact RPI. Thirty-year data were reviewed and 14 120 BCCs were identified. Three hundred ten of 14 120 were reported as BCCs with PI. Twenty sporadic case reports of BCCs with PI were also identified. RPI was noted to be in 63.2% of BCC cases with PI and in 85% of sporadic case reports. The authors did meet their hypothesis and showed that most BCC with PI were indeed cases of RPI. The authors suggestion is valid in that pathologists should be aware of the existence of RPI to avoid misdiagnosis as invasive carcinoma.

S. Bhambri, DO

Effect of dosing frequency on the safety and efficacy of imiquimod 5% cream for treatment of actinic keratosis on the forearms and hands: a phase II, randomized placebo-controlled trial
Gebauer K, Shumack S, Cowen PSJ (Fremantle Dermatology, Western Australia; St George Hosp, Sydney, New South Wales, Australia; Monash Med Centre, Clayton, Victoria, Australia)
Br J Dermatol 161:897-903, 2009

Background.—Clinical studies in cutaneous conditions other than actinic keratosis (AK) have revealed that the safety and efficacy profile of imiquimod is influenced by dosing frequency.

Objectives.—To evaluate dosing frequency response of imiquimod 5% for treatment of AK.

Methods.—This was a phase II, multicentre, randomized, double-blind, placebo-controlled study. Adults with ≥ 10 but ≤ 50 clinical AKs, one of which was histologically confirmed, were randomized (4 : 1) to 2–6 packets of imiquimod or placebo cream applied to the dorsum of the forearms and hands once daily 2, 3, 5 or 7 times per week for 8 weeks. The primary endpoint was complete clearance of AKs in the treatment area at 8 weeks post-treatment.

Results.—One hundred and forty-nine (94 men and 54 women) white subjects, with a mean ± SD age of 71 ± 10·2 years, were enrolled. Twenty-eight subjects (18·8%) discontinued from study: 0%, 3·1%, 6·9%, 30·0% and 33·3% withdrew for local skin reactions or adverse events in the combined placebo, and in the imiquimod 2, 3, 5 or 7 times per week groups, respectively. Seven serious adverse events occurred;

none was related to the study drug. Median baseline lesions ranged from 38 to 40 for the treatment groups. Complete clearance was achieved in 0%, 3·2%, 6·9%, 3·3% and 6·7% of subjects, and partial clearance (≥ 75% lesion reduction) in 0%, 22·6%, 24·1%, 20·0% and 36·7% of subjects for the placebo and imiquimod 2, 3, 5 or 7 times per week regimens, respectively.

Conclusions.—Imiquimod 5% applied more frequently than 3 times per week to AKs was not well tolerated. Complete clearance rates were low; however, partial clearance rates increased with increased dosing frequency ($P = 0·002$).

▶ Imiquimod is an immune modifier that stimulates innate cells to produce cytokines and has been used in the treatment of actinic keratosis (AK). This is a phase 2, randomized, placebo-controlled trial using imiquimod 5% cream for the treatment of AK on the forearms and hands in 149 (94 men and 54 women) Australian and New Zealand subjects with a mean age of 71. Patients were all Caucasian with skin type I or II. Patients were randomized to either imiquimod 5% cream or placebo (4:1) to be applied once daily 2, 3, 5, or 7 times a week. All patients had not been treated with imiquimod or systemic retinoids within 2 years. Efficacy was evaluated by clinical AK lesional counts within the target area performed from baseline. Subjects were instructed to apply the study drug at night and wash it off the following day. There was an increase in proportion of subjects with adverse events observed more frequent in imiquimod dosing groups (5-7 times per week) compared with the less frequent dosing group (2 times per week). This was also reflected with an increase in proportion of subjects requiring rest periods (> 80% vs 22.6%). Complete clearance rates were low in all groups, ranging from 0% to 6.7% of subjects, without evidence of a dosing frequency response. There was an increase in partial clearance with increase in dose frequency ($P = .0034$). The mean percentage lesion reduction was 21.2% for placebo and 44.6% to 65.3% for imiquimod. In addition, more than 50% of subjects required rest periods, and 25% of those patients missed doses because of these needed rest periods. Eleven subjects had considerable inflammation, and 28 subjects (18.8%) discontinued the study: 0%, 3.1%, 6.9%, 30%, and 33.3%. Limitations included imiquimod use restricted to the arm and hands. Additionally, because imiquimod causes erythema and inflammation, it may result in hyperpigmentation in other ethnic groups such as Asians and African American groups and should be studied with other skin types. Also investigators had to rely on self-reports to assess whether patients were following directions and washing off the study drug at the appropriate time. Also, resolution of AK lesions was done on a clinical basis without histological confirmation. Although authors noted that there was an increase in partial clearance with increase in dose frequency, a histological confirmation may be more telling. Additionally it would answer other questions concerning erythema and adverse effects. It may be misleading that erythema may not correlate with clearance of AK lesions when examined histologically. In conclusion, imiquimod 5% applied more frequently than 3 times per week for the treatment of AKs was not well tolerated in this study.

J. Q. Del Rosso, DO

G. K. Kim, DO

Topical 3.0% diclofenac in 2.5% hyaluronic acid gel induces regression of cancerous transformation in actinic keratoses
Dirschka T, Bierhoff E, Pflugfelder A, et al (Dermatological Practice Ctr, Wuppertal, Germany; Inst of Dermatopathology, Bonn, Germany; Eberhard Karls Univ Tübingen, Germany)
J Eur Acad Dermatol Venereol 24:258-263, 2010

Background.—Actinic keratoses (AKs) are frequently diagnosed in dermatological patients. As they represent *in situ* carcinomas, effective treatment is required.

Objectives.—We investigated the effect of topical 3.0% diclofenac in 2.5% hyaluronic acid gel on AK.

Methods.—Sixty-five patients with AKs were clinically evaluated before and after 3 months' treatment with topical 3.0% diclofenac in 2.5% hyaluronic gel. Biopsy specimens were taken and stained with haematoxylin-eosin and immunohistological markers. Specimens were evaluated by histological type of AKs using the AK classification scheme suggested by Röwert-Huber *et al.* [(early) *in situ* squamous cell carcinoma type AK Grade I–III], number of mitoses per high-power field and expression of immunohistological markers.

Results.—Complete clinical resolution was observed in 11 patients (16.9%). A significant ($P < 0.001$) downgrading of AK grade was observed. Complete histological resolution was achieved in 15 patients (23.1%). The number of mitoses per high-power field was reduced significantly ($P < 0.001$). The expression of anti-p53-antibody decreased significantly ($P = 0.009$), as did the expression of anti-MiB-1 antibody ($P = 0.021$).

Conclusions.—3.0% diclofenac in 2.5% hyaluronic acid gel causes regression of signs of cancerous transformation after 3 months' therapy.

▶ Actinic keratosis (AK) is a common sun-induced skin condition that may progress into squamous cell carcinoma. This is an open-label, randomized, multicenter phase IV trial evaluating the clinical and histological effects of topical 3.0% diclofenac in 2.5% hyaluronic gel (Solaraze, Almirall S.A., Barcelona, Spain) applied twice daily to AKs located on the face and/or scalp for 3 months. There were 2-mm punch biopsies that were taken before and 3 months after treatment. Studies comprised 65 Caucasian patients (skin type I and II) from the study center in Wuppertal ($n = 36$) and Tübingen ($n = 29$) who were diagnosed with AKs on face or scalp (51 males and 14 females; age range 51-81 years; average age of 67.5 years; and median age of 69 years). Before and after treatment, routine histology showed various histological types of AK (type I and II). Significant changes in AK types were seen for bowenoid AKs ($P < .001$) and unclassified AKs. Complete clinical resolution was observed in 11 patients (16.9%). Adnexal involvement of AK was reduced from 46 patients (70.77%) before treatment to 9 patients (13.85%) after treatment ($P < .001$). The number of mitoses decreased significantly after treatment ($P < .001$). The expression of anti-p53 antibody decreased significantly ($P = .009$) as did the expression of anti-MiB-1 antibody ($P = .021$). Complete histological resolution was achieved in 15 patients (23.1%). A significant ($P < .001$) downgrading of AK grade was also observed. Five patients (7.7%) showed either AK I or AK II by histological investigation after treatment. These findings suggest the importance of histological evaluation of AKs and emphasize that clinical findings alone may be misleading, especially with drying agents that may produce scaling that mimics AK lesions. However, without mapping each AK lesion on the face before and after treatment and following them through treatment, it may be difficult to differentiate new AK lesions that develop throughout the study. The authors also suggest that changes in histological types of AKs (bowenoid to unclassified) after 3 months of treatment convey that the lesion may respond better to other treatments such as cryosurgery or may need further treatment with topical 3.0% diclofenac in 2.5% hyaluronic acid gel. An interesting concept that was observed in this study was with hypertrophic AKs and atrophic AKs responding well to topical 3.0% diclofenac in 2.5% hyaluronic acid gel. This challenged the argument that hypertrophic AKs do not respond well to topical therapy. Limitations to this study were short follow-up period and all patients being Caucasian. This study was conducted only on the face and scalp, and response may be different in other areas such as the forearms. Another limitation was that although there were patients with unresolved AK lesions, the authors did not proceed to treatment for longer than 3 months to examine the response rates and discuss which types of AKs responded with longer treatment. This study showed a histologically significant downgrade with regard to the AK I-III classification scheme after topical treatment observed in the histopathological level.

J. Q. Del Rosso, DO

G. K. Kim, DO

Combination Therapy with Imiquimod, 5-Fluorouracil, and Tazarotene in the Treatment of Extensive Radiation-Induced Bowen's Disease of the Hands
Modi G, Jacobs AA, Orengo IF, et al (Baylor College of Medicine, Houston, TX)
Dermatol Surg 36:694-700, 2010

Background.—Squamous cell carcinoma (SCC) accounts for 20% of all cases of nonmelanoma skin neoplasia, making it the second most common skin cancer. Treatment is designed to eradicate the tumor while preserving surrounding tissues, function, and cosmetic results. Mohs micrographic surgery (MMS) technique has the highest cure rate, margin control, and tissue conservation, but may cause significant disfigurement and compromise function. Tumors that are multifocal, extensive, or in cosmetically sensitive areas may require an alternative approach. Imiquimod is an immune response modifier successfully used for SCC in situ (SCCIS), invasive SCC, condyloma, molluscum contagiosum, and actinic keratoses. Seldom used on hand lesions, it has been beneficial in SCCIS on the penis, perianal region, face, eyelids, trunk, and legs. 5-Fluorouracil (5-FU) targets cancer cells and has successfully treated SCCIS, basal cell carcinoma (BCC), and actinic keratoses, achieving cure rates of 87% to 92%. The retinoid tazarotene has been used alone or in combination to manage psoriasis and acne. It has limited success topically for SCCIS and superficial BCC. A patient with multifocal SCCIS on the hands was managed using a topical combination of these three agents.

> *Case Report.*—Man, 56, had biopsy-confirmed SCCIS on the right index finger, with multiple erythematous crusted plaques, ulcerations, and hyperkeratotic lesions on the dorsal and palmar aspects of both hands. He was a nuclear pharmacy technician who had not worn radiation-protective gear early in his 30-year career. His father also had had SCC. The right index finger had been amputated. Biopsy of three representative lesions demonstrated epithelial hyperkeratosis. SCCIS was diagnosed in two locations and focal severe squamous cell atypia at the third. Clinicopathologic evaluation confirmed the presence of radiation-induced extensive multifocal SCCIS of both hands. Computed tomography and sentinel lymph node biopsy revealed no evidence of metastasis.

The diffuse nature of the lesions and prospective loss of hand function mitigated against surgery, so topical treatment was begun using 5% imiquimod each evening 7 days a week for 6 weeks. The lesions were not responding as desired after 4 weeks, so topical tazarotene 0.1% cream was added for morning application and imiquimod continued. After 2 weeks there was increased erythema and scattered shallow erosions. After 6 weeks a 1-month break was taken for healing to occur. After 3 months the size and appearance of the lesions had improved markedly, but multiple persistent nonresponding lesions remained. 5-FU was added, so the patient applied tazarotene in the morning, 5-FU in the afternoon, and occluded imiquimod at night for 6 weeks, then a 1-month hiatus was observed. The patient experienced pain and burning of the hands with this regimen, so 5-FU was discontinued when the pain was intolerable. Marked, brisk reactive changes occurred, including hyperkeratosis, fissuring, erythema, erosion, and frank ulceration. Over monthly evaluations the remaining lesions gradually resolved and no new lesions developed. A suspected superimposed infection of an ulcer complicated the course, but responded to oral antibiotics. After 18 months a verrucae remained and was treated with cryotherapy. No new lesions have developed over the past 28 months.

Conclusions.—Combining a local immune stimulant, a chemotherapeutic agent, and a retinoid offered synergistic benefit for extensive, severe, multifocal SCCIS of the hands. Studies of each agent alone are needed to determine the best combination.

▶ This is a single case report of a multifocal squamous cell carcinoma in situ (SCCIS) on the dorsal hands treated with a combination of imiquimod, 5-fluorouracil (5-FU), and tazarotene in a patient with prior radiation exposure to the affected area. A 56-year-old man presented with biopsy-proven SCCIS affecting the dorsum of both hands. Although surgery is an option, if lesions are large and/or extend over a joint, topical treatment may be preferred because of the histologically diffuse nature of SCCIS and the potential for loss of critical motor and/or sensory function. Treatment was initiated with imiquimod 5% cream applied to the hands twice daily for 2 weeks. However, the lesion was not responding clinically, and topical tazarotene 0.1% was added with daily application in the morning and imiquimod at night. However, after 3 months, there were still multiple persistent nonresponsive focal lesions on both hands. Topical 5-FU was added once daily in the afternoon to the regimen with a cycle of 6 weeks of treatment. The hands showed marked and brisk reaction after adding 5-FU application to the regimen. At 18 months after topical treatment, only a solitary hyperkeratotic papule persisted, and the patient was free of new lesions over 28 months of follow-up. A biopsy of the solitary papule may be helpful to determine the actual histologic diagnosis of that persistent, recurrent, or new focus. In cases where there is no visible evidence of residual involvement after therapy, a posttreatment biopsy demonstrating clearance may help to give some assurance of a therapeutic response; however, it would not definitely indicate eradication of SCCIS as it would provide a very small peek at the actual histologic clearance of SCCIS within the field treated topically. Rather, a negative biopsy posttreatment may give a false sense of security to the clinician and/or patient that SCCIS is completely gone when it may not be or that it may arise from a contiguous area of radiation-treated skin or actinic damage adjacent to the topically treated field. Ultimately, long-term clinical follow-up is of paramount importance, as has been shown with follow-up of superficial basal cell carcinoma after clearance with topical therapy. Also, because the patient was on a multidrug regimen, it is unknown what relative contribution to lesion clearance each agent provided. There are multiple case reports and series demonstrating therapeutic response of SCCIS with topical imiquimod 5%, used over a variety of treatment durations, for SCCIS involving a variety of anatomic sites including face, extremities, and genitalia. The usual suggested starting frequency with topical imiquimod 5% is 1 daily application every other day. If no visible inflammation occurs within the first 2 to 3 weeks, application frequency may be increased; however, daily or twice daily use should definitely initiate visible inflammation. If not, it is unlikely that the SCCIS will be responsive to topical imiquimod monotherapy. Typically, a brisk inflammatory response occurs with SCCIS treatment indicating a cytokine dermatitis, which suggests that at least partial or complete clearance will occur. There are little data in the literature on combination topical therapy for nonmelanoma skin cancers such as SCCIS, with only a few reports of combined topical use of imiquimod and 5-FU. This case report adds to our therapeutic consideration list in difficult cases such as this one. However, large-scale controlled studies would be helpful.

J. Q. Del Rosso, DO

G. K. Kim, DO

Current pathology work-up of extremity soft tissue sarcomas, evaluation of the validity of different techniques
Verheijen P, Witjes H, van Gorp J, et al (Diakonessenhuis, Utrecht, The Netherlands; Meander Hosp, Postbus, Amersfoort, The Netherlands; et al)
Eur J Surg Oncol 36:95-99, 2010

Objective.—In patients with extremity soft tissue sarcomas (STSs) a correct histopathological diagnosis is considered important before surgical treatment. We evaluated the preoperative use and sensitivity of the various pathology techniques.

Methods.—In a population-based study in patients operated for a newly diagnosed extremity STS between January 2000 and December 2003 the preoperative pathology work-up was evaluated. Data were retrieved from a national pathology database (PALGA). The sensitivity of the three techniques was assessed considering an examination affirmative when the conclusion of the pathology report stated the presence of mesenchymal malignancy.

Results.—The pathology reports of 573 patients were identified in the database. In 177 patients (31%) no pathology examination was done before resection of the tumour. In the remaining 396 patients the pathology procedure of first choice had been an incisional biopsy (IB) in 195 patients (49%), a core-needle biopsy (CNB) in 90 patients (23%) and a fine needle aspiration (FNA) in 111 patients (28%). An affirmative diagnosis was established in 95% of the patients following an IB, in 78% after a CNB and in 38% following FNA. After an initial CNB an additional IB was performed in 18 of the 90 patients improving the yield to 89%. After an initial FNA a subsequent histological biopsy was done in 53 of the 111 patients, increasing the sensitivity to 71%.

Conclusions.—In this population-based study in patients treated for extremity STS, the proportion of patients operated without preoperative pathology evaluation was high. In the remaining patients an incisional biopsy was still the most commonly performed technique with the highest yield.

▶ This article examines a category of disease tangential but wholly aligned with most of dermatology and dermatopathology, namely the pathologic diagnosis of soft tissue sarcomas (liposarcoma, leiomyosarcoma, malignant fibrous histiocytoma, sarcoma not otherwise specified, fibrosarcoma, and other sarcomatous entities).

The authors note, and dermatologists, even for the basis of rational referral, should be aware, that the principle means for making such a diagnosis is magnetic resonance imaging and histopathologic examination.

However, using the Dutch Network and National Database and Pathology, the authors examined extremity soft tissue sarcomas diagnosed during January 2000 to December 2003 and found that 31% had no biopsy at all before definitive surgery. Also, the investigators found that incisional biopsy was superior to core needle biopsy, and both were markedly superior to fine-needle aspiration in rendering a diagnosis.

Perhaps this latter finding is not a particular surprise, because in the world of dermatopathology (and pathology in a larger sense), there is a constant desire for a greater amount of tissue. In clinical medicine, there is continued pressure to render a diagnosis with the least amount of tissue necessary.[1] In sum, evidence suggests actual incisional biopsy is superior to core needle biopsy for diagnosis of soft tissue sarcoma. It should be stressed, however, that even in 9 of 20 cases in which core needle biopsy rendered a false-negative result, the histopathology was still at least suspicious enough to prompt a later and larger sampling that resulted in affirmative diagnosis. Hence, a graded approach may sometimes be appropriate, and its employment should, perhaps, not surprise the dermatologist as a referee, but one should always remember the general advice, "Tissue is the issue, when cancer is the [expected] answer."

W. A. High, MD, JD, MEng

Reference

1. Fernandez EM, Helm T, Ioffreda M, Helm KF. The vanishing biopsy: the trend toward smaller specimens. *Cutis.* 2005;76:335-339.

Dermatofibrosarcoma Protuberans of the Vulva: A Clinicopathologic and Immunohistochemical Study of 13 Cases
Edelweiss M, Malpica A (Univ of Texas, M D Anderson Cancer Ctr, Houston)
Am J Surg Pathol 34:393-400, 2010

Dermatofibrosarcoma protuberans (DFSP) is a low-grade sarcoma seldom seen in the vulva with only 29 cases reported. We present the clinicopathologic and immunohistochemical features of 13 such cases seen in our institution over a period of 29 years (1978 to 2007). Patient age ranged from 23 to 76 years (mean, 46 y). Twelve patients had a vulvar mass. One patient presented with a pigmented skin lesion. Tumor size ranged from 1.2 to 15 cm (median, 4 cm). Microscopically, all the cases showed typical features of DFSP. In 1 case, myxoid changes were also noted; 3 cases showed fibrosarcomatous transformation. Of interest, in 7 of our 13 cases, a variety of diagnoses, such as cellular dermatofibroma, cellular leiomyoma, neurofibroma, low-grade leiomyosarcoma, fibrosarcoma, low-grade malignant schwannoma, desmoplastic melanoma, cellular neurofibroma, and low-grade malignant peripheral nerve sheet tumor were initially considered. All 11 cases tested for CD34 were positive, whereas 7/9 cases, 8/9 cases, and 9/9 cases were positive for PDGFR-α, PDGFR-β, and c-abl, respectively. All patients were initially treated with excisional biopsy, wide local excision, or radical vulvectomy. Local recurrences occurred in 7 cases. One patient also developed distant metastases. All recurrences were treated surgically; 1 patient also received chemotherapy and radiotherapy and another received imatinib (Gleevec). Follow-up data ranging from 2 to 444 months was available for all patients. Nine patients had no evidence of disease, 2 patients were alive with disease, 1 patient had died of disease, and 1 patient had died of other causes. DFSP affects women of a wide age range and has a propensity to recur locally. The frequent expression of PDGFR-α, PDGFR-β, and c-abl in these cases agrees with the findings of other investigators and supports the use of imatinib (Gleevec) in cases that are recurrent or not amenable to surgery.

▶ Dermatofibrosarcoma protuberans (DFSP) of the vulva is a rare entity, affecting women usually in their 4th to 5th decade in life. Vulvar DFSP usually presents as an indurated mass, with a diagnosis of DFSP not clinically suspected in most cases. This is a study examining the clinical and immuno-histochemical features of 13 cases of vulvar DFSP. Most of the tumors in this report involved dermis and subcutaneous fat with 2 cases extending into the skeletal muscle. Eleven cases tested positive for CD34, and estrogen receptor staining was positive in 1 case. However, the significance of testing positive for the estrogen receptor was not discussed in regards to treatment options because most of the tumors were locally excised. Immunohistochemical studies for platelet derived growth factor receptor-α and platelet derived growth factor receptor-β, c-kit, and c-abl were also conducted in 9 cases to determine if systemic imatinib (Gleevac) would be of use. However, only 1 patient in this study was treated with imatinib for a recurrent tumor not suitable for surgery, with good response. Fibrosarcomatous changes were observed in 3 of the cases; however, the significance of these features is still debatable in regards to tumor progression, which was not explored in this study. Follow-up ranged from 2 to 444 months, with 7 patients experiencing recurrences. This study was not a randomized case-controlled study. It would have been interesting if the authors compared DFSP of vulva with those involving the head and neck region and discussed the different clinicopathologic and immunohistochemical features of both. It would have also been interesting to note if there are higher rates of recurrence according to location of the tumor, which would provide clinicians valuable information when addressing treatment options. However, with vulvar DFSP being so rare, this report provided valuable insight into the histologic features, immunohistochemical findings, and treatment of this disease.

J. Q. Del Rosso, DO

G. K. Kim, DO

Dermatofibrosarcoma protuberans: Recurrence is related to the adequacy of surgical margins
Heuvel ST, Suurmeijer A, Pras E, et al (Univ of Groningen, The Netherlands)
Eur J Surg Oncol 36:89-94, 2010

Introduction.—The aim of the study was to investigate the results of surgical treatment in primary and recurrent dermatofibrosarcoma protuberans (DFSP), with respect to local tumor control.

Patients and Methods.—Thirty-eight patients were treated between 1971 and 2005 at the University Medical Center Groningen (UMCG). Thirty patients presented with primary disease (79%) and 8 patients with locally recurrent disease (21%). The treatment consisted of surgical resection and in case of marginal or positive resection margins (R1 resection) adjuvant radiotherapy.

Results.—Adequate surgical margins as a single modality was associated with 100% local control in all primary DFSPs. Two patients whose resection specimens had microscopically positive resection margins had withdrawn from adjuvant radiotherapy and developed local recurrence (LF rate 7%). Two of the 8 patients referred with a local recurrence developed a second recurrence (LF rate 25%); one of these patients developed distant disease and ultimately died of systemic disease. None of the five patients with DFSP-FS developed LF after treatment at the UMCG.

After a median follow-up of 89 (12–271) months, the 10-year disease-free survival was 85% and the 10-year disease specific survival was 100%.

Conclusion.—After wide surgical resection of a DFSP or DFSP-FS, or an R1 resection combined with adjuvant radiotherapy the risk of local recurrence is extremely low.

▶ Dermatofibrosarcoma protuberans (DFSP) is a rare soft tissue sarcoma that has a cutaneous origin. The goal of this article was to look at the recurrence rate of DFSP after surgical excision. A total of 38 patients (30 with primary disease and 8 with recurrent disease) were enrolled. Of the 30 patients treated for primary disease, 24 had negative margins after surgical resection and 5 received adjuvant radiotherapy. The DFSP was resected using a 2 to 3 cm margin. The 10-year disease-free survival was 85%, and 10-year disease-specific survival was 100%. The study size was small with 38 patients, but given the relative rarity of the cancer, it does provide some additional support for surgical excision using wide surgical margins (2-3 cm).

S. Bhambri, DO

Detection of Merkel cell polyomavirus DNA in Merkel cell carcinomas

Varga E, Kiss M, Szabó K, et al (Univ of Szeged, Hungary)
Br J Dermatol 161:930-932, 2009

Background.—Merkel cell carcinoma (MCC) is a rare, aggressive tumour for which an increasing incidence has been reported. A new human polyomavirus, Merkel cell polyomavirus (MCV), was recently isolated from these tumours by applying digital transcriptome subtraction methodology.

Objectives.—To detect the presence or absence of MCV in MCCs and other, randomly selected neoplasms.

Methods.—Nine primary or recurrent MCCs from seven patients were examined; 29 other tumours (squamous cell, basal cell and basosquamous carcinomas and malignant melanomas) were examined for comparative purposes. Viral large T protein (LT1 and LT3), and viral capsid protein (VP1) were detected by primer-directed amplification, using a polymerase chain reaction (PCR)-based method, and the amplified PCR products were analysed by agarose gel electrophoresis and subsequent sequence analysis.

Results.—The presence of viral T antigen and/or viral capsid DNA sequences was demonstrated in seven of the eight MCC lesions. None of the comparative samples contained MCV DNA.

Conclusions.— Our findings strongly support the hypothesis that MCV infection may well be specific for MCC, and MCV may play a role in the pathogenesis of MCC.

▶ In January 2008, using digital transcriptome subtraction methodology, Feng et al were the first to report on an association between Merkel cell polyomavirus (MCV) and Merkel cell carcinoma (MCC).[1] Independent epidemiological evidence suggests MCV is a ubiquitous infection of older children and adults, likely transmitted by an aerorespiratory route, but the MCV virus found in MCC appears to have undergone monoclonal genomic integration and the viral T antigen has truncation mutations that prohibit viral propagation.

In the original study, 8 of 10 MCCs tested were found to be infected with MCV. Additional studies from other laboratories yielded surprisingly similar results, with 75% to 85% of MCC demonstrating evidence of MCV using polymerase chain reaction—based techniques and a general lack of any such evidence in other nonmelanoma skin cancer.[2-4] This study agrees with those general results.

Nevertheless, it seems likely that additional events lead to a multifactorial means of cancer acquisition. For example, MCC is also associated with exposure to ultraviolet light and ionizing radiation, and these exposures may increase mutations within the virus, leading to oncogene formation. Furthermore, why 20% of MCC is negative for MCV is completely unknown, but speculation focuses on the possibility that MCC is actually a larger subcategory of multiple cancers, which appear similar histologically and clinically but are not necessarily etiologically related.

At present, there is no widely available test for the presence of the virus nor is treatment impacted by the presence or absence of MCV. In this regard, a more notable test is the presence or absence of p63 expression by immunohistochemistry, a widely available testing methodology, which may afford prognostic benefit.[5]

W. A. High, MD, JD, MEng

References

1. Feng H, Shuda M, Chang Y, Moore PS. Clonal integration of a polyomavirus in human Merkel cell carcinoma. *Science.* 2008;319:1096-1100.
2. Kassem A, Schöpflin A, Diaz C, et al. Frequent detection of Merkel cell polyomavirus in human Merkel cell carcinomas and identification of a unique deletion in the VP1 gene. *Cancer Res.* 2008;68:5009-5013.
3. Becker JC, Houben R, Ugurel S, Trefzer U, Pföhler C, Scharam D. MC polyomavirus is frequently present in Merkel cell carcinoma of European patients. *J Invest Dermatol.* 2008;129:248-250.
4. Reisinger DM, Shiffer JD, Cognetta AB Jr, Chang Y, Moore PS. Lack of evidence for basal or squamous cell carcinoma infection with Merkel cell polyomavirus in immunocompetent patients with Merkel cell carcinoma. *J Am Acad Dermatol.* 2010;63:400-403.
5. Asioli S, Righi A, Volante M, Eusebi V, Bussolati G. p63 expression as a new prognostic marker in Merkel cell carcinoma. *Cancer.* 2007;110:640-647.

Diagnostic imaging in Merkel cell carcinoma: Lessons to learn from 16 cases with correlation of sonography, CT, MRI and PET
Peloschek P, Novotny C, Mueller-Mang C, et al (Med Univ of Vienna, Austria)
Eur J Radiol 73:317-323, 2010

Objective.—The authors report imaging findings in a series of 16 patients with MCC, a rare tumour which is often managed primarily by a dermatologist. To our knowledge, no equivalent series of MCC has been described in the nuclear medicine literature.

Material and Methods.—In this IRB-approved retrospective noncomparative case series 16 patients with biopsy-proven Merkel cell carcinoma were included between January 1999 and October 2007. Twenty-nine whole body PET scans (18F-FDG $n = 24$, 18F-FDOPA $n = 5$) in 16 patients were retrospectively reviewed with regard to tracer uptake in six anatomical sites per patient. For 127/144 of FDG-PET evaluated regions and 68/144 of regions depicted by conventional imaging methods, a valid standard of reference could be obtained. A combined standard of reference was applied, which consisted of histopathology (lymphadenectomy or biopsy) or clinical or radiological follow-up for at least 12 months. Results: the mean FDG uptake over the clinicopatholigical verified FDG avid areas was 4.7 SUV (1.5–9.9 SUV). The region based assessment of diagnostic value, in consideration of the standard of reference, resulted in a sensitivity of 85.7% and a specificity of 96.2% of FDG-PET ($n = 127$) and in a combined sensitivity of 95.5% and a specificity of 89.1% for morphological imaging methods

($n = 68$). Differences between methods did not reach statistical significance ($p = 1.00$, $p = 0.18$).

Conclusions.—FDG-PET is a highly useful whole body staging method of comparable value compared to conventional imaging methods with restricted field of view. The lessons learned from case series are discussed.

▶ Merkel cell carcinoma (MCC) is a rare malignancy with a high mortality rate often with regional lymph node involvement upon discovery. In this study, the authors wanted to evaluate whether positive emission tomography (PET) imaging would be useful in the staging of MCC. This is a retrospective study of 16 patients with MCC evaluated with 29 whole-body PET scans. Results revealed that in 3 of 16 patients, the primary tumor was in situ, and in 13 of 16 patients, the lesion was resected at the date of imaging. In 4 of 16 (25%) patients, the MCC had already affected regional lymph nodes at initial presentation (stage II), and in 5 of 16 (31.2%) patients, the MCC had spread to distant sites (stage III). Results revealed that the primary sites were the face (n = 5), the upper extremities (n = 5), lower extremity (n = 4), the trunk (n = 1), and the oral mucosa (n = 1). Authors concluded that sonography can be cost-effective for initial staging. For those who have lymph node metastasis, ^{18}F fluoro-2-deoxy-D-glucose (FDG)-PET is performed because of the high risk of distant metastasis. Authors advocated that when FDG uptake is abnormal, CT or MRI may give higher resolution when planning for palliative surgery or radiation therapy. MRI is recommended for tumor spread in regions where sonography is not accessible deep into the fascia of the head and neck region. Overall impact of survival rates when using FDG-PET imaging was unknown, but this approach may help in early detection. A limitation to this study was that it was a retrospective case series, and impact on management and outcome was not assessed. Histopathological correlation with imaging studies was not performed to validate FDG-PET as a useful tool in detecting distant metastasis. This was also a small patient population. This study assisted the authors in summarizing the role of FDG-PET in the staging of MCC.

J. Q. Del Rosso, DO

G. K. Kim, DO

Diameter of Involved Nerves Predicts Outcomes in Cutaneous Squamous Cell Carcinoma with Perineural Invasion: An Investigator-Blinded Retrospective Cohort Study

Ross AS, Miller Whalen F, Elenitsas R, et al (Vanderbilt School of Medicine, Nashville, TN; Temple Univ, Philadelphia, PA; Univ of Pennsylvania, Philadelphia; et al)
Dermatol Surg 35:1859-1866, 2009

Background.—Perineural invasion (PNI) has been associated with poor prognosis in cutaneous squamous cell carcinoma (CSCC), but it is unclear how different degrees of nerve involvement affect prognosis.

Objective.—To determine whether the diameter of nerves invaded by CSCC affects outcomes of recurrence, metastasis, and disease-specific and overall survival.

Methods.—A retrospective cohort study was conducted of patients with CSCC with PNI. Dermatopathologists blinded to subject outcomes determined the diameter of the largest involved nerve.

Results.—Data were obtainable for 48 patients. Small-caliber nerve invasion (SCNI) of nerves less than 0.1 mm in diameter was associated with significantly lower risks of all outcomes of interest. Disease-specific death was 0% in subjects with SCNI, versus 32% in those with large-caliber nerve invasion (LCNI) ($p = .003$). Other factors associated with significantly worse survival were recurrent or poorly differentiated tumors or tumor diameter of 2 cm or greater or depth of 1 cm or greater. On multivariate analysis, only tumor diameter and age predicted survival.

Conclusions.—The individual prognostic significance of factors associated with poor survival remains uncertain. Small-caliber nerve invasion may not adversely affect outcomes. Defining PNI as tumor cells within the nerve sheath and routine recording of diameter of involved nerves, tumor depth, and histologic differentiation on pathology reports will facilitate further study.

▶ Cutaneous squamous cell carcinoma (CSCC) is usually associated with a good prognosis if there is no nodal or distant metastasis. Perineural invasion (PNI) can be a marker for local recurrence, distant metastasis, and poor prognosis. In this study, the authors wanted to investigate whether CSCC with PNI involving larger diameter nerves would be associated with a worse outcome as compared with smaller diameter nerves with PNI. This is a retrospective cohort study of 48 patients with CSCC with PNI diagnosed at the University of Pennsylvania between 1996 and 2005, with a follow-up of 3 months. All patients were Caucasians, with 34 (71%) of them being male. The median diameter of involved nerves was 0.09 mm. Small-caliber nerves are the nerves with diameter less than 0.1 mm, whereas large-caliber nerves are the nerves with diameter greater than 0.1 mm. Tumors involving small-caliber nerves had significantly smaller tumor diameter ($P = .009$), were more superficial ($P < .001$), were more likely to be primary tumors ($P < .001$), and were more likely to occur in women ($P < .04$). Seventeen percent of patients died from CSCC with PNI. These 8 deaths were due to lung metastasis and not due to intracranial extension of CSCC. In addition, lower overall survival was also associated with poorly differentiated tumors ($P = .02$). The risk of death was 83% lower for those with clinical tumor diameters less than 2 cm. Limitations included a short follow-up period of 3 months and the small study size. Also, when nerves were cut tangentially and appeared ovid, the shortest diameter of the oval was recorded, which could have over- or underestimated nerve sizes. In conclusion, poor prognostic factors in this study included larger caliber size nerves and poorly differentiated tumors.

J. Q. Del Rosso, DO

G. K. Kim, DO

Distinct progression-associated expression of tumor and stromal MMPs in HaCaT skin SCCs correlates with onset of invasion

Vosseler S, Lederle W, Airola K, et al (German Cancer Res Ctr [DKFZ], Heidelberg, Germany; Helsinki Univ Central Hosp, Finland; et al)
Int J Cancer 125:2296-2306, 2009

Matrix metalloproteinases (MMPs) are critically involved in tumor invasion and metastasis. However, failure of broad spectrum MMP inhibitors in clinical trials emphasizes the need for detailed analyses of the specific role of different MMPs in tumor malignancy. Using HaCaT-keratinocyte clones representing distinct stages in skin squamous cell carcinoma (SCC) progression, we demonstrate the expression of specific tumor and stroma-derived MMPs with the onset and maintenance of tumor invasion. Although MMP-9-positive leukocytes are present in benign and malignant tumor transplants at the onset of stromal activation and angiogenesis, mRNA expression of stroma-derived MMP-9 as well as MMP-2, −13 and −14 is exclusively found in enhanced malignant tumor transplants. Their expression initiates with the onset of invasion, whereas being absent in early noninvasive stages of malignant transplants. In addition, a high expression of tumor-derived MMP-1, −2 and −14 contributes to malignant and invasive tumor growth. However, stroma-derived MMP-3 is exclusively restricted to very late-stage invasive and malignant transplants. The functional contribution of these proteases to invasive growth is supported by the gelatinolytic activity in the tumor transplants that again initiates with the onset of invasive growth suggesting a crucial role of MMP-2, −9, −13 and −14 for the establishment of a reactive stroma that promotes tumor invasion. These data demonstrate a complex cooperation of distinct tumor and stroma-derived MMPs in the establishment of malignant tumors and provide the basis for a more specific use of highly selective MMP inhibitors during distinct stages of tumor progression.

▶ The last few years have brought forward many new insights into the role of cathelicidins in diseases such as acne, rosacea, psoriasis, and skin cancer. Matrix metalloproteinases (MMPs) and other antimicrobial peptides have been targeted as important operators both in maintaining host integrity and pathogenesis of these disease states.

Although confusing at first, the authors' implication of a role of MMPs in progression of carcinogenesis can be initially prefaced by the observation that, "In squamous epithelia, expression of MMPs is generally restricted to malignant tumors, whereas benign or premalignant lesions lack MMP expression. In contrast, MMPs are expressed by many benign or premalignant cell types under culture conditions *in vitro*." Another important finding to distinguish the activity of benign MMPs is that "loss of contact with intact basement membrane that occurs during wound healing and cancer growth and exposure of the cells to interstitial collagen as seen in early-stage organotypic cultures stimulate collagenase production." These are important concepts when we consider the fact that the potential to inhibit these processes comes with the price of altering normal dermal stroma integrity.

Using these observations as a template, the role of MMPs in carcinogenesis takes on a new meaning when we think of these as important host defense enzymes as well as proteases important in maintaining homeostasis in the dermis, for example, the finding of the authors that MMP-2 (gelatinase) is activated by MMP-14 (other membrane-type MMP) to facilitate tumor progression through dermal stromal elements. MMP-13 and MMP-3 are also implicated in promoting tumor invasion, tumor-related angiogenesis, and metastasis, prompting the concept of targeted therapy for controlling their activity, but a balance must exist to prevent impacting normal host defense systems involving these MMPs as well as baseline functions of dermal stroma integrity.

Although this article is involved and somewhat complicated, the points introduced regarding the potential roles of MMPs in carcinogenesis and promotion of tumor invasion and metastasis are necessary to review to avoid confusion when we hear about how MMPs affect the progression of other dermatoses.

N. Bhatia, MD

Epidermotropic Merkel cell carcinoma: A case series with histopathologic examination

D'Agostino M, Cinelli C, Willard R, et al (Warren Alpert Med School of Brown Univ, Providence, RI)
J Am Acad Dermatol 62:463-468, 2010

Background.—Merkel cell carcinoma (MCC), an aggressive malignancy that has been increasing in incidence, rarely presents with an epidermotropic pattern.

Objective.—We conducted an immunohistochemical evaluation of 6 previously unpublished cases of epidermotropic MCC, focusing particularly on the staining characteristics of epithelial membrane antigen and cytokeratin-20 in the hope of providing insight into the mechanism of epidermotropism in MCC.

Methods.—This study is a retrospective evaluation using light microscopy and immunohistochemistry.

Results.—Forty cases of MCC with pathology at Rhode Island Hospital and the Miriam Hospital in Providence, RI, from 1983 through 2009 were reviewed. Following exclusion criteria, 6 patients (5 men, 1 woman) with a mean age of 82.5 years (range, 72-92) demonstrated epidermotropism. Three of 6 patients had MCC of the eyelid. In cases 1, 3, and 6, the perinuclear dot pattern observed with cytokeratin-20 in the epidermotropic MCC cells was less pronounced than the pattern observed in the dermis, and in all 6 of the tumors, the epidermal staining pattern observed with epithelial membrane antigen was not more or less prominent than the staining observed in the dermis.

Limitations.—The small total number of cases of epidermotropic MCC is a limitation.

Conclusion.—The data presented reinforce the differential diagnosis of tumors with an epidermotropic growth pattern and the importance of immunohistochemical staining in the histologic workup of such tumors: squamous cell carcinoma in situ, melanoma, mycosis fungoides, eccrine porocarcinoma, sebaceous carcinoma of the eyelid, mammary and extramammary Paget disease, MCC, and epidermotropic metastases. It is notable that 3 of 6 identified tumors were located on the eyelid; further study of epidermotropic MCC may shed more light on this finding, either as an unusual coincidence or a finding with unexplained significance.

▶ Certainly, a query to trainees in dermatology as to the common cutaneous malignancies with epidermotropism will trigger near-mindless recital of squamous cell carcinoma in situ, melanoma, mammary/extramammary Paget disease, periocular sebaceous carcinoma, and mycosis fungoides. In this study, the authors reinforce the need to include Merkel cell carcinoma within that list.

It is intriguing to note that 50% of the 6 cases in this small series, which spanned 26 years (1983-2009), occurred in a periocular location as well and that while staining with epithelial membrane antigen was similar in the dermal and epidermal components, the expression of a cytokeratin-20–positive perinuclear dot was less pronounced in the epidermal component in one-half of cases. Purists sometimes note that it is likely more proper to refer to this immunostaining pattern as a paranuclear dot (meaning immediately next to the nucleus).

Lastly, it should be recalled that there is decided tendency of squamous cell carcinoma, and squamous cell carcinoma in situ, to occur and/or overlie Merkel cell carcinoma on occasion, and therefore, this phenomenon of concurrent malignancies must be distinguished from what seems to be the exceptional epidermotropic variant of Merkel cell carcinoma alone.[1]

W. A. High, MD, JD, MEng

Reference

1. Sirikanjanapong S, Melamed J, Patel RR. Intraepidermal and dermal Merkel cell carcinoma with squamous cell carcinoma in situ: a case report with review of literature. *J Cutan Pathol.* 2010;37:881-885.

Expression of hedgehog signaling molecules in Merkel cell carcinoma
Brunner M, Thurnher D, Pammer J, et al (Med Univ of Vienna, Austria; et al)
Head Neck 32:333-340, 2010

Background.—The Hedgehog signaling pathway is important for human development and carcinogenesis in various malignancies.

Methods.—One tissue microarray with triplets of 28 samples from 25 patients with Merkel cell carcinoma (MCC) was constructed. Six samples of normal skin and 5 samples of normal oral mucosa served as controls.

All samples were analyzed immunohistochemically with antibodies directed against Sonic hedgehog, Indian hedgehog, Patched, Smoothened, Gli-1, Gli-2, and Gli-3.

Results.—All investigated proteins were frequently and intensely over-expressed in MCCs (Sonic hedgehog, 93%; Indian hedgehog, 84%; Patched, 86%; Smoothened, 79%; Gli-1, 79%; Gli-2, 79%; Gli-3, 86%) compared with control samples. High levels of Patched and Indian hedgehog were significantly associated with an increase in patients overall ($p = .015$) and recurrence-free survival ($p = .011$), respectively.

Conclusions.—Our results indicate that the Hedgehog signaling pathway is strongly activated in MCC and thus may play a role in carcinogenesis.

▶ Although the roles and interactions of Sonic Hedgehog, Smoothened, Patched receptor, and Gli proteins are well elucidated in the pathogenesis of basal cell carcinoma (BCC), their roles in the development of Merkel cell carcinoma (MCC) is not clear and may not have any impact based on the findings in this article. In the development of BCC, Hedgehog binds to Patched receptor, which inhibits Smoothened when Hedgehog is absent but continues the activation cascade in Hedgehog's presence, which in turn is further activated by Gli-1 and Gli-2 proteins, while Gli-3 protein attempts to serve as a suppressor. This process is further enhanced in BCC progression, among other tumors, by mutations to important regulator proteins, such as p53 and Patched, which are the mechanisms that the authors attempt to elucidate for MCC.

Although the study found an elevation in the expression of these important signal proteins, especially important given the similarities in BCC and MCC in terms of clinical presentations and locations in heavily photodamaged skin, there was no clear demonstration of the pathways and interactions among the proteins to suggest similarities in tumor promotion and activity. However, it does suggest to the reader that the expression of more targets may lead to other avenues to control disease progression. MCC is one of the diseases in dermatology that lacks a current standard of nonsurgical management and further understanding of these steps in pathogenesis may help in this unmet need.

N. Bhatia, MD

Expression of p53 and p16 in actinic keratosis, bowenoid actinic keratosis and Bowen's disease
Bagazgoitia L, Cuevas J, Juarranz Á (Universidad de Alcalá de Henares, Madrid, Spain; Hosp Universitario de Guadalajara, Spain; Universidad Autónoma de Madrid, Spain)
J Eur Acad Dermatol Venereol 24:228-230, 2010

Introduction.—Bowen's disease (BD) and bowenoid actinic keratosis (bAK) have traditionally been differentiated according to the presence or absence of dysplasia in the follicular epithelium. p16 has been suggested to be a useful tool to make the differential diagnosis between BD and AK and as a marker of bad prognosis.

Materials.—Five biopsies of BD, five of AK and five of bAK where stained for p53 and p16.

Results.—All lesions showed positive immunostaining of p53, affecting to the lower two thirdss of the epidermis in BD and bAK, and only the basal layer in non-bAK. All the BD and bAK cases were positive for p16, showing a similar immunostaining pattern, whereas no staining was observed in non-bAK.

Discussion and Conclusion.—These findings suggest a common pathogenic mechanism for BD and bAK. bAK might have worse prognosis than AK. p16 might not be useful as a tool for differential diagnosis between AK and BD because bAK and BD show an extremely similar immunohistochemical pattern.

▶ The results of this small study suggest a common pathogenic mechanism for Bowen's disease (BD) and bowenoid actinic keratosis (bAK) according to the immunohistochemical detection and distribution of p16 in both lesions. AK represents the initial manifestation of a continuum toward the development of squamous cell carcinoma (SCC), and at this stage, AKs have shown the potential to spontaneously regress when the main cause (ie, ultraviolet radiation) is reduced or discontinued, conferring AKs unique features that separate them biologically from bAKs. In addition, the authors state that bAK might have a worse prognosis than AK, which correlates with both loss of maturation of keratinocytes and the p16 pattern found in bAK, resembling the BD pattern but not the AK pattern. Although no positive or negative predictive values were provided, the immunohistochemical patterns reported in this study correlate with previous studies, suggesting p16's role in the irreversible transformation of AKs into SCC. However, according to these findings, p16 as a tool failed to differentiate bAK from BD beyond morphological features, which may be related to the common pathogenic pathway mentioned by the authors.

B. Berman, MD, PhD

Factors Contributing to Incomplete Excision of Nonmelanoma Skin Cancer by Australian General Practitioners

Hansen C, Wilkinson D, Hansen M, et al (Univ of Queensland, Brisbane, Australia)
Arch Dermatol 145:1253-1260, 2009

Objective.—To study rates of incomplete excision of basal (BCC) and squamous (SCC) cell cancer by Australian general practitioners with a special interest.

Design.—Records review.

Setting.—A network of 15 primary care skin cancer clinics across Australia.

Participants.—Fifty-seven physicians performing excisions of 9417 BCCs and SCCs in a single network of 15 primary care skin cancer clinics across Australia between 2005 and 2007.

Main Outcome Measures.—Rates of incomplete excision according to physician, clinic, anatomic location of the lesion, and whether a previous biopsy had been performed.

Results.—Four hundred forty-three of 6881 BCCs (6.4%) and 159 of 2536 SCCs (6.3%) were excised incompletely. Incomplete BCC and SCC excisions were more frequent on the head and neck (282 of 2872 excisions [9.8%] and 97 of 861 [11.3%], respectively) than elsewhere. Ears (74 of 388 excisions [19.1%]) and nose (78 of 546 [14.3%]) had the highest rates of incompletely excised BCCs, and ears (26 of 144 excisions [18.1%]) and forehead (20 of 157 [12.7%]) had the highest rates of incompletely excised SCCs. Of all BCC excisions, 67.3% were once-off excisions with no previous biopsy, and these excisions were more likely to be incomplete (odds ratio, 1.73; 95% confidence interval, 1.36-2.20) than those with a previous biopsy. There was, however, substantial variation in frequency of incomplete excision between clinics for BCC (ranging from 3.3% to 24.7%) and SCC (ranging from 0% to 17.2%) and between physicians within clinics (BCC ranging from 0% to 31.1%, and SCC ranging from 0% to 23.5%).

Conclusions.—Overall frequency of incomplete excision is low and similar to that in other reports. However, high frequency in high-risk sites, low rates of previous biopsy, and substantial variation in performance between physicians and clinics suggests there is significant opportunity to further improve health outcomes.

▶ So here is an instance that the term "consider the source" is appropriate. We have a review of performance of nonspecialists with less training than dermatologists, who are in sparse numbers and less accessible, who are forced by the necessity of the epidemic of skin cancer in Australia to perform aggressive surgeries. These might require training that exceeds what the average primary care physician there receives, but we have to question several things before making a conclusion: (1) Is there an avenue for these nondermatologists to get the training that they need or want, for them to improve their efficiency of surgery? (2) Is there adequate quality assurance for them to perform excisions of malignant tumors? and (3) Does the health system in place in Australia allow for the patient to have a choice on who performs the surgery? The access to a dermatologist might vary between Darwin, Alice Springs, and Sydney, but the quality of training that a primary care physician has to treat skin cancer should not because they are on the front lines. Then the questions become about the role of the dermatologist as a teacher as well as the ability and technical skills of the surgeon, which can only be refined and not necessarily taught. In a crude comparison to golf, where each golfer has a set point of how good they could be despite all the lessons possible, the skills of surgery work in a very parallel fashion. And with that come these statistics of incomplete excision margins, poor wound healing and postsurgical management, and more importantly, poor recognition of limitations for performing surgery under the pressure of controlling an epidemic that is rolling downhill fast. So again, this is a good time to take a step back and consider the source of the message here because it will vary based on geography among other factors.

N. Bhatia, MD

Follow-up of actinic keratoses after shave biopsy by *in-vivo* reflectance confocal microscopy — a pilot study
Richtig E, Ahlgrimm-Siess V, Koller S, et al (Med Univ Graz, Austria)
J Eur Acad Dermatol Venereol 24:293-298, 2010

Background.—Monitoring of treatment efficacy after shave biopsy of actinic keratoses (AK) is often difficult, as clinical and dermoscopic features may not be reliable.

Objectives.—We investigated the applicability of *in-vivo* reflectance confocal microscopy (RCM) for the follow-up of AK after shave biopsy.

Methods.—A total of 10 lesions were investigated by RCM before shave biopsy, after 3 and 12 months by two observers in agreement blinded to location, patients and time interval.

Results.—At baseline all lesions showed typical clinical, dermoscopic and RCM criteria of AK. Three months after shave biopsy, all lesions presented clinically as normal skin (NS), but two lesions showed features suspicious for AK by RCM. After 12 months, one lesion of these two lesions changed into NS in RCM, whereas the other lesion progressed into clinical visible AK. At baseline, the two observers diagnosed 10 of 10 lesions correctly in RCM, after 3 months eight of 10 lesions and after 12 months all lesions were diagnosed correctly.

Conclusions.—Our results suggest that RCM might be a useful tool in the follow-up of AK after shave biopsy and might be used in inconclusive clinical and dermoscopic presentations of lesions after surgery or other treatment modalities.

▶ This article confirms what many clinicians have long suspected, that is, even if clinically resolved, an actinic keratosis (AK) lesion may still be present subclinically. This lends credence to the concept that new AKs seen after initial successful destructive or topical therapy may in fact be residual lesions rather than actual new lesions. It should encourage dermatologists to consider a more aggressive multimodality therapy for AKs to account for clinical and subclinical lesions that can persist yet not be physically evident. The study also supports the use of reflectance confocal microscopy for the management of inconclusive lesions. It is a good pilot study that warrants follow-up with a larger, prospective, blinded study.

A. Torres, MD, JD

Fractional Cryosurgery for Skin Cancer

Gonçalves JCA (District Hosp, Santarém, Portugal)
Dermatol Surg 35:1788-1796, 2009

Background.—Cryosurgical treatment of facial skin cancers 10 mm or larger in diameter can originate retractile scars that may alter physiognomic features.

Objectives.—To treat skin cancers 10 mm or larger in diameter on the face with a cryosurgical method that prevents retractile scars. Also, to clarify the differences between this method and Zacarian's segmental cryosurgery.

Methods and Materials.—Fractional cryosurgery is performed in stages. First, the center of the lesion is frozen, reducing its size, then this procedure is repeated as necessary until the tumor diameter is smaller than 10 mm, at which point the standard cryosurgical procedure is performed. Eighty-seven basal cell carcinomas (BCCs) and nine squamous cell carcinomas (SCCs) of the face (65 of which were orbital or periocular) measuring between 9 and 45 mm were treated.

Results.—The cure rate of BCCs was related to tumor size. All SCCs were cured without recurrence. Global mean follow-up was 4.5 years.

Conclusion.—Fractional cryosurgery does not cause deformity, and the final scar has no relation to the mass of the original tumor but instead corresponds to the size of the lesion preceding the last cryosurgical procedure.

▶ This is an interesting article in which cryosurgery was used to treat skin cancers, primarily basal cell carcinoma (BCC) and squamous cell carcinoma (SCC). A total of 96 facial BCC and SCC patients were treated with most cancers located in the orbital and periocular regions (65 of 96). The results were impressive, but this modality has limited practical value in the United States where Mohs micrographic surgery (MMS) is the standard of care for treating skin cancers on the face. Treatment of facial skin cancers with cryosurgery may serve as an option in those patients in whom MMS is not an option.

S. Bhambri, DO

Guidelines for practical use of MAL-PDT in non-melanoma skin cancer

Christensen E, Warloe T, Kroon S, et al (Norwegian Univ of Science and Technology (NTNU), Trondheim, Norway; Oslo Univ Hosp Rikshospitalet, Norway; Stavanger Univ Hosp, Norway; et al)
J Eur Acad Dermatol Venereol 24:505-512, 2010

Methyl aminolaevulinate photodynamic therapy is increasingly practiced in the treatment of actinic keratoses, Bowen's disease and basal cell carcinomas. This method is particularly suitable for treating multiple lesions, field cancerization and lesions in areas where a good cosmetic outcome is of importance. Good treatment routines will contribute to a favourable result. The Norwegian photodynamic therapy (PDT) group consists of medical specialists with long and extensive PDT experience. With support in the literature, this group presents guidelines for the practical use of topical PDT in non-melanoma skin cancer.

▶ This article is an excellent reference on the use of methylaminolevulinic acid photodynamic therapy (MAL-PDT) for the treatment of actinic keratoses (AKs), basal cell carcinoma (BCC), and Bowen disease (squamous cell carcinoma in situ). It provides a detailed practical step-by-step approach and guidelines for the use of MAL-PDT. To that end this article is a must read and key reference for PDT practitioners.

If we put aside the fact that PDT is not approved in the United States for the treatment of nonmelanoma skin cancers (NMSC), there are several additional practical considerations which merit discussion. These include staffing issues, dedicated office/clinic space in which to perform PDT, reimbursement issues, and efficacy compared with other treatment modalities. The widespread adoption of PDT has been limited in large part because of the cost of additional staffing to perform PDT and the required dedicated office space to perform it must be balanced by medical reimbursement. The economics of PDT has made it difficult for physicians to put down their prescription pad, cryosurgery unit, or curette and scalpel when it comes to treating AKs and NMSC using PDT. Additionally, the therapeutic efficacy of MAL-PDT for treating superficial and nodular (< 2 mm) BCC has reported to be in the 80% clearance range. While offering superior aesthetic outcomes in most cases, the tumor clearance rates of PDT are significantly less than that ($\geq$90%) reported overall for Mohs micrographic surgery, wide excisional surgery, ionizing radiation, and cryosurgery, while roughly equivalent to curettage and electrodessication.[1] Despite these issues, PDT is a safe and effective modality with a high level of patient satisfaction for the treatment of AKs and NMSC.

G. Martin, MD

Reference

1. Love WE, Bernhard JD, Bordeaux JS. Topical imiquimod or fluorouracil therapy for basal and squamous cell carcinoma: a systematic review. *Arch Dermatol.* 2009;145:1431-1438.

Imiquimod 2.5% and 3.75% for the treatment of actinic keratoses: Results of two placebo-controlled studies of daily application to the face and balding scalp for two 2-week cycles
Swanson N, Abramovits W, Berman B, et al (Oregon Health and Science Univ, Portland; Baylor Univ Med Ctr and Univ of Texas Southwestern School of Medicine, Dallas; Univ of Miami, FL; et al)
J Am Acad Dermatol 62:582-590, 2010

Background.—The approved imiquimod 5% cream regimen for treating actinic keratoses requires a long treatment time and is limited to a small area of skin.

Objective.—We sought to evaluate imiquimod 2.5% and 3.75% for short-course treatment of the full face or balding scalp.

Methods.—In two identical studies, adults with 5 to 20 lesions were randomized to placebo, imiquimod 2.5%, or imiquimod 3.75% (1:1:1). Up to two packets (250 mg each) were applied per dose once daily for two 2-week treatment cycles, with a 2-week, no-treatment interval between cycles. Efficacy was assessed at 8 weeks posttreatment.

Results.—A total of 479 patients were randomized to placebo, or imiquimod 2.5% or 3.75%. Complete and partial clearance (≥75% lesion reduction) rates were 6.3% and 22.6% for placebo, 30.6% and 48.1% for imiquimod 2.5%, and 35.6% and 59.4% for imiquimod 3.75%, respectively (*P* < .001 vs placebo, each; *P* = .047, 3.75% vs 2.5% for partial clearance). Median reductions from baseline in lesion counts were 25.0% for placebo, 71.8% for imiquimod 2.5%, and 81.8% for imiquimod 3.75% (*P* < .001, each active vs placebo; *P* = .048 3.75% vs 2.5%). There were few treatment-related discontinuations. Patient rest period rates were 0% for placebo, 6.9% for imiquimod 2.5%, and 10.6% for imiquimod 3.75%.

Limitations.—Local pharmacologic effects of imiquimod, including erythema, may have limited concealment of treatment assignment in some patients.

Conclusions.—Both imiquimod 2.5% and 3.75% creams were more effective than placebo and were well tolerated when administered daily as a 2-week on/off/on regimen to treat actinic keratoses.

▶ Imiquimod 5% cream, first introduced in 1997 and approved for actinic keratosis (AK) treatment in 2004, has been a significant part of the dermatologist's armamentarium in treating patients with multiple AKs. Problems with the 5% formulation were primarily length of treatment (16 weeks) based on the Food and Drug Administration (FDA)-approved regimen, limited treatment area (< 25 cm²), dosing schedule (2 times per week), and compliance due to length of treatment.

The newer formulations, 2.5% and 3.75%, evaluated in this study proved more effective than placebo. Yet, more importantly, the newer formulations, particularly the 3.75% strength, and the short-course cyclical therapy provided statistically significant reduction in AKs. Complete clearance rates and partial clearance rates were both improved. Global improvement of treated areas was noted by patients and physician investigators. The shortened cyclical treatment regimen (2 weeks on, 2 weeks off, and 2 weeks on) was well tolerated by patients overall. Efficacy data of imiquimod 3.75% formulation, particularly median AK lesion reduction, were almost identical to imiquimod 5% cream (82% vs 83%), keeping in mind that the 3.75% cream was used to treat an entire anatomic region (face or scalp) as compared with a target area of 5 cm × 5 cm with the 5% cream. The incidence of adverse skin reactions in this study was 6.3% for imiquimod 2.5% and 10.6% for imiquimod 3.75%.

Field therapy is becoming a standard of treatment in patients with multiple AKs. The newer FDA-approved formulation of imiquimod (3.75%) with cyclical therapy was well tolerated by patients and highly effective in treating multiple AKs of face and scalp.

J. L. Smith, MD

Imiquimod 2.5% and 3.75% for the treatment of actinic keratoses: Results of two placebo-controlled studies of daily application to the face and balding scalp for two 3-week cycles
Hanke CW, Beer KR, Stockfleth E, et al (Laser and Skin Surgery Ctr of Indiana, Carmel; Palm Beach Esthetic Dermatology and Laser Ctr, West Palm Beach, FL; Charité Univ Hosp, Berlin, Germany; et al)
J Am Acad Dermatol 62:573-581, 2010

Background.—Imiquimod 5% cream is approved as a 16-week regimen for the treatment of actinic keratoses involving a 25-cm^2 area of skin.

Objective.—We sought to evaluate imiquimod 2.5% and 3.75% creams for short-course treatment of the entire face and scalp.

Methods.—In two identical studies, adults with 5 to 20 lesions were randomized to placebo, or imiquimod 2.5% or 3.75% cream (1:1:1). Up to two packets (250 mg each) were applied per dose once daily for two 3-week treatment cycles, with a 3-week, no-treatment interval. Efficacy was assessed at 8 weeks posttreatment.

Results.—In all, 490 subjects were randomized to placebo, or imiquimod 2.5% or 3.75% cream. Median baseline lesion counts for the treatment groups were 9 to 10. Complete and partial clearance rates were 5.5% and 12.8% for placebo, 25.0% and 42.7% for imiquimod 2.5%, and 34.0% and 53.7% for imiquimod 3.75% ($P < .001$, each imiquimod vs placebo; $P = .034$, 3.75% vs 2.5% for partial clearance). Median reductions from baseline in lesion count were 23.6%, 66.7%, and 80.0% for the placebo, imiquimod 2.5%, and imiquimod 3.75% groups, respectively ($P < .001$ each imiquimod vs placebo). There were few treatment-related discontinuations. Temporary treatment interruption (rest) rates were 0%, 17.1%, and 27.2% for the placebo, imiquimod 2.5%, and imiquimod 3.75%, respectively.

Limitations.—Local effects of imiquimod, including erythema, may have led to investigator and subject bias.

Conclusions.—Both imiquimod 2.5% and 3.75% creams were more effective than placebo and had an acceptable safety profile when administered daily as a 3-week on/off/on regimen.

▶ To understand immune response modifiers such as imiquimod is to understand the mechanisms of action and where they apply clinically. Unlike other therapies for actinic keratoses, or similar conditions requiring these management strategies such as skin cancers, warts, and molluscum contagiosum, it is essential to recognize the interactions among dendritic cells, lymphocytes, cytokines, and other players in the game. Controlled trials have always been limited by the reporting of perceived adverse events and local site reactions, which in the case of imiquimod are actually the reflected impact on the immune system by promoting recognition of antigenic components of the target lesions. Keeping in mind that application of a cream that stimulates an immune response is going to result in a visible and tangible reaction, the reader should place this class of drugs in a different mind-set when comparing tolerability at different strengths when efficacy is the key goal.

This article, along with a similar publication using a 2-week regimen instead of 3 weeks,[1] represents the quest for the new imiquimod: the attempt to take the old imiquimod 5% cream, which had its benefits at a perceived price of local and rarely systemic reactions, and try to find if the impact of therapy can still be gained at a lower dose to increase tolerability. At the time of the publication of this article, there was significant variability in the dosage frequency of imiquimod despite the label regimen of twice weekly for 16 weeks, which prompted a search for a more simplified and uniform dosage that would have some predictability for expectations for outcomes of patients and dermatologists. As the authors discovered, there was a balance struck with the 3.75% dosage showing equal tolerability to the 2.5% dose. In the phase III studies done with 5% imiquimod[2] as well as the anecdotal studies comparing daily dosage of imiquimod 5% for superficial basal cell carcinoma,[3] issues were found with surface area and daily dosage along with discontinuation rates (30% in the daily use of 5% imiquimod cream compared with fewer in either the 2-week or 3-week studies).

Eventually, the story concludes with the finding of imiquimod 3.75% at a dosage cycle of 2 weeks on, 2 weeks off, and 2 weeks on totaling 6 weeks of therapy to be most effective. Per the authors, providing a more refined, predictable, and tolerable regimen would eventually lead to better efficacy and less recurrence, which is where the story is left to be told. As a consultant for the manufacturer of imiquimod (3M Pharmaceuticals and Graceway Pharmaceuticals), it has been an interesting decade watching the purification of the dosage regimen for actinic keratosis come to an attempted consensus. But as I stated, to understand imiquimod is to understand its mechanism of action, so that patient compliance is maintained, efficacy is achieved, and reactions are managed.

N. Bhatia, MD

References

1. Swanson N, Abramovits W, Berman B, Kulp J, Rigel DS, Levy S. Imiquimod 2.5% and 3.75% for the treatment of actinic keratoses: results of two placebo-controlled studies of daily application to the face and balding scalp for two 2-week cycles. *J Am Acad Dermatol.* 2010;62:582-590.
2. Lebwohl M, Dinehart S, Whiting D, et al. Imiquimod 5% cream for the treatment of actinic keratosis: results from two phase III, randomized, double-blind, parallel group, vehicle-controlled trials. *J Am Acad Dermatol.* 2004;50:714-721.
3. Geisse JK, Rich P, Pandya A, et al. Imiquimod 5% cream for the treatment of superficial basal cell carcinoma: a double-blind, randomized, vehicle-controlled study. *J Am Acad Dermatol.* 2002;47:390-398.

Imiquimod Enhances IFN-γ Production and Effector Function of T Cells Infiltrating Human Squamous Cell Carcinomas of the Skin

Huang SJ, Hijnen D, Murphy GF, et al (Brigham and Women's Hosp, Boston, MA; Utrecht Univ Med Ctr, The Netherlands; et al)
J Invest Dermatol 129:2676-2685, 2009

Squamous cell carcinomas (SCCs) are sun-induced skin cancers that are particularly numerous and aggressive in patients taking T-cell immunosuppressant medications. Imiquimod is a topical immune response modifier and Toll-like receptor 7 (TLR7) agonist that induces the immunological destruction of SCC and other skin cancers. TLR7 activation by imiquimod has pleiotropic effects on innate immune cells, but its effects on T cells remain largely uncharacterized. Because tumor destruction and formation of immunological memory are ultimately T-cell-mediated effects, we studied the effects of imiquimod therapy on effector T cells infiltrating human SCC. SCC treated with imiquimod before excision contained dense T-cell infiltrates associated with tumor cell apoptosis and histological evidence of tumor regression. Effector T cells from treated SCC produced more IFN-γ, granzyme, and perforin and less IL-10 and transforming growth factor-β (TGF-β) than T cells from untreated tumors. Treatment of normal human skin with imiquimod induced activation of resident T cells and reduced IL-10 production but had no effect on IFN-γ, perforin, or granzyme, suggesting that these latter effects arise from the recruitment of distinct populations of T cells into tumors. Thus, imiquimod stimulates tumor destruction by recruiting cutaneous effector T cells from blood and by inhibiting tonic anti-inflammatory signals within the tumor.

▶ The battle between tumors and our immune system is fought with multiple weapons: Fas ligand binding to receptors on cells (hand-to-hand combat), pro-cellular cytokines by type 1 helper T lymphocytes versus downregulation by interleukin (IL)-10 and tumor growth factor beta (TGF-β) (chemical warfare), direct cytotoxicity by natural killer cells (biologic warfare), and regulation of responses by FOXP3 suppressor cells (intelligence). Promotion of cellular responses appropriate for the battle is maximized in the face of imiquimod, which acts to shift the balance against cytokines, IL-10, and TGF-β. This article provides some very clear results that support how immune response modifiers, such as imiquimod, affect the war, not just the battle, against tumors. This is also one of many excellent articles from the same group working on the subject.

N. Bhatia, MD

Incidence and Clinical Predictors of a Subsequent Nonmelanoma Skin Cancer in Solid Organ Transplant Recipients With a First Nonmelanoma Skin Cancer: A Multicenter Cohort Study

Tessari G, Naldi L, Boschiero L, et al (Univ of Verona, Italy; Ospedali Riuniti di Bergamo, Italy; Azienda Ospedaliera di Verona, Italy)

Arch Dermatol 146:294-299, 2010

Objective.—To compare the long-term risk of primary nonmelanoma skin cancer (NMSC) and the risk of subsequent NMSC in kidney and heart transplant recipients.

Design.—Partially retrospective cohort study.

Setting.—Two Italian transplantation centers.

Patients.—The study included 1934 patients: 1476 renal transplant recipients and 458 heart transplant recipients.

Main Outcome Measures.—Cumulative incidences and risk factors of the first and subsequent NMSCs.

Results.—Two hundred patients developed a first NMSC after a median follow-up of 6.8 years after transplantation. The 3-year risk of the primary NMSC was 2.1%. Of the 200 patients with a primary NMSC, 91 (45.5%) had a second NMSC after a median follow-up after the first NMSC of 1.4 years (range, 3 months to 10 years). The 3-year risk of a second NMSC was 32.2%, and it was 49 times higher than that in patients with no previous NMSC. In a Cox proportional hazards regression model, age older than 50 years at the time of transplantation and male sex were significantly related to the first NMSC. Occurrence of the subsequent NMSC was not related to any risk factor considered, including sex, age at transplantation, type of transplanted organ, type of immunosuppressive therapy, histologic type of the first NMSC, and time since diagnosis of the first NMSC. Histologic type of the first NMSC strongly predicted the type of the subsequent NMSC.

Conclusions.—Development of a first NMSC confers a high risk of a subsequent NMSC in transplant recipients. Intensive long-term dermatologic follow-up of these patients is advisable.

▶ This study is the first to look at risk factors for both first and subsequent nonmelanoma skin cancer (NMSC) in organ transplant patients. Several notable findings are presented, and data confirm what we see in our daily practice. Patients with NMSC are frequently seen for subsequent NMSC, both in the immunocompetent and immunocompromised populations. The 3-year risk for subsequent NMSC in immunocompetent patients is 35% to 60%. Euvrard et al reported a 5-year risk of 71% for developing an NMSC after an index squamous-cell carcinoma (SCC) in the transplant population.[1] In this study, the 3-year risk of a second NMSC was 32.2%, and it was 49 times higher than that in patients with no previous NMSC. When these patients present with their first skin cancer, they should immediately be educated about the need for sun protection, self-examination, and routine follow-up.

When they looked specifically at the risk factors associated with development of a subsequent skin cancer, none of the clinical risk factors that are associated with first NMSC, such as age at transplantation and male sex, are predictors for a second NMSC. What is not addressed and would be an interesting study is to evaluate changes in sun-protective behavior within the group developing the second skin cancer and compare it with those who did not develop another cancer or who had a longer time period till the second cancer.

The significance of this article is that it emphasizes the need for continued education for prevention and early detection of skin cancer in this patient population. When a transplant patient presents with the first NMSC, the need for intense education regarding sun protection and his/her risk for skin cancer cannot be overemphasized. Although most patients are educated before their transplant about their increased risk of skin cancer, they often do not consider it to be an important issue. Presenting this information again when the patient develops skin cancer for the first time may have more significant and effective impact because the risk suddenly seems real. This may be especially important in regard to SCC, for the data do support that the histologic type of the first NMSC strongly predicted the subsequent NMSC of the same type. Patients with a primary SCC may need to be followed-up more closely for subsequent SCC, as these tumors can be more aggressive in this patient population, and early detection and treatment can be lifesaving.

E. M. Billingsley, MD

Reference

1. Euvrard S, Kanitakis J, Claudy A. Skin cancers after organ transplantation. *N Engl J Med.* 2003;348:1681-1691.

Incidence Estimate of Nonmelanoma Skin Cancer in the United States, 2006
Rogers HW, Weinstock MA, Harris AR, et al (Advanced Dermatology, Norwich, CT; Brown Med School, Providence, RI; Alpert Med School at Brown Univ, Providence, RI; et al)
Arch Dermatol 146:283-287, 2010

Objectives.—To estimate the incidence of nonmelanoma skin cancer (NMSC) in the US population in 2006 and secondarily to indicate trends in numbers of procedures for skin cancer treatment.

Design.—A descriptive analysis of population-based claims and US Census Bureau data combined with a population-based cross-sectional survey using multiple US government data sets, including the Centers for Medicare and Medicaid Services Fee-for-Service Physicians Claims databases, to calculate totals of skin cancer procedures performed for Medicare beneficiaries in 1992 and from 1996 to 2006 and related parameters. The National Ambulatory Medical Care Service database was used to estimate NMSC-related office visits. We combined these to estimate totals of new skin cancer diagnoses and affected individuals in the overall US population.

Results.—The total number of procedures for skin cancer in the Medicare fee-for-service population increased by 76.9% from 1 158 298 in 1992 to 2 048 517 in 2006. The age-adjusted procedure rate per year per 100 000 beneficiaries increased from 3514 in 1992 to 6075 in 2006. From 2002 to 2006 (the years for which the databases allow procedure linkage to patient demographics and diagnoses), the number of procedures for NMSC in the Medicare population increased by 16.0%. In this period, the number of procedures per affected patient increased by 1.5%, and the number of persons with at least 1 procedure increased by 14.3%. We estimate the total number of NMSCs in the US population in 2006 at 3 507 693 and the total number of persons in the United States treated for NMSC at 2 152 500.

Conclusions.—The number of skin cancers in Medicare beneficiaries increased dramatically over the years 1992 to 2006, due mainly to an increase in the number of affected individuals. Using nationally representative databases, we provide evidence of much higher overall totals of skin cancer diagnoses and patients in the US population than previous estimates. These data give the most complete evaluation to date of the under-recognized epidemic of skin cancer in the United States.

▶ The incidence of nonmelanoma skin cancer continues to rise, and despite technological advances in diagnosis and treatment as well as the advent of computers in the office, the true incidence still eludes us. The numbers given every year are only estimations. Nonmelanoma skin cancer is not typically reported in most cancer registries.

As health care policy changes with new laws being implemented over the next several years, it is vitally important for dermatologists to achieve accurate estimations of nonmelanoma skin cancer. By doing so, it may strengthen our position with policymakers of the burden of nonmelanoma skin cancer. In addition, increased emphasis may be placed on skin cancer programs, such as education, prevention, and treatment.

The authors used 2 Medicare databases to estimate current nonmelanoma skin cancer incidence. Their conclusion is that the incidence from 1992 to 2006 has dramatically increased to epidemic proportions.

J. L. Smith, MD

Incidence of Merkel cell carcinoma in renal transplant recipients

Koljonen V, Kukko H, Tukiainen E, et al (Helsinki Univ Hosp, Finland; et al)
Nephrol Dial Transplant 24:3231-3235, 2009

Background.—The risk factors for Merkel cell carcinoma (MCC), a rare type of skin cancer, are poorly understood. Some evidence suggests that MCC is more common in individuals with abnormal immune function resulting from viral infection, autoimmune disease or organ transplantation.

Methods.—The national Renal Transplant Registry and the Finnish Cancer Registry data were searched for recipients of a renal transplant who were diagnosed with MCC. The MCC diagnoses were confirmed using immunohistochemistry.

Results.—Three cases of MCC were detected among 4200 individuals who underwent renal transplantation from 1967 to 2005 [expected number 0.05, standardized incidence ratio (SIR) 66, 95% CI 14–194, $P < 0.001$]. The latency period between the transplant and detection of MCC ranged from 6 to 19 years. In all three cases, the cause of transplantation was an autoimmune disease. All three died from aggressive MCC with a survival time ranging from 0.5 to 2.1 years.

Conclusions.—The results indicate that the risk of MCC is greatly increased among subjects who have undergone renal transplantation. The course of the disease appears aggressive in this patient population. The physicians who treat recipients of a kidney transplant should be aware of the substantially increased risk of MCC.

▶ Merkel cell carcinoma (MCC) is an aggressive skin cancer that is sometimes seen in immunosuppressed patients. The purpose of this study was to investigate the incidence of MCC among patients with renal transplant in a nationwide population-based Finnish Cancer Registry (FCR). A total of 4200 individuals received a renal transplant during the study period of 1967-2005, with 60% of them being men aged between 45 years and 59 years (36%). All patients were Caucasian and elderly. Subjects were diagnosed with MCC from the files of the FCR and the national transplant registry, with histological diagnoses reviewed. The presence of MCC polyoma virus (MCPyV) DNA was analyzed from tumor sections. The number of MCC cases was compared with the expected number of cases based on cancer incidence in the national population, stratified by age and gender. There were 3 cases of MCC identified, with all patients having undergone organ transplant because of autoimmune renal disease. The mean age of MCC diagnosis was 59 years. All patients were treated with methylprednisolone posttransplant—2 received azathioprine, and 2 received cyclosporin. The latency period between a renal transplant and the MCC diagnosis ranged from 6 years to 19 years. All MCCs occurred on the head, with 2 involving the cheeks and 1 on the earlobe. The standardized incidence ratio was as high as 66 (95% confidence interval 14-194) for a diagnosis of MCC among individuals who had undergone kidney transplant. In this study, only 1 of the 3 MCC cases was MCPyV positive, suggesting that MCPyV may not be uniformly associated with development of MCC in patients with a renal transplant. However, there were only 3 MCC cases, and a larger study population is needed to evaluate if MCPyV is truly not a factor just in renal transplant patients, but also overall. All affected patients expired from progressive MCC, with a survival time ranging from 0.5 years to 2.1 years. A limitation of this study was that it was site specific only to the Finnish population, with all patients being Caucasian. MCPyV-positive MCC may be found at a higher incidence in other patients with organ transplant and in other populations around the world. It may be that MCC found in patients with renal organ transplants may not be similar to those that occur in the general population. All patients in this study were previously on immunosuppressive agents and had underlying autoimmune disease. In future studies, it may be relevant to evaluate if these 2 factors also relate to development of MCC as compared with the general population. In conclusion, the risk for development of aggressive MCC in renal transplant may be increased, with additional studies needed.

J. Q. Del Rosso, DO
G. K. Kim, DO

Mechanisms of Inactivation of *PTCH1* Gene in Nevoid Basal Cell Carcinoma Syndrome: Modification of the Two-Hit Hypothesis

Pan S, Dong Q, Sun L-S, et al (Peking Univ School and Hosp of Stomatology, Beijing, China)
Clin Cancer Res 16:442-450, 2010

Purpose.—*PTCH1* has been identified as the gene responsible for nevoid basal cell carcinoma syndrome (NBCCS). Keratocystic odontogenic tumors (KCOT) are aggressive jaw lesions that may occur in isolation or in association with NBCCS. The aim of this study was to investigate the genetic and/or epigenetic mechanisms of inactivation of the *PTCH1* gene in patients with NBCCS and related sporadic KCOTs.

Experimental Design.—Loss of heterozygosity was analyzed in 44 patients (15 NBCCS-related and 29 sporadic KCOTs), all of whom were previously analyzed for *PTCH1* mutations. Allelic location was established in tumors carrying two coincident mutations. *PTCH1* mRNA expression and promoter methylation status were analyzed in a panel of KCOTs to define the possible role of epigenetic effects on *PTCH1* inactivation.

Results.—Although mutations and loss of heterozygosity of *PTCH1* were frequently detected in both syndromic and nonsyndromic cases, hypermethylation of the *PTCH1* promoter was not identified in the present series. Of all the 44 cases examined, 13 were identified to fit the two-hit model, 14 to conform to a one-hit model, and the remaining 17 cases showing no alteration in *PTCH1*. The distribution of two-hit, one-hit, and non-hit cases was significantly different between syndrome and nonsyndrome patients ($P < 0.02$).

Conclusions.—This study indicates that *PTCH1* gene alternation may play a significant role in the pathogenesis of NBCCS and the related sporadic tumors. Not only the standard two-hit model, but also haploinsufficiency or dominant-negative isoforms may be implicated in the inactivation of the *PTCH1* gene.

► Although somewhat intimidating, the article is an excellent resource for the review of carcinogenesis in cutaneous oncology. The role of the two-hit hypothesis is not as pervasive in discussion of skin cancer in comparison to other visceral tumors, but it makes sense to the application of skin cancer after reading this study. The issue of how mutations can impact the disease process brings the concepts of one-hit and two-hits hypotheses to light, especially in basal cell nevus syndrome where the predisposition is in place due to the genetic defects. At the end of the discussion is an excellent review of the roles of PTCH1, SMO, and Sonic Hedgehog and how they all interact, which is important not just for board examinations but for how the disease process can be targeted. One day, the therapy standards might not just stop at excision or topical chemotherapy but involve a biologic target against the mutated gene products, so fundamental understanding of the disease mechanisms is still essential.

N. Bhatia, MD

Merkel cell polyomavirus DNA detection in lesional and nonlesional skin from patients with Merkel cell carcinoma or other skin diseases
Foulongne V, Dereure O, Kluger N, et al (Univ of Montpellier I, France; et al)
Br J Dermatol 162:59-63, 2010

Background.—A novel polyomavirus, the Merkel cell polyomavirus (MCPyV), has recently been identified in Merkel cell carcinoma (MCC).

Objectives.—To investigate the specificity of this association through the detection, quantification and analysis of MCPyV DNA in lesional and non-lesional skin biopsies from patients with MCC or with other cutaneous diseases, as well as in normal skin from clinically healthy individuals.

Methods.—DNA was extracted from lesional and nonlesional skin samples of patients with MCC or with other cutaneous diseases and from normal-appearing skin of clinically healthy subjects. MCPyV DNA was detected by polymerase chain reaction (PCR) and quantified by real-time PCR. Additionally, the T antigen coding region was sequenced in eight samples from seven patients.

Results.—MCPyV DNA was detected in 14 of 18 (78%) patients with MCC, five of 18 (28%) patients with other skin diseases $(P = 0.007)$ and one of six (17%) clinically healthy subjects. In patients with MCC, viral DNA was detected in nine of 11 (82%) tumours and in 10 of 14 (71%) nontumoral skin samples $(P = 0.66)$. MCPyV DNA levels were higher in MCC tumours than in nontumoral skin from patients with MCC, and than in lesional or nonlesional skin from patients with other cutaneous disorders. Signature mutations in the T antigen gene were not identified in the two MCC tumour specimens analysed.

Conclusions.—High prevalence and higher levels of MCPyV DNA in MCC supports a role for MCPyV in tumorigenesis. However, the high prevalence of MCPyV in the nontumoral skin and in subjects without MCC suggests that MCPyV is a ubiquitous virus.

▶ The Merkel cell polyomavirus (MCPyV) has recently been identified in the pathogenesis of Merkel cell carcinoma (MCC). This was a study to investigate

MCPyV DNA presence in lesional and nonlesional skin biopsies from patients with MCC and with other cutaneous diseases and in normal skin from healthy individuals. DNA was extracted from lesional and nonlesional skin samples of patients with MCC or with other cutaneous diseases and from normal-appearing skin of clinically healthy subjects. MCPyV DNA was detected by polymerase chain reaction. There were 18 patients with MCC involved in the study (median age of 72.5 years). From 7 of these patients, there were also nontumoral skin biopsies obtained at a distance from the tumor at the opposite extremity of the body. Nontumoral skin biopsies were also taken from 7 additional patients for whom tumoral material was unavailable or inappropriate for molecular biology testing. There were 18 patients with other benign or malignant skin diseases that were investigated with both lesional and nonlesional skin biopsies obtained. There were psoriasis (n = 10), Kaposi sarcoma (n = 3), porokeratosis (n = 1), melanoma (n = 1), Sézary syndrome (n = 1), keratoacanthoma (n = 1), and squamous cell carcinoma (n = 1). There was MCPyV DNA detected in 14 of 18 (78%) patients with MCC. Among these patients, viral DNA was detected in 9 of 11 (82%) tumors and in 10 of 14 (71%) distant nontumoral skin samples ($P = .66$). MCPyV DNA was also detected in 5 of 18 (28%) patients with other skin diseases, with an equal frequency in lesional and nonlesional skin biopsies. The overall MCPyV DNA detection rate was then significantly higher in patients with MCC than in those with other skin diseases ($P = .007$). The highest MCPyV DNA levels were observed in fresh MCC samples. Overall, no statistically significant difference was observed between MCPyV DNA levels in MCC samples compared with nontumoral skin from patients with MCC and lesional and nonlesional skin samples from patients with other skin conditions ($P = .54$). Moreover, viral DNA may be detected in both lesional and distant normal skin in about 30% of patients with non-MCC cutaneous disorders and in normal-appearing skin of healthy individuals. There was a high prevalence and higher levels of MCPyV DNA in MCC, supporting a role for MCPyV in tumorigenesis. The authors suggest that MCPyV DNA detection does not represent a specific marker for MCC and that the presence of MCPyV by itself is not a sufficient condition for developing MCC, which differs from other studies. However, this study does not address the origin of MCPyV. It may be an organism that is ubiquitous in the environment, and more studies need to be performed to learn more about MCPyV. Also, patients who develop MCCs may have a localized cutaneous immune suppression, and other factors such as chronic sun exposure may account for why MCCs are seen in high frequency in the head and neck region. To add, MCPyV may be among 1 of the many components in the pathogenesis of MCC development.

J. Q. Del Rosso, DO
G. K. Kim, DO

Merkel Cell Polyomavirus: A Specific Marker for Merkel Cell Carcinoma in Histologically Similar Tumors
Duncavage EJ, Le B-M, Wang D, et al (Washington Univ School of Medicine, St Louis, MO)
Am J Surg Pathol 33:1771-1777, 2009

The recently described Merkel cell polyomavirus (MCPyV) is reportedly present in 50% to 80% of Merkel cell carcinomas (MCC). Although the virus has been shown to be absent from other cutaneous neoplasms, its association with malignancies that are histologically similar to MCC, specifically small cell carcinoma of the lung and other high-grade neuroendocrine tumors, has yet to be thoroughly investigated. To address this issue, we identified a set of 74 cases of visceral high-grade neuroendocrine tumors from a variety of anatomic sites, including 32 cases from the lung, 16 cases from the gastrointestinal tract, 20 cases from the female reproductive system, 3 cases from soft tissue, 2 cases from the head and neck region, and 1 case from the bladder. Using a set of primers optimized to detect MCPyV in formalin-fixed tissue, polymerase chain reaction (PCR)-based testing showed evidence of MCPyV DNA in only 1 of the 74 tumors; however, clinicopathologic review of the positive case (a neuroendocrine tumor of the small intestine) disclosed that the patient had a history of primary MCC of the buttock. PCR-based testing also showed no evidence of the related WU and KI polyomaviruses in the set of 74 cases. We conclude that, when evaluated by PCR-based testing, MCPyV is a specific marker for MCC that can be helpful in distinguishing cases of metastatic MCC from other high-grade neuroendocrine tumors. Our results also suggest that MCPyV does not have a role in the oncogenesis of visceral high-grade neuroendocrine tumors.

▶ Merkel cell polyomavirus (MCPyV) was first described by Feng et al in January 2008, and it is highly suspected to cause most cases of Merkel cell carcinoma (MCC). This article sought to test the strength of that association by screening for the presence of the virus in 74 tumors that are histologically similar to MCC, specifically small-cell carcinoma of the lung and other high-grade neuroendocrine tumors, using polymerase chain reaction—based technology. While only 1 of 74 tumors showed evidence of MCPyV DNA, even this case was confounded by the fact that the patient had had MCC of the buttock previously.

MCPyV is monotypically integrated within the DNA of the MCC cells, suggesting that this integration occurred before clonal expansion as a malignant population, and it is associated with other viral T antigen mutations that leave the virus unable to propagate, but it is thought that it promotes carcinogenesis by altering the activity of tumor suppressor and cell cycle regulatory proteins, possibly acting in collusion with other procarcinogenic events, such as exposure to ultraviolet light or ionizing radiation. Absences of detection in a variety of neuroendocrine malignancies and small-cell lung carcinoma highlight the likelihood of a causal role in MCC.

W. A. High, MD, JD, MEng

Organ transplant recipients and skin cancer: assessment of risk factors with focus on sun exposure
Terhorst D, Drecoll U, Stockfleth E, et al (Charité Universitätsmedizin, Berlin, Germany)
Br J Dermatol 161:85-89, 2009

Background.—Organ transplant recipients (OTRs) have an increased risk of developing skin cancer, especially epithelial tumours. A number of factors such as immunosuppression, age, ultraviolet radiation and skin type are considered as important in aetiology.

Objectives.—The purpose of this study was to further evaluate the risk factors for OTRs regarding skin cancer after transplantation. A detailed investigation of the specific compounds of sun exposure was realised.

Methods.—A questionnaire-based study was performed in a specialist OTR dermatology clinic from January to April 2009. The subjects were 70 organ transplanted patients who had developed some form of skin cancer after transplantation. As controls served 69 organ transplanted patients who had no history of skin cancer. The controls were matched concerning age, transplanted organ and gender. Photo protection, sun exposure and transplantation data were part of the questionnaire. Statistical analysis was performed with Mann—Whitney-U-test, chi-square test or Fisher's exact test.

Results.—The total sun burden (TSB) and the recreational sun exposure in particular attained higher scores in the skin cancer group (TSB-score: mean $11 \cdot 8$ vs. $10 \cdot 0$, $P < 0 \cdot 05$; recreational sun exposure: mean $6 \cdot 3$ vs. $5 \cdot 1$, $P < 0 \cdot 05$). The skin cancer group had fairer skin types than the control group (median skin type 2 vs. 3, $P < 0 \cdot 05$). The OTRs who developed skin cancer have been more likely to have a history or present intake of azathioprine (mean 42% vs. 21%, $P < 0 \cdot 05$). Also, the skin cancer group has been transplanted for a longer time (mean $12 \cdot 3$ vs. $7 \cdot 2$ years, $P < 0 \cdot 001$), analogously had a younger age at transplantation (mean $49 \cdot 5$ vs. $52 \cdot 7$ years, $P < 0 \cdot 001$).

Conclusions.—Recreational sun exposure is of central importance for OTRs. A long period of transplantation and thus immunosuppression presents a main risk factor for the development of skin cancer in OTRs. A multi disciplinary management with the best medication and a focus on sun protection is needed to prevent skin cancer in OTRs.

▶ This article reveals that the old principle of the "pound of cure," or protection against ultraviolet radiation for the organ transplant recipient, might actually be the "ounce of prevention," or ounce of sunscreen necessary on a daily basis. In the face of immunosuppression, the potential for progression of carcinogenesis and acceleration of mutations that impact tumor suppressor genes, such as *p53*, initiation of oncogenes, such as *Ras* and *p16*, and the conversion of normal keratinocyte progression into dyskeratosis and sunburn cells, all lead to the development of actinic keratoses and squamous cell carcinoma at a much faster rate in patients undergoing organ transplants.[1-3] As a result, it has to be the responsibility of the dermatologist, the transplant team, and most importantly, the patient to make sure that sunscreens and limitation of excessive solar exposure are part of a daily routine. In many ways, the use of sunscreens to the skin is similar to the use of toothpaste for prevention of cavities, and especially in the case of someone at high risk for dental caries, that risk escalates in the patient with an organ transplant and immunosuppression.

N. Bhatia, MD

References

1. Levine AJ, Momand J, Finlay CA. The p53 tumour suppressor gene. *Nature*. 1991; 351:453-456.
2. Ling G, Ahmadian A, Persson A, et al. PATCHED and p53 gene alterations in sporadic and hereditary basal cell cancer. *Oncogene*. 2001;20:7770-7778.
3. Spencer JM, Kahn SM, Jiang W, DeLeo VA, Weinstein IB. Activated ras genes occur in human actinic keratoses, premalignant precursors to squamous cell carcinomas. *Arch Dermatol*. 1995;131:796-800.

Patients With Merkel Cell Carcinoma Tumors ≤ 1.0 cm in Diameter Are Unlikely to Harbor Regional Lymph Node Metastasis
Stokes JB, Graw KS, Dengel LT, et al (Univ of Virginia Health System, Charlottesville; Salem Veterans Affair's Med Ctr, VA)
J Clin Oncol 27:3772-3777, 2009

Purpose.—Merkel cell carcinoma (MCC) is a rare, aggressive neuroendocrine cutaneous malignancy. Current recommendations include offering regional lymph node evaluation by either sentinel lymph node biopsy (SLNB) or complete lymph node dissection (CLND) to all patients with MCC; however, we hypothesized a cohort of low-risk patients may exist for whom regional nodal metastasis would be unlikely.

Methods.—A retrospective review of the Department of Veterans Affairs national health care database was performed. Patients undergoing resection of primary MCC were identified; and demographic, medical, and social history; tumor characteristics; nodal status; and recurrence events were recorded.

Results.—Between 1995 and 2006, 346 patients were diagnosed with MCC. Of these, 213 underwent resection of the primary lesion and evaluation of the draining lymph node basin. Fifty-four patients (25%) had tumors ≤ 1.0 cm in diameter. Average tumor diameter was 0.7 cm, and 63% were located on the head or neck. Only two patients (4%) with tumors ≤ 1.0 cm had regional lymph node metastasis, compared with 51

(24%) of 213 patients with tumors more than 1.0 cm ($P \leq .0001$). Both patients had clinically evident nodal disease at presentation and underwent CLND. Both have remained recurrence-free for 40 months. Thirteen (25%) of 51 patients with nodal metastasis and tumors more than 1 cm had occult nodal metastasis.

Conclusion.—In this series, patients with MCC $\leq$ 1.0 cm were unlikely to have regional lymph node metastasis, suggesting that regional nodal evaluation may reasonably be avoided in these patients. However, these data support SLNB for MCC more than 1 cm in diameter.

▶ The object of this study was to retrospectively analyze patients who presented to the Veterans Administration with Merkel cell carcinoma (MCC) in a period between 1995 and 2006 and to assist the current recommendations including offering lymph node evaluations by either sentinel lymph node biopsy or complete lymph node dissections. Specifically, the study looked at a cohort of apparently lower risk patients who may exist for whom regional nodal metastasis would be unlikely, and complete lymphadenectomy may not be beneficial.

The study is a retrospective analysis and for a practicing dermatologist is recommended reading. This study demonstrates an analysis of 346 patients who were diagnosed with MCC. Of these, 213 patients underwent resection of the primary tumor and evaluation of the draining lymph node basin. Fifty-four patients had tumors $\leq$1.0 cm in diameter, and the average tumor diameter was 0.7 cm, with 63% located on the head and neck. Only 2 patients (4%) with tumors $\leq$1.0 cm had regional lymph node metastasis, compared with 51 (24%) of 213 patients with tumors > 1.0 cm ($P < .0001$). These patients had clinically evident nodal disease on presentation and underwent complete lymph node dissection.

Compared with other forms of skin cancer, MCC is an aggressive neuroendocrine tumor, which is rare, 100 times less prevalent than melanoma. The incidence has tripled recently increasing from 0.15 per 100 000 in 1986 to 0.44 per 100 000 in 2001. Some of the rise in the incidence may be because of an increased use of immunostaining procedures, which are valuable diagnostic tools for diagnosing of MCC since the mid 1990s. Other factors that may contribute to the increase of MCC include a rise in the aging patient population, increased sun exposure, and a greater number of immunosuppressed patients.

The overall prognosis of MCC is poor. MCC is characterized by its high incidence of local recurrence and the propensity for regional lymph node and distant metastasis. The recent results of the Surveillance, Epidemiology, and End Results Program database reported 5-year survival rates of 75% for localized disease, 59% for regional disease, and only 25% for distant MCC. Five years survival with advanced disease with nodal involvement ranges from 22% to 65%. In patients with node-negative disease, the survival is 80% to 88%. The completion of dissection with adjuvant radiation therapy is noted to decrease regional failure rates from 50% to 70%, down to 20% in MCC.

The overall recurrence rate of this group is 21%, which is significantly less than the recurrence rates of 52% to 54%. It appears that the group of patients with MCC who have tumors less than or equal to 1.0 cm can be identified with low enough risk of regional lymph node metastasis that regional lymph node evaluation by sentinel lymph node biopsy or complete lymph node dissection could be reasonably and safely omitted. Patients with tumors less than or equal to 1.0 cm may safely avoid surgical intervention of regional lymph node basins, and further revision of staging schemes for MCC should consider them as a subset.

L. Cleaver, DO

Prevalence of a History of Skin Cancer in 2007: Results of an Incidence-Based Model
Stern RS (Beth Israel Deaconess Med Ctr, Boston, MA)
Arch Dermatol 146:279-282, 2010

Objectives.—To estimate the 2007 person prevalence of common types of nonmelanoma skin cancer (NMSC), basal cell carcinoma (BCC) and squamous cell carcinoma (SCC), or both, in the United States using an incidence-based mathematical model; and to compare the prevalence of skin cancer with that of other common cancers.

Design.—I developed a mathematical model to estimate the prevalence of NMSC in the United States in 2007. This model used age-specific incidence data adjusted to reflect changes in incidence from 1957 to 2006, the age distribution of the population from 1957 to 2006, and the likelihood that an incident tumor was the first ever for that person. I performed sensitivity analyses that varied my assumption about change in incidence over time and proportion of incident tumors that were a first-ever NMSC for an individual. I used standard methods for analysis of survey data to calculate the number of persons who report a history of the selected cancers and published Surveillance, Epidemiology, and End Results (SEER) estimates for incidence-based estimates for prevalence of cancers other than NMSC.

Setting.—National Health Interview Survey (NHIS) 2007 data, National Cancer Institute Skin Cancer Incidence data (1977-1978), and SEER data.

Main Outcome Measure.—Incidence-based estimate of prevalence of NMSC and melanoma and patient reports of a history of skin and selected other cancers.

Results.—Approximately 13 million white non-Hispanics living in the United States at the beginning of 2007 have had at least 1 NMSC. About 1 in 5 seventy-year-olds have had NMSCs, and most of those affected have had multiple NMSCs. In the 2007 NHIS estimates, only 5 million persons report a history of skin cancer, less than half the number estimated based on incidence and survival data.

Conclusions.—My incidence-based model indicates that the prevalence of a skin cancer history is about 5 times higher than that of breast or prostate cancer and greater than the 31-year prevalence of all other cancers combined. Despite their high frequency, population-based incidence and burden data for BSC and SCC are largely lacking (Table 2).

▶ The objective of this study is to estimate the prevalence of the common types of nonmelanoma skin cancer (NMSC) using an incidence-based mathematical model to compare the prevalence of skin cancer with that of other common cancers. The design is a mathematical model that uses age-specific incidence data reflecting changes in the incidences of NMSC from 1957 to 2006. The age distribution out of this group and the likelihood that an incident tumor was the first ever for that person are assumptions. The sensitivity analysis was obtained and calculated using the Surveillance, Epidemiology, and End Results (SEER) estimates for incidence-based prevalence of cancers other than NMSCs. Skin cancer rates were compared with other forms of cancer using the published SEER data. This study shows information based on the mathematical model, and these conclusions may be more valid than this reported data for skin cancers. Approximately 13 million white non-Hispanics living in the United States at the beginning of 2007 have had at least 1 NMSC, and approximately 20% of 70-year olds have had NMSCs. Many of those have had multiple NMSCs. In the 2007 National Health Interview Survey, only 5 million people report a history of skin cancer, less than half the number estimated on incidence and survival data. A mathematical model uses a number of estimates and assumptions that are variable. Using assumptions at the rate of 3% per year from 1997 rather than the approximation of a 2% incidence of NMSC would translate 1.8 million, which is substantially higher than the most recent estimates. Ultimately, the problem with NMSC is that reporting of cases is not mandatory, so the exact number of cases of NMSC in the United States is very difficult to ascertain. By using the annual incidence and increased prevalence data, it is estimated in the study that approximately 14 million persons or nearly 5% of the US population have a history of NMSC. By the age of 70 years, nearly 1 in 5 white US residents have had at least 1 NMSC,

TABLE 2.—Number of Persons With Cancer History by Site and Data Source

Site	NHIS 2007, in 100 000s (95% CI)	Population Prevalence Based on Incidence, 100 000s	Prevalence Ratio, NHIS to Incidence Estimate
Breast	26 (23-29)	25[a]	1.04
Prostate	20 (17-23)	22[a]	0.91
Skin			
Melanoma	11 (9-13)	8[a]	1.45
NMSC[b]	38 (33-43)	13[b]	0.29
Unknown	12 (11-13)	NC	NC
Total NMSC, known and unknown type skin cancer	50 (45-55)	13[b]	0.39
Total skin cancers	61 (55-67)	137[ab]	0.45

Abbreviations: CI, confidence interval; NC, not calculated; NHIS, National Health Interview Survey; NMSC, nonmelanoma skin cancer.
Editor's Note: Please refer to original journal article for full references.
[a]Surveillance, Epidemiology, and End Results[8] (31-year prevalence).
[b]See "Methods" section for calculation of prevalence of NMSC among non-Hispanic whites 2007.

or about a million current US residents aged 50 years already have had at least 1 NMSC. About 30% of the US white population who have survived to age of 90 years have had at least 1 NMSC. This study is based upon a mathematical model, and the precision is unknown. There are sensitivity analyses, which indicate that there are a wide range of assumptions based on estimates, and in 2007, at least 10 million, but probably less than 15 million US residents, have had at least 1 NMSC.

L. Cleaver, DO

Primary cutaneous myxoid spindle cell squamous cell carcinoma: a clinicopathologic study and review of the literature
Yang A, Hanley A, Velazquez EF, et al (Kaiser Permanente, Mission Viejo, CA; Global Pathology Laboratory, Miami Lakes, FL; Brigham and Women's Hosp Harvard Med School, Boston, MA; et al)
J Cutan Pathol 37:465-474, 2010

Mucocutaneous squamous cell carcinoma (SCC) may rarely exhibit intracellular mucin production. Extracellular mucin production is an even rarer finding in SCC that is not well documented in the literature. Here, we report six cases of primary cutaneous and mucocutaneous SCC with prominent extracellular stromal mucin deposition and an epithelial spindle cell component. We propose the term 'myxoid spindle cell SCC' (MSC SCC) to describe the histologic characteristics of these six cases. We also propose a set of histologic and immunohistochemical findings for distinguishing MSC SCC from primary cutaneous and metastatic spindle cell neoplasms including other sarcomatoid carcinomas, myxoid sarcomas and the spindle cell variant of atypical fibroxanthoma (AFX). The criteria can also help discern MSC SCC from spindle cell melanomas, which may rarely show a prominent myxoid stroma. Given the small numbers of cases reported to date, the presence of prominent myxoid stroma in primary cutaneous spindle cell SCC has unknown prognostic significance at this time.

▶ This is a well-reviewed article demonstrating 6 cases of a rare tumor, cutaneous myxoid spindle cell squamous cell carcinoma, and distinguishing it clinically and histologically from other malignancies, such as primary and metastatic cutaneous sarcomatoid carcinomas, myxoid atypical fibrous xanthoma, myxofibrosarcoma, malignant peripheral nerve sheath tumor, and spindle cell melanoma with myxoid changes. The histologic criteria that were used for inclusion in this series were: (1) predominant population of poorly differentiated spindle cells, (2) more than 50% of the lesion showing prominent myxoid stromal changes, (3) neoplastic spindle and squamous cells positive for at least 1 cytokeratin, especially high-molecular-weight cytokeratin, and (4) neoplastic cells negative for melanocytic and mesenchymal markers. This article also demonstrates the importance of performing broad immunohistochemical markers to determine the lineage of these poorly differentiated neoplastic cells.

S. B. Momin, DO

Reflectance Confocal Microscopy for Noninvasive Monitoring of Therapy and Detection of Subclinical Actinic Keratoses

Ulrich M, Krueger-Corcoran D, Roewert-Huber J, et al (Charité Univ Medicine, Berlin, Germany)
Dermatology 220:15-24, 2010

Background.—Actinic keratoses (AK) represent cutaneous carcinoma in situ and have previously been evaluated by reflectance confocal microscopy (RCM). Treatment of AK with imiquimod (IMIQ) 5% cream has been shown to 'highlight' subclinical lesions.

Objective.—The aim of this study was to test the applicability of RCM for noninvasive monitoring of actinic field cancerization and detection of subclinical AK.

Subjects and Methods.—AK and surrounding skin sites with no apparent AK of 11 volunteers were selected for imaging and subsequently classified as 'clinical' and 'subclinical' AK. IMIQ was used 3 times weekly for 4 weeks.

Results.—RCM was able to detect morphologic features of AK in both clinical and subclinical AK; features were more pronounced in clinical lesions. The immunomodulatory response induced by IMIQ was visualized by RCM.

Conclusion.—Our findings indicate that RCM allows noninvasive monitoring of treatment response in vivo and permits early detection of subclinical AK, thus substantiating the incentive for therapy.

▶ The authors are to be commended for their persistence and documentation of the inflammatory response observed in the treatment of actinic keratoses (AKs). This is not an easy feat because any crusting makes reflectance confocal microscopy (RCM) difficult. Yet one of the more valuable contributions they make in this study is confirmation that after noninvasive topical therapy with imiquimod, the initial abnormal changes seen in lesional and perilesional skin with RCM normalize as previously described by Torres, Storey, Anders, et al … "Microarray analysis of aberrant gene expression in actinic keratosis: effect of the Toll-like receptor-7 agonist imiquimod," which included confocal microscopy analysis of AK, and surrounding sun-exposed nonlesional skin before and after therapy, published in the May 2007 issue of the *British Journal of Dermatology*. The concept that this can be used to guide the need for additional therapy even if there is no clinical lesion present is very important but has to be tempered by the fact that the persistence of severe atypia may in fact indicate residual lesion, but this is not known for sure and could alternatively indicate ultraviolet light—induced damage not necessarily premalignant in nature. Nevertheless, it seems that either the lesions or the sun-induced changes improve with some therapies and can be documented with RCM.

A. Torres, MD, JD

Single-Institution Series of Early-Stage Merkel Cell Carcinoma: Long-Term Outcomes in 95 Patients Managed with Surgery Alone
Bajetta E, Celio L, Platania M, et al (Fondazione IRCCS, "Istituto Nazionale Tumori", Milan, Italy)
Ann Surg Oncol 16:2985-2993, 2009

Aim.—To determine the long-term outcomes of early-stage Merkel cell carcinoma (MCC) patients managed with surgery alone.

Methods.—Ninety-five consecutive patients were reviewed. Patients were treated by wide local excision. Clinically negative regional nodes were either followed up ($n = 42$) or staged with sentinel lymph node biopsy ($n = 21$), and clinically positive nodes underwent lymph node dissection ($n = 32$).

Results.—Median follow-up was 65 months. A total of 45 (47%) patients relapsed, with 80% of the recurrences occurring within 2 years and 96% within 5 years. The 5-year crude cumulative incidence (CCI) of recurrence and disease-specific survival (DSS) were 52% and 67%, respectively. CCI of local 5-year recurrence was 5% for the study cohort. Patients with MCC in the head and neck region had a 5-year local-recurrence CCI of 19%, and patients with MCC in the extremity and trunk region had a 5-year local-recurrence CCI of 2% ($P = 0.007$). Comparing patients with ≤ 2 versus > 2 metastatic lymph nodes, the 5-year regional-recurrence CCI was 0% versus 39% ($P = 0.004$). The 5-year distant-recurrence CCI was higher in clinically node-positive patients compared with node-negative patients (37% versus 12%; $P = 0.005$). Patients with MCC in the head and neck region experienced no distant recurrences, patients with MCC in the extremity and trunk region had a 5-year distant-recurrence CCI of 22%, and patients with occult primary had a 5-year distant-recurrence CCI of 49% ($P = 0.023$). The 5-year DSS rate was 80% for pathologically node-negative patients.

Conclusion.—The prognosis for surgically managed early-stage MCC is variable. Thus multidisciplinary tumor-board consultation is needed to optimize individual patient management.

▶ Merkel cell carcinoma (MCC) is a malignant tumor with a high potential for morbidity and mortality. Data regarding long-term surgical outcomes in the literature are sparse. Long-term retrospective studies and randomized trials are needed to further delineate the clinical course and appropriate management of this highly aggressive tumor.

The authors in this article adequately describe their findings in a group of 45 patients with MCC, with a median follow-up period of 65 months. Given the rarity of MCC, this is a relatively large patient population, although the authors admit that this study may not be large enough to accurately reflect true surgical outcomes.

The data in this article suggest that lymph node status is an extremely important predictor of future outcome and, much like melanoma management, may warrant discussions regarding sentinel lymph node biopsy in these patients. Obtaining clear margins with surgical management is important, although it may be difficult in certain areas such as the face. Additional long-term follow-up studies are needed for comparative data regarding treatment strategies, excision margins, postoperative radiation, and lymph node dissection.

R. I. Ceilley, MD
J. Wilson, MD

Skin cancer: preventive photodynamic therapy in patients with face and scalp cancerization. A randomized placebo-controlled study
Apalla Z, Sotiriou E, Chovarda E, et al (Aristotle Univ, Thessaloniki, Greece; et al)
Br J Dermatol 162:171-175, 2010

Background.—Patients with a previous medical history of nonmelanoma skin cancers (NMSCs) often develop multiple or recurrent malignant lesions around the site of the primary tumour. This finding led to the field cancerization theory, which suggests that the entire epithelial surface of the regional skin has an increased risk for the development of malignant lesions. Management of field change is challenging, taking into account the high impact of NMSCs on public health and healthcare costs.

Objectives.—We sought to investigate whether field-photodynamic therapy (PDT) of extreme photodamaged skin would prevent new NMSCs, in comparison with a control area receiving placebo-PDT, in patients with clinical and histological signs of field cancerization.

Methods.—Forty-five patients, previously diagnosed as having NMSCs of the face or scalp, with actinic keratoses symmetrically distributed over the same regions, were randomized for field treatment with 20% aminolaevulinic acid (ALA)-PDT on one side and placebo-PDT on the other. During the next 12-month period of follow up, patients were clinically evaluated for new NMSCs.

Results.—A significant delay in the mean time of appearance and a reduction in the total number of new lesions were observed in the field-PDT protocol, when compared with the control.

Conclusions.—The results obtained showed that field therapy with ALA-PDT confers a significant preventive potential against the formation of new NMSCs in patients with field changes.

▶ This study adds further support for the role of photodynamic therapy (PDT) as a safe and highly effective field therapy in the treatment of actinic keratosis

(AK) of the face and scalp. In comparison with other topical field therapies such as 5-fluorouracil, imiquimod, and diclofenac, it has a shorter treatment cycle and hence less patient downtime overall. Additionally, because it is delivered as an in-office procedure, PDT guarantees patient compliance. Future development of PDT treatment parameters for AK of the trunk and extremities will hopefully take place and expand its use.

It is interesting to note in Fig 3 in the original article that after a 6-month delay in the development of new lesions on the PDT-treated side, the rate of lesion development continued at roughly the same rate as the placebo-treated side. These data suggest that there is an inadequate sustained (12 months) field clearance response evoked by PDT. In light of new evidence surrounding the role of HPV in the development of AK, efforts to enhance the immune responsiveness of PDT with immunomodulator therapy would provide a future area of study.[1]

G. Martin, MD

Reference

1. Harwood CA, Proby CM. Human papillomaviruses and non-melanoma skin cancer. *Curr Opin Infect Dis.* 2002;15:101-114.

Skin cancers associated with HIV infection and solid-organ transplantation among elderly adults

Lanoy E, Costagliola D, Engels EA (Natl Cancer Inst, Rockville, MD; INSERM, Paris, France)

Int J Cancer 126:1724-1731, 2010

Immunosuppression may be etiologic for some skin cancers. We investigated the impact of human immunodeficiency virus (HIV) infection and solid-organ transplantation on skin cancer risk. We conducted a population-based case—control study among elderly U.S. adults (non-Hispanic whites, age 67 years or older), using Surveillance, Epidemiology and End Results Medicare linked data. The study comprised 29,926 skin cancer cases (excluding basal cell and squamous cell carcinomas) and 119,704 controls, frequency-matched by gender, age and calendar year (1987—2002). Medicare claims identified solid-organ transplantation or HIV infection before cancer diagnosis/control selection. As negative controls, we evaluated other medical conditions (*e.g.*, hypertension and depression) and cancers (breast, colon and prostate) not linked to immunosuppression. Odds ratios (ORs) compared prevalence in cases and controls, adjusted for matching factors and number of prior physician claims. Risks of Kaposi sarcoma ($N = 602$) and cutaneous non-Hodgkin lymphoma ($N = 1,836$) were increased with solid-organ transplantation (OR [95%CI]: 11.06 [5.27—23.23] and 2.27 [1.00—5.15], respectively) and HIV infection (21.58 [11.94—38.99] and 2.41 [1.05—5.52], respectively). Solid-organ transplantation was also associated with increased risks of Merkel cell carcinoma ($N = 1,286$; OR [95%CI] 4.95 [2.62—9.34]) and other cutaneous sarcomas ($N = 972$; 4.19 [1.83–9.56]). Solid-organ transplantation was nonsignificantly associated with melanoma ($N = 23,974$; (OR 1.36 [95%CI 0.98–1.88]). Null or weak associations were observed for negative control medical conditions and cancers. Solid-organ transplantation and HIV infection were followed by increased risk for some skin cancer subtypes among elderly adults. These results highlight the potential role of immunity in development of skin cancers.

▶ For many skin cancers, immunosuppression is thought to be an important risk factor. The higher incidence of cancers in human immunodeficiency virus (HIV)-infected people and in solid organ transplant recipients is considered to possibly be related to infection with oncogenic viruses, such as polyomavirus.

Using data from the Surveillance, Epidemiology, and End Results Medicare database linkage, the study investigated immunosuppression as a risk factor for the development of skin cancers among elderly adults in the United States. Skin cancers other than basal cell carcinoma (BCC) and squamous cell carcinoma (SCC) were evaluated, as these data were not captured in the database used. The cancers included were melanoma, Merkel cell carcinoma, appendageal carcinoma, cutaneous non-Hodgkin lymphoma, and other sarcomas. The immunosuppressed patients were elderly patients with solid organ transplants and those with HIV infection.

This case-control study had a very large database, including almost 30 000 cases of skin cancer and almost 120 000 controls. The data and statistical analyses are complex and very detailed.

Melanoma was the most common cancer seen, with a modest increased risk after organ transplant. Much significantly, stronger associations were seen for both HIV and transplant patients with Kaposi sarcoma and cutaneous non-Hodgkin lymphoma. Merkel cell carcinoma was also seen more frequently in both patient groups but of statistical significance only for the transplant group. Of note, this is the first study to formally quantify the increased risk for Merkel cell carcinoma with solid organ transplantation.

For dermatologists involved in the care of transplant patients and HIV-infected patients, we often think of BCC and SCC. This study demonstrates the need to also be aware of the increased risk of Kaposi sarcoma in these patients, and also non-Hodgkin lymphoma, Merkel cell carcinoma, appendageal cancers, such as sebaceous carcinoma, and other skin sarcomas, such as fibrous histiocytoma, dermatofibrosarcoma, hemangiosarcoma, and leiomyosarcoma. This study looked only at elderly adults, and it may not be generalizable to younger patients.

E. M. Billingsley, MD

Sunburns, Sun Protection and Indoor Tanning Behaviors, and Attitudes Regarding Sun Protection Benefits and Tan Appeal among Parents of U.S. Adolescents—1998 Compared to 2004
Bandi P, Cokkinides VE, Weinstock MA, et al (American Cancer Society, Atlanta, GA; Rhode Island Hosp and Brown Univ, Providence)
Pediatr Dermatol 27:9-18, 2010

This study presents nationally representative trends (1998–2004) and patterns in skin cancer risk behaviors, including sunburns, sun protection, and indoor tanning behaviors, and attitudes regarding ultraviolet radiation exposure among parents of U.S. adolescents. Data were from the American Cancer Society Sun Surveys I and II, telephone-based random digit dialed cross-sectional surveys of U.S. adolescents and their parents conducted in the summers of 1998 and 2004. Between 1998 and 2004, use of sunscreen, wide-brimmed hats and composite use of three to five behaviors increased significantly; concurrently, indoor tanning use increased significantly and sunburn prevalence changed a little. In 2004, 47% reported summer sunburns and more than half of those received painful sunburns. Parents continued to report low compliance with recommended behaviors; sunscreen use was most frequently reported, but many followed inappropriate application practices. About 13% practiced indoor tanning in the past year. Parents reported high levels of positive attitudes toward sun protection benefit, but at the same time, significant proportions reported positive tan appeal and outdoor sun exposure attitudes. The low rates and mixed progress in safe ultraviolet radiation exposure behaviors demand more attention for primary skin cancer prevention among parents of adolescents that focuses on changing beliefs about tanning appeal and promotes comprehensive ultraviolet radiation exposure protection.

▶ This was a study in pediatric dermatology looking at the trends and patterns in skin cancer risk behaviors comparing the parents of adolescents from 1998 to 2004. This article looks at a number of measurable outcomes and is able to show a consensus of change from 1998 to 2004. This information shows an increasing trend toward more sun protection and looks at the overall risk factors of this group. The validity of this test information from 1998 to 2004 is certainly interesting, but these data are already somewhat timed.

The research is sound, and the investigators used the American Cancer Society Sun Surveys in a telephone random digit dialed national representative survey of a noninstitutionalized population. This article looks at a number of risk factors, which include sunburns and behaviors reducing the chance of sunburn. The classic sunburn is the summer sunburn, and 41.7% parents reported being sunburned at least once; 14% reported that they had been sunburned 3 or more times. More than half, 57% of those sunburned, reported that they received at least 1 painful sunburn. Regular sun protection behaviors were most commonly noted as the use of sunscreen, but seeking shade and using umbrellas were noted in 40% of those surveyed. The use of protective clothing such as long pants was reported by 25% interviewed. A wide brim hat was reported as being used by 14%, and a long sleeve shirt was reported from 7.7%. The use of sunscreen irrespective of the sun protection factor (SPF) value was 47.4%, and 41.4% reported the use of sunscreen of an SPF value of 15 or higher. There was no significant change in the prevalence of the frequency of sunburns between 1998 and 2004. Other protective options such as avoidance of sun between 10 AM and 4 PM did not change significantly, and the use of wide brim hats did increase by 7.2% with a P value of less than .001. Use of long sleeves and long pants did not change significantly. The use of sunscreen in the general public in outdoor settings did increase by 9.7% and had a P value of less than .001.

A significant finding of the study shows that the final knowledge, attitudes, and beliefs regarding the sun exposure are certainly directly related to the practice of protective ultraviolet radiation protection among parents themselves, and they are also correlated with their children's behaviors. This study emphasizes the need for an educational message to parents, targeting ultraviolet protection needs to reduce these risk factors and excessive outdoor sun exposure.

L. Cleaver, DO

Topical nicotinamide modulates cellular energy metabolism and provides broad-spectrum protection against ultraviolet radiation-induced immunosuppression in humans
Sivapirabu G, Yiasemides E, Halliday GM, et al (Univ of Sydney at Royal Prince Alfred Hosp, Camperdown, New South Wales, Australia)
Br J Dermatol 161:1357-1364, 2009

Background.—Ultraviolet (UV) radiation can profoundly suppress the cutaneous immune system, thus enhancing carcinogenesis. Agents that prevent UV-induced immunosuppression may thus reduce skin cancer. Nicotinamide (vitamin B3) prevents UV-induced immunosuppression and carcinogenesis in mice, and solar-simulated (ss) UV-induced immunosuppression in humans. Its effectiveness against different UV wavebands and mechanism of action is as yet unknown.

Objectives.—To determine the effects and mechanisms of topical nicotinamide on UV-induced suppression of delayed type hypersensitivity (DTH) responses in humans.

Methods.—Healthy Mantoux-positive volunteers in four randomised, double-blinded studies were irradiated with solar-simulated (ss)UV (UVB + UVA) or narrowband UVB (300 nm) or UVA (385 nm). Topical nicotinamide (0·2% or 5%) or its vehicle were applied immediately after each irradiation. Mantoux testing was performed at irradiated sites and adjacent unirradiated control sites 48 h after the first irradiation and measured 72 h later. Immunosuppression was calculated as the difference in Mantoux-induced erythema and induration at test sites compared to control sites. Human keratinocyte cell cultures, with and without ssUV and nicotinamide, were used for quantitative real-time reverse transcriptase-polymerase chain reaction assessment of TP53 and enzymes that regulate oxidative phosphorylation.

Results.—Nicotinamide cooperated with ssUV to increase enzymes involved in cellular energy metabolism and p53, and significantly protected against immunosuppression caused by UVB, longwave UVA and single and repeated ssUV exposures.

Conclusions.—Longwave UVA, which is poorly filtered by most sunscreens, was highly immune suppressive even at doses equivalent to 20 min of sun exposure. Nicotinamide, which protected against both UVB and UVA, is a promising agent for skin cancer prevention.

▶ In a world that is becoming obsessed with the benefits of anti-inflammatory agents, it is not a surprising twist that the immunosuppressive effects of ultraviolet (UV) light from sun exposure are correlated with increased skin carcinogenesis. This is an excellent randomized, intraindividual comparison study demonstrating the effectiveness of nicotinamide in reducing the immunosuppressive effects of UV light from sunlight up to 5 days after sun exposure. The immunosuppressive effects were measured by Mantoux reactions, minimal erythemal dose, the expression of tumor suppressor genes, and the body's own antioxidant mechanisms.

While the participant numbers for each group is on the low side, this is a very well-designed study using multiple methods for scientifically measuring the immunosuppression and stimulation as mentioned above.

The results of this study show diminished immunosuppression with the use of topical niacinamide; however, long-term follow-up is still necessary to prove that the reduced immunosuppression provided by topical nicotinamide actually reduces the rate and progression of cutaneous carcinogenesis.

J. Levin, DO

Viral DNA detection and *RAS* mutations in actinic keratosis and nonmelanoma skin cancers

Zaravinos A, Kanellou P, Spandidos DA (Univ of Crete, Greece)
Br J Dermatol 162:325-331, 2010

Background.—Actinic keratosis (AK) is a well-established precancerous skin lesion that has the potential to progress to squamous cell carcinoma (SCC). Basal cell carcinoma (BCC) is a locally aggressive slowly growing tumour that rarely metastasizes. A number of viruses have been proposed to play a role in the development of nonmelanoma skin cancers (NMSC), but the most plausible evidence to date suggests that cutaneous human papillomavirus (HPV) is the key instigating factor.

Objectives.—To evaluate the prevalence of HPV, cytomegalovirus (CMV), herpes simplex virus (HSV) and Epstein–Barr virus (EBV) and investigate their relationship with the presence of RAS gene mutations in cutaneous lesions obtained from nonimmunosuppressed patients.

Methods.—HPV, CMV, HSV and EBV detection was performed using polymerase chain reaction (PCR) in skin biopsies (26 AK, 12 SCC and 15 BCC samples) that were collected from immunocompetent patients. The RAS mutation incidence was also investigated in all cutaneous lesions by use of PCR/restriction fragment length polymorphism and direct DNA sequencing.

Results.—Seventeen out of 53 (32%) skin lesions were found to be positive for HPV DNA. The highest incidences of HPV infection were five of 15 (33%) in BCC and four of 12 (33%) in SCC specimens. The HPV incidence was eight of 26 (31%) in AK and eight of 53 (15%) in normal skin tissue. Twelve out of 53 (23%) skin lesions were CMV-positive. The highest incidence of CMV infection was six of 15 (40%), observed in BCC specimens. The CMV incidence was two of 26 (8%) in AK and four of 12 (33%) in SCC. No normal skin biopsy was found to be positive for CMV. All cutaneous samples were negative for HSV and EBV DNA, as assessed by our PCR-based assays. Only three samples, one AK (4%), one BCC (6%) and one SCC (8%), were found to carry a G>T transversion at the second position of *HRAS* codon 12. Both *HRAS* mutant SCC and BCC biopsies were HPV- and CMV-positive, as well.

Conclusions.—HPV DNA is detected in NMSC, AK and normal skin biopsies. Our results also indicate that CMV is involved in NMSC at higher levels than in premalignant lesions, whereas the virus was not detected in normal skin biopsies. HSV and EBV do not appear to be involved in the pathogenesis of cutaneous lesions. Moreover, we suggest that the *HRAS* codon 12 mutation is not a very common event in AK or NMSC. Finally, both viral infection and *HRAS* activation appear to represent independent factors in the aetiology of NMSC, samples of which were obtained from immunocompetent patients.

▶ Zaravinos et al present data confirming what was found in a similar study in 2003[1]: an increased prevalence of cytomegalovirus (CMV) in nonmelanoma skin cancer (NMSC) and no increase in the prevalence of Epstein-Barr virus (EBV) and herpes simplex virus (HSV). The specific subtypes of NMSC, such as basal cell carcinoma (BCC), squamous cell carcinoma (SCC), and actinic keratosis (AK), with the highest incidence of CMV varied between these 2 studies, with 1 showing the greatest incidence of CMV infections to be in premalignant lesions and the other showing the greatest incidence to be in BCC specimens. Therefore, Zaravinos et al's study further supports the idea that CMV may play a role in the pathogenesis of NMSC, and prevention of this infection may represent a future target for the prevention of NMSC. Studies to further characterize the specific role of CMV in NMSC are necessary. In addition, a larger sample size may help to settle some of the inconsistencies between data obtained in the 2 studies.

The role of both human papillomavirus (HPV) and *RAS* mutations in cutaneous oncogenesis has been studied in the past with varying results and was examined by Zaravinos et al. This study came to the important conclusion that although both HPV infection and *RAS* mutations were seen in the NMSC lesions, there is no direct relationship between these factors.

B. Berman, MD, PhD

Reference

1. Zafiropoulos A, Tsentelierou E, Billiri K, Spandidos DA. Human herpes viruses in non-melanoma skin cancers. *Cancer Lett.* 2003;198:77-81.

Photodynamic therapy with BF-200 ALA for the treatment of actinic keratosis: results of a prospective, randomized, double-blind, placebo-controlled phase III study
Szeimies R-M, Radny P, Sebastian M, et al (Regensburg Univ Hosp, Germany; Private Practice, Friedrichshafen, Germany; Private Practice, Mahlow, Germany; et al)
Br J Dermatol 163:386-394, 2010

Background.—Photodynamic therapy (PDT) with 5-aminolaevulinic acid (ALA) provides a therapeutic option for the treatment of actinic keratosis (AK). Different strategies are applied to overcome the chemical instability of ALA in solution and to improve skin penetration. A new stable nanoemulsion-based ALA formulation, BF-200 ALA, is currently in clinical development for PDT of AK.

Objectives.—To evaluate the efficacy and safety of PDT of AK with BF-200 ALA.

Methods.—The study was performed as a randomized, multicentre, double-blind, placebo-controlled, interindividual, two-armed trial with BF-200 ALA and placebo. A total of 122 patients with four to eight mild to moderate AK lesions on the face and/or the bald scalp were included in eight German study centres. The efficacy of BF-200 ALA after one and two PDT treatments was evaluated. BF-200 ALA was used in combination with two different light sources under illumination conditions defined by European competent authorities.

Results.—PDT with BF-200 ALA was superior to placebo PDT with respect to patient complete clearance rate (per-protocol group: 64% vs. 11%; $P < 0.0001$) and lesion complete clearance rate (per-protocol group: 81% vs. 22%) after the last PDT treatment. Statistically significant differences in the patient and lesion complete clearance rates and adverse effect profiles were observed for the two light sources, Aktilite® CL128 and PhotoDyn® 750, at both time points of assessment. The patient and lesion complete clearance rates after illumination with the Aktilite® CL128 were 96% and 99%, respectively.

Conclusions.—BF-200 ALA is a very effective new formulation for the treatment of AK with PDT. Marked differences between the efficacies and adverse effects were observed for the different light sources used.

Thus, PDT efficacy is dependent both on the drug and on the characteristics of the light source and the illumination conditions used.

▶ Over the past decade, photodynamic therapy (PDT) has emerged as a mainstream field therapy with efficacy and safety data comparable or superior to traditional field therapies, such as 5-fluorouracil, imiquimod, and diclofenac. What makes PDT particularly attractive is the limited downtime (generally 1 week in duration) associated with treatment side effects, such as scaling, significant irritation, crusting, weeping, and erosions compared with other field therapies whose visible cutaneous side effects can last weeks to months. The development of the nanoemulsion gel formulation containing 10% 5-aminolaevulinic acid (ALA) offers an easy-to-use gel alternative with the potential for improved epidermal penetration, short incubation times (3 hours), and efficacy and safety equivalent to the currently approved 20% ALA solution. The selection of ALA instead of methyl-ALA as the prodrug in the gel formulation avoids potential sensitization issues involving methylated ALA formulations. This formulation looks to be a promising addition to the PDT arsenal. A very important aspect of the study was its demonstration of the importance of carefully choosing which activating light source to use. Your choice of activating light sources can significantly alter your PDT outcomes.

G. Martin, MD

14 Nevi and Melanoma

A Multimarker Prognostic Assay for Primary Cutaneous Melanoma

Kashani-Sabet M, Venna S, Nosrati M, et al (Univ of California-San Francisco; et al)

Clin Cancer Res 15:6987-6992, 2009

Purpose.—To determine the prognostic significance of a multimarker assay incorporating expression levels of three molecular markers in primary cutaneous melanoma.

Experimental Design.—We assessed expression levels of NCOA3, SPP1, and RGS1 using immunohistochemical analysis in a tissue microarray cohort of 395 patients. For each marker, we identified optimal cut-points for expression intensity to predict disease-specific survival (DSS) and, as a secondary endpoint, sentinel lymph node (SLN) status. The cumulative overexpression of all three markers was embodied in a multimarker index, and its prognostic effect on DSS and SLN status was assessed using Cox regression, Kaplan-Meier analysis, and logistic regression. The prognostic effect of this multimarker assay on DSS was assessed in an independent cohort of 141 patients, in which marker expression levels were scored using immunohistochemical analysis of stained tissue sections.

Results.—Increasing multimarker index scores were significantly predictive of reduced DSS and increased SLN metastasis in the 395-patient cohort. Multivariate logistic regression analysis revealed multimarker expression scores as an independent predictor of SLN status ($P = 0.001$). Multivariate Cox regression analysis showed the independent effect of the multimarker index on DSS ($P < 0.001$). The multimarker index was the most significant factor predicting DSS when compared with other clinical and histologic factors, including SLN status ($P = 0.002$). Multimarker expression scores were also the most significantly predictive of DSS in the independent cohort ($P = 0.01$).

Conclusions.—These results describe a multimarker assay with independent prognostic effect on the prediction of survival associated with melanoma in two distinct cohorts (Table 4).

▶ In this interesting article, the authors developed and optimized 3 molecular markers—NCOA3, SPP1 (osteopontin), and RGS1—using a cohort of 395 patients. This cohort possessed at least 2 years of follow-up or a documented recurrence after sentinel lymph node examination, and it was, as expected, weighted toward melanoma of greater depth.

TABLE 4.—Multivariate Cox Regression Analysis of the Effect of Various Factors on DSS—Effect of the Digital Multimarker Index ($n = 255$)

Prognostic Factor	χ^2	Risk Ratio	P
Multimarker index	10.63	1.34	0.001
SLN status	9.12	2.09	0.003
Clark level	6.80	1.66	0.009
Ulceration	6.38	1.91	0.01
Sex	1.83	1.43	0.18
Tumor thickness	1.10	1.21	0.29
Age	0.95	1.08	0.33
Site	0.85	1.25	0.36

The authors then compared the expression level of this multimarker assay to an independent cohort of 141 patients from a completely different institution to assess its prognostic use. The multimarker assay was an independent predictor of both disease-specific survival and, in the latter cohort, a predictor of the likelihood of sentinel lymph node involvement.

Perhaps the most interesting aspect of this article was that the multimarker assay was a predictor of disease-specific survival even when sentinel lymph node status was included in the multivariate model because the determination of this expression level is made from simple immunohistochemical analysis of the primary tumor, without the risk or cost of an additional sentinel node procedure.

While this study is small and isolated in comparison with the large numbers of patients who are involved in the development of prognostic factors for inclusion in the American Joint Cancer Committee guidelines, it is extremely interesting to think that we are at the edge of developing immunohistochemical markers to be used upon tissue sections from the primary tumor, which might allow for a customized prognostic index and even customized therapy, to be developed without a need for additional surgical sampling.

W. A. High, MD, JD, MEng

Accuracy of teledermatology for pigmented neoplasms
Warshaw EM, Lederle FA, Grill JP, et al (Minneapolis Veterans Affairs Med Ctr, MN; et al)
J Am Acad Dermatol 61:753-765, 2009

Background.—Accurate diagnosis and management of pigmented lesions is critical because of the morbidity and mortality associated with melanoma.

Objective.—We sought to compare accuracy of store-and-forward teledermatology for pigmented neoplasms with standard, in-person clinic dermatology.

Methods.—We conducted a repeated measures equivalence trial involving veterans with pigmented skin neoplasms. Each lesion was evaluated by a clinic dermatologist and a teledermatologist; both generated a primary diagnosis, up to two differential diagnoses, and a management plan. The primary outcome was aggregated diagnostic accuracy (match of any chosen diagnosis with histopathology). We also compared the severity of inappropriately managed lesions and, for teledermatology, evaluated the incremental change in accuracy when polarized light dermatoscopy or contact immersion dermatoscopy images were viewed.

Results.—We enrolled 542 patients with pigmented lesions, most were male (96%) and Caucasian (97%). The aggregated diagnostic accuracy rates for teledermatology (macro images, polarized light dermatoscopy, and contact immersion dermatoscopy) were not equivalent (95% confidence interval for difference within ±10%) and were inferior (95% confidence interval lower bound <10%) to clinic dermatology. In general, the addition of dermatoscopic images did not significantly change teledermatology diagnostic accuracy rates. In contrast to diagnostic accuracy, rates of appropriate management plans for teledermatology were superior and/or equivalent to clinic dermatology (all image types: all lesions, and benign lesions). However, for the subgroup of malignant lesions (n = 124), the rate of appropriate management was significantly worse for teledermatology than for clinic dermatology (all image types). Up to 7 of 36 index melanomas would have been mismanaged via teledermatology.

Limitations.—Nondiverse study population and relatively small number of melanomas were limitations.

Conclusions.—In general, the diagnostic accuracy of teledermatology was inferior whereas management was equivalent to clinic dermatology. However, for the important subgroup of malignant pigmented lesions, both diagnostic and management accuracy of teledermatology was generally inferior to clinic dermatology and up to 7 of 36 index melanomas would have been mismanaged via teledermatology. Teledermatology and teledermatoscopy should be used with caution for patients with suspected malignant pigmented lesions.

▶ Even in very primitive trials of teledermatology, there appeared to be inherent limitations in dealing with malignant processes and specifically, pigmented lesions.[1] In this study, the authors seek to investigate directly the use of teledermatology, augmented not only by simple clinical photography but also with polarized light dermatoscopy and contact immersion dermatoscopy, with classic clinical examination.

While the study is relatively small and dominated by elderly white men (also the population is mostly affected by melanoma), there was clear superiority to clinical examination with regard to diagnostic accuracy. Perhaps most importantly, even with incorporation of dermatoscopy images, analyzed by experienced dermatologists (> 5 years experience with dermatoscopy), teledermatology alone would have resulted in mismanagement of over 20% of melanomas included in the study.

Does this diminish or doom employment of teledermatology? No, certainly not. It does point out a repeatable weakness, at least using current technology, but perhaps it even opens to debate the possibility of using teledermatology in *other* areas, outside of the evaluation of pigmented lesions, if for no other reason then to free clinic resources for the evaluation of pigmented processes, thereby leading to better overall resource utilization.

W. A. High, MD, JD, MEng

Reference

1. High WA, Houston MS, Calobrisi SD, Drage LA, McEvoy MT. Assessment of the accuracy of low-cost store-and-forward teledermatology consultation. *J Am Acad Dermatol.* 2000;42:776-783.

Characteristics Associated With Early and Late Melanoma Metastases
Brauer JA, Wriston CC, Troxel AB, et al (Univ of Pennsylvania, Philadelphia)
Cancer 116:415-423, 2010

Background.—Differences in risk factors for metastases at different time intervals after treatment have been described in several malignancies; however, to the authors' knowledge, no extensive study examining this issue in melanoma has been conducted to date.

Methods.—The authors performed a nested case-control study of patients with melanoma who presented with only local disease. Patients in the case group included 549 patients who developed metastases ≥6 months after surgery. Of these, 320 patients developed metastasis within 3 years after undergoing definitive surgery (early metastases [EM]), and 70 patients developed metastasis ≥8 years after undergoing definitive surgery (late metastases [LM]). For each case, a control patient was chosen who had melanoma but who did not develop metastases in the same interval. Univariate and conditional multivariate logistic regression were used in the analysis of 34 clinical and tumor characteristics.

Results.—Multivariate analysis confirmed previously established risk factors for metastases, such as increasing tumor thickness. In addition, the authors discovered that a personal history of nonmelanoma skin cancer ($P = .006$) and a history of cancer other than skin cancer ($P = .020$) also were associated with metastasis. In comparing the 320 EM patients with the 70 LM patients, EM patients were more likely to have thicker lesions ($P < .001$), ulcerated lesions ($P = .016$), and a history of nonmelanoma skin cancer ($P = .024$).

Conclusions.—In this study, 2 potentially novel risk factors for melanoma metastases were identified, and different profiles of risk factors were constructed for EM versus LM. These differences may be important in future risk identification and stratification for clinical trials and for the management and treatment of patients with melanoma.

▶ The incidence of melanoma continues to increase in the United States. It has been estimated that in 2009, 8650 Americans died of melanoma.[1] In light of these staggering and frightening statistics, investigators studied the characteristics involved in metastases of this deadly skin cancer. More specifically, the authors prospectively studied a cohort of 4196 patients with invasive melanoma confined to a primary site in their Pigmented Lesion Clinic from 1972 to 2005. Subsequently, 13.1% of the melanoma patients developed metastases. Investigators confirmed previously reported clinical risk factors for metastases, including male gender, older age, and the primary lesion being located on a site other than extremities. Histologically, lesions with vertical growth phase, increased thickness, ulceration, and microscopic satellites were at greater risk for metastases. Two previously unreported risk factors were patients having a history of nonmelanoma skin cancer and a history of cancer other than skin cancer. When comparing early metastasis (EM) with late metastasis (LM), the only statistically significant risk factor was patients with EM had thicker primary lesions than patients with LM. Results were obtained from a referral center and therefore may not be applicable to the general population due to selection bias.

S. Bellew, DO
J. Q. Del Rosso, DO

Reference

1. Rigel DS. Trends in dermatology: melanoma incidence. *Arch Dermatol.* 2010;146: 318.

Classifying ambiguous melanocytic lesions with FISH and correlation with clinical long-term follow up
Gaiser T, Kutzner H, Palmedo G, et al (Univ of Heidelberg, Germany; Dermatopathologie Friedrichshafen, Bodensee, Germany; et al)
Mod Pathol 23:413-419, 2010

Recently, initial studies describing the use of multicolor fluorescence *in situ* hybridization (FISH) for classifying melanocytic skin lesions have been published demonstrating a high sensitivity and specificity in discriminating melanomas from nevi. However, the majority of these studies included neither histologically ambiguous lesions nor a clinical long-term follow up. This study was undertaken to validate a special multicolor FISH test in histologically ambiguous melanocytic skin lesions with known clinical long-term follow up. FISH was scored by three independent pathologists in a series of 22 melanocytic skin lesions, including 12 ambiguous cases using four probes targeting chromosome 6p25, centromere 6, 6q23, and 11q13. The FISH results were compared with array comparative genomic hybridization data and correlated to the clinical long-term follow up (mean: 65 months). Pair-wise comparison between the interpretations of the observers showed a moderate to substantial agreement (κ 0.47–0.61). Comparing the FISH results with the clinical behavior reached an overall sensitivity of 60% and a specificity of 50% ($\chi^2 = 0.25$; $P = 0.61$) for later development of metastases. Comparison of array comparative genomic hybridization data with FISH analyses did not yield significant results but array comparative genomic hybridization data demonstrated that melanocytic skin lesions with the development of metastases showed significantly more chromosomal aberrations ($P < 0.01$) compared with melanocytic skin lesions without the development of metastases. The FISH technique with its present composition of locus-specific probes for *RREB1/MYB* and *CCND1* did not achieve a clinically useful sensitivity and specificity. However, a reassessment of the probes and better standardization of the method may lead to a valuable diagnostic tool.

▶ The authors used multicolored fluorescent in situ hybridization (FISH) studies to evaluate 12 ambiguous melanocytic lesions in patients with long-term clinical follow up. Recent articles have suggested that FISH may be helpful in distinguishing benign pigmented lesions from melanoma. The authors of this study elected to see if FISH could be useful in distinguishing ambiguous melanocytic lesions. After comparing the FISH results to the clinical outcomes, they determined that the FISH studies showed an overall sensitivity of 60% and a specificity of 50%. Thus, it appears that these particular FISH studies would not be very helpful in identifying the clinical outcome of ambiguous melanocytic lesions. The article suggests, however, that the promise of chromosomal analysis for determining clinical outcome of ambiguous melanocytic lesions remains open but that further refinement of the FISH probes is necessary.

S. M. Purcell, DO

Clinical responses observed with imatinib or sorafenib in melanoma patients expressing mutations in *KIT*
Handolias D, Hamilton AL, Salemi R, et al (Peter MacCallum Cancer Centre, East Melbourne, Victoria, Australia; Royal Prince Alfred Hosp, Camperdown, New South Wales, Australia)
Br J Cancer 102:1219-1223, 2010

Background.—Mutations in *KIT* are more frequent in specific melanoma subtypes, and response to KIT inhibition is likely to depend on the identified mutation.

Methods.—A total of 32 patients with metastatic acral or mucosal melanoma were screened for mutations in *KIT* exons 11, 13 and 17.

Results.—*KIT* mutations were found in 38% of mucosal and in 6% of acral melanomas. Three patients were treated with imatinib and one with sorafenib. All four patients responded to treatment, but three have since progressed within the brain.

Conclusions.—The observed clinical responses support further investigation of KIT inhibitors in metastatic melanoma, selected according to *KIT* mutation status.

▶ This is an interesting study where *KIT* mutation tumor characteristics, and predicted sensitivity to tyrosine kinase inhibitors, were able to guide therapy in patients expressing *KIT* mutations in mucosal melanomas with impressive results, including symptom improvement within days in 50% of the cases and significant reduction in the sum of target lesions. However, for some reason yet to be elucidated, the efficacy of tyrosine kinase inhibitors seems to be truncated by resistance and substantially decreases over time to the point of allowing the development of fatal brain metastasis in 3 out of 4 cases. Resistance was addressed by the authors as possibly related to pharmacokinetic changes including increased drug clearance and conformational alterations of the kinase preventing the appropriate drug-kinase interaction. In the case of brain disease, tyrosine kinase inhibitors seem to work initially according to the cases reported where the metastasis tended to develop only over time, which cannot be explained by limited penetration to the brain. We hypothesize that some degree of local tolerance and/or antidrug antibody formation, which depends on time to develop, cannot be disregarded because further increases in dosage failed to generate any response. The authors also mention the need for a multidrug approach in case of less-sensitive mutations. This study represents a step in the right direction toward the molecular-targeted approach for the treatment of melanomas.

B. Berman, MD, PhD

Dermoscopy of pigmented lesions on mucocutaneous junction and mucous membrane
Lin J, Koga H, Takata M, et al (Shinshu Univ School of Medicine, Asahi, Matsumoto, Japan)
Br J Dermatol 161:1255-1261, 2009

Background.—The dermoscopic features of pigmented lesions on the mucocutaneous junction and mucous membrane are different from those on hairy skin. Differentiation between benign lesions and malignant melanomas of these sites is often difficult.

Objective.—To define the dermoscopic patterns of lesions on the mucocutaneous junction and mucous membrane, and assess the applicability of standard dermoscopic algorithms to these lesions.

Patients and Methods.—An unselected consecutive series of 40 lesions on the mucocutaneous junction and mucous membrane was studied. All the lesions were imaged using dermoscopy devices, analysed for dermoscopic patterns and scored with algorithms including the ABCD rule, Menzies method, 7-point checklist, 3-point checklist and the CASH algorithm.

Results.—Benign pigmented lesions of the mucocutaneous junction and mucous membrane frequently presented a dotted-globular pattern (25%), a homogeneous pattern (25%), a fish scale-like pattern (18·8%) and a hyphal pattern (18·8%), while melanomas of these sites showed a multi-component pattern (75%) and a homogeneous pattern (25%). The fish scale-like pattern and hyphal pattern were considered to be variants of the ring-like pattern. The sensitivities of the ABCD rule, Menzies method, 7-point checklist, 3-point checklist and CASH algorithm in diagnosing mucosal melanomas were 100%, 100%, 63%, 88% and 100%; and the specificities were 100%, 94%, 100%, 94% and 100%, respectively.

Conclusion.—The ring-like pattern and its variants (fish scale-like pattern and hyphal pattern) are frequently observed as well as the dotted-globular pattern and homogeneous pattern in mucosal melanotic macules. The algorithms for pigmented lesions on hairy skin also apply to those on the mucocutaneous junction and mucous membrane with high sensitivity and specificity.

▶ This article concludes that the algorithms for pigmented lesions on hair-bearing skin also apply to those on the mucocutaneous junction and mucous membranes with high sensitivity and specificity. This is helpful information because there is a paucity of studies involving dermoscopy and lesions of the mucous membranes. However, an important message that we can also draw is to be cautious about how we interpret dermoscopic images on mucocutaneous membranes because the changes may not have the same significance they have in hair-bearing skin. Emphasized in this regard is how color changes, such as hues of red, may not have the same significance because of naturally increased vascularity on mucous membranes. More important was the observation that what may appear to be new or different dermoscopic patterns may simply vary with the vantage point of the observer/evaluator. Such was the case of the new hyphal and fish scale patterns described, which at first appeared to be very meaningful and on closer observation were simply variations of the ring-like pattern viewed from a different angle. The latter emphasizes the old adage that beauty is in the eye of the beholder and sometimes we see what we want to see, so we need to be careful not to read our bias or wishes into dermoscopic patterns.

A. Torres, MD, JD

Discordance in the histopathologic diagnosis of melanoma at a melanoma referral center
Shoo BA, Sagebiel RW, Kashani-Sabet M (Univ of California, San Francisco)
J Am Acad Dermatol 62:751-756, 2010

Background.—Histopathologic analysis remains the gold standard for the pathologic diagnosis of melanoma. Numerous histologic criteria are used to diagnose melanoma, but none alone are sufficient to establish this diagnosis. Therefore, differentiating between benign pigmented lesions and melanoma may be controversial. Although several studies have examined the interobserver variability in the pathological diagnosis of melanoma, the prevalence of discordant diagnoses of melanocytic neoplasms is unknown.

Objective.—We sought to examine the discordance rate of melanoma diagnoses referred to our pigmented lesion clinic, a subset of the University

of California, San Francisco (UCSF) Department of Dermatology and Comprehensive Cancer Center Melanoma Center during a 2-year period.
Methods.—A total of 392 new patients given a diagnosis of thin melanoma (melanoma in situ, stage IA, stage IB) or benign nevus were referred in 2006 and 2007, with initial diagnoses rendered by an outside dermatopathologist or surgical pathologist. Subsequently, these specimens were re-evaluated by routine histopathologic examination at the UCSF Dermatopathology Service and a distinct diagnosis was rendered. The two available diagnoses were compared, and discordance was defined as the lack of agreement between two pathologists when rendering a benign versus malignant versus ambiguous diagnosis.
Results.—The discordance rate of melanomas and nevi between the referring centers and UCSF was 14.3%.
Limitations.—This review was limited in that there were few patients with benign pigmented lesions referred to the pigmented lesion clinic at UCSF.
Conclusion.—The level of discordance in the routine histopathologic interpretation of melanocytic neoplasms can be high.

▶ The gold standard for diagnosis of melanoma is histopathologic diagnosis. While there are numerous histopathologic criteria for the diagnosis of melanoma, they are, by nature, subjected to interpretation by the reading pathologist. This qualitative interpretation of criteria may lead to discordance (disagreement) of diagnosis. Several studies have clearly established that discordance does exist in the diagnosis of pigmented lesions. This article is a retrospective study from the University of California, San Francisco (UCSF) designed to determine the discordance rate of pigmented lesion diagnoses referred to their center. Overall, the discordance rate (difference in the diagnosis of the referred case to the diagnosis rendered at UCSF) was 14.3%. Of 392 cases referred to their center, they established that 56 cases had discordant diagnoses. The authors suggest that this rate may be underestimated, particularly because benign pigmented lesions are not generally referred to their center. Furthermore, they suggest that discordance is most important because a patient with a melanoma may receive a diagnosis of benign nevus with potential fatal implications, or a patient with a benign lesion may receive a diagnosis of melanoma resulting in long-term surveillance or insurance problems. Interestingly, when reviewing the discordant cases, it is clear that the greatest number of cases were those initially diagnosed as malignant and reviewed as benign or ambiguous (33 benign and 3 ambiguous) versus those initially diagnosed as benign or ambiguous and subsequently reviewed as malignant (5 benign and 5 ambiguous). As a clinician, I am somewhat comforted that the tendency in the discordance is toward diagnosing benign lesions as malignant rather than toward diagnosing malignant lesions as benign.

S. M. Purcell, DO

Disparity in Melanoma: A Trend Analysis of Melanoma Incidence and Stage at Diagnosis Among Whites, Hispanics, and Blacks in Florida

Hu S, Parmet Y, Allen G, et al (Univ of Miami Miller School of Medicine, FL; Ben-Gurion Univ of the Negev, Beer-Sheva, Israel)
Arch Dermatol 145:1369-1374, 2009

Objective.—To examine and compare the temporal trends in melanoma incidence and stage at diagnosis among whites, Hispanics, and blacks in Florida from 1990 to 2004.

Design.—Cross-sectional and retrospective analysis.

Setting.—Florida Cancer Data System.

Patients.—Melanoma cases with known stage and race/ethnicity reported from 1990 to 2004.

Main Outcome Measures.—Age-adjusted melanoma incidence and stage at diagnosis.

Results.—Of 41 072 cases of melanoma, 39 670 cases were reported for white non-Hispanics (WNHs), 1148 for white Hispanics (WHs), and 254 for blacks. Melanoma incidence rates increased by 3.0% per year among WNH men ($P < .001$), 3.6% among WNH women ($P < .001$), 3.4% among WH women ($P = .01$), and 0.9% among WH men ($P = .52$), while remaining relatively stable among black men and women. Both WHs and blacks had significantly more advanced melanoma at presentation: 18% of WH and 26% of black patients had either regional or distant-stage melanoma at diagnosis compared with 12% of WNH patients. The proportion of distant-stage melanoma diagnosed among WHs and blacks changed little from 1990 to 2004, compared with a steady decrease in the percentage of melanoma cases diagnosed at distant stage among WNHs ($P < .001$). Such differences in the time trends of the proportion of distant-stage melanoma remained after excluding in situ cases.

Conclusions.—The rising melanoma incidence among WNHs and WHs emphasizes the need for primary prevention. The persistence of disparity in melanoma stage at diagnosis among WHs, blacks, and WNHs warrants closer examination of secondary prevention efforts in minority groups.

▶ The authors of this study successfully demonstrate that ethnic minority groups are suffering not only delayed and primarily late diagnosis of melanoma but also of decreased odds of survival because of this delay.

The study itself only vaguely quantifies the reasons for this occurring, but the inference is clear—socioeconomic and cultural/social reasons are most likely behind this. The authors describe the disparity in diagnosis between white, Hispanic (including white Hispanic), and blacks and rightly describe that existing public and health care education reaches the white or nonethnic populations with greater frequency and success.

This point is the main success of the article. In describing the vast difference between ethnic groups in their early stage diagnosis and the consequential results of that, the need for an improved and focused education program is indisputable.

For practitioners this information is tantamount to a wake-up call. Past thoughts on skin pigment and prevalence of skin cancer and melanoma may need to be re-thought. Although it is true that darker pigmented individuals are statistically at a lower risk, by not educating all patients, regardless of race, on the importance of self-examination and occasional professional examination, we risk putting an increasingly larger segment of our population at greater risk.

Through clinical practice and with the aid of professional societies, a new message needs to be developed in order to permeate social, cultural, and socio-economic boundaries preventing the message from being heard and understood.

R. I. Ceilley, MD

Efficacy of Skin Self-Examination Practices for Early Melanoma Detection

Pollitt RA, Geller AC, Brooks DR, et al (Stanford Univ School of Medicine, CA; Harvard School of Public Health, Boston, MA; Boston Univ School of Public Health, MA; et al)

Cancer Epidemiol Biomarkers Prev 18:3018-3023, 2009

Although skin self-examination (SSE) may increase rates of early melanoma detection, the efficacy of different SSE practices has not been thoroughly studied. We examined associations between SSE practices and tumor thickness in patients with recently diagnosed melanoma.

Methods.—321 melanoma patients at three hospitals completed questionnaires on demographics and SSE practices. Patient-reported SSE was measured by routine examination of 13 specific body areas, frequency of mole examination, and use of a melanoma picture aid to assist with SSE. Histologic diagnoses and Breslow depth were confirmed by dermatopathologists. Regression analyses were used to calculate ratios of geometric mean tumor thickness and odds ratios for having thicker versus thinner tumors for different SSE behaviors.

Results.—Rates of SSE varied considerably by SSE item. Patients routinely examining at least some of their skin had thinner melanomas [adjusted geometric mean tumor ratio, 0.73; 95% confidence interval (95% CI), 0.50-0.94]. Frequency of mole examination did not predict tumor thickness. Using a melanoma picture as a SSE aid was strongly associated with reduced tumor thickness (adjusted ratio, 0.75; 95% CI, 0.66-0.85 for ever versus never use). A composite measure of thoroughness of SSE was the best predictor of thickness (adjusted ratio, 0.58; 95% CI, 0.36-0.75) for high versus low thoroughness.

Conclusions.—SSE was associated with decreased tumor thickness by most measures. However, the diverse rates of SSE practices and the distinct associations between these practices and melanoma thickness suggest a complexity in SSE that should be addressed in future studies. SSE should be evaluated by more than one measure.

▶ The authors take a close look at skin self-examination (SSE) and its potential effectiveness in early melanoma detection as well as the relationships between

SSE, tumor thickness, and overall melanoma survival rates. The stratification of SSE into different subtypes (eg, specific and different SSE behaviors) has not previously been evaluated to the extent demonstrated in this study.

The study is well designed, and the authors meet their objectives to obtain an improved understanding of the effectiveness of SSE, which has previously been limited by variable study definitions (eg, number or percent body sites examined, frequency and method of examination, and use of supplemental techniques to SSE, such as the use of photographs).

The authors used a questionnaire to evaluate the specific SSE-associated behaviors and practices performed by newly diagnosed melanoma patients before their confirmed diagnosis. The authors examined the effect of 3 specific SSE practices on the level of melanoma severity (eg, by tumor thickness) at diagnosis.

The study is of adequate sample size. The duration (2 years) is more than ample to assure its accuracy. The stratification of SSE into 3 specific measures (routine examination of 13 specific body areas, frequency of mole examination, and use of photographs of the melanoma) clearly demonstrates an advance from previous studies providing greater detail for statistical analysis. The authors used linear and logistic multivariate regression analyses to assess the effect of SSE on tumor thickness. The data obtained provide unique and practical information for both the academic-based and the community-based clinicians (eg, patients who had never used a melanoma photograph to help with SSE in the past had higher odds of having a thicker tumor when compared with those who had [odds ratio, 2.02; 95% confidence interval, 0.86-4.74 for more than 4 mm vs lesser than or equal to 1 mm tumor thickness]). A composite measure assessing the thoroughness of SSE by combining first and third techniques was the strongest predictor of tumor thickness.

A major limitation to the study is the use of patient-reported SSE as opposed to the use of an outside source for such evaluation. Positive aspects of this study include the timely completion of study surveys within 3 months of melanoma diagnosis, the use of 3 SSE practices, and the correlation of these practices with a dermatopathologist-confirmed diagnosis of melanoma.

B. P. Glick, DO, MPH

Factors Associated with False-Negative Sentinel Lymph Node Biopsy in Melanoma Patients
Scoggins CR, Martin RCG, Ross MI, et al (Univ of Louisville School of Medicine, KY; Univ of Texas M.D. Anderson Cancer Ctr, Houston; et al)
Ann Surg Oncol 17:709-717, 2010

Introduction.—Some melanoma patients who undergo sentinel lymph node (SLN) biopsy will have false-negative (FN) results. We sought to determine the factors and outcomes associated with FN SLN biopsy.

Methods.—Analysis was performed of a prospective multi-institutional study that included patients with melanoma of thickness > 1.0 mm who underwent SLN biopsy. FN results were defined as the proportion of node-positive patients who had a tumor-negative sentinel node biopsy. Kaplan—Meier survival analysis and univariate and multivariate analyses were performed.

Results.—This analysis included 2,451 patients with median follow-up of 61 months. FN, true-positive (TP), and true-negative (TN) SLN results were found in 59 (10.8%), 486 (19.8%), and 1,906 (77.8%) patients, respectively. On univariate analysis comparing the FN with TP groups, respectively, the following factors were significantly different: age (52.6 vs. 47.6 years, $p = 0.004$), thickness (mean 2.1 vs. 3.1 mm, $p = 0.003$), lymphovascular invasion (LVI; 3.7 vs. 13.7%, $p = 0.037$), and local/in-transit recurrence (LITR; 32.2 vs. 12.4%, $p < 0.0001$); these factors remained significant on multivariate analysis. Overall 5-year survival was greater in the TN group (86.7%) compared with the TP (62.3%) and FN (51.3%) groups ($p < 0.0001$); however, there was no significant difference in overall survival comparing the TP and FN groups ($p = 0.32$).

Conclusions.—This is the largest study to evaluate FN SLN results in melanoma, with a FN rate of 10.8%. FN results are associated with greater patient age, lower mean thickness, less frequent LVI, and greater risk of LITR. However, survival of patients with FN SLN is not statistically worse than that of patients with TP SLN.

▶ Although not perfect, the sentinel lymph node (SLN) biopsy in patients with melanoma is used by clinicians to provide clinically relevant prognostic information. As noted by the article, false-negative results do occur. To that end, Scoggins et al performed an impressive, large, prospective, multi-institutional study involving 2451 patients to try to identify both the factors and the outcomes associated with false-negative SLN biopsies. The study included patients with melanoma and Breslow thickness of > 1.0 mm who underwent SLN biopsy. The conclusions of the study found that when comparing false-negative and true-positive patient groups, the following factors were associated with false-negative results: greater patient age, lower mean thickness, less frequent lymphovascular invasion, and local/in-transit recurrence. Overall, false negatives were identified in 10.8% of the patients. Interestingly, both surgical error and pathological assessment of the nodal specimen were mentioned in the article; however, they were not identified as conclusive factors. The article noted that the vast majority of patients in the study were admitted by centers with ample experience in SLN biopsies. It would be interesting to note whether an element, such as surgical error, would become a significant factor for false-negative SLNs if conducted in other less experienced centers, but further studies would be needed. Also of interest was the conclusion that even in patients with false-negative results, there was no significant difference in overall survival comparing the true positives with the false negatives. Overall, the article achieved its objective and provides further insight into an interesting topic in the use of SLN biopsy in melanoma management.

B. D. Michaels, DO
J. Q. Del Rosso, DO

Histological regression in primary melanoma: not a predictor of sentinel lymph node metastasis in a cohort of 397 patients
Socrier Y, Lauwers-Cances V, Lamant L, et al (Paul Sabatier-Toulouse III Univ, Toulouse; et al)
Br J Dermatol 162:830-834, 2010

Background.—Regression has been proposed as a potential marker of dissemination in thin melanomas. Previous studies have shown conflicting results.

Objective.—To determine if regression in melanoma is associated with an increased risk of sentinel lymph node (SLN) metastasis.

Methods.—A cohort analysis was conducted. Data on all patients were collected on a standardized case report form during 10 years. A total of 397 consecutive patients with melanoma who underwent a SLN biopsy were analysed. All cases of melanoma and SLN biopsies were examined by the same two pathologists. Differences between melanomas with and without SLN metastasis were compared using Fisher's exact test or the two-sample *t*-test and the χ^2 test. Multivariable logistic regression was used to adjust for possible confounding factors.

Results.—We analysed 397 patients (411 melanomas) who underwent a SLN biopsy. The median Breslow index was $1 \cdot 8$ mm (interquartile range $1 \cdot 1-3$). Regression was observed in 23% ($n = 94$). SLN metastases were observed in 26% ($n = 106$). The frequency of SLN metastasis was 16% in melanomas with regression and 29% without regression ($P = 0 \cdot 012$). The adjusted odds ratio (OR) for regressive melanoma was $0 \cdot 9$ [95% confidence interval (CI) $0 \cdot 4-1 \cdot 9$; $P = 0 \cdot 777$]. The risk of SLN metastasis was increased in melanoma cases with a Breslow index from $1 \cdot 5$ to $< 2 \cdot 0$ mm (adjusted OR $3 \cdot 1$; 95% CI $1 \cdot 4-7 \cdot 1$; $P = 0 \cdot 006$) and $\geq 2 \cdot 0$ mm (adjusted OR $3 \cdot 5$; 95% CI $1 \cdot 7-7 \cdot 4$; $P = 0 \cdot 001$) and ulceration of the melanoma (adjusted OR $1 \cdot 8$; 95% CI $1 \cdot 1-3 \cdot 2$; $P = 0 \cdot 03$).

Conclusion.—Regression is not an independent predictor of the risk of SLN metastasis in melanoma.

▶ The prognostic role of regression in melanoma has been unclear, with several studies suggesting a worse prognosis for patients with a regressed melanoma and others indicating that regression is not associated with an increased risk of lymphatic metastasis. In many centers, regression is used as criteria for patients to undergo sentinel lymph node (SLN) examination in thin melanomas.

This article strongly suggests that histologic regression is not associated with an increased risk of SLN metastasis and that histologic regression should not be used as an independent reason for SLN biopsy.

This study is strengthened by the facts that 10 years of data involving 397 consecutive patients undergoing SLN biopsy were evaluated and by the same 2 pathologists. The criteria for SLN biopsy referral included Breslow thickness ≥ 1 mm, histological signs of regression, ulceration, and Clark level $> III$. As a result, many thin melanomas were evaluated. Positive SLN biopsies were seen less frequently in the patients with regression. This was especially noted in the thinner melanomas. When strictly statistically analyzed, the effect of regression on the risk of SLN metastasis was nonsignificant. The risk of SLN metastasis was increased in intermediate and thick melanomas and if ulceration was present.

The authors offer an explanation that regression in thicker melanomas may be a result of a feedback mechanism where melanoma cells may have reached a lymph node, stimulating activated lymphocytes against melanoma cells, whereas regression in thinner melanomas may be a result of a locally triggered immune response.

This article is helpful in further clarifying the criteria for referral for SLN biopsy. Regression is not supported as a factor with prognostic significance for SLN metastasis.

The 2 prognostic criteria remain tumor thickness and ulceration.

E. M. Billingsley, MD

Increased Melanoma Risk in Parkinson Disease: A Prospective Clinicopathological Study

Bertoni JM, for the North American Parkinson's and Melanoma Survey Investigators (Univ of Nebraska Med Ctr and Veterans Affairs Med Ctr, Omaha; et al)
Arch Neurol 67:347-352, 2010

Objective.—To evaluate the possible association of Parkinson disease (PD) and melanoma in North America.

Design, Setting, and Patients.—Thirty-one centers enrolled patients with idiopathic PD. At visit 1, a neurologist obtained a medical history. At visit 2, a dermatologist recorded melanoma risk factors, performed a whole-body examination, and performed a biopsy of lesions suggestive of melanoma for evaluation by a central dermatopathology laboratory. We compared overall prevalence of melanoma with prevalence calculated from the US Surveillance Epidemiology and End Results (SEER) cancer database and the American Academy of Dermatology skin cancer screening programs.

Results.—A total of 2106 patients (mean [SD] age, 68.6 [10.6] years; duration of PD, 7.1 [5.7] years) completed the study. Most (84.8%) had received levodopa. Dermatology examinations revealed 346 pigmented lesions; dermatopathological findings confirmed 20 in situ melanomas (0.9%) and 4 invasive melanomas (0.2%). In addition, histories revealed 68 prior melanomas (3.2%). Prevalence (5-year limited duration) of invasive malignant melanoma in the US cohort of patients with PD (n = 1692) was 2.24-fold higher (95% confidence interval, 1.21-4.17) than expected in age- and sex-matched populations in the US SEER database. Age- or sex-adjusted relative risk of any melanoma for US patients was more than 7 times that expected from confirmed cases in American Academy of Dermatology skin cancer screening programs.

Conclusions.—Melanoma prevalence appears to be higher in patients with PD than in the general population. Despite difficulties in comparing other databases with this study population, the study supports increased melanoma screening in patients with PD.

▶ This large prospective study evaluated the possible association of Parkinson disease and melanoma. The prevalence of melanoma in Parkinson disease this North American study reported is 1.1% and suggests that the risk of melanoma may be higher than in comparable populations.

A concern might be that the increased melanoma prevalence is because of the use of levodopa in Parkinson patients. However, this study found no evidence that levodopa increases the incidence of melanoma.

However, this study supports increased melanoma screenings in patients with Parkinson disease.

J. L. Smith, MD

Is There a Benefit to Sentinel Lymph Node Biopsy in Patients With T4 Melanoma?
Gajdos C, Griffith KA, Wong SL, et al (Univ of Michigan Health System, Ann Arbor; Univ of Michigan Comprehensive Cancer Ctr, Ann Arbor)
Cancer 115:5752-5760, 2009

Background.—Controversy exists as to whether patients with thick (Breslow depth >4 mm), clinically lymph node-negative melanoma require sentinel lymph node (SLN) biopsy. The authors examined the impact of SLN biopsy on prognosis and outcome in this patient population.

Methods.—A review of the authors' institutional review board-approved melanoma database identified 293 patients with T4 melanoma who underwent surgical excision between 1998 and 2007. Patient demographics, histologic features, and outcome were recorded and analyzed.

Results.—Of 227 T4 patients who had an SLN biopsy, 107 (47%) were positive. The strongest predictors of a positive SLN included angiolymphatic invasion, satellitosis, or ulceration of the primary tumor. Patients with a T4 melanoma and a negative SLN had a significantly better 5-year distant disease-free survival (DDFS) (85.3% vs 47.8%; $P < .0001$) and overall survival (OS) (80% vs 47%; $P < .0001$) compared with those with metastases to the SLN. For SLN-positive patients, only angiolymphatic invasion was a significant predictor of DDFS, with a hazard ratio of 2.29 ($P = .007$). Ulceration was not significant when examining SLN-positive patients but the most significant factor among SLN-negative patients, with a hazard ratio of 5.78 ($P = .02$). Increasing Breslow thickness and mitotic rate were also significantly associated with poorer outcome. Patients without ulceration or SLN metastases had an extremely good prognosis, with a 5-year OS >90% and a 5-year DDFS of 95%.

Conclusions.—Clinically lymph node-negative T4 melanoma cases should be strongly considered for SLN biopsy, regardless of Breslow depth. SLN lymph node status is the most significant prognostic sign among these patients. T4 patients with a negative SLN have an excellent prognosis in the absence of ulceration and should not be considered candidates for adjuvant high-dose interferon.

▶ The management of melanoma with Breslow depth greater than 1 mm remains nonstandardized. Most experts recommend consideration of sentinel lymph node (SLN) biopsy for Breslow depth between 1 and 4 mm. However, many clinicians argue that for deeper lesions, SLN biopsy may not be necessary because of the relatively high rate of regional and systemic metastases.

This article reports a significant prognostic advantage for melanoma lesions with Breslow depth > 4 mm with a negative SLN biopsy. As discussed, consideration for adjuvant interferon therapy may be undertaken in patients with evidence of systemic disease or with deeper Breslow depth lesions. The authors argue that lymph node-negative patients have a much more favorable prognosis and therefore should not be considered for adjuvant therapy, offering clinicians better information with regard to entertaining systemic therapy.

The results of this study add to the large amount of literature regarding SLN biopsy and its prognostic value to clinicians and patients. This is vital information for clinicians to be aware of, as patients with melanoma lesions > 4 mm in Breslow depth have historically been thought to have a poor prognosis. The decision for SLN biopsy should be considered and discussed thoroughly in this subset of patients.

R. I. Ceilley, MD

J. B. Wilson, MD

Large congenital melanocytic nevi and neurocutaneous melanocytosis: One pediatric center's experience
Lovett A, Maari C, Decarie J-C, et al (Sainte-Justine Hosp Ctr, Montreal, Quebec, Canada)
J Am Acad Dermatol 61:766-774, 2009

Background.—Large congenital melanocytic nevi (LCMN) predispose to neurocutaneous melanocytosis (NCM), which is associated with significant morbidity and mortality.

Objective.—To identify risk factors for NCM in patients with LCMN and suggest guidelines for their management.

Methods.—Medical records of patients with LCMN were reviewed at Sainte-Justine Hospital between 1980 and 2006. Presence of multiple satellite nevi and posterior midline location were evaluated as risk factors for NCM using chi-square test. Magnetic resonance imaging scans were reviewed by a neuroradiologist.

Results.—Twenty-six of 52 patients underwent radiologic investigation. Six of 26 (23%) had NCM. Patients with this condition are more likely to have multiple satellite nevi (100% vs 50%, $P = .03$) and have a trend to posterior midline location of their LCMN (100% vs 60%, $P = .08$).

Patients with NCM are more likely to have both multiple satellite nevi and posterior midline location (100% vs 25%, $P = .002$). Radiologic findings are also presented.

Limitations.—This was a retrospective case series with imprecise chart data in 38% of cases.

Conclusion.—The presence of multiple satellite nevi alone or with associated posterior midline location of LCMN is associated with a higher risk of NCM. We recommend magnetic resonance imaging testing before 4 months of age in patients with these features.

▶ Lovett et al sought to determine if there were notable risk factors predisposing patients to neurocutaneous melanocytosis (NCM). To this end, the article achieves its objective. This both informative and largely persuasive article found that there is a statistically significant correlation between NCM and the presence of multiple satellite nevi (MSN) alone (P value = .03) or in association with posterior midline location of large congenital melanocytic nevi (PML with LCMN) (P value = .002). If such findings are present, the authors recommend magnetic resonance imaging (MRI) before 4 months of age in these patients. It should be noted that this study was not without its limitations. First and foremost, the study was based on a retrospective analysis, which was limited in size. Considering the relative rarity of LCMN, the study population was considerable in number. Of the 200 patients reviewed, 52 patients met qualifying criteria for the study, and only 26 of those patients had radiographic analysis for NCM. Of these 26 patients evaluated radiographically, 6 patients had NCM. Thus, 20 of the 26 criteria-eligible patients did not have NCM. A future study with a larger sample size may be necessary to lend additional confirmation to the identified correlation. Until then, based on the patients identified, the study provides a statistically convincing correlation and one that is hard for the dermatologist to ignore given the pediatric population that NCM affects and its potential sequelae. Thus, without contrary evidence, practitioners should consider conducting MRI testing for NCM before 4 months of age in all patients with MSN and PML with LCMN, based on the findings in this article.

B. D. Michaels, DO
J. Q. Del Rosso, DO

Low rates of clinical recurrence after biopsy of benign to moderately dysplastic melanocytic nevi
Goodson AG, Florell SR, Boucher KM, et al (Univ of Utah Health Sciences Ctr, Salt Lake City)
J Am Acad Dermatol 62:591-596, 2010

Background.—Little is known about the recurrence/persistence rates of dysplastic nevi (DN) after biopsy, and whether incompletely removed DN should be re-excised to prevent recurrence.

Objective.—Our purpose was to determine the recurrence rates of previously biopsied DN, and to assess whether biopsy method, margin involvement, congenital features, epidermal location, and degree of dysplasia are associated with recurrence.

Methods.—Patients having a history of a "nevus biopsy" at least 2 years earlier were assessed for clinical recurrence. Slides of original lesions were re-reviewed by a dermatopathologist.

Results.—A total of 271 nevus biopsy sites were assessed in 115 patients. Of 195 DN with greater than 2 years of follow-up, 7 (3.6%) demonstrated recurrence on clinical examination. In all, 98 DN had a follow-up period of at least 4 years with no clinical recurrence. Of 61 benign nevus biopsy sites examined, clinical recurrence was observed in two (3.3%). For all nevi, recurrence was significantly associated with shave biopsy technique but not with nevus dysplasia or subtype, or the presence of positive margin or congenital features.

Limitations.—Most biopsies were performed in a pigmented lesion clinic at a single tertiary referral center. Determinations of nevus recurrence were made on clinical rather than histologic grounds, and follow-up times were limited in some cases.

Conclusion.—In this cohort, rates of clinical recurrence after biopsy of DN and benign nevi were extremely low. Re-excision of nevi, including mildly to moderately DN with a positive margin, may not be necessary.

▶ The significance of dysplastic melanocytic nevi is in its relation to melanoma. Dysplastic nevi may mimic melanoma, be risk factors for developing melanoma, and occasionally be precursors to melanoma. Although most clinicians will agree that severely dysplastic nevi warrant re-excision, controversy still exists on whether there is a need to completely re-excise nevi with mild to moderate dysplasia. Current practice by clinicians according to 1 survey study indicates that dermatologists routinely re-excise incompletely removed dysplastic nevi with moderate or greater atypia or when recommended by the pathologist.[1] The dilemma lies in whether there is likelihood of recurrence in incompletely excised mild to moderately dysplastic nevi. This retrospective study assessed 271 nevus biopsies in 115 patients in an effort to determine recurrence rates in these melanocytic lesions. In fact, researchers found very low recurrence rates (3%-4%) regardless of nevus subtype, positive margins, or congenital features. The only statistically significant association found was in biopsy technique. Shave biopsies were more significantly associated ($P = .045$) with recurrence of nevi. The difference was accentuated when punch biopsies were compared with shave biopsies. It is unclear whether this is because of recurrence being more likely to develop from deep rather than lateral margins or if results are because of the fact that punch biopsies are often done on smaller lesions.

Clearly, further research with longer duration of follow-up is needed to develop clear guidelines on management of dysplastic nevi. This study lends support to the option of conservative monitoring of these lesions in light of results that indicate low likelihood of recurrence. The decision to observe over re-excision should be made on individual basis as personal or family history of melanoma may be a factor. However, the main goal of treating patients with dysplastic nevi continues to be modifying potential risk factors for skin cancer, including recommendation of sun-protective measures and regular monitoring of patients for early detection.

S. Bellew, DO

J. Q. Del Rosso, DO

Reference

1. Fung MA. Terminology and management of dysplastic nevi: responses from 145 dermatologists. *Arch Dermatol.* 2003;139:1374-1375.

Melanoma and Melanocytic Tumors of Uncertain Malignant Potential in Children, Adolescents and Young Adults—The Stanford Experience 1995–2008
Berk DR, Labuz E, Dadras SS, et al (Stanford Univ Med Ctr, CA)
Pediatr Dermatol 27:244-254, 2010

Pediatric melanoma is difficult to study because of its rarity, possible biological differences in preadolescents compared with adolescents, and challenges of differentiating true melanoma from atypical spitzoid neoplasms. Indeterminant lesions are sometimes designated as melanocytic tumors of uncertain malignant potential (MelTUMPs). We performed a retrospective, single-institution review of melanomas, MelTUMPs and Spitz nevi with atypical features (SNAFs) in patients at 21 years of age and younger from 1995 to 2008. We identified 13 patients with melanoma, seven with Mel-TUMPs, and five with SNAFs. The median age for melanoma patients was 17 years, 10 for MelTUMPs, and six for SNAFs. Of the 13 melanoma patients, only four were younger than 15 years, while six were adolescents, and three were young adults. Nine melanoma patients (69%) were female. The most common histologic subtype was superficial spreading. The median depth for melanomas was 1.2 mm, and 3.4 mm for MelTUMPs. Microscopic regional nodal involvement detected on elective or sentinel lymph node (SLN) dissection was present in 2/10 (20%) of primary melanomas and 2/6 (33%) of Mel-TUMPs. Complete lymphadenectomy was performed on four melanoma patients, with three positive cases. Patient outcome through March 31, 2009 revealed no in-transit or visceral metastasis in patients with MelTUMPs or SNAFs. One SLN-positive patient (8%) with melanoma developed recurrent lymph node and liver metastasis and died 15 months after primary diagnosis. Our data highlight the rarity, female predominance, and significant rate of SLN positivity of pediatric melanoma. The high rate of MelTUMPs with regional nodal disease reinforces the need for close follow-up.

▶ A retrospective analysis from Stanford evaluated pediatric melanoma and melanocytic tumors of uncertain malignant potential (MelTUMP) over a 13-year period from 1995-2008. The authors evaluated melanoma, Mel-TUMPs, and Spitz nevi with atypical features (SNAF) in patients aged 21 years and younger. Over that 13-year time frame, they identified 13 melanomas, 7 MelTUMPs, and 6 SNAFs. Although they did not state how many pediatric cases were seen over that 13-year period, it can be surmised that pediatric melanoma is rare. However, the authors cite evidence that the incidence of pediatric melanoma is increasing. Thus, they urge that practitioners be aware of melanoma in the pediatric population. Particularly, dermatologists should be aware that pediatric melanomas predominate in females, may be amelanotic or present with pyogenic granuloma features, and have a predilection for trunk and extremities.

S. M. Purcell, DO

Melanoma Thickness Trends in the United States, 1988–2006
Criscione VD, Weinstock MA (The Warren Alpert Med School of Brown Univ, Providence, RI)
J Invest Dermatol 130:793-797, 2010

Over the past two decades, numerous efforts have been initiated to improve screening and early detection of melanoma both in the United States and worldwide. It is commonly believed that these efforts have contributed to the stabilization of melanoma mortality, and that the proportion of thick melanoma with unfavorable prognosis is on the decline. Data obtained from 17 population-based cancer registries of the Surveillance Epidemiology and End Result (SEER) program of the National Cancer Institute for 1988–2006 were used to examine trends in melanoma tumor thickness. For malignant melanoma cases with recorded thickness, the proportionate distribution among four thickness categories (≤1, 1.01–2, 2.01–4, and 4 mm) remained relatively stable over the 19-year study period, however, for melanomas resulting in death, the proportion of thick tumors increased. The most substantial change occurred in the proportion of melanoma *in situ*, which nearly doubled from 1988 to 2006. Surveillance and early detection efforts in the United States have not resulted in a substantial reduction in the proportion of tumors with prognostically unfavorable thickness. Continued improvement and new methods of screening, especially among demographics with higher incidence of thick tumors, is necessary.

▶ Invasive melanoma incidence rates are continuing to rise in the United States despite efforts to elevate public awareness and improve screening methods. Concurrently, many other cancer incidences are shown to be decreasing.[1] This article investigates the trend in melanoma thickness in the United States by evaluating 153 124 melanoma patients registered with the Surveillance Epidemiology and End Result (SEER) program of the National Cancer Institute for 1988 to 2006. In general, results indicate that melanoma thickness has remained relatively stable during this period. However, for fatal melanomas with known thickness, there was an increase in the proportion of thick tumors. As mentioned by authors, there are apparent limitations to the study that involves SEER data. There is not only underreporting of tumor thickness but also ambiguity and inconsistencies in reporting of tumor thickness, which all limit the analysis of melanoma thickness trends. Results highlight the need for new expanded melanoma screening modalities.

S. Bellew, DO

J. Q. Del Rosso, DO

Reference

1. Rigel DS. Trends in dermatology: melanoma incidence. *Arch Dermatol.* 2010;146: 318.

Non-Steroidal Anti-Inflammatory Drugs and Melanoma Risk: Large Dutch Population-Based Case—Control Study

Joosse A, Koomen ER, Casparie MK, et al (Leiden Univ Med Ctr, The Netherlands; Foundation PALGA, Utrecht, The Netherlands; et al)
J Invest Dermatol 129:2620-2627, 2009

This case—control study investigates the potential chemoprophylactic properties of non-steroidal anti-inflammatory drugs (NSAIDs) on the incidence of cutaneous melanoma (CM). Data were extracted from the Dutch PHARMO pharmacy database and the PALGA pathology database. Cases had a primary CM between 1991 and 2004, were ≥18 years, and were observed for 3 years in PHARMO before diagnosis. Controls were matched for date of birth, gender, and geographical region. NSAIDs and acetylsalicylic acids (ASAs) were analyzed separately. Adjusted odds ratio (OR) and 95% confidence interval (CI) were calculated using multivariable logistic regression, and the results were stratified across gender. A total of 1,318 CM cases and 6,786 controls were eligible to enter the study. CM incidence was not significantly associated with ever ASA use (adjusted OR: 0.92, 95% CI: 0.76−1.12) or ever non-ASA NSAID use (adjusted OR: 1.10, 95% CI: 0.97−1.24). However, continuous use of low-dose ASAs was associated with a significant reduction of CM risk in women (adjusted OR: 0.54, 95% CI: 0.30−0.99) but not in men (OR: 1.01, 95% CI: 0.69−1.47). A significant trend ($P=0.04$) from no use, non-continuous use to continuous use was observed in women. Continuous use of low-dose ASAs may be associated with a reduced incidence of CM in women, but not in men.

▶ The chemoprophylactic properties of nonsteroidal antiinflammatory drugs (NSAIDs) are being increasingly investigated, as evidenced by more reporting in recent literature. This large case-control study purports decreased incidence rates of cutaneous melanoma (CM) in female patients who were found to have used continuous low-dose aspirin (ASA) over a 3-year period. Similar findings have been reported showing a protective effect on prostate cancer but not on colorectal, breast, or lung cancer.

This study has many potential limitations and does not adequately address the major confounding variable in their study, namely, that patients who are compliant with everyday ASA use are likely to be compliant with other aspects of preventative health maintenance, including photoprotection. This is further evidenced by the fact that intermittent users of ASA and users of non-ASA NSAIDs were not strongly associated with decreased CM incidence, as the use of medications on such an interval is not consistent with preventative health maintenance.

The results of this study, as the authors admit, are in direct conflict with a recent randomized control trial, which is better able to control for such confounding factors. Analysis of the possible benefit of long-term low-dose ASA and 3-hydroxy-3-methyl·glutaryl coenzyme A reductase inhibitors (statins) would be of interest as well.

R. I. Ceilley, MD
J. B. Wilson, MD

Plantar Melanoma: Is the Prognosis Always Bad?
Baumert J, Schmidt M, Kunte C, et al (Ludwig Maximilian Univ Munich, Germany)
Dermatol Surg 36:1325-1327, 2010

Background.—Patients in various age groups, with various tumor sites, and having different cutaneous melanoma subtypes can demonstrate variations in biological behavior. There is no positive time trend with diminished tumor thickness for melanoma of the feet or nodular or acrolentiginous melanoma (ALM). Patients with plantar melanoma were screened for factors that may be predictive of progression or death.

Methods.—The 92 patients (mean age 59 years) had invasive plantar melanomas. Clinical data were collected, noting site of the lesion(s), histopathological features, and tumor thickness in millimeters. Follow-up extended a mean of 8.9 years for overall survival (OS) data and 7.8 years for disease-free survival (DFS). Hazard ratios (HRs) for tumor thickness were estimated.

Results.—Tumor thickness was 1.00 mm or less in 44.6% of patients, between 1.01 and 2.00 mm in 22.8% of patients, and over 2.00 mm in 32.6% of patients. Disease progressed in 27 patients, with 13 dying from melanoma and 12 from other causes. Greater tumor thickness had substantially worse prognosis for OS and DFS. Follow-up at 10 years showed that 79% of the patients who had a tumor thickness of 1.00 mm or less and 50% of patients with a tumor thickness greater than 1.00 mm were still living. Thus patients with a tumor thickness over 2.00 mm had a significantly greater risk of mortality than patients with a tumor thickness of 1.00 mm or less.

Conclusions.—Plantar melanomas were rare in the sample population, affecting only 0.9% of the patients. Tumor thickness was the most important prognostic factor for both DFS and OS. Improving the early and effective detection of plantar melanoma should be a goal to improve mortality data.

▶ The objective of this study is to look at the survival of plantar melanoma patients. This article achieves those objectives but could use more extensive comparative data. The article is a good study with a reasonable patient population.

This study was completed in Germany, where the authors looked at patients in the department of dermatology from 1978-2006. They selected out the 92 patients who had a disease-free interval average of 7.8 years and a 8.9% overall survival. Of the 92 patients with plantar melanoma, 44.6% had Breslow tumor thickness of 1.00 mm or less, 22.8% had thickness of 1.01 to 2 mm, and 32.6% had thickness more than 2 mm. After 10 years, 79% of the patients with Breslow thickness of 1.00 mm or less were still alive compared with 50% of patients with thickness greater than 1.0 mm. In the original collection of melanoma patients, there were 10 704 patients, with only 0.9% (92 patients) found to have invasive plantar melanoma. The plantar melanoma subset appears to be rare. As with other studies of melanoma, the tumor thickness appears to be the most important prognostic indicator in patients with plantar melanomas. There did not appear to be a variation of prognosis with the plantar tumor site. The universal conclusion is that early detection of melanoma is important. Inspection of the plantar surface for melanoma is important. Through stressing the importance to patients and their relatives of examination of difficult-to-see areas, such as the bottom of the foot, lesions may be caught earlier.

L. Cleaver, DO

Predictors of Occult Nodal Metastasis in Patients With Thin Melanoma
Faries MB, Wanek LA, Elashoff D, et al (Saint John's Health Ctr, Santa Monica, CA)
Arch Surg 145:137-142, 2010

Hypothesis.—Thin primary lesions are largely responsible for the rapid increase in melanoma incidence, making identification of appropriate candidates for nodal staging in this group critically important. We hypothesized that common clinical variables may accurately estimate the risk of nodal metastasis after wide excision and determine the need for sentinel node biopsy.

Design.—Review of prospectively acquired data in a large melanoma database.

Setting.—A tertiary referral center.

Patients.—A total of 2211 patients with thin melanoma treated by wide local excision alone were identified in the database between January 1, 1971, and December 31, 2005. Of those, 1732 met entry criteria.

Main Outcome Measures.—We examined the rate of regional nodal recurrence and the impact of clinical and demographic variables by univariate and multivariate analyses.

Results.—The overall nodal recurrence rate was 2.9%; median time to recurrence was 38.3 months. Univariate analysis of 1732 patients identified male sex ($P < .001$), increased Breslow thickness ($P < .001$), and increased Clark level ($P < .001$) as significant for nodal recurrence. Multivariate analysis identified male sex (hazard ratio, 3.5; 95% confidence interval, 1.8-7.0; $P < .001$), younger age (0.45; 0.24-0.86; $P = .001$), and increased Breslow thickness (2.5; 1.6-3.7; categorical $P < .001$) as significant for nodal recurrence. The Clark level was no longer significant ($P = .63$). Breslow thickness, age, and sex were used to develop a scoring system and nomogram for the risk of nodal involvement. Predictions ranged from 0.1% in the lowest-risk group to 17.4% in the highest-risk group.

Conclusions.—Many patients with thin melanoma will have nodal recurrence after wide excision alone. Three simple clinical variables may be used to estimate recurrence risk and select patients for sentinel node biopsy.

▶ Most new cases of malignant melanoma are thin lesions, depth of invasion less than 1 millimeter. Patients with thin lesions have a low incidence of nodal disease and subsequent metastasis leading to death. Assigning nodal basin involvement by sentinal lymph node dissection is widely accepted for intermediate thicker lesions. However, a small percentage of patients with thin melanomas do experience disease recurrence and risk death from melanoma. By using univariate analysis, Breslow thickness and Clark level were significant predictors of nodal disease.

By using multivariate analysis, Breslow thickness, age of the patient (younger greater than older), and sex of patient (male greater than female) were significant predictors of disease recurrence. Clark level and primary tumor site were not predictors.

In addition, ulceration has a 7.7% nodal recurrence rate compared with 2.7% without ulceration.

Overall, the nodal recurrence rate of 1732 patients with thin melanomas was 2.9%, and median time to tumor recurrence was 38.3 months. While sentinel lymph node dissection is not uniformly recommended for thin melanomas, 3 common clinical variables (Breslow thickness, age, and sex) may be helpful in estimating recurrence risk.

J. L. Smith, MD

Predictors of sentinel lymph node metastasis in melanoma

Cadili A, Dabbs K (Univ of Alberta, Edmonton, Alta)
Can J Surg 53:32-36, 2010

Background.—Several studies have examined the correlation between patient and tumour characteristics and sentinel lymph node (SLN) metastasis in patients with melanoma. Although most studies have identified Breslow thickness as an important factor, results for other variables have been conflicting. Much of this variability is probably because of differences in measurement techniques and reporting practices at different institutions. We sought to identify the predictors of SLN melanoma metastasis in our institution and patient population.

Methods.—We performed a retrospective chart review of 348 patients with malignant melanoma who underwent SLN biopsy at a single institution from January 1999 to April 2007. We compared multiple variables related to patient demographics, primary tumour characteristics and SLN characteristics between patients in the positive and negative SLN groups.

Results.—Breslow thickness and nodular tumour type were independent factors significantly correlated with a positive SLN biopsy result in our study. Head and neck tumour location correlated with a lower likelihood of positive SLN status in univariate but not multivariate analyses.

Conclusion.—This study confirms the status of Breslow thickness as a reproducible predictor of positive SLN status. We also found that nodular type was predictive of positive SLN status, an outcome that has not been reported by others.

▶ This study was a retrospective chart review that analyzed 8 years of data from patients with melanoma who underwent sentinel lymph node (SLN) biopsy. This article was helpful in analyzing the clinical and tumor features that were significantly correlated with a positive SLN biopsy. This study, like previous studies, confirmed that the Breslow thickness is a significant independent predictor of SLN metastasis. A new and interesting finding was that nodular histology was a significant predictor of positive SLN status. I appreciated the authors' hypothesis for this finding, including the explanation of distinguishing features of nodular melanoma that impact the prognosis, namely the delayed presentation, greater tumor thickness, and low likelihood to develop in pre-existing nevi.

This article, published in February 2010 (but accepted June 2008), was not up to date regarding the new American Joint Committee on Cancer melanoma staging system. There was no reference to mitotic rate and its impact on SLN status. In addition, it was unclear in the results section whether or not head and neck tumor location was correlated with a positive SLN biopsy result. In 1 sentence, the authors state that head and neck tumor location was correlated with a negative SLN result; however, they subsequently state that the odds of a positive SLN biopsy result were 20-fold higher among patients with a head or neck tumor than among those with a nonhead or neck tumor. This was confusing to the reader and should be clarified.

T. Nino, MD

A. Torres, MD, JD

Prevalence and distribution of melanocytic naevi on the scalp: a prospective study
De Giorgi V, Sestini S, Grazzini M, et al (Univ of Florence, Italy)
Br J Dermatol 162:345-349, 2010

Background.—Few studies have examined the incidence and characteristics of naevi on the scalp. Most studies of scalp naevi have been performed in children, whose incidence of scalp naevi is relatively high, at about 0·5—11·7% of the total body count of common naevi.

Objectives.—To investigate the prevalence and distribution of scalp melanocytic naevi in patients of all ages. To our knowledge, ours is the first study to analyse in detail the relationships between melanocytic naevi on the scalp and total body naevi and total body atypical naevi.

Methods.—We conducted a prospective study of patients visiting the dermatology outpatient clinic at the University of Florence, for examinations unrelated to the presence of naevi or melanoma. The study enrolled 795 subjects (417 females; 52·4%), with a median age of 35 years (range 4—80).

Results.—The number of melanocytic naevi on the scalp increased significantly ($r = 0·2057$, $P = 0·0008$) as the number of total body melanocytic naevi increased and a correlation was found between the number of clinically atypical total body naevi and the number of scalp naevi. Relatively few naevi (15·5%) were located at the frontal region compared with other regions of the scalp, although the frontal region is more exposed to ultraviolet (UV) rays. Compared with subjects without alopecia, whose hair shields the scalp from UV rays, subjects with androgenetic alopecia showed no significant increase in number of scalp naevi.

Conclusions.—Despite practical difficulties, early diagnostic screening for melanoma or screening during follow-up examination for previous melanoma should involve examination of the entire skin surface, scalp included.

▶ Past studies have revealed that atypical nevi can increase the risk for developing melanomas. The scalp and genital regions are anatomical sites least explored during ordinary screening examinations for skin cancer and may be hidden sites associated with low public awareness. This is a prospective study of 209 suspicious lesions from 795 subjects (mean age 35 years) evaluated by 17 dermatologists from the outpatient clinic of Dermatology at the University of Florence, Italy between 2005-2007. Twenty-one subjects (2.6%) were phototype I, 435 subjects (54.8%) were phototype II, 318 subjects

(40%) were phototype III, and 21 subjects (2.6%) were phototype IV. Sixty-six subjects (8.3%) reported a family history of melanoma, and 21 subjects (2.6%) reported a personal history of melanoma. The total body count of atypical nevi was < 5 in 696 subjects (87.5%), 72 subjects (9.1%) had 6 to 10 atypical nevi, and 27 subjects (3.4%) had > 10. Almost two-thirds of the study (66.4%) had no scalp nevi. The number of melanocytic nevi on the scalp increased significantly ($r = 0.2057$, $P = .008$) as the number of total body melanocytic nevi increased and a correlation was found between the number of clinically atypical total body nevi and the number of scalp nevi. Only 4 subjects had atypical scalp nevi, located on the right parietal region (2 nevi), the frontal region (1 nevus), and the left parietal region (1 nevus). Authors diagnosed androgenic alopecia in 249 subjects, with 54 of the patients being female. An association between personal history of melanoma and presence of scalp nevi approached did not reach statistical significance ($P = .059$). The pattern of nevi distribution was unaffected by sex or phenotypic features, such as skin color or degree of freckling. These results revealed that the number of melanocytic nevi present on the scalp increased significantly ($P = .0008$) with the increase of total body melanocytic nevi and atypical total body nevi, indicating that the scalp should always be explored carefully, especially in patients with high-risk melanoma or in patients with > 30 melanocytic nevi. In this study, relatively few scalp nevi (15.5%) were located at the frontal region compared with other regions of the scalp and may indicate that ultraviolet rays may play a relatively insignificant role in nevogenesis on the scalp, compared with other anatomical areas. Compared with subjects without alopecia, subjects with androgenetic alopecia showed no statistically significant increase in the number of scalp nevi. Limitations included short follow-up period and a single institutional site. This study represents a snap shot in time, and patients may develop melanomas in areas that were once considered benign. Also, dermoscopy was used to establish a definitive diagnosis of atypical nevi along with the clinical ABCDE rule, and biopsies would have yielded more definitive results. Authors concluded that melanoma screening should include the entire scalp along with other skin surface areas.

J. Q. Del Rosso, DO

G. K. Kim, DO

Prognostic Significance of a Positive Nonsentinel Lymph Node in Cutaneous Melanoma
Ghaferi AA, Wong SL, Johnson TM, et al (Univ of Michigan Health System, Ann Arbor)
Ann Surg Oncol 16:2978-2984, 2009

Purpose.—Sentinel lymph node (SLN) biopsy provides important prognostic information for patients with cutaneous melanoma. There may be additional prognostic significance to melanoma spreading from the SLN to nonsentinel lymph nodes (NSLN). We examined the implications of a positive NSLN for overall and distant disease-free survival.

Methods.—Using a prospectively maintained, Institutional Review Board-approved melanoma database we studied patients who had a cutaneous melanoma, a positive SLN, and a completion lymph node dissection (CLND). Survival was determined using a combination of hospital records and the Social Security Death Index (SSDI). Univariate and multivariate Cox regression analysis was performed to further characterize predictors of overall and distant disease-free survival. Kaplan—Meier analysis was used to generate survival curves.

Results.—A total of 429 patients with positive SLN biopsies were identified, with at least one positive NSLN identified in 71 (17%). Median follow-up time was 36.8 months. Presence of a positive NSLN was significantly associated with poor outcome, although long-term survival was possible. Presence of ulceration, high mitotic rate, angiolymphatic invasion, total number of positive nodes, and volume of disease >1% in the SLN were significant predictors of survival on univariate analysis, but lost significance on multivariate. Multivariate Cox analysis revealed several predictors of overall survival: increasing age [hazard ratio (HR) 1.04, $P < 0.01$], Breslow depth (HR 1.76, $P < 0.01$), presence of extracapsular extension in the SLN (HR 2.39, $P < 0.01$), and positive NSLN (HR 1.92, $P < 0.01$).

Conclusion.—Among node-positive melanoma patients, presence of a positive NSLN is a highly significant poor prognostic sign, even after considering the total number of positive nodes and volume of disease in the SLN. CLND after a positive SLN provides this important prognostic information.

▶ This study offers some valuable insight in the management of patients with melanoma in that a positive nonsentinel lymph node (NSLN) in a patient with positive SLNs appears not to be related to the total number of nodes involved and thus may be a useful independent prognostic factor. This would support complete lymph node dissection in patients with a positive SLN biopsy for reasons other than to reduce the risk of local recurrence with its attendant morbidity. However, as the authors noted, we must be careful before jumping to this conclusion because the NSLNs were only sectioned by bivalve and stained with hematoxylin and eosin leaving the possibility that serial sectioning and/or immunostaining might have picked up the presence of disease in other nodes, thus making it an issue of the volume of disease predicting outcome as opposed to NSLN being a special prognostic factor. Nevertheless, NSLN status seems to be highly predictive of worse overall and distant disease-free survival, and a prospective study that includes serial sectioning and/or immunostaining would be most interesting and have the potential to yield very helpful information.

L. Meadows, MD

A. Torres, MD, JD

Reflectance Confocal Microscopy and Features of Melanocytic Lesions: An Internet-Based Study of the Reproducibility of Terminology

Pellacani G, Vinceti M, Bassoli S, et al (Univ of Modena and Reggio Emilia, Modena, Italy; et al)
Arch Dermatol 145:1137-1143, 2009

Objective.—To test the interobserver and intraobserver reproducibility of the standard terminology for description and diagnosis of melanocytic lesions in in vivo confocal microscopy.

Design.—A dedicated Web platform was developed to train the participants and to allow independent distant evaluations of confocal images via the Internet.

Setting.—Department of Dermatology, University of Modena and Reggio Emilia, Modena, Italy.

Participants.—The study population was composed of 15 melanomas, 30 nevi, and 5 Spitz/Reed nevi. Six expert centers were invited to participate at the study.

Intervention.—Evaluation of 36 features in 345 confocal microscopic images from melanocytic lesions.

Main Outcome Measure.—Interobserved and intraobserved agreement, by calculating the Cohen κ statistics measure for each descriptor.

Results.—High overall levels of reproducibility were shown for most of the evaluated features. In both the training and test sets there was a parallel trend of decreasing κ values as deeper anatomic skin levels were evaluated. All of the features, except 1, used for melanoma diagnosis, including roundish pagetoid cells, nonedged papillae, atypical cells in basal layer, cerebriform clusters, and nucleated cells infiltrating dermal papillae, showed high overall levels of reproducibility. However, less-than-ideal reproducibility was obtained for some descriptors, such as grainy appearance of the epidermis, junctional thickening, mild atypia in basal layer, plump bright cells, small bright cells, and reticulated fibers in the dermis.

Conclusion.—The standard consensus confocal terminology useful for the evaluation of melanocytic lesions was reproducibly recognized by independent observers.

▶ This is a timely article, as more individuals and institutions are exploring the value and usefulness of reflectance confocal microscopy (RCM). Of note is that this study shows that independent observers can achieve a good level of concordance after undergoing a short web-based RCM interpretation training program. Granted, all participants were skilled in RCM use but so are pathologists similarly situated, and yet there is often discordance among pathologists as to a malignant melanoma histopathological diagnosis. Thus, this study should stimulate dermatologists to keep abreast of RCM developments, as it races to become a standard tool.

A. Torres, MD, JD

Reflectance confocal microscopy of facial lentigo maligna and lentigo maligna melanoma: a preliminary study

Ahlgrimm-Siess V, Massone C, Scope A, et al (Med Univ of Graz, Austria; Memorial Sloan-Kettering Cancer Ctr, NY)
Br J Dermatol 161:1307-1316, 2009

Background.—Facial lentigo maligna (LM) and lentigo maligna melanoma (LMM) may be difficult to diagnose clinically and dermoscopically. Reflectance confocal microscopy (RCM) enables the in vivo assessment of equivocal skin lesions at a cellular level.

Objectives.—To assess cytomorphological and architectural RCM features of facial LM/LMM.

Methods.—Four women and eight men aged 58—88 years presenting with facial skin lesions suspicious of LM/LMM were included. In total, 17 lesion areas were imaged by RCM before biopsy. The histopathological diagnosis of LM was made in 15 areas; the other two were diagnosed as early LMM.

Results.—A focal increase of atypical melanocytes and nests surrounding adnexal openings, sheets of mainly dendritic melanocytes, cord-like rete ridges at the dermoepidermal junction (DEJ) and an infiltration of adnexal structures by atypical melanocytes were found to be characteristic RCM features of facial LM/LMM. Areas with a focal increase of atypical melanocytes and nests surrounding adnexal openings were observed at the basal layer in three cases. The remaining cases displayed these changes at suprabasal layers above sheets of mainly dendritic melanocytes. Cord-like rete ridges at the DEJ and an infiltration of adnexal structures by atypical melanocytes were observed in all cases. Previously described criteria for RCM diagnosis of melanoma, such as epidermal disarray, pleomorphism of melanocytes and pagetoid spreading of atypical melanocytes, were additionally observed.

Conclusions.—We observed a reproducible set of RCM criteria in this case series of facial LM/LMM.

▶ This article is limited by the small number of cases evaluated, but it does attempt to provide new information that supports the concept that increased adnexal or periadnexal involvement by atypical melanocytes may be a reflectance confocal microscopy (RCM) clue to aid in the diagnosis of lentigo maligna and lentigo maligna melanoma. The data also confirm that the previously reported RCM criteria for the diagnosis of melanoma apply as well to lentigo maligna. It waits to be seen if the findings of this study can be duplicated in future larger studies, but in the meantime, it provides a good starting point for dealing with difficult melanocytic skin lesions.

A. Torres, MD, JD

Sentinel Lymph Node Biopsy in Pediatric and Adolescent Cutaneous Melanoma Patients

Howman-Giles R, Shaw HM, Scolyer RA, et al (Royal Prince Alfred and Mater Hosps, Sydney, New South Wales, Australia; et al)
Ann Surg Oncol 17:138-143, 2010

Background.—The rarity of melanoma in young patients, particularly pediatric ones, has to date precluded any valid comparisons being made between young patients and adults undergoing sentinel lymph node biopsy (SLNB) for intermediate thickness localized melanoma. The present study takes advantage of the large Sydney Melanoma Unit (SMU) database to clarify this issue.

Materials and Methods.—Clinical and pathologic data on pediatric and adolescent AJCC Stage I and II cutaneous melanoma patients aged <20 years undergoing SLNB at the SMU between January 1993 and February 2008 were reviewed. SLNB positivity rates and outcomes in these patients were compared with adult SMU patients.

Results.—In 55 young patients, overall median tumor thickness was 1.7 mm (range, 0.6–5.2 mm) and overall SLNB positivity rate was 14 of 55 (25%), tumors tending to be thicker (median, 2.6 mm), and SLNB positivity rate higher (2 of 6; 33%) in patients aged <10 years. Of the 14 patients, 13 underwent immediate completion lymph node dissection (CLND); 2 patients had non-SLN metastases (15.4%). Only 0.7% of a total of 295 lymph nodes removed at CLND were involved with melanoma. In 14 SLNB-positive patients with follow-up data, 3 (21%) have died from melanoma after a median follow-up of 60 months, compared with 42% of 356 SLNB positive adults.

Conclusions.—Although the SLNB positivity rate was higher in pediatric and adolescent melanoma patients than in adults (25% vs. 17%, respectively), non-SLN positivity and melanoma-specific death rates were low.

▶ Although the incidence of childhood melanoma is increasing, it remains an uncommon pediatric malignancy. Because of this, large-scale prognostic and therapeutic studies in childhood melanoma have been difficult to perform, and therapeutic standards for childhood melanoma are based on adult protocols. In adults, sentinel lymph node (SLN) biopsies are indicated for all melanomas greater than 1 mm thick and for melanomas less than 1 mm with histological features associated with a poor prognosis, such as ulceration, Clark level III or IV invasion, and high mitotic rate. Management of childhood melanoma includes these same criteria for SLN biopsies even though previous studies have suggested that lymph node involvement does not correlate with prognosis in childhood melanoma.[1,2]

The goal of this study is to further characterize childhood melanoma and determine the use of SLN biopsy in patients with childhood melanoma. The study gathered 55 cases of childhood melanoma with SLN biopsy treated at the Sydney Melanoma Unit. They found that pediatric and adolescent patients tended to have deeper melanomas (median 1.7 mm), with younger patients (< 10 years of age) having thicker lesions at diagnosis than older patients (> 10 years of age). The younger patients also had a higher incidence of positive SLN than older patients, with the overall incidence of positive SLN being higher in childhood melanoma patients than in adults. Overall, patients with childhood melanoma had a better prognosis than adult patients despite the thicker tumors and higher frequency of positive SLN, but patients with poor outcomes all had positive SLN biopsies.

Clearly, the biology of childhood melanoma is different than adult melanoma and more research is needed to further elucidate these differences and guide clinical practice. Based on the conclusion from this study, SLN biopsy is still indicated in childhood melanoma. A positive SLN in these patients does not indicate as poor a prognosis as adults with positive SLN, but those patients should be followed closely for metastatic disease.

M. Jen, MD

References

1. Roaten JB, Partrick DA, Bensard D, et al. Survival in sentinel lymph node-positive pediatric melanoma. *J Pediatr Surg.* 2005;40:988-992.
2. Bütter A, Hui T, Chapdelaine J, Beaunoyer M, Flageole H, Bouchard S. Melanoma in children and the use of sentinel lymph node biopsy. *J Pediatr Surg.* 2005;40:797-800.

Sentinel Lymph Node Dissection in Primary Melanoma Reduces Subsequent Regional Lymph Node Metastasis as Well as Distant Metastasis After Nodal Involvement
Leiter U, Buettner PG, Bohnenberger K, et al (Eberhard-Karls-Univ, Tuebingen, Germany; James Cook Univ, Townsville, Queensland, Australia)
Ann Surg Oncol 17:129-137, 2010

Background.—In many countries sentinel lymph node dissection (SLND) followed by complete lymphadenectomy if positive is routinely performed treatment for primary cutaneous melanoma. However, the potential survival benefit of SLND is still controversial.

Methods.—Patients with primary cutaneous melanoma (tumor thickness 1.00 mm or greater) diagnosed in the Department of Dermatology, University of Tuebingen, Germany between 1991 and 2000 were included in the study. A total of 439 patients who received SLND were compared retrospectively with 440 patients without SLND with regards to occurring patterns of metastases and disease-free and overall survival. SLND-positive cases and SLND-negative patients with subsequent development of regional lymph node metastasis (SLND-LN+) were compared with non-SLND patients who had developed regional lymph node metastasis (non-SLND-LN+).

Results.—Regional lymph node metastases as the first recurrence occurred more frequently in the non-SLND collective (16.5%) compared with the SLND group (7.3%; $P = 0.001$), whereas satellite/in-transit metastases and distant metastases did not differ. Driven by the reduction of regional lymph node metastases, disease-free survival was improved in the SLND collective ($P = 0.003$). No significant difference in overall survival was observed ($P = 0.090$). The risk of dying from melanoma was 2.2 times higher in the non-SLND-LN+ group than in the SLND-LN+ group ($P = 0.009$), while the risk of developing distant metastasis was 2.3 times higher ($P = 0.002$).

Conclusions.—SLND reduced subsequent regional lymph node metastases and improved disease-free survival, while overall survival remained unaffected. SLND reduced distant metastases and improved overall survival in the subgroups of patients with regional lymph node involvement.

▶ Controversy still exists regarding the benefit of sentinel lymph node (SLN) biopsy other than for prognostic purposes. The benefit of complete lymphadenectomy if SLN dissection (SLND) is positive is unclear. The risk of complications, morbidity, and cost of the procedures are not insignificant. The only apparent benefit of SLND followed by complete lymphadenectomy in positive patients is improved disease-free survival with fewer regional lymph node metastases in patients with primary cutaneous melanoma having tumor thickness of 1 mm or greater.

This is a well-done article that further confirms many of the findings of the Multicenter Selective Lymphadenectomy Trial. Most importantly, it confirms that SLND increases the likelihood of disease-free survival, although overall survival is unchanged. Its importance as a prognostic indicator cannot be understated, as there is clearly a more favorable outcome and disease-free survival for SLND-negative patients. It should be offered to all patients with a melanoma between 1 and 4 mm thickness.

The weak point of the article is the retrospective design and differences between the 2 groups. Despite this, the article does add to a growing list of studies supporting the use of SLND for better prognosis, more accurate staging, and improved regional disease. The lack of improved survival, fewer in-transit metastases, and distant metastases is notable. Further studies are needed before SLND should be recommended for reasons other than prognostic benefit or to guide adjuvant therapy.

R. I. Ceilley, MD

B. A. Kopitski, DO

Serum 25-Hydroxyvitamin D₃ Levels Are Associated With Breslow Thickness at Presentation and Survival From Melanoma
Newton-Bishop JA, Beswick S, Randerson-Moor J, et al (St James's Univ Hosp, Leeds, UK; Univ Hosp Birmingham Natl Health Service Foundation Trust, UK; Univ of Pennsylvania, Philadelphia)
J Clin Oncol 27:5439-5444, 2009

Purpose.—A cohort study was carried out to test the hypothesis that higher vitamin D levels reduce the risk of relapse from melanoma.

Methods.—A pilot retrospective study of 271 patients with melanoma suggested that vitamin D may protect against recurrence of melanoma.

We tested these findings in a survival analysis in a cohort of 872 patients recruited to the Leeds Melanoma Cohort (median follow-up, 4.7 years).

Results.—In the retrospective study, self-reports of taking vitamin D supplements were nonsignificantly correlated with a reduced risk of melanoma relapse (odds ratio = 0.6; 95% CI, 0.4 to 1.1; $P = .09$). Nonrelapsers had higher mean 25-hydroxyvitamin D_3 levels than relapsers (49 v 46 nmol/L; $P = .3$; not statistically significant). In the cohort (prospective) study, higher 25-hydroxyvitamin D_3 levels were associated with lower Breslow thickness at diagnosis ($P = .002$) and were independently protective of relapse and death: the hazard ratio for relapse-free survival (RFS) was 0.79 (95% CI, 0.64 to 0.96; $P = .01$) for a 20 nmol/L increase in serum level. There was evidence of interaction between the vitamin D receptor (VDR) BsmI genotype and serum 25-hydroxyvitamin D_3 levels on RFS.

Conclusion.—Results from the retrospective study were consistent with a role for vitamin D in melanoma outcome. The cohort study tests this hypothesis, providing evidence that higher 25-hydroxyvitamin D_3 levels, at diagnosis, are associated with both thinner tumors and better survival from melanoma, independent of Breslow thickness. Patients with melanoma, and those at high risk of melanoma, should seek to ensure vitamin D sufficiency. Additional studies are needed to establish optimal serum levels for patients with melanoma.

▶ The hypothesis that adequate vitamin D levels is associated with thin Breslow melanomas and ultimately significantly lower relapse rate is not clearly proven in this retrospective and prospective cohort study. Patients included in this study had a melanoma with Breslow thickness greater than 0.75 and disease-free interval of at least 3 years. The prospective cohort study had a median follow-up of 4.7 years. Factors influencing vitamin D levels inclusively were younger adults and patients with higher body mass index (BMI). Interestingly, patients with intermediate BMI (between 24.9 and 29.9) had the best survival rate and highest vitamin D levels.

Although the findings are suggestive of a possible link between sufficient vitamin D levels and long-term survival of melanoma, the author concludes that further studies are needed to establish optimal vitamin D levels in patients with melanoma.

J. L. Smith, MD

Should All Patients With Melanoma Between 1 and 2 mm Breslow Thickness Undergo Sentinel Lymph Node Biopsy?
Mays MP, Martin RCG, Burton A, et al (Univ of Louisville, KY; et al)
Cancer 116:1535-1544, 2010

Background.—Sentinel lymph node (SLN) biopsy generally is recommended for patients who have melanoma with a Breslow thickness ≥ 1 mm. Most patients with melanoma between 1 mm and 2 mm thick have tumor-negative SLNs and an excellent long-term prognosis. The objective of the current study was to evaluate prognostic factors in this subset of patients and determine whether all such patients require SLN biopsy.

Methods.—Patients with melanoma between 1 mm and 2 mm in Breslow thickness were evaluated from a prospective multi-institutional study of SLN biopsy for melanoma. Disease-free survival (DFS) and overall survival (OS) were evaluated by Kaplan-Meier analysis to compare patients with melanoma that measured from 1.0 mm to 1.59 mm (Group A) versus patients with melanoma that measured from ≥1.6 mm to 2.0 mm thick (Group B). Univariate and multivariate analyses were performed to evaluate factors predictive of tumor-positive SLN status, DFS, and OS.

Results.—The current analysis included 1110 patients with a median follow-up of 69 months. SLN status was tumor-positive in 133 of 1110 patients (12%) including 66 of 762 patients (8.7%) in Group A and 67 of 348 patients (19.3%) in Group B ($P < .0001$). On multivariate analysis, age, Breslow thickness, and lymphovascular invasion were independently predictive of a tumor-positive SLN ($P < .05$). DFS ($P < .0001$) and OS ($P = .0001$) were significantly better for Group A than for Group B. When tumor thickness was treated as either a continuous variable ($P < 0.0001$) or a categorical variable ($P < .0001$), it was significantly predictive of DFS and OS. On multivariate analysis, Breslow thickness, age, ulceration, histologic subtype, regression, Clark level, and SLN status were significant factors predicting DFS; and Breslow thickness, age, primary tumor location, sex, ulceration, and SLN status were significant factors predicting OS ($P < .05$). A subgroup of patients who had tumors <1.6 mm in Breslow thickness, had no lymphovascular invasion, and were aged ≥59 years had a low risk (5%) of tumor-positive SLN.

Conclusions.—The current findings indicated that there is significant diversity in the biologic behavior of melanoma between 1 mm and 2 mm in Breslow thickness. SLN biopsy is recommended for all such patients to identify those with lymph node metastasis who are at the greatest risk of recurrence and mortality.

▶ Sentinel lymph node biopsy (SLNB) has emerged in the past 2 decades as a valuable prognostic tool for assessing regional lymph node status in patients with clinical stage I or II melanoma. The status of the SLN is the most sensitive and specific staging tool available today and is an important indicator of long-term prognosis. Current recommendations suggest SLNB in patients with clinically negative nodes and >1-mm thickness tumors.[1,2] This multi-institutional prospective study evaluated 1110 melanoma patients with median follow-up of 69 months with an objective to see whether certain clinicopathologic factors can predict a low risk of SLN metastasis in a subset of patients. Results, however, were to the contrary. The study did not identify any group of thin melanoma patients (>1 mm but <2 mm thickness) who had negligible risk for lymph node metastasis. Therefore, authors continue to recommend SLNB for most patients who have melanoma measuring between 1 and 2 mm in thickness.

S. Bellew, DO

J. Q. Del Rosso, DO

References

1. Current (2009) American Joint Committee recommendations for SLNB include patients who have T1b, T2, T3, and T4 melanomas and clinically negative regional lymph nodes. http://www.cancerstaging.org/. Accessed March 17, 2011.
2. Stebbins WG, Garibyan L, Sober AJ. Sentinel lymph node biopsy and melanoma: 2010 update Part II. *J Am Acad Dermatol.* 2010;62:737-748.

Small and Medium-Sized Congenital Nevi in Children: A Comparison of the Costs of Excision and Long-Term Follow-Up
Roldán FA, Hernando AB, Cuadrado A, et al (Hosp Gregorio Marañon, Madrid, Spain; Universidad Autónoma de Madrid, Spain; et al)
Dermatol Surg 35:1867-1872, 2009

Background.—Clinical decisions on whether to follow up or remove small and medium congenital melanocytic nevi (SMCMN) in children have cost implications that have not been studied.

Objectives.—To compare the costs of excision of SMCMN in children with lifelong follow-up in a tertiary center.

Methods and Materials.—We elaborated models for the evaluation of the costs of excision and long-term follow-up. We retrospectively collected data on 113 consecutive excised SMCMN (105 single-step interventions and 8 multiple-step interventions) from the medical records of our pediatric dermatology unit from 2001 to 2007 and calculated and compared the costs (direct and indirect) of surgery and follow-up.

Results.—The mean ± standard deviation and total cohort costs for single-step interventions were €1,504.73 ± 198.33 and 157,996.20, respectively. Median and cohort lifelong follow-up costs were similar if performed every 4 years (1,482.66 ± 34.98 and 156,679.63). For multiple-step interventions (3 or 4 steps), surgery costs were similar to those of annual lifelong follow-up. In the case of two-step surgery, costs were similar to lifelong follow-up every 2 years.

Conclusions.—An analysis of the costs of surgery and long-term follow-up in children with SMCMN is possible. Although the clinical judgment of the dermatologist and parental opinion are the main determinants in the management of SMCMN, costs should also be taken into account. The authors have indicated no significant interest with commercial supporters.

▶ Congenital melanocytic nevi (CMN) occur in 1% of newborns, classified according to their size. Giant CMN is defined as nevi > 20 cm, medium-sized CMN between 1.5 and 19.9 cm, and small CMN are defined as < 1.5 cm.[1] Most clinicians agree that giant CMN should be removed early, as the risk of malignancy is higher for those patients. However, management of small or medium-sized nevi is not as clear-cut. This study evaluated the cost-effectiveness in observing small and medium-sized CMN (SMCMN) in follow-up visits versus surgical excision of nevus. Results indicate median cost of excision is comparable to a lifelong follow-up for every 4 years, 2-step surgery similar to a 2-year follow-up, and in a 3-step or 4-step excision cost is equal to annual lifelong follow-up. Although cost can be a consideration, the decision should largely depend on the collaboration of the clinician and the parents and/or patient if old enough. Management of SMCMN should depend on individual factors, which may include history of changing nevus, functional or cosmetic issues, anxiety of patients or parents, and ease of monitoring depending on location, degree, and regularity of color.[2] The risk of melanoma in SMCMN is low (< 1% over a lifetime).[2] Therefore, routine prophylactic surgical removal of SMCMN in the absence of above features is not recommended. Furthermore, elective surgical removal should be delayed until puberty, if possible.

S. Bellew, DO

J. Q. Del Rosso, DO

References

1. Tannous ZS, Mihm MC Jr, Sober AJ, Duncan LM. Congenital melanocytic nevi: clinical and histopathologic features, risk of melanoma, and clinical management. *J Am Acad Dermatol*. 2005;52:197-203.
2. Price HN, Schaffer JV. Congenital melanocytic nevi-when to worry and how to treat: facts and controversies. *Clin Dermatol*. 2010;28:293-302.

Staged Excision of Lentigo Maligna and Lentigo Maligna Melanoma: A 10-Year Experience
Bosbous MW, Dzwierzynski WW, Neuburg M (Medical College of Wisconsin, Milwaukee)
Plast Reconstr Surg 124:1947-1955, 2009

Background.—The treatment of lentigo maligna and lentigo maligna melanoma presents a difficult problem for clinicians. Published guidelines recommend a 5-mm excision margin for lentigo maligna and a 1-cm margin for lentigo maligna melanoma, yet these are often inadequate. The authors' purpose is to report their 10-year experience using staged excision for the treatment of lentigo maligna and lentigo maligna melanoma of the head and neck.

Methods.—Staged excision was performed on 59 patients over a 10-year period. Data on patient demographics, lesion characteristics, and treatment were collected through an institutional review board—approved chart review.

Results.—Using staged excision, 62.7 percent of patients required a 10-mm or greater margin to achieve clearance of tumor. Two or more stages of excision were required in 50.9 percent of patients. Invasive melanoma (lentigo maligna melanoma) was identified in 10.2 percent of patients initially diagnosed with lentigo maligna. There was one (1.7 percent) documented recurrence during a median 2.25-year follow-up period (range, 0 to 10.17 years).

Conclusions.—Staged excision is an effective treatment for lentigo maligna and lentigo maligna melanoma. Previously published recommendations of 5-mm margins for wide local excision are inadequate for tumors located on the head and neck.

▶ Margin control surgery for lentigo maligna (LM) and lentigo maligna melanoma (LMM) has been reported in the literature but with few studies reporting the long-term follow-up. Staged excision has been shown to be a simple and effective alternative to Mohs micrographic surgery for LM and LMM without the need for sometimes difficult interpretation of melanocytic lesions with frozen sections.

The authors of this study have added very beneficial knowledge to the treatment of LM and LMM. Their 10-year retrospective review eliminates the possible variance in the procedure of staged excision and focuses only on the outcomes. During a period of time when the standard of care was a 5-mm margin (National Institutes of Health Consensus Conference on Melanoma), their practice was showing that degree of margin was insufficient.

Previous studies have demonstrated similar outcomes. Whether by Mohs micrographic surgery or geometric excision of the lesion, 5-mm margins are indicative of substantially higher recurrence rates and the need for more stages/layers being performed.

The finding that 62.7% of patients required a greater than 10-mm margin supports the need for margin control with these tumors, as standard 5-mm margins for melanoma in situ are inadequate for most patients. Further studies with longer follow-up are needed to reflect the true recurrence rates with staged excision.

The importance of this cannot be understated. The earlier LM is evaluated and treated, the less likely that it will progress to LMM. If a standard for treatment can be established and more clinicians can evaluate LM at its earliest stages, morbidity and mortality rates as well as cosmesis will be greatly improved.

The weak link in the article is that of the short-term median follow-up of only 2.25 years. The recurrence rate was 1.7%, which was lower than previously reported rates in the literature. However, this may not represent the true recurrence rates for staged excision, as most recurrences of LM and LMM occur later, often within a 3- to 5-year period or longer. Their results were not compared with study results from other geographic regions where sun exposure and strength thereof may impact invasion levels. Altogether, their results are very enlightening on the need for larger margin resection and the use of permanent sections. However, much larger and more inclusive studies need to be undertaken to underscore the authors' results.

R. I. Ceilley, MD

J. B. Wilson, MD

Sun and Solarium Exposure and Melanoma Risk: Effects of Age, Pigmentary Characteristics, and Nevi

Veierød MB, Adami H-O, Lund E, et al (Univ of Oslo, Norway; Karolinska Institutet, Stockholm, Sweden; Univ of Tromsø, Norway; et al)

Cancer Epidemiol Biomarkers Prev 19:111-120, 2010

Background.—Few prospective studies have analyzed solar and artificial (solarium) UV exposure and melanoma risk. We investigated these associations in a Norwegian-Swedish cohort study and addressed effect modification by age, pigmentary characteristics, and nevi.

Methods.—The cohort included women ages 30 to 50 years at enrollment from 1991 to 1992. Host factors and exposure to sun and solariums in life decades were collected by questionnaire at enrollment. Relative risks (RR) with 95% confidence intervals (CI) were estimated by Poisson regression.

Results.—Among 106,366 women with complete follow-up through 2005, 412 melanoma cases were diagnosed. Hair color and large, asymmetric nevi on the legs were strongly associated with melanoma risk ($P_{trend} < 0.001$), and the RR for ≥ 2 nevi increased from brown/black to blond/yellow to red-haired women (RRs, 1.72, 3.30, and 4.95, respectively; $P_{interaction} = 0.18$). Melanoma risk increased significantly with the number of sunburns and bathing vacations in the first three age decades ($P_{trend} \leq 0.04$) and solarium use at ages 30 to 39 and 40 to 49 years [RRs for solarium use ≥ 1 time/mo 1.49 (95% CI, 1.11-2.00) and 1.61 (95% CI 1.10-2.35), respectively; $P_{trend} \leq 0.02$]. Risk of melanoma associated with sunburns, bathing vacations, and solarium use increased with accumulating exposure across additional decades of life.

Conclusions.—Melanoma risk seems to continue to increase with accumulating intermittent sun exposure and solarium use in early adulthood. Apparently, super-multiplicative joint effects of nevi and hair color identify people with red hair and multiple nevi as a very high risk group and suggest important gene-gene interactions involving *MC1R* in melanoma etiology.

▶ This is one of those articles that makes you want to hang a copy in the waiting room or give to every patient. Even though the conclusions and some other information are somewhat obvious to dermatologists, the way that it is presented and designed for discussion and review really stimulates conversation about setting screening guidelines and prevention strategies with all of our patients, not just those at higher risk of skin cancer or with a history of extensive sun exposure. The risk criteria are broken down to not just skin type but hair color, incidence of nevi on legs, and cumulative years in tanning beds (solarium) and warm weather vacations. This would be a great article to formulate either a patient questionnaire or a simple summary for patients to understand risk factors aside from how fair they are or whether they burn or tan. And to back it up, there are over 100 000 patients reviewed over nearly 30 years in a part of the world where most patients are with skin types I to III. I think it is a great article for review and for the journal it was published in, despite being "master of the obvious."

N. Bhatia, MD

The Importance of Attached Nail Plate Epithelium in the Diagnosis of Nail Apparatus Melanoma
Ruben BS, McCalmont TH (Univ of California, San Francisco)
J Cutan Pathol 37:1028-1029, 2010

Background.—Achieving an accurate histopathological diagnosis of any melanoma is challenging, but the diagnosis of nail unit melanoma is especially difficult. The condition is rare, so many physicians are unfamiliar with it. It is also highly subject to misinterpretation, and the nail plate presents a physical barrier to be overcome. Distorted and fragmented biopsies are common when samples are obtained through the inflexible ungual shield. With a poor prognosis under the best circumstances, missing the diagnosis becomes an extremely serious problem, permitting the lesion to thicken, the stage at ultimate diagnosis to become more advanced, and survival to diminish. An alternate source for sampling was suggested.

Diagnostic Approach.—Most physicians rely on traditional criteria to make the diagnosis. This involves an assessment of circumscription, determination of the ratio of single cells to nests, cytologic appraisal of atypia and level of intraepithelial scatter, and assessment of junctional/subjunctional lymphocytes. These are all predicated on obtaining an adequate specimen, which is often not the case.

Obtaining Samples.—Closely examining epithelium attached to or dangling from the nail plate may offer a way to diagnose nail unit melanoma. This may contain the desired nail epithelium and matrix needed for diagnostic purposes.

Conclusions.—Often the diagnosis of nail unit melanoma is missed, causing serious consequences. Using attached ungual epithelium may improve diagnoses and help the patient and clinician.

▶ Nail biopsy specimens are often difficult to process and interpret by the dermatophathologist. Specimens may be crushed or possibly misoriented because of the complexities of the nail unit and the challenges that nail biopsy present. The dermatopathologists give tips on reading difficult nail slides by suggesting that the tissue that is adhered to the undersurface of the specimen be evaluated. There is often a fragment of attached nail plate epithelium which when evaluated can be useful in arriving at the correct diagnosis. Clear communication between the pathologist and the nail surgeon regarding the orientation and origin of the nail specimen (nail bed vs nail matrix) is very useful.

P. Rich, MD

Targeted High-Resolution Ultrasound Is Not an Effective Substitute for Sentinel Lymph Node Biopsy in Patients With Primary Cutaneous Melanoma

Sanki A, Uren RF, Moncrieff M, et al (Royal Prince Alfred and Mater Hosps, Sydney, New South Wales, Australia; Royal Prince Alfred Hosp, Sydney, New South Wales, Australia; Univ of Sydney, New South Wales, Australia; et al)
J Clin Oncol 27:5614-5619, 2009

Purpose.—To reassess traditional ultrasound descriptors of sentinel lymph node (SLN) metastases, to determine the minimum cross-sectional area (CSA) of an SLN metastasis detectable by ultrasound (US), and to establish whether targeted, high-resolution US of SLNs identified by lymphoscintigraphy before initial melanoma surgery can be used as a substitute for excisional SLN biopsy.

Methods.—US was performed on SLNs identified in 871 lymph node fields in 716 patients. SLN biopsy was performed within 24 hours of lymphoscintigraphy and US examination. The CSA of each SLN metastatic deposit was determined sonographically and histologically.

Results.—The sensitivity of targeted US in the detection of positive SLNs was 24.3% (95% CI, 19.5% to 28.7%), and the specificity was 96.8% (95% CI, 95.9% to 97.7%). The sensitivity was highest for neck SLNs (45.8%) and improved with greater Breslow thickness. The median histologic CSA of the SLN metastatic deposits was 0.39 mm^2 (12.75 mm^2 for US true-positive results and 0.22 mm^2 for US false-negative results). True-positive, US-detected SLNs had significantly greater CSAs (*t* test $P < .001$) than undetected SLN metastases and were more likely to be spherical in cross-section. More than two sonographic descriptors of SLN metastases or rounding of the node alone were factors highly suggestive of a melanoma deposit.

Conclusion.—US is not an appropriate substitute for SLN biopsy, but it is of value in preoperative SLN assessment and postoperative monitoring.

▶ Just how far has high-resolution ultrasound come in detecting nodal melanoma metastasis was answered in this well-controlled study: a long way. However, it has a long way to go before its sensitivity rivals histological confirmation via sentinel lymph node biopsy. Studies such as this one are vital in developing parameters for determining the presence of nodal melanoma metastasis. As ultrasonic technology evolves, devices such as high-resolution ultrasound either alone or in combination with other noninvasive imaging technologies will hopefully lessen the need for more invasive surgical techniques. For the present time, the role of high-resolution ultrasound in nodal melanoma metastasis has value as a preoperative assessment and postoperative monitoring tool.

G. Martin, MD

The impact of dermoscopy on the management of pigmented lesions in everyday clinical practice of general dermatologists: a prospective study

van der Rhee JI, Bergman W, Kukutsch NA (Leiden Univ Med Ctr, the Netherlands)

Br J Dermatol 162:563-567, 2010

Background.—Dermoscopy greatly improves the clinical diagnosis of pigmented lesions. Few studies have investigated, however, how dermoscopy is guiding management decisions in everyday clinical practice. In addition, most studies have been performed in the setting of dermoscopy experts working in pigmented lesion clinics.

Objectives.—To assess the impact of dermoscopy on clinical diagnosis and management decisions for pigmented lesions in everyday practice of general dermatologists.

Methods.—We performed a prospective study in general dermatology clinics in community hospitals run by dermatologists with intermediate dermoscopy experience and expertise. Each clinician independently included suspicious lesions from consecutive patients. Pre- and postdermoscopy diagnoses and management decisions were recorded. Pathology was used as reference diagnosis.

Results.—In total, 209 suspicious lesions were included in the study by 17 dermatologists. Fourteen lesions were histologically proven *in situ* or invasive malignant melanomas. Based on clinical diagnoses, dermoscopy improved sensitivity from 0·79 to 0·86 ($P = 1·0$). All 14 melanomas were intended to be excised based on naked eye examination alone, independent of dermoscopic evaluation. Specificity increased from 0·96 to 0·98 ($P = 0·22$). Dermoscopy resulted in a 9% reduction of the number of excisions.

Conclusions.—Dermoscopy reduced the number of excisions, but did not improve the detection of melanomas. Our results suggest that in everyday clinical practice of general dermatologists the main contribution of dermoscopy is a reduction of unnecessary excisions.

▶ Dermoscopy can aid in the clinical diagnosis of pigmented lesions and may be better in discriminating between melanoma and benign pigmented lesions. The aim of this study was to assess prospectively the impact of dermoscopy on the clinical diagnosis and management of pigmented lesions. This study included 17 general dermatologists with a median experience in dermoscopy of 7.5 years (range, 6 months to 14 years). Twelve clinicians (71%) reported a methodology similar to consecutive sampling. Five clinicians (29%) stated that they had followed inclusion instructions but with no detailed description of their method of sampling. Participants judged a mean number of 12 lesions (range 4-20) with a total of 209 lesions. Data on clinical diagnosis and management were complete for 207 (99%) and 196 (94%) lesions, respectively. There were a total of 99 lesions that were biopsied: 72 for diagnostic purposes, 10 were invasive, and 4 were in situ melanomas. Dermoscopy improved sensitivity from 0.79 to 0.86 ($P = 1.0$). All 14 melanomas were intended to be excised based on naked eye examination alone, independent of dermoscopic evaluation. Sensitivity was calculated to be 0.79 (11/14) for naked eye examination alone and 0.86 (12/14) for naked eye examination aided by dermoscopy. Specificity was 0.96 (186/193) before and 0.98 (190/193) after dermoscopy had been performed ($P = .22$) and resulted in a 9% reduction in the number of excisions. Statistical analysis demonstrated that the improvements of sensitivity and specificity by the addition of dermoscopy were not statically significant ($P = 1.0$ and $P = .22$, respectively). In 13% (n = 25) of the lesions, management changed after dermoscopy had been performed: for 16 lesions (8%), a diagnostic biopsy was abandoned and for 9 lesions (5%), a diagnostic biopsy was induced. Before dermoscopy, 40% (79/196) of included lesions were intended to be excised (diagnostic biopsy). After dermoscopy, 37% (72/196) of the lesions were excised. The malignant:benign ratio of excised lesions decreased from 1:5.6 (14/79) before to 1:5.1 lesions (14/72) after dermoscopy had been performed. In addition, dermoscopy did not improve the detection of melanomas, and all 14 melanomas in this study were intended to be excised before dermoscopy was performed. A limitation to this study was that examiners did not have a uniform method for identifying suspicious lesions. Although in this study authors suggest that dermoscopy may prevent unnecessary excisions, if a clinician has a strong clinical suspicion for melanoma, they may consider a biopsy of the lesion because of dire consequences of leaving a possible melanoma on a patient. Also, it may be of value if investigators had a baseline dermoscopy examination for suspicious lesions including evaluation of changes that indicate malignancy.

J. Q. Del Rosso, DO

G. K. Kim, DO

The Impact of Partial Biopsy on Histopathologic Diagnosis of Cutaneous Melanoma: Experience of an Australian Tertiary Referral Service

Ng JC, Swain S, Dowling JP, et al (Monash Univ, Melbourne, Victoria, Australia; The Alfred Hosp, Prahran, Melbourne, Australia)
Arch Dermatol 146:234-239, 2010

Objective.—To compare partial and excisional biopsy techniques in the accuracy of histopathologic diagnosis and microstaging of cutaneous melanoma.

Design.—Prospective case series.

Setting.—Tertiary referral, ambulatory care, institutional practice.

Patients.—Consecutive cases from 1995 to 2006.

Interventions.—Partial and excisional biopsy. Other factors considered were anatomic site, physician type at initial management, hypomelanosis, melanoma subtype, biopsy sample size, multiple biopsies, and tumor thickness.

Main Outcome Measures.—Histopathologic diagnosis (false-negative misdiagnosis—overall or with an adverse outcome—and false-positive misdiagnosis) and microstaging accuracy. Odds ratios (ORs) and 95% confidence intervals (CIs) obtained from multinomial logistic regression.

Results.—Increased odds of histopathologic misdiagnosis were associated with punch biopsy (OR, 16.6; 95% CI, 10-27) ($P < .001$) and shave biopsy (OR, 2.6; 95% CI, 1.2-5.7) ($P = .02$) compared with excisional biopsy. Punch biopsy was associated with increased odds of misdiagnosis with an adverse outcome (OR, 20; 95% CI, 10-41) ($P < .001$). Other factors associated with increased odds of misdiagnosis included acral lentiginous melanoma (OR, 5.1; 95% CI, 2-13) ($P < .001$), desmoplastic melanoma (OR, 3.8; 95% CI, 1.1-13.0) ($P = .03$), and nevoid melanoma (OR, 28.4; 95% CI, 7-115) ($P < .001$). Punch biopsy (OR, 5.1; 95% CI, 3.4-7.6) ($P < .001$) and shave biopsy (OR, 2.3; 95% CI, 1.5-3.6) ($P < .001$) had increased odds of microstaging inaccuracy over excisional biopsy. Tumor thickness was the most important determinant of microstaging inaccuracy when partial biopsy was used (odds of significant microstaging inaccuracy increased 1.8-fold for every 1 mm increase in tumor thickness; 95% CI, 1.4-2.4) ($P < .001$).

Conclusions.—Among melanoma seen at a tertiary referral center, histopathologic misdiagnosis is more common for melanomas that have been assessed with punch and shave biopsy than with excisional biopsy. Regardless of biopsy method, adverse outcomes due to misdiagnosis may occur. However, such adverse events are more commonly associated with punch biopsy than with shave and excisional biopsy. The use of punch and shave biopsy also leads to increased microstaging inaccuracy.

▶ The misdiagnosis of melanoma can be devastating to both the patient and physician. This is a prospective case series study comparing partial and excisional biopsy as well as examining the histopathologic diagnosis and microstaging accuracy in both general practitioners and dermatologists. This study sets out to assess the accuracy of histopathologic diagnosis and microstaining of a partial biopsy compared with excisional biopsy for melanoma in a tertiary referral center. Of the 2470 referrals included in the study (2127 excisional biopsies, 163 punch biopsies, and 180 shave biopsies), there were 83 false-negative misdiagnoses (3.4%), including 37 associated with an adverse outcome (1.5%); 135 false-positive misdiagnoses (5.5%); and 2252 correct diagnoses (91.5%). The odds of misdiagnosis were very much higher with punch biopsy than with excisional biopsy, whereas shave biopsy was only weakly associated with misdiagnoses. This study found increased odds for misdiagnosis, and adverse outcomes remained significant for punch biopsy (odds ratio [OR] for misdiagnosis, 14.7 [$P < .01$]; OR for adverse outcome, 13.2 [$P < .001$]). The delay in diagnosis was shorter following misdiagnosis with punch and shave biopsies (median delay 30.6 months) than with excisional biopsies (median delay 49.1 months). Increased odds of misdiagnosis were associated with initial management by general practitioners (compared with dermatologist), acral lentiginous melanoma, desmoplastic melanoma, and nevoid melanoma. General practitioners remained at increased odds for misdiagnosing ($P < .001$) and adverse outcomes ($P < .001$) compared with dermatologists. Inaccurate microstaging was present in 34% of cases misdiagnosed with punch biopsy (41 of 122), 19% with shave biopsy (31 of 1630), and 9.1% with excisional biopsy (179 of 1967). For every 1-mm increase in tumor thickness, the risk of inaccurate microstaging increased 1.8-fold ($P < .001$). This study demonstrated the increased risks of melanoma histopathologic misdiagnosis and microstaging inaccuracy by punch and shave biopsy compared with excisional biopsy. The fact that general practioners had more adverse outcomes compared with dermatologists may be explained by a more difficult spectrum of presenting lesions, differences in clinical skills, lesion selection, or sending of specimens to less experienced pathologists. Nevertheless, this study builds a case for precaution in the use of partial biopsy, especially with general practitioners. Although adverse outcomes may be because of external factors that are not in the control of the clinician, this article stresses an excellent point that adverse events have been associated with punch biopsy compared with shave and excisional biopsy. To add, the use of punch and shave biopsy also leads to an increase in microstaging inaccuracy. Another important consideration is that the term shave is poorly descriptive of the nature of the technique needed to properly biopsy pigmented skin lesions. Overall (there may always be occasional rational exceptions), with a lesion that is clinically macular or a very thin papule or plaque (without nodularity), a saucerization is what is truly needed to ensure the best chance of encompassing the full lesion by breadth and depth. Saucerization allows for inclusion of the entire breadth of the lesion based on evaluation of the visible lesion margins and includes extension through reticular dermis, to avoid transection of the lesion, which would then preclude accurate evaluation of Breslow thickness if a melanoma is present. The term shave conceptually implies a procedure that is likely to be too superficial to fully encompass the lesion histologically. If the lesion is a thick plaque or nodule, excisional biopsy is preferred.

J. Q. Del Rosso, DO

G. K. Kim, DO

The Nodal Location of Metastases in Melanoma Sentinel Lymph Nodes
Riber-Hansen R, Nyengaard JR, Hamilton-Dutoit SJ, et al (Aarhus Univ Hosp, Aarhus C, Denmark; Aarhus Univ, Aarhus C, Denmark; et al)
Am J Surg Pathol 33:1522-1528, 2009

Background.—The design of melanoma sentinel lymph node (SLN) histologic protocols is based on the premise that most metastases are found in the central parts of the nodes, but the evidence for this belief has never been thoroughly tested.

Methods.—The nodal location of melanoma metastases in 149 prospectively analyzed, completely step sectioned, positive SLNs from 96 patients was examined using 3 theoretical protocols, evaluating respectively: (1) the 3 most central step sections only; (2) the 3 most peripheral step sections only; and (3) 3 step sections evenly distributed throughout the individual SLNs. In addition, the size of the metastases located exclusively outside the 2 regional protocols (ie, 3 central sections, and 3 peripheral sections) were measured and compared with each other.

Results.—The metastasis detection rates of the central, the peripheral, and the evenly distributed protocols were 77%, 79%, and 78%, respectively. No difference in either the mean volume or the maximum diameter of the metastases located exclusively outside the central and the peripheral protocols was found (volume: 0.036 vs. 0.031 mm^3 and diameter: 0.320 vs. 0.332 mm).

Conclusions.—In SLNs, melanoma metastases are located throughout the nodes. Metastases located exclusively outside the peripheral or the central protocol are equally sized. Complete step sectioning of all SLNs will ensure both high metastasis detection rates and detection of all large metastases, and allow for performance of unbiased size estimates.

▶ The sentinel lymph node (SLN) biopsy status in the absence of clinical metastatic disease is generally considered to be the most important factor in predicting prognosis for survival in patients with melanomas with Breslow depths between 1 and 4 mm. Given the heavy emphasis this test is given, it is imperative to look at how it is performed and ways of making it as accurate as possible.

This article reviews how the SLN is examined histologically and attempts to determine whether a pattern can be found indicating the most likely site of metastasis within the lymph node. If this were to be determined, then it could help guide pathologists with where to start and perhaps stop their sectioning if the findings were negative. The goal would be to develop sentinel sectioning as it were.

The authors conclude by saying that it remains that the more sections of a lymph node that are examined the more likely that the metastases will be found. While this conclusion will not likely change the course of how SLNs are histologically examined, it is a point well made and worth further examination. Essentially, the authors are looking to develop a highly sensitive test or screening test for the histological examination of the SLN. What they are looking to develop is a regimented way to examine lymph nodes with an acceptable rate of false negative tests (type II error). The most important factor in decreasing the possibility of type II error in a study is to increase the power. Therefore, before any conclusions are reached regarding this concept, it will be essential to have a much larger sample number. This would seem a worthwhile goal toward developing an even better test.

A. Smith, MD
A. Torres, MD, JD

The Role of Circumstances of Diagnosis and Access to Dermatological Care in Early Diagnosis of Cutaneous Melanoma: A Population-Based Study in France

Durbec F, Vitry F, Granel-Brocard F, et al (Hôpital Robert Debré, Reims France; Hôpital Maison Blanche, Reims, France; Hôpital Fournier, Nancy, France; et al)

Arch Dermatol 146:240-246, 2010

Objectives.—To describe circumstances of the diagnosis and access to dermatological care for patients with cutaneous melanoma (CM) and to investigate factors associated with early detection.

Design.—Retrospective population-based study of incident cases of invasive CM in 2004, using questionnaires to physicians and a survey of cancer registries and pathology laboratories.

Setting.—Five regions in northeastern France.

Patients.—Six hundred fifty-two patients who were referred to dermatologists by general practitioners (group 1) or by other specialists (group 2), who directly consulted a dermatologist for CM (group 3), or who were diagnosed as having CM during a prospective follow-up of nevi (group 4) or when consulting a dermatologist for other diseases (group 5).

Main Outcome Measures.—Characteristics of patients, tumors, and patients' residence in each group, including the geographical concentration of dermatologists. We performed multivariate analysis of these factors to determine association with Breslow thickness.

Results.—Age, tumor location, Breslow thickness, ulceration, histological type, and geographical concentration of dermatologists significantly differed among groups. Patients consulting dermatologists directly formed the largest group (45.1%). Those referred by general practitioners (26.1%) were the oldest and had the highest frequency of thick (>3 mm), nodular, and/or ulcerated CM. Patients from groups 4 (8.4%) and 5 (14.1%) had the thinnest CMs. Ulcerated and/or thick tumors were absent in group 4. In multivariate analysis, histological types superficial spreading melanoma and lentigo maligna melanoma, younger age, high concentration of dermatologists, and detection by dermatologists were significantly associated with thinner CMs.

Conclusion.—Easy access of patients to dermatologists, information campaigns targeting elderly people, and education of general practitioners are complementary approaches to improving early detection.

▶ The authors provide a high quality retrospective population-based analysis of the incidence of cutaneous melanoma (CM) and how the severity and demographics of this malignancy vary based on who (eg, physician type, primary care vs dermatology) makes the initial diagnosis. Their objective was to describe circumstances related to the diagnosis of and access to dermatological care for patients with CM and to investigate factors associated with early detection. The type of CM associated with the lowest mortality was correlated most frequently with a diagnosis made by a dermatologist. Another significant finding associated with a potential decrease in mortality was the demographic component, residing within a close proximity to a dermatologist.

The study appears to be well done. The 652 patient sample size provides an ample number. The limitations are primarily geographic in that only 5 regions in Northeast France were included. It is challenging to conclude that the same applies for the entire country, or world; however, the authors do discuss similar previous study results in Italy and North America. The other limiting factor was time. They only examined data from a 1-year period. This may not account for changes in governmental health care policies or other variations that could become apparent over a longer period of time.

The relevance of this article is the direct demonstration of the need for skin cancer screenings by dermatologists. The article also shows the importance of ease of access of patients to dermatologists and its potential to decrease morbidity, mortality, and health care costs. The authors demonstrate further the need to promote melanoma-screening education for primary care physicians to further diminish the morbidity associated with this disease.

B. P. Glick, DO, MPH

A. Wiener, DO

T. J. Singer, DO

The Use of High-Resolution Ultrasonography for Preoperative Detection of Metastases in Sentinel Lymph Nodes of Patients with Cutaneous Melanoma

Kunte C, Schuh T, Eberle JY, et al (Ludwig-Maximilian-Univ Munich, Germany)
Dermatol Surg 35:1757-1765, 2009

Background.—Sentinel lymph node biopsy (SLNB) reliably assesses the status of the regional lymph node basins and provides prognostic information in patients with cutaneous melanoma, but is logistically demanding and expensive.

Objective.—The aim of this study was to evaluate the ability of high resolution B-mode ultrasonography (US) for pre-operative identification and characterization of sentinel lymph nodes (SLN) in patients with cutaneous melanoma.

Patients and Methods.—In a prospective trial, the use of high resolution US was assessed in 25 consecutive patients with cutaneous melanoma identified for SLNB, first, for its value in primary detection of SLN, and, second, for its value in the correct assessment of SLN after lymphoscintigraphic mapping.

Results.—High resolution B-mode US correctly identified two of 6 positive SLN. The sensitivity, specificity, positive predictive value, and negative predictive value of US were 33.3% (95% CI 43.3−77.7), 100.0% (95% CI 88.1−100.0), 100.0% (95% CI 15.8−100.0) and 87.9% (95% CI 71.8−96.6), respectively.

Conclusion.—High resolution B-mode US cannot replace SLNB, especially in the detection of micrometastases, but it remains the most important method to assess the lymph node status for macrometastases presurgically.

▶ Management of patients with intermediate risk melanomas has been a challenging and controversial topic. Sentinal lymph node biopsy (SLNB) has proven to provide useful prognostic information as well as guiding the decision to perform regional lymph node dissection. However, SLNB is an invasive technique with potential morbidity as well as adding to the increasing cost of melanoma patient management. The development of noninvasive techniques in the detection of lymph node metastases is an important and admirable enterprise. As the authors mention, results have been mixed in the detection of lymph node metastases < 4-5 mm.

In this study, ultrasonography (US) would have identified 2 out of 6 positive lymph node basins and spared the patient a SLNB. While this is important from the perspective of patient convenience (sparing 1 surgical procedure) and reducing the cost of health care and potential morbidity, these patients would still have received lymph node dissection with a positive US and, therefore, they would still have been subject to the morbidity associated with this procedure.

Obviously, the ultimate goal would be to have a test sensitive enough to rule out micrometastases and spare patients at intermediate risk further invasive procedures, such as SLNB. The negative predictive value of 87.9% reported in this study, while encouraging, may still not be high enough to avoid SLNB for many dermatologists and oncologic surgeons. The sensitivity is admittedly much too low for B-mode US to be considered a screening test for micrometastases.

The utility of US in detection of macrometastases is certainly of value as an adjunct to physical examination. This commendable study provides useful clinical information, namely, that B-mode US cannot replace SLNB as a means to detect micrometastases but can be used as a useful adjunct to physical examination in detecting macrometastases and that further technologic advances are needed for less invasive screening of micrometastases. The addition of color Doppler analysis of the sentinel lymph nodes (SLNs) looking for alterations in vascular pattern, addition of fine needle aspirate to preoperative screening, and other technologic advances may provide quality tests high enough to help avoid surgical procedures.

Finally, given medical-legal implications, many oncologic surgeons may not be willing to perform lymph node dissection of the regional basin without a biopsy-proven lymph node, given the substantial morbidity associated with this procedure. This issue would potentially be addressed with US-guided fine needle aspirate cytology but would need to be part of the routine armamentarium and practice to substantially limit the amount of SNLB procedures performed.

R. I. Ceilley, MD

Thick Melanoma: Prognostic Value of Positive Sentinel Nodes

Vermeeren L, van der Ent FWC, Sastrowijoto PSH, et al (Maaslandhospital Sittard, Sittard-Geleen, The Netherlands)
World J Surg 33:2464-2468, 2009

Background.—Sentinel lymph node biopsy (SNB) is a widely accepted procedure used to accurately stage patients with melanoma. Its value in patients with thick melanoma (Breslow thickness >4 mm) is reason for discussion because of the generally poor prognosis of these patients. The purpose of this study was to report on the incidence of SNB positivity in patients with thick melanoma and to analyze the prognostic value of SNB in these patients.

Methods.—The prospective database of 248 patients with cutaneous melanoma, who underwent SNB in the Maaslandhospital Sittard between January 1994 and August 2007, was reviewed and completed. In 31 patients, SNB was performed for a thick melanoma. We analyzed survival (Kaplan—Meier) and survival differences (log-rank) in this group.

Results.—In 64.5% of the patients with a thick melanoma, the SNB was positive. In our patients, SNB result was the only predictor for overall survival in patients with a thick melanoma ($P = 0.045$).

Conclusions.—To be accurately informed about a patient's prognosis and to decide whether subsequent completion lymph node dissection is indicated, SNB should not be omitted in patients with a primary thick melanoma.

▶ If there is one disease that commands close attention to guidelines and protocols, it is melanoma. However, that is also the same disease that, more often than not, refuses to play by the rules. Therefore, if there is a tendency to diagnose and treat melanoma more aggressively, it is because there is a tendency not to want to let melanoma win.[1-3]

As the authors suggest, sentinel lymph node biopsy (SLNB) is performed less commonly in thicker melanomas because of the potential for high mortality rates at that stage. So to justify the procedure, there needs to be a value to what the information will tell us in the management of these more advanced patients. The underlying theme is to make dermatologists question why we have not been doing SLNBs in everyone with more advanced melanoma, which in today's age of interferons and ipilimumab makes perfect sense...this is because many patients with even distant metastasis have a better survival chance than they did in the days when sentinel lymph node dissection was first becoming accepted, yet dermatologists might still be hanging on to those messages rather than giving patients their best chance to win.

There is an important observation that the authors share, "Our results indicate that SLNB is the only prognostic factor of importance for survival in patients with a thick melanoma." From there, they also conclude that, "thickness of melanomas >4 mm Breslow should not be a reason to omit SNB, because it is an important, and in our series the only, prognostic factor in this patient group." But this is again to establish disease-free survival and recurrence potential, which in terms of the study is important; so what clinicians need from this information is in terms of who should receive treatment based on ordering the one test that might either make a huge difference in their outcomes or give one more scar for no reason. This comes back to the most important question: does determination of prognostic factors in deep melanoma also determine who will receive treatment? Because we now have newer therapies that have been available since the article's publication date, this is an important step in the critical evaluation of the results.

So when the next patient who walks into the clinic and unfortunately receives a diagnosis of melanoma, ulcerated and Breslow depth 4.3 mm, what should we do? Based on the conclusions of the authors, we need to weigh SLNB findings as just an important prognostic factor as the others.

N. Bhatia, MD

References

1. Morris KT, Busam KJ, Bero S, Patel A, Brady MS. Primary cutaneous melanoma with regression does not require a lower threshold for sentinel lymph node biopsy. *Ann Surg Oncol.* 2008;15:316-322.
2. Gershenwald JE, Mansfield PF, Lee JE, Ross MI. Role for lymphatic mapping and sentinel lymph node biopsy in patients with thick ($\geq$4 mm) primary melanoma. *Ann Surg Oncol.* 2000;7:160-165.
3. Verma S, Quirt I, McCready D, Bak K, Charette M, Iscoe N. Systematic review of systemic adjuvant therapy for patients at high risk for recurrent melanoma. *Cancer.* 2006;106:1431-1442.

15 Lymphoproliferative Disorders

Drug-associated reversible granulomatous T cell dyscrasia: a distinct subset of the interstitial granulomatous drug reaction
Magro CM, Cruz-Inigo AE, Votava H, et al (Weill Cornell Med College, NY; New York Univ; et al)
J Cutan Pathol 37:96-111, 2010

Background.—A cutaneous T-cell infiltrate exhibiting cytologic and architectural atypia, an aberrant phenotypic profile and clonal restriction would fall under the rubric of a T-cell dyscrasia. Although such an infiltrate could represent a lymphoma, this constellation of findings can also be seen in drug-associated pseudolymphoma.

Methods.—In 2001, two of the authors (CMM and AEC) proposed the term *reversible T-cell dyscrasia* to describe atypical T-lymphocytic infiltrates that manifest a light microscopic, phenotypic and molecular profile that closely parallels cutaneous T-cell lymphoma but regress when the causal drug is withdrawn.

Results.—Herein we report our 10 cases of drug-associated pseudolymphoma resembling granulomatous mycosis fungoides.

Conclusions.—We term this reaction pattern *drug-associated reversible granulomatous T-cell dyscrasia* and consider it a distinct subset of the interstitial granulomatous drug reaction.

▶ The description of interstitial granulomatous drug reaction, occurrence of which was also described by Magro et al in 1999, was an important contribution to the literature, and I agree with the assertion that based upon how often the pattern is encountered in dermatopathology, it is likely underreported in the literature. In this submission, Magro et al again describe a related interstitial lymphogranulomatous process, without sarcoidal qualities, which resembles a lymphoproliferative disorder, namely granulomatous mycosis fungoides. This semblance occurs not only by light microscopy but also through immunohistochemcial and genotypic features, including T-cell clonality.

Drugs involved in the 10 cases described include statins, angiotensin-converting enzyme inhibitors, calcium channel blockers, antidepressants, anticonvulsants, and synthetic estrogens, medications that are rather ubiquitous in our aging US population. It is equally important to mention that in nearly each case, cessation of the drug led to regression of the condition. Lastly,

423

this article reiterates that the diagnosis of mycosis fungoides remains, at its most fundamental level, a diagnosis that requires clinicopathologic correlation. The adage "clonality is not necessarily or absolutely indicative of malignancy," is an apt concept to be mindful of in an era when genotypic studies are so widely and readily available.

Other entities recently described to manifest T-cell clonality include pigmented purpuric dermatoses[1] and some cases of lymphomatoid papulosis,[2] but again, clonality in these conditions seems either to be not truly malignant in nature or the population is held under close check by immunosurveillance. Future reporting and larger series will be useful in studying the applicability of this latest entity to the clinical situation.

W. A. High, MD, JD, MEng

References

1. Plaza JA, Morrison C, Magro CM. Assessment of TCR-beta clonality in a diverse group of cutaneous T-Cell infiltrates. *J Cutan Pathol.* 2008;35:358-365.
2. Schultz JC, Granados S, Vonderheid EC, Hwang ST. T-cell clonality of peripheral blood lymphocytes in patients with lymphomatoid papulosis. *J Am Acad Dermatol.* 2005;53:152-155.

Paucity of intraepidermal FoxP3-positive T cells in cutaneous T-cell lymphoma in contrast with spongiotic and lichenoid dermatitis
Wada DA, Wilcox RA, Weenig RH, et al (Mayo Clinic, Rochester, MN)
J Cutan Pathol 37:535-541, 2010

Background.—FoxP3 is the most specific available marker for regulatory T cells (Tregs). Tumor-associated FoxP3-positive Tregs have been identified in various neoplasms, including cutaneous T-cell lymphoma (CTCL). FoxP3 expression in CTCL varies across groups; few studies have compared CTCL with inflammatory conditions.

Methods.—Lesional skin biopsies from 20 patients with CTCL [13 mycosis fungoides (MF); 7 Sézary syndrome (SS)] and 22 with inflammatory dermatoses (11 spongiotic; 11 lichenoid or interface) were examined for FoxP3 expression by immunohistochemistry. Epidermal FoxP3-positive lymphocytes were counted as a percentage of the total epidermal CD3-positive T-cell population.

Results.—FoxP3-positive T cells composed the minority of infiltrate in all major categories. Lower numbers of epidermal FoxP3-positive T cells were observed in CTCL, particularly MF, than in inflammatory dermatoses (P < .001). CTCL neoplastic T cells did not express FoxP3.

Conclusion.—FoxP3-positive T cells are less frequently encountered in MF than in inflammatory dermatoses. FoxP3-positive T cells occur in higher proportions in the dermis than in the epidermis and probably correlate with coexisting inflammatory components. CTCL neoplastic cells do not typically express a Treg phenotype and are associated with low numbers of FoxP3-positive Tregs in the infiltrate. FoxP3 expression by immunohistochemistry may aid histologic evaluation of these conditions.

▶ It has been established that FoxP3 is a regulator of regulatory T cells (Tregs) and plays a central role in self-tolerance by suppressing the immune response. Tumor-associated Tregs have been studied in various malignancies, including cutaneous T-cell lymphoma (CTCL) with an increase in FoxP3-positive T cells in skin biopsies from patients who had mycosis fungoides (MF). Some research has implicated using Tregs as a diagnostic marker for CTCL and MF. This is a study of 20 cases of CTCL (13 MF and 7 Sezary syndrome [SS]) and 22 cases of inflammatory dermatoses (11 cases of spongiotic dermatitis and 11 cases of lichenoid or interface dermatitis) comparing FoxP3 expression by immunohistochemistry in lesional skin biopsies. Cases of spongiotic and lichenoid dermatitis were confirmed with histological features and clinical impression. FoxP3-positive cells composed 5% or less of the intraepidermal infiltrate in 8 of 12 cases of MF in contrast to only 3 of 22 cases of inflammatory disorders. The intraepidermal FoxP3-positive lymphocytes observed in patients with CTCL (MF and SS) were lower than those observed in patients with spongiotic and lichenoid or interface dermatoses ($P < .001$). However, in SS alone, the percentage of epidermal FoxP3-positive lymphocytes was observed to be 20% greater in 3 of 7 patients. Dermal FoxP3-positive cells were also more common in the inflammatory group than in CTCL ($P = .003$). FoxP3-positive cells made up 15% of the epidermal infiltrate in both cases of spongiotic dermatitis with atypical histologic features. This study was consistent with previous theories that neoplastic cells in CTCL do not express detectable FoxP3 cells and are thus not characterized as having a Treg phenotype. This study showed a lower percentage (< 10%) of FoxP3-positive T cells in the epidermis of lesions from patients with MF compared with previous studies. Limitations included small sample size and no controls of normal skin. To add, markers such as FoxP3 may change over time, especially in a neoplastic dermatosis, and a baseline FoxP3 population study comparing over a disease course may indicate progression of the disease. This study revealed that FoxP3 expression is not usually observed in the neoplastic population of CTCL patients and may not be a useful diagnostic tool from immunohistochemical analysis. However, the paucity of FoxP3-positive epidermal T cells observed in MF is of unknown significance. To add, there may be other contributing factors, such as ligand expression and other regulatory cells, that are involved in this disease process. Therefore, the presence or absence of FoxP3-positive T cells may not be reliable in MF, but this study showed that it may be seen more frequently in spongiotic and lichenoid dermatitis.

J. Q. Del Rosso, DO
G. K. Kim, DO

T-cell receptor γ gene rearrangement in cutaneous T-cell lymphoma: comparative study of polymerase chain reaction with denaturing gradient gel electrophoresis and GeneScan analysis

Goeldel AL, Cornillet-Lefebvre P, Durlach A, et al (Hôpital Robert Debré, Reims Cedex, France)

Br J Dermatol 162:822-829, 2010

Background.—The usefulness of T-cell receptor gene rearrangement (TCR-GR) analyses for differentiating cutaneous T-cell lymphoma (CTCL) from benign inflammatory disorders (BID) has been insufficiently studied to date.

Objectives.—To evaluate the diagnostic value of TCR-GR analyses, comparing polymerase chain reaction (PCR) with denaturing gradient gel electrophoresis (DGGE) analysis and BIOMED-2 standardized protocol PCR with GeneScan analysis (BIOMED-2-GS).

Methods.—Both types of PCR were performed in 157 patients evaluated for initial features suggestive of CTCL between 1996 and 2007. After clinical and histological review, the final diagnosis was CTCL in 77 cases and BID in 80 cases.

Results.—DGGE and BIOMED-2-GS had a similar diagnostic value for distinguishing CTCL from BID, with a sensitivity of 74% and 77%, respectively, and a specificity of 86%. The observed concordance between both methods was 90% and the kappa coefficient was 0·79. Positivity rates did not depend on the PCR method but varied according to the type of CTCL (73–75% in mycosis fungoides, 90–100% in Sézary syndrome, 40–60% in lymphomatoid papulosis and 100% in other types). The positivity rate in BID was 14% with both methods. The most frequent BID with a monoclonal pattern were drug-induced cutaneous lymphoid hyperplasia, erythrodermic psoriasis and pityriasis lichenoides chronica.

Conclusions.—BIOMED-2-GS analysis of the TCRγ gene is as sensitive and specific as DGGE for CTCL diagnosis. In addition, BIOMED-2-GS is less time-consuming and gives more information concerning the size and nature of TCR-GR.

▶ Standardization of polymerase chain reaction (PCR) techniques and primers used to detect malignancy is very important when comparing studies and collating data. There are many studies published about the efficacy of PCR for diagnosing malignant lymphoproliferations in skin, but unfortunately, each study differs in their methods and choice in primers. The objective of this study was to evaluate the diagnostic value of T-cell receptor gene rearrangement (TCR-GR) analysis using PCR with denaturing gradient gel electrophoresis versus BIOMED-2—standardized PCR protocol with GeneScan (GS) analysis in 157 patients with initial features suggestive of cutaneous T-cell lymphoma (CTCL). The results of this study demonstrate that both methods are relatively equivalent in detecting monoclonality in both patients with CTCL and patients with benign inflammatory disease. However, the

BIOMED-2 protocol with GS is far less time consuming and may give us more information regarding the clonal T-cell population.

The authors did an excellent job showing the equivalence of the 2 methods presented for detecting monoclonal and polyclonal populations. This study may perhaps lead the way for the BIOMED-2 protocol with GS in the routine evaluation for patients suspected for CTCL.

However, the problem still remains that monoclonality does not always equate to malignancy just as the absence of monoclonality does not always rule out malignancy, which should enforce the fact that TCR-GR analysis is an adjunctive diagnostic tool and not an independent diagnostic method.

J. Levin, DO

J. Q. Del Rosso, DO

Cutaneous type adult T-cell leukemia/lymphoma is a characteristic subtype and includes erythema/papule and nodule/tumor subgroups
Miyata T, Yonekura K, Utsunomiya A, et al (Aichi Cancer Ctr Res Inst, Nagoya, Japan; Kagoshima Univ Graduate School of Med and Dental Sciences, Japan; Imamura Bun-in Hosp, Kagoshima, Japan; et al)
Int J Cancer 126:1521-1528, 2010

We first analyzed the genomic profile of cutaneous type adult T-cell leukemia/lymphoma (ATLL) in an attempt to clarify its clinical and biological characteristics. Genomic gains of 1p, 7q and 18q and loss of 13q were frequently detected. Gain of 1p36.33-32 or loss of 13q33.1-3 indicated poor prognosis. Among cases with generalized lesions, erythema/papule or nodule/tumor cases showed a distinct genomic profile, indicating that these 2 groups were biologically different and developed via different genetic pathways. Furthermore, cases with generalized nodule/tumor lesions tended to progress to aggressive ATLL.

▶ Adult T-cell leukemia/lymphoma (ATLL) is caused by the human T-cell leukemia virus type I (HTLV1), which can remain latent for decades, but ultimately, approximately 2.5% of HTLV1 carriers develop ATLL. The authors describe a cutaneous type of ATLL characterized by skin lesions and low viral load in peripheral blood.

DNA was extracted from frozen skin biopsy samples, and array comparative genomic hybridization analysis was performed on 22 cutaneous-type ATLL cases. Eight patients' skin lesions were characterized by erythema, 3 by papules, 3 by nodules, and 8 by tumors. Seven patients had localized disease, and 15 had generalized skin lesions. Many were elderly males.

Cutaneous-type ATLL had specific genomic aberrations (such as 1p36 gain) that distinguished it from lymphoma-type ATLL that contained other genomic aberrations (such as 14q32 gain), which were less frequent in cutaneous-type ATLL. Most generalized cutaneous-type ATLL cases had genomic aberrations. The genomic profiles for patients with erythema or papules were distinct from those with nodules or tumors. In patients with localized cutaneous-type ATLL, genomic aberrations were detected in the 3 patients with tumors but in none of the patients with erythema or papules.

There are several difficulties with the information reported here. The term cutaneous-type ATLL is not universally accepted, as half of all ATLL cases have some skin lesions. Despite distinct genomic profiles demonstrated in this study, survival rate was not affected by the different profiles. Nevertheless, a distinct genomic profile detected in this study suggests that the different groups be studied separately when therapies are introduced or patients are studied for clinical outcomes.

M. Lebwohl, MD

16 Miscellaneous Topics in Cosmetic and Laser Surgery

A Comparative Study of Topical 5-Aminolevulinic Acid Incubation Times in Photodynamic Therapy with Intense Pulsed Light for the Treatment of Inflammatory Acne
Oh SH, Ryu DJ, Han EC, et al (Yonsei Univ College of Medicine, Seoul, Korea)
Dermatol Surg 35:1918-1926, 2009

Background.—Photodynamic therapy (PDT) with topical 5-aminolevulinic acid (ALA) is used for effective treatment of facial acne vulgaris.

Objectives.—To determine which of two different incubation times (30 minutes and 3 hours) is more effective in PDT with intense pulsed light (IPL) for acne vulgaris.

Methods & Materials.—Twenty Korean subjects with moderate to severe acne were enrolled for a randomized, half-facial treatment study. Three sessions with short incubation with ALA plus IPL (30 minutes, $n = 9$) or long incubation with ALA plus IPL (3 hours, $n = 11$) on one side of the face and IPL alone on the other side were performed at 1-month intervals.

Results.—All subjects showed improvement in inflammatory acne lesions after three sessions of ALA-PDT or IPL alone ($p < .001$ in all groups). The degree of improvement in inflammatory acne lesions was greater in the long incubation time group than the short incubation time group or the IPL-alone group, although the mean reduction of inflammatory acne lesions was statistically different only between the long incubation group and the IPL-only group ($p = .01$). There were no statistical differences between the short incubation group and IPL-alone group. All three groups had decreased sebum secretion after three sessions ($p < .001$ in all groups), but the differences between groups were not statistically significant. Only transient erythema and mild edema were reported for all treatment groups.

Conclusion.—PDT with a long ALA incubation time might be more adequate for a pronounced outcome with inflammatory acne.

▶ New treatments, such as photodynamic therapy (PDT) with topical 5-aminolevulinic acid (ALA), have been shown to be an effective treatment for facial acne vulgaris. Intense pulsed light (IPL) is commonly used as a PDT light source for acne treatment. Incubation time for ALA ranges from 30 to 60 minutes, with optimal contact time for ALA still unknown. This is a randomized, prospective, evaluator-blinded, split-face comparative study (n = 20) using IPL comparing 2 different incubation times: 1 at short incubation group, 30 minutes (n = 9), compared with long incubation group, 3 hours (n = 11). Controls were IPL alone (n = 20) performed at 1-month intervals with 3 sessions. Patients were skin type III/IV with moderate to severe acne. Patients who had been on oral antibiotics isotretinoin within 6 months, history of keloids, photosensitivity, or were pregnant were excluded. No other antiacne therapies were continued with treatment with light therapy. Clinical improvement was assessed globally according to the patient's subjective response and also by a blinded investigator at 4, 8, and 12 weeks. Sebum secretion was measured using a Sebumeter. The mean reduction in lesions at 12 weeks was 89.5% (3 hours ALA), 83.0% (30 minutes ALA), and 74.0% (IPL alone) and $P < .001$ in all cases. The degree of improvement in inflammatory lesions was greater in the long incubation time group compared with short and IPL alone. However, there was a statistical difference only between long incubation group and IPL-alone group ($P = .01$). Mean reduction in sebum secretion at 12 weeks was 46.7%, 31.5%, and 37.5%, respectively ($P < .001$ in all cases), with no statistical differences between the 3 groups. Authors state that all patients tolerated treatment without application of topical anesthesia and showed no noticeable side effects except for transient erythema and edema lasting from hours to days. A patient in the short incubation time experienced hyperpigmentation, and another developed acneiform eruption in the same group. It was unknown which group had the most associated side effects. Limitations included small study size with skin type III/IV group and short follow-up period of 12 weeks after the third treatment. Other incubation times with ALA are needed in future studies and longer follow-up for a definitive conclusion on optimal ALA contact time. PDT with long incubation time (3 hours) with ALA may be more adequate for inflammatory acne lesions.

J. Q. Del Rosso, DO

G. K. Kim, DO

A Five-Patient Satisfaction Pilot Study of Calcium Hydroxylapatite Injection for Treatment of Aging Hands

Marmur ES, Al Quran H, de Sa Earp AP, et al (The Mount Sinai Med Ctr, NY)
Dermatol Surg 35:1978-1984, 2009

Background.—The process of skin aging is not limited to the face but involves every part of the body, including the hands. A common manifestation of aging of the hands is the loss of volume, which occurs as the skin loses its subcutaneous fat. Injectable dermal fillers have surfaced as a popular method to address such deficiencies.

Objectives.—To report the use of calcium hydroxylapatite (CaHA) to address lost volume.

Methods.—Five female subjects with soft tissue deficiency of the dorsa of the hands were enrolled at Mount Sinai Medical Center. A solution of CaHA with 2% lidocaine in amounts of 0.3 to 1.0 mL was injected interdigitally at each of three to five insertion sites; the sites were massaged and molded up to three times to ensure an optimal cosmetic end point. Subjects were seen for a follow-up visit after 1, 4, 16, and 24 weeks.

Results.—With a single injection, all subjects reached their correction goals without requiring any touch-ups. At the 24-week visit, the subjects retained the filling effect, with no adverse events and high patient satisfaction.

Conclusion.—CaHA, a new, easily injectable, safe dermal filler, has emerged as an excellent option for soft tissue augmentation in aging hands.

▶ This is an important pilot study showing that CaHA can be used successfully in rejuvenation of the aging hands—often an area of aesthetic medicine overlooked. Although only a small number of patients were enrolled, the end results and longevity of the therapy reveal useful information that should translate into a larger clinical trial. The only concern is minimizing the adverse events—swelling and edema were common, and could be a hindrance to some wanting this procedure, although they can be minimized with appropriate aftercare, as was done here.

M. H. Gold, MD

A Retrospective Review of Calcium Hydroxylapatite for Correction of Volume Loss in the Infraorbital Region
Hevia O (Private Practice, Miami, FL)
Dermatol Surg 35:1487-1494, 2009

Background.—The correction of infraorbital volume loss with dermal fillers results in a natural, youthful, rested appearance. Defects in this facial region should be treated for optimal patient satisfaction.

Objective.—This retrospective review describes large-scale use of injection of calcium hydroxylapatite (CaHA) and a technique for injection into the infraorbital region.

Methods and Materials.—Using a 30-gauge, 0.5 needle, CaHA was injected into the infraorbital region of 301 patients. Neat CaHA was initially twice diluted with lidocaine 2% solution in 85 patients. Subsequently, 216 patients were treated with single-dilution CaHA and 0.15 mL of 2% lidocaine.

Results.—Injection of CaHa through a 30-gauge, 0.5 needle resulted in minimal bruising, discomfort, or pain. Infraorbital volume restoration was achieved efficiently and effectively, with natural results. Patients were satisfied with the longevity of correction. Adverse events were few and confined to ecchymosis (10%), edema (2%), and erythema (1%). Three of six patients reported edema lasting beyond 7 days. No overcorrection was observed.

Conclusion.—Using a 30-gauge, 0.5 needle, diluted CaHA can be safely injected into the infraorbital region with minimal adverse events and high patient satisfaction.

▶ This was a retrospective review of using calcium hydroxylapatite (CaHA) in the infraorbital area of the face for aesthetic correction. This review shows that through different dilutions of CaHA and enhanced injection techniques, the satisfaction rates were very high in aesthetic correction. Several comments appear warranted, including that this appears to be an advanced injection technique and should be used, as the author notes, only by skilled injectors and those very familiar with CaHA, as this material has no antedote if not injected correctly. This review is a little less scientific than traditional prospective studies, but with enough patients it appears, from a power point, to be significant. I would have liked to see some charts showing what was performed for each patient and the breakdown of the dilution amounts given to each patient. That being said, as the author notes, this area has been sort of off-limits to many with aesthetic concerns, which can be successfully treated using CaHA with good long-term results, but only by skilled injectors.

M. H. Gold, MD

A Safety and Feasibility Study of a Novel Radiofrequency-Assisted Liposuction Technique

Blugerman G, Schavelzon D, Paul MD (Clínica B&S de Excelencia en Cirugía Plástica, Buenos Aires, Argentina; Univ of California, Irvine)
Plast Reconstr Surg 125:998-1006, 2010

Background.—The feasibility, safety, and efficacy of a novel radiofrequency device for radiofrequency-assisted liposuction were evaluated in various body areas.

Methods.—From July to December of 2008, 23 subjects underwent radiofrequency-assisted liposuction using the BodyTite system. Information regarding aesthetic results and local and systemic complications was collected immediately after the procedure and at 6- and 12-week follow-up.

Results.—The mean age of the patients was 38.8 ± 12.4 years, and 87 percent were women. Radiofrequency-assisted liposuction was performed successfully in all cases; volume aspirated per patient was 2404 ± 1290 ml, whereas operative time was 158 ± 44 minutes. All patients underwent liposuction at the hip and low abdominal areas, bilaterally. Body contour improvement was observed postoperatively in all patients and there were no severe systemic or local complications, although postoperative pain was minimal in all patients. Weight and circumference reductions were significant at both 6-week and 3-month follow-up. Skin tightening was judged optimal by the surgeon in all patients.

Conclusions.—The authors' study suggests that the removal of moderate volumes of fat with concurrent subdermal tissue contraction can be performed safely and effectively with radiofrequency-assisted liposuction. Additional benefits of this technique are excellent patient tolerance and fast recovery time. Nonetheless, a larger sample is required to confirm the authors' results and guarantee the efficacy and safety of the procedure. Direct comparison with traditional liposuction or energy-assisted liposuction techniques may provide some insights to tailor future indications of this novel technique.

▶ This is a fascinating article with a new laser-assisted liposuction device, which recently has become available in the laser-assisted liposuction world. It uses an internal and an external bipolar radiofrequency electrode, which are designed to generate fat liquefaction, blood vessel coagulation, and skin tightening. In this clinical trial, the authors studied 23 individuals with this device and followed a variety of parameters over time, up to 3 months following the procedure. Linear skin contraction was also measured. The mean volume of aspirate per patient was 2404 ± 1290 ml. Histologic examination showed coagulation of the small vessels in the fatty tissue; rupture and fragmentation of the adipocytes; and development of fatty channels, collagen fragmentation with edema, and disarray. Linear contraction was noted to be 13.9% at 6 weeks and 24.3% at 12 weeks. Skin tightening varied from 9% to 42%. MRI studies performed in 5 patients showed significant reduction of the subcutaneous fat in the treated areas. Through this study, the authors demonstrated that this new bipolar radiofrequency laser-assisted liposuction device was useful in removing fat and providing the skin tightening and skin contracture, which was significant during the course of the study. Many people recommend laser-assisted liposuction to speed the skin tightening process—this clinical study confirmed that use and makes this a significant contribution to the laser liposuction literature.

M. H. Gold, MD

Advanced Laser Techniques for Filler-Induced Complications

Cassuto D, Marangoni O, De Santis G, et al (Univ of Catania, Italy; Fondazione Glauco Bassi, Trieste, Italy; Univ of Modena and Reggio Emilia, Italy; et al)
Dermatol Surg 35:1689-1695, 2009

Background.—The increasing use of injectable fillers has been increasing the occurrence of disfiguring anaerobic infection or granulomas. This study presents two types of laser-assisted evacuation of filler material and inflammatory and necrotic tissue that were used to treat disfiguring facial nodules after different types of gel fillers.

Materials and Methods.—Infectious lesions after hydrogels were drained using a lithium triborate laser at 532 nm, with subsequent removal of infected gel and pus (laser assisted evacuation). Granuloma after gels containing microparticles were treated using an 808-nm diode laser using intralesional laser technique. The latter melted and liquefied the organic and synthetic components of the granulomas, facilitating subsequent evacuation. Both lasers had an easily controllable thin laser beam, which enabled the physician to control tissue damage and minimize discomfort and pain.

Results.—All 20 patients experienced reduction or complete resolution, the latter increasing with repeated treatments.

Conclusion.—Laser-assisted treatment offers a successful solution for patients who have been suffering from disfiguring nodules from injected fillers—often for many years. The procedure broadens the range of treatment options in cases of untoward reactions to fillers, in line with surgical removal but with lower morbidity and less cosmetic disfigurement.

▶ Filler-induced complications are a major problem—especially as more and more fillers are becoming available and more and more people are injecting fillers—from physicians and nurse injectors using them under the direct supervision of a physician to others with little clinical training and no supervision. With this increasing use, the varieties available, and not everyone understanding those fillers, complications are on the rise. With the more permanent fillers adverse events can be more severe in that the material will not absorb, and the currently available therapies for these complications with permanent fillers are not all that efficacious. The authors introduce 2 lasers that they have used successfully to treat complications from permanent fillers—something that is quite important for us to be aware of. More of an explanation on these lasers and mechanisms would have made the article even better, but with 20 patients studied and the impressive results obtained, we should be aware that we have increased options when dealing with these difficult complications from permanent fillers.

M. H. Gold, MD

Ageing appearance in China: biophysical profile of facial skin and its relationship to perceived age
Mayes AE, Murray PG, Gunn DA, et al (Unilever Discover, Bedford, UK; et al)
J Eur Acad Dermatol Venereol 24:341-348, 2010

Background.—Perceived age is important to women and is a primary driver for topical product use and facial cosmetic surgery. Changes in facial features and biophysical skin parameters with chronological age and their associations with perceived age have not been described in Asian populations.

Objective.—To investigate the relationship between biophysical properties of the skin, visual features of skin ageing and perceived facial age in Chinese women.

Methods.—Facial photographs were collected of 250 Chinese women, aged 25−70 years in Shanghai, China. The perceived facial age was determined and related to the chronological age for each participant and to a range of visual assessments of skin appearance and objective biophysical measurements of the skin. The profile of changes in these parameters with age was investigated together with the differences in those parameters for women judged to look younger than their chronological age and those judged to look older than their chronological age.

Results.—Large discrepancies in perceived age (up to 29 years) were found in women of the same chronological age. Each objective skin measure and visual assessment parameter had a stronger correlation with perceived age than with chronological age. The strongest relationships to perceived age were for wrinkles and hyperpigmentation. Skin colour, hydration and trans-epidermal water loss (TEWL) had weaker associations with perceived age. Women judged to look older than their chronological age had significantly higher scores than those judged to look younger for coarse wrinkles and hyperpigmentation across all age groups. The appearance differences between these groups were evident in composite facial images of the same average chronological age.

Conclusions.—We have identified the skin attributes which differ with perceived age in Chinese women. Perceived age is a better measure of the biological age of facial skin than is chronological age in this population.

▶ Skin aging differences between Asians and Caucasians is well known. One study reported a 10-year delay in onset of facial wrinkles for Chinese women as compared with French women.[1] With the recent explosion in the field of cosmetic dermatology, it is increasingly important to identify specific features of skin aging in different populations to better target cosmetic therapies and skin care products. This study investigated age-related changes in 250 Chinese women aged between 25 and 70 years living in Shanghai. Authors found greater range of perceived ages at an older chronological age for Chinese patients. In addition, the strongest correlation to perceived age was fine lines and course wrinkles along with overall photodamage. Hyperpigmentation or more specifically, the evenness of skin tone was also highly correlated with perceived age, although not as strong as for skin wrinkling. In summary, authors found the perceived age to be a better measure of a person's biological age of facial skin in the Chinese population.

Limitations of this study are that participants were all of Chinese descent and cannot be generalized to other Asian groups. In fact, a study by Tsukahara et al[2] reported age-related differences between Japanese, Chinese, and Thai women.

S. Bellew, DO
J. Q. Del Rosso, DO

References

1. Nouveau-Richard S, Yang Z, Mac-Mary S, et al. Skin ageing: a comparison between Chinese and European populations. A pilot study. *J Dermatol Sci.* 2005;40:187-193.
2. Tsukahara K, Sugata K, Osanai O, et al. Comparison of age-related changes in facial wrinkles and sagging in the skin of Japanese, Chinese and Thai women. *J Dermatol Sci.* 2007;47:19-28.

Anatomic Concepts for Brow Lift Procedures

Knize DM (Univ of Colorado Health Sciences Ctr)
Plast Reconstr Surg 124:2118-2126, 2009

Background.—Brow lifting became a component of the facialplasty procedure 45 years ago, and the original brow-lifting technique incorporating a coronal incision approach is still practiced by many surgeons today. Over the past 15 years, however, the endoscope-assisted procedure and the limited incision, nonendoscopic techniques have evolved as alternate procedures for brow lifting. The level of artistry in performing any brow lift technique is raised when the surgeon acquires knowledge of upper facial anatomy and integrates that knowledge into a working concept of the aging process of the upper face.

Methods.—This article presents one surgeon's concepts of the process that culminate in the typical appearance of the aged upper face. The same understanding of upper facial anatomy that can be called upon to explain the steps in this aging process can also be applied to the technical steps of any foreheadplasty procedure. Those anatomic structures that play a role in this process are examined here.

Results.—The typical appearance of the aged upper face is the product of muscle action and gravitational forces acting on the unique anatomy of the human face. Interestingly, the appearance of the typical aged upper face exhibits much the same characteristics as one might observe in the face of an individual experiencing the emotions of sadness or grief. It is an inappropriate facial expression of sadness or grief that most often motivates the patient to schedule a consultation with the plastic surgeon.

Conclusion.—Any of the brow lift procedures used in current clinical practice can provide a successful cosmetic result in selected patients if the procedure incorporates technical steps based on sound anatomic principles.

▶ Regardless of one's interest in cosmetic procedures or surgical expertise, this is an excellent review of the fundamentals of facial anatomy and an overview of the dynamics of facial muscle actions and their impact on appearance of the aging face. Even if you don't perform any cosmetic surgery or have a limited patient base for facial aesthetics, this article is a good reference for anyone independent of specialty or experience to grasp some of the mechanics of photoaging. This is also a useful review for a clinician unfamiliar with facial anatomy issues that affect minor cosmetic procedures such as fillers and injection of botulinum toxin.

N. Bhatia, MD

Changes in Eyebrow Position and Shape with Aging

Matros E, Garcia JA, Yaremchuk MJ (Massachusetts General Hosp, Boston;
Harvard Med School, Boston, MA)

Plast Reconstr Surg 124:1296-1301, 2009

Background.—Lack of an objective goal for brow-lift surgery may explain why several articles in the plastic surgery literature conclude that brow lifts produce eyebrows with shape and position that are not aesthetically pleasing. By comparing eyebrow shape and position in both young and mature women, this study provides objective data with which to plan forehead rejuvenating procedures.

Methods.—Two cohorts of women aged 20 to 30 years and 50 to 60 years were photographed to determine eyebrow position. Measurements were made from a horizontal plane between the medial canthi to three points at the upper eyebrow margin. Exclusion criteria included prior surgery, plucked eyebrows, and botulinum toxin.

Results.—The eyebrow in the 20- to 30-year-old group ($n = 36$) was 15.7, 19.8, and 21.3 mm above the medial canthus, pupil, and lateral canthus, respectively. Lateral brow position was significantly higher than the mid brow ($p < 0.05$). In the 50- to 60-year-old group ($n = 34$), the brow was 19.1, 22.4, and 22.4 mm above the medial canthus, pupil, and lateral canthus, respectively. At all three points, the brow was higher in older compared with younger subjects. This difference was significant at the medial and mid brow ($p < 0.05$).

Conclusions.—Unlike other areas of the body where there is descent of soft tissues, there is paradoxical elevation of eyebrows with aging. These findings explain why surgical elevation of the mid and medial brow provides results that are neither youthful nor aesthetically pleasing. Techniques that selectively elevate the lateral brow are more likely to have a rejuvenating effect on the upper third of the female face.

▶ Youthful looking eyebrows is the goal of many cosmetic rejuvenating procedures. However, past brow-lift procedures have created brows with unnatural shape and position, resulting in patients looking more surprised than younger. This is a study of 2 cohorts of women aged 20 to 30 years and 50 to 60 years photographed with measurements taken at the medial, mid, and lateral brow positions, and it examines the eyebrow height differences between younger and older individuals. The position of the upper brow margin was 15.7, 18.8, and 21.3 mm ($n = 36$) above the medial canthus, pupil, and lateral canthus, respectively, in the younger group. The lateral brow position was significantly higher than the mid brow position ($P < .05$) in the younger group. In older subjects ($n = 34$), the upper brow was 19.1, 22.4, and 22.4 mm. For each of the 3 points measured, the brow was positioned higher in the older subjects than in the younger subjects. This difference was statistically significant at the medial and mid brow positions ($P < .05$). These findings are contrary to the mainstream thinking that eyebrows descend over time. There is evidence that eyebrows may elevate over time. A limitation of this study was that the study group was evaluated only in women, and ethnic backgrounds were not discussed. Study results may vary among different ethnicities and between genders. Additionally, some individuals may have naturally higher medial and mid brow positions, and baseline measurements of older individuals were unknown. More longitudinal studies are needed with a larger study group comparing the same individual over a longer period of time to unveil the natural eyebrow aging process. To conclude, this was an interesting study suggesting that the eyebrow height may elevate over time, and this may change the thinking behind brow-lift procedures.

J. Q. Del Rosso, DO

G. K. Kim, DO

Clinical Experience in the Treatment of Different Vascular Lesions Using a Neodymium-Doped Yttrium Aluminum Garnet Laser

Civas E, Koc E, Aksoy B, et al (Civas Clinic, Ankara, Turkey; Gulhane School of Medicine, Ankara, Turkey; et al)

Dermatol Surg 35:1933-1941, 2009

Background.—A neodymium-doped yttrium aluminum garnet (Nd:YAG) laser has been used with good results for the treatment of various vascular lesions.

Objective.—To report our experience with a variable long-pulsed Nd:YAG laser for the treatment of different vascular lesions.

Materials and Methods.—One hundred ten patients with different vascular skin lesions were included. Patients were examined before the treatment; 1 week after each treatment session; and 1, 2, and 3 months after the last treatment session. Improvement was judged according to clinical examination of the patients and by comparing pre- and post-treatment photographs. Results were graded in four groups using percentage resolution (0–25%, 26–50%, 51–75%, and 76–100%.

Results.—One hundred five patients (19 port wine stains, 48 telangiectasias, 25 hemangiomas, and 13 other vascular lesions) completed the study; 71.5% of patients showed greater than 50% improvement. Good to excellent (more than 50%) results were achieved in 63.2% of patients with port wine stain, 80.0% of patients with hemangioma, 66.7% of patients with telangiectasia, and 84.6% of patients with other vascular lesions; 71.5% of all patients were very satisfied or satisfied with the results.

Conclusion.—A variable long-pulsed Nd:YAG laser was found to be effective in the treatment of different vascular lesions ranging from easy to difficult to treat.

▶ This article appears to be a better exposé on why we should not be using long-pulsed neodymium-doped yttrium aluminum garnet (Nd:YAG) laser routinely to treat vascular lesions. Significant side effects were noted in 12.4% of the patients. This device can be carefully used to treat telangiectasia, blebs, port wine stains, and leg veins. However, it is not always as well suited to treat port wine stains as some other laser systems. Even with careful use, the side effects can be unpredictable.

E. A. Tanghetti, MD

Enhanced Efficacy of Photodynamic Therapy with Methyl 5-Aminolevulinic Acid in Recalcitrant Periungual Warts After Ablative Carbon Dioxide Fractional Laser: A Pilot Study
Yoo KH, Kim BJ, Kim MN (Chung-Ang Univ, Seoul, Korea)
Dermatol Surg 35:1927-1932, 2009

Background.—Photodynamic therapy (PDT) with aminolevulinic acid (ALA) has been used to improve recalcitrant periungual warts, but most lesions achieved complete remission after more than four sessions, and some lesions did not respond to the method. In this pilot study, the potential for synergistic effects of the combination of ablative carbon dioxide (CO_2) fractional laser and methyl 5-ALA (MAL)-PDT for the treatment of recalcitrant periungual warts was examined.

Materials and Methods.—Twelve Korean patients (8 women and 4 men aged 20–45, mean age 27.9) with a total of 40 periungual warts were enrolled in the present study. The lesions were treated using an ablative CO_2 fractional laser. Immediately after each fractional treatment, MAL was applied on the periungual warts, and 3 hours later, such areas were illuminated with a red light at a dose of 50 J/cm^2 for 15 minutes.

Results.—After a mean of 2.2 treatments per wart, a mean clearance of 100% was achieved in 36 (90%) warts. Two warts (5%) had 50% clearance, and two (5%) showed no response after three treatments. There were no recurrences of the warts that had achieved 100% clearance during the follow-up period of 6 months. Most of the treatments had no severe side effects during or after their administration.

Conclusion.—A potential for enhanced clinical results when using combined ablative CO_2 fractional laser and MAL-PDT for the treatment of periungual warts was shown in this pilot study.

▶ This article addresses a very complex problem. The investigators demonstrate very impressive clearances using a fractional ablative carbon dioxide (CO_2) laser and methyl 5-aminolevulinic acid photodynamic therapy (MAL-PDT). The CO_2 laser in this fractional mode could provide a channel to deliver the MAL to deeper areas than would be available by topical applications alone. This is a nice proof of concept article that should be repeated in a double-blind controlled fashion. Unfortunately, children were not included in this study. Pain was controlled in most cases by topical eutectic mixture of lidocaine anesthetic (EMLA) with a 10% drop out due to discomfort. This would be something to keep in mind for those difficult patients with periungual warts.

E. A. Tanghetti, MD

Low-Fluence Q-Switched Neodymium-Doped Yttrium Aluminum Garnet (1,064 nm) Laser for the Treatment of Facial Melasma in Asians

Wattanakrai P, Mornchan R, Eimpunth S (Ramathibodi Hosp, Phayathai, Bangkok, Thailand)
Dermatol Surg 36:76-87, 2010

Background.—Pigment lasers have been used in melasma with unsatisfactory results.

Objective.—To determine the effectiveness and safety of 1,064-nm Q-switched neodymium-doped yttrium aluminum garnet (QS-Nd:YAG) laser treatment of melasma in Asians.

Materials and Methods.—Split-face randomized study comparing combination QS-Nd:YAG laser and 2% hydroquinone with topical treatment in dermal or mixed-type melasma. Twenty-two patients were treated with 1,064-nm QS-Nd:YAG laser, 6-mm spot size, 3.0- to 3.8-J/cm^2 fluence for five sessions at 1-week intervals. Pigmentation was objectively recorded using a colorimeter (lightness index score), and subjective assessments were evaluated using the modified Melasma Area and Severity Index (mMASI) score.

Results.—After five laser treatments, statistically significant improvement of melasma from baseline was observed in colorimeter ($p<.001$) and mMASI score ($p<.001$) on the laser side. The laser side achieved an average 92.5% improvement in relative lightness index and 75.9% improvement in mMASI, compared with 19.7% and 24%, respectively, on the control side ($p<.001$). Mottled hypopigmentation developed in three patients. During follow-up, four of 22 patients developed rebound hyperpigmentation, and all patients had recurrence of melasma.

Conclusion.—QS-Nd:YAG laser treatment for melasma in Asians produced only temporary improvement and had side effects. Common complications were hypopigmentation, melasma recurrence, and rebound hyperpigmentation.

▶ Facial melasma is a perplexing problem with no easy fix. An initial promising report by Polnikorn[1] strongly suggested that weekly treatment with 1064-nm low-fluence Q-switched neodymium-doped yttrium aluminum garnet laser provided significant reduction in melasma, without recurrences on follow-up. This well-done study shows a nice response during treatment, but 13.6% of patients developed mottled hyperpigmentation, and 18% had rebound hyperpigmentation. Finally, all patients had recurrence of their melasma. This careful study sets the record straight. We are still lacking a good treatment device for melasma.

E. A. Tanghetti, MD

Reference

1. Polnikorn N. Treatment of refractory dermal melasma with the MedLite C6 Q-switched Nd:YAG laser: two case reports. *J Cosmet Laser Ther.* 2008;10: 167-173.

Needle Preference in Patients Receiving Cosmetic Botulinum Toxin Type A

Price KM, Williams ZY, Woodward JA (Duke Eye Ctr, Durham, NC; Mount Sinai School of Medicine, NY)

Dermatol Surg 36:109-112, 2010

Background.—Patients often complain of pain and bruising from needle injections. Some clinicians believe smaller gauge needles cause less pain. Thirty-gauge needles are currently the standard needles employed for administering botulinum toxin type A (BTX-A).

Objective.—This study sought to determine whether patients receiving BTX-A have a preference for 30-gauge or 32-gauge needles based on the amount of pain and bruising experienced.

Methods.—Thirty-seven subjects received BTX-A on the right side of the face using a 30-gauge needle and on the left side using a 32-gauge needle. Subjects were masked to needle size. They were then asked to rate injection pain on an 11-point numerical rating scale and to note any bruising. Physician preference was also evaluated.

Results.—There were no statistically significant differences in the amount of intra-procedural pain ($p = .37$) or the level of post-procedural pain and discomfort ($p = .76$) experienced. Twenty-seven percent of subjects reported greater bruising with the 32-gauge needle, versus 29.7% with the 30-gauge needle. The physician injector did not have a preference. Lastly, 83.8% of subjects did not detect a difference in BTX-A paralysis effect.

Conclusion.—We do not recommend using 32-gauge needles in place of 30-gauge needles for administering BTX-A.

► Botulinum toxin type A (BTX-A) has increased in popularity in recent years and is widely used by cosmetic dermatologists. BTX-A is produced by an anaerobic bacterium, *Clostridium botulinum*. The toxin exerts its therapeutic effect by blocking neuromuscular activity and thus causing muscular weakness. When used properly by experienced injectors, BTX-A is considered a safe and effective treatment for facial rejuvenation with relatively little adverse effects.[1] The most common patient complaint is pain and bruising, and this can be limited by using a topical anesthetic prior to injection and using smaller gauge needles.[1] This study investigated the patient-perceived difference between using the 32-gauge versus the 30-gauge needle during injection, and if this difference is significant enough for clinicians to change to the more expensive 32-gauge needle in an effort to decrease patient discomfort. Results of the study indicate no significant difference in the 2 sizes. In addition, the physician injector did not have a needle preference. Limitations to the study include small number of subjects (37) with only 1 male enrolled, as there may be differences in pain tolerance in men and women. And although the patients were blinded to the needle size, the physician was not. In summary, authors do not suggest changing the size of needle to the more costly 32-gauge, as there was no significant difference found between the 2 sizes.

S. Bellew, DO
J. Q. Del Rosso, DO

Reference

1. Klein AW. Contraindications and complications with the use of botulinum toxin. *Clin Dermatol.* 2004;22:66-75.

Outcomes of Childhood Hemangiomas Treated with the Pulsed-Dye Laser with Dynamic Cooling: A Retrospective Chart Analysis

Rizzo C, Brightman L, Chapas AM, et al (New York Univ Skin and Cancer Unit; Laser & Skin Surgery Ctr of New York)
Dermatol Surg 35:1947-1954, 2009

Background.—Laser treatment of childhood hemangiomas remains controversial. Previous studies have used outdated technology, resulting in a potential overrepresentation of adverse outcomes.

Objective.—To evaluate outcomes of hemangiomas treated with the most current laser technology.

Methods.—A retrospective chart analysis of 90 patients with a median age of 3.0 months and a total of 105 hemangiomas were enrolled over a 2.5-year period. All were treated with the 595-nm long-pulse pulsed-dye laser (LP-PDL) with dynamic epidermal cooling at 2- to 8-week intervals depending on the stage of growth. Exclusion criteria were previous laser, surgical, or corticosteroid treatment. Three reviewers assessed outcomes.

Results.—Near-complete or complete clearance in color were achieved for 85 (81%) and in thickness for 67 (64%) hemangiomas. There was no scarring or atrophy. Ulceration occurred in one case and resolved during treatment. Hyperpigmentation and hypopigmentation occurred in 4% and 14% of hemangiomas, respectively.

Conclusion.—Early treatment of childhood hemangiomas with the 595-nm LP-PDL with dynamic cooling may reduce the proliferative phase and result in excellent rates of clearing and few adverse events.

▶ This is a useful examination of the treatment of childhood hemangiomas with the modern pulse dye laser with cooling. This article suggests in a retrospective manner that this laser does result in improvement in color and, in some instances, thickness of hemangiomas. There is a suggestion that this device might also improve the proliferative phase of this problem. It is clear from this article that in expert hands this device is useful in improving the appearance of childhood hemangiomas. It is difficult to say absolutely that this device will result in resolution that might have occurred naturally. Randomized trials of this condition would be difficult since no 2 patients or lesions would be exactly the same. The safety of this device in expert hands is well demonstrated in this investigation.

E. A. Tanghetti, MD

Perioral Wrinkles: Histologic Differences Between Men and Women

Paes EC, Teepen HJLJM, Koop WA, et al (Univ Med Ctr, Utrecht, The Netherlands; St Elisabeth Hosp, Tilburg, The Netherlands; Univ Med Ctr, Leeuwarden, The Netherlands)

Aesthet Surg J 29:467-472, 2009

Background.—Women tend to develop more and deeper wrinkles in the perioral region than men. Although much is known about the complex mechanisms involved in skin aging, previous studies have described histologic differences between men and women with respect to skin aging only incidentally and have not investigated the perioral region.

Objective.—The purpose of this study was to investigate gender-specific differences in the perioral skin.

Methods.—To determine wrinkle severity, skin surface replicas of the upper lip region in 10 male and 10 female fresh cadavers were analyzed by using the dermaTOP blue three-dimensional digitizing system (Breuckmann, Meersburg, Germany). In 30 fresh male and female cadavers, three full-thickness lip resections were investigated in a blinded fashion for specific histologic features. All results were statistically analyzed in a linear regression model with SPSS software (version 15.0; SPSS, Chicago, IL).

Results.—The female replicas showed more and deeper wrinkles than the male replicas ($P < .01$). Histologic analysis revealed that the perioral skin of men displayed a significantly higher number of sebaceous glands ($P = .000$; 95% confidence interval [CI] 23.6–53.2), sweat glands ($P = .002$; 95% CI 2.1–8.1), and a higher ratio between vessel area and connective tissue area in the dermis ($P = .009$; 95% CI 0.003–0.021). The amount of hair follicles did not significantly differ between men and women, although the average number of sebaceous glands per hair follicle was greater in men ($P = .002$; 95% CI 0.33–1.28).

Conclusions.—Women exhibit more and deeper wrinkles in the perioral region and their skin contains a significantly smaller number of appendages than men, which could be a feasible explanation for why women are more susceptible to development of perioral wrinkles.

▶ In the world of aesthetic dermatology dominated by dermal fillers and neurotoxins, it is fascinating that the authors took a step back to examine gender-specific differences in perioral wrinkles at the microscopic level. Documented differences could conceivably lead to targeted antiwrinkle therapies. In the case of perioral wrinkles, women have more and deeper wrinkles than men. Of interest is that the genesis of these wrinkles appears to be in large part a dermal phenomenon as there was little difference in epidermal thickness between the genders. The dermis in men contains more sebaceous glands, sweat glands, and a higher ratio between blood vessel area and connective tissue area. While there was no difference in the number of hair follicles between men and women, the hair follicles in men had more sebaceous glands associated with each follicle. How these findings will ultimately translate into antiwrinkle therapy over time should prove to be interesting.

G. Martin, MD

Photorejuvenation with Topical Methyl Aminolevulinate and Red Light: A Randomized, Prospective, Clinical, Histopathologic, and Morphometric Study
Issa MCA, Piñeiro-Maceira J, Vieira MTC, et al (Federal Univ of Rio de Janeiro, Brazil; Fluminense Federal Univ, Rio de Janeiro, Brazil; et al)
Dermatol Surg 36:39-48, 2010

Background.—Photodynamic therapy (PDT) is an option for skin rejuvenation. Although many studies report clinical improvement with PDT in photodamaged skin, histologic and morphometric evidence is not documented in most cases.

Objective.—To evaluate clinical and histopathologic changes induced by methyl aminolevulinate (MAL)-PDT and to morphometrically quantify collagen and elastic fibers in skin remodeling induced by MAL-PDT in photodamaged skin.

Methods and Materials.—Fourteen patients were treated with two sessions of MAL-PDT. The light source was a light-emitting diode: 635 nm, 37 J/cm^2. Skin biopsies were performed before and 3 and 4 months after treatment. All fragments were stained using the hematoxylin-eosin, orcein, and picrosirius techniques. Morphometric studies were done of three samples from each patient.

Results.—Global clinical improvement was observed in 10 of 14 patients. The histopathologic study showed increased collagen fibers 3 and 6 months after treatment. The decrease in the amount of elastic fiber was statistically significant 3 ($p = .016$) and 6 ($p = .008$) months after treatment. The increase in the amount of collagen fiber was statistically significant 6 months after treatment ($p = .048$).

Conclusion.—Clinical improvement with regard to texture, firmness, wrinkle depth, skin coloration, and clearance of actinic keratoses was observed. Histopathologic and morphometric studies were consistent with the clinical findings.

▶ This study demonstrates that a vigorous treatment with topical methyl aminolevulinate and red light does have a rejuvenative effect on photodamaged skin. However, this comes at a price. "Side effects resembling those from a superficial peeling occurred in 11 patients and resembled TCA 35% peeling in three patients" out of 14 total patients treated. The degree of improvement seen 6 months after treatment could have been achieved by the use of a topical retinoid. This study demonstrates that methyl aminolevulinate can be considered as a useful treatment in patients with photodamage but may not offer advantages over other therapeutic options.

E. A. Tanghetti, MD

Pulsed Dye Laser in the Treatment of Nail Psoriasis

Oram Y, Karincaoğlu Y, Koyuncu E, et al (American Hosp, İstanbul, Turkey; İnönü Univ, Malatya, Turkey; et al)
Dermatol Surg 36:377-381, 2010

Background.—The treatment options for nail psoriasis have been limited, and the management of nail psoriasis has been challenging for physicians.

Objectives.—To evaluate the effect of pulsed dye laser (PDL) in the treatment of nail psoriasis.

Methods.—Psoriatic nails of five patients were treated using PDL (595 nm) once monthly for 3 months. The pulse duration was 1.5 ms, the beam diameter was 7 mm, and the laser energy was 8.0 to 10.0 J/cm^2. Clinical efficacy was statistically evaluated according to Nail Psoriasis Severity Index (NAPSI) score differences before and after the treatment.

Results.—Statistical analysis of NAPSI scores before and after treatment showed significant difference ($p < .05$, paired t-test). The nail bed lesions, particularly onycholysis and subungual hyperkeratosis, responded best to the treatment.

Limitations.—Limitations include the lack of blinding and comparison and the small number of patients.

Conclusion.—PDL might be an alternative treatment for nail psoriasis.

▶ Treatment of nail psoriasis is often challenging for patient and physician alike. This brief report evaluates 5 patients with nail psoriasis treated with pulsed dye laser (PDL) 595 nm monthly for 3 months. The National Psoriasis Severity Index score used to evaluate the efficacy of treatment showed significant improvement before and after treatment. The nail bed lesions responded better to treatment than the nail matrix lesion. This study is very small, open label, noncontrolled, yet it does suggest a beneficial effect of PDL, which warrants further exploration.

P. Rich, MD

Randomized, Placebo-Controlled Study of a New Botulinum Toxin Type A for Treatment of Glabellar Lines: Efficacy and Safety

Brandt F, Swanson N, Baumann L, et al (Dermatology Res Inst LLC, Coral Gables, FL; Oregon Health and Science Univ, Portland; Univ of Miami, FL; et al)
Dermatol Surg 35:1893-1901, 2009

Background.—A new botulinum toxin type A (BoNT-A) has been assessed in the United States for treatment of glabellar lines. In April 2009, the US FDA approved the Biologics License Application for a new US formulation of BoNT-A (Dysport [abobotulinumtoxinA]; Medicis Aesthetics Inc., Scottsdale, AZ).

Objective.—To compare efficacy and safety of a single treatment of BoNT-A with placebo in subjects with moderate to severe glabellar lines. *Methods and Materials.*—One hundred fifty-eight subjects with moderate to severe glabellar lines were randomized 2:1 to receive 50 U of BoNT-A ($n = 105$) or placebo ($n = 53$). Responders were defined as having no or mild glabellar lines at 30 days posttreatment according to investigator and subject assessments (co-primary endpoint) using the validated Glabellar Line Scale Score at maximum frown. Subject diaries were used to document onset of effect. When conducting the research, the authors conformed to the ethical guidelines of the 1975 Declaration of Helsinki.

Results.—According to investigator assessment, the proportion of responders to BoNT-A at Day 30 was 89.5%, versus 7.5% for placebo ($p < .001$); according to subject assessment, the proportion of responders was 75.7%, versus 9.8% for placebo ($p < .001$).

Conclusion.—A single treatment with BoNT-A (50 U) was significantly superior to placebo in the correction of moderate to severe glabellar lines, with comparable tolerability.

▶ This is a well-performed, randomized, placebo-controlled study demonstrating the statistically significant effectiveness of a new type of botulinum toxin type A (Dysport) for treating glabellar lines. In this study, the placebo and treatment groups were well matched in terms of age, sex, race, and subject investigator evaluation. Interestingly, the article reports a similar percentage of treatment-induced adverse effects for both placebo and botulinum toxin type A treatment groups, demonstrating that most of the side effects seen in this study were because of injection rather than the botulinum toxin type A itself. The few adverse effects that were seen in the actively treated group consisted of ptosis and local injection site reaction. Given that this brand of botulinum toxin type A contains a hemagglutin protein complex with its botulinum toxin, it may not be surprising that some of the population will have injection site reactions similar to many vaccines. Ptosis is also not a surprising adverse effect, given the mechanism of the active ingredient. However, this is a side effect that could usually be avoided in most patients with slight variation of technique and injection location.

By comparing these results with a double-blinded, placebo-controlled study by Carruthers et al[1] using another brand of botulinum toxin type A (Botox) for treating glabellar lines, similar efficacy results and moderately differing side effect profiles were noted. The Botox-treated group showed significantly less injection site reactions than the Dysport-treated group, which may indeed have something to do with our above-mentioned hypothesis.

J. Levin, DO

Reference

1. Carruthers JD, Lowe NJ, Menter MA, Gibson J, Eadie N, Botox Glabellar Lines II Study Group. Double-blind, placebo-controlled study of the safety and efficacy of botulinum toxin type A for patients with glabellar lines. *Plast Reconstr Surg.* 2003;112:1089-1098.

Reduced Pain with Use of Proprietary Hyaluronic Acid with Lidocaine for Correction of Nasolabial Folds: A Patient-Blinded, Prospective, Randomized Controlled Trial

Monheit GD, Campbell RM, Neugent H, et al (Univ of Alabama at Birmingham; Total Skin and Beauty Dermatology Ctr, Birmingham, AL; Georgia Skin Cancer and Aesthetic Dermatology, Athens, GA; et al)
Dermatol Surg 36:94-101, 2010

Background.—Pain during and after implantation of dermal gel fillers is a consistent complaint of patients undergoing soft tissue augmentation. Reduction of pain during injection would increase patient comfort and improve the overall patient experience.

Objective.—To evaluate pain at the injection site during and after the injection of Prevelle SILK or Captique and to evaluate outcomes after 2 weeks.

Methods & Materials.—In a patient-blinded, prospective, randomized, split-face design trial, a nonanimal-derived hyaluronic acid based filler formulated with lidocaine (Prevelle SILK) was injected in one nasolabial fold (NLF), and the same filler without lidocaine (Captique) was injected in the contralateral NLF of 45 enrolled patients. Injection site pain was measured using a visual analogue scale at injection (time 0) and 15, 30, 45, and 60 minutes after injection. Patients were asked to return for an evaluation after 2 weeks and to complete a self-assessment questionnaire during the follow-up visit.

Results.—There was more than 50% less pain associated with the dermal gel with lidocaine than with the same filler without lidocaine at all time points ($p < .05$). The greatest difference in pain was recorded at the time of injection, and then the effect gradually declined over the 60-minute period. Both fillers were well tolerated, and there was no difference in outcome after 2 weeks.

Conclusion.—Addition of lidocaine to a filler resulted in significantly less pain associated with the procedure without compromising outcomes.

▶ This study demonstrated the use of lidocaine added to an hyaluronic acid (HA) filler—once lidocaine is added, the pain associated with HA injections can be significantly reduced. This is the first lidocaine clinical trial performed and is extremely important in aesthetic medicine. And now, almost every HA filler is either available or being studied with lidocaine—so the future of all fillers will be with the addition of lidocaine for better pain control. This was a very well-thought and well-performed study.

M. H. Gold, MD

Skin Tightening Effect Using Fractional Laser Treatment: I. A Randomized Half-Side Pilot Study on Faces of Patients with Acne

Dainichi T, Kawaguchi A, Ueda S, et al (Kurume Univ, Fukuoka, Japan; Ueda-Setsuko Clinic, Fukuoka, Japan; et al)
Dermatol Surg 36:66-70, 2010

Background.—Fractional laser resurfacing is a new procedure for skin rejuvenation.

Objective.—To assess the skin remodeling effect of fractional laser treatment.

Methods.—Twelve Asian patients with acne were irradiated using a fractional 1,540-nm erbium glass laser on a random half of the face twice with a 4-week interval.

Results.—The faces were contoured on the treated side of most patients. Statistical analyses of the facial images showed that the skin tightening effect was significant 4 weeks after the first and second irradiation ($p < .001$ after both treatments).

Conclusion.—These results suggest that fractional laser resurfacing is a possible alternative to nonsurgical skin tightening of the face.

▶ This article suggests that there is some tightening that is observed by comparing pixel changes from a treated and untreated side of the face. Unfortunately, there is no grading of the pictures from a visual perspective. For most patients and physicians, if the change is not visible it is not significant. Unfortunately, we have no idea from independent graders whether these patients' changes were significant for independent viewers. It is unlikely that clinically significant tightening will occur with a nonablative device. We have done tests with a nonablative combination 1440-nm fractional laser and 1320-nm laser device and have found at most 3% tissue shrinkage with 3 treatments measured by tattooing on buttocks skin. This is compared to 3-6 times that amount with traditional ablative treatments. Most patients do not appreciate a 3% tissue shrinkage. This 1540-nm fractional nonablative device more likely wounds tissue resulting in tissue remodeling and improvement in acne scars and textural changes in the skin. It is interesting to note that this study was done on patients with acne. No mention is made of the changes in acne with treatment. My experience with nonablative treatments on patients with active acne suggests that it makes acne worse. This is not unexpected since there is a significant amount of swelling associated with this treatment, which would further occlude follicular orifices. It is also problematic that the tightening noted was not permanent and appeared to disappear after 6 months. Laser surgeons generally feel that the ablative fractional devices provide a more noticeable level of skin tightening.

E. A. Tanghetti, MD

Successful Treatment of Atrophic Postoperative and Traumatic Scarring With Carbon Dioxide Ablative Fractional Resurfacing: Quantitative Volumetric Scar Improvement

Weiss ET, Chapas A, Brightman L, et al (Laser & Skin Surgery Ctr of New York)
Arch Dermatol 146:133-140, 2010

Objective.—To assess the safety and efficacy of ablative fractional resurfacing (AFR) for nonacne atrophic scarring.

Design.—In this before-and-after trial, each scar received 3 AFR treatments and 6 months of follow-up.

Setting.—Private academic practice.

Patients.—Fifteen women with Fitzpatrick skin types I to IV, aged 21 to 66 years, presented with 22 nonacne atrophic scars between June 1 and November 30, 2007. Three patients (3 scars) were excluded from the study after receiving 1 AFR treatment and not returning for follow-up visits. The remaining 12 patients (19 scars) completed all 3 treatments and 6 months of follow-up.

Interventions.—Each scar received 3 AFR treatments at 1- to 4-month intervals.

Main Outcome Measures.—Erythema, edema, petechiae, scarring, crusting, and dyschromia were graded after treatment and through 6 months of follow-up. Skin texture, pigmentation, atrophy, and overall appearance were evaluated after treatment and through 6 months of follow-up by the patient and a nonblinded investigator. A 3-dimensional optical profiling system generated high-resolution topographic representations of atrophic scars for objective measurement of changes in scar volume and depth.

Results.—Adverse effects of treatment were mild to moderate, and no scarring or delayed-onset hypopigmentation was observed. At the 6-month follow-up visit, patient and investigator scores demonstrated improvements in skin texture for all scars (patient range, 1-4 [mean, 2.79]; investigator range, 2-4 [mean, 2.95]), pigmentation for all scars (patient range, 1-4 [mean, 2.32]; investigator range, 1-4 [mean, 2.21]), atrophy for all scars (patient range, 1-4 [mean, 2.26]; investigator range, 2-4 [mean, 2.95]), and overall scar appearance for all scars (patient range, 2-4 [mean, 2.89]; investigator range, 2-4 [mean, 3.05]). Image analysis revealed a 38.0% mean reduction of volume and 35.6% mean reduction of maximum scar depth.

Conclusion.—The AFR treatments represent a safe, effective treatment modality for improving atrophic scarring due to surgery or trauma.

► This well-done study demonstrates that ablative fractional resurfacing can provide benefits to atrophic facial scars that are the results of surgery or trauma. The author suggests that a lower setting and care must be taken in off-face treatments. The flaws of this study are that this was not rated by blinded non-investigators. In performing a study, the investigators and subjects all have a bias. The improvement after 2 treatments suggests that waiting 6 months after 2 treatments might produce a similar result to 3 treatments. The literature on ablative resurfacing for scarring provides ample evidence that it takes at least 6 to 12 months after a procedure to see optimal results. It would be interesting to see a prospective study comparing nonablative with ablative resurfacing for this indication. The data would suggest that the volume of ablative tissue should result in more wound contraction and a better clinical outcome. Finally, it would be ideal to evaluate 2 ablative settings, 1 more superficial and 1 deep, to see if the depth of ablation really matters. If the density was increased in the more superficial treatments, the volume of area would be constant and would be a good indication as to whether deeper is really better.

E. A. Tanghetti, MD

The Efficacy and Safety of 10,600-nm Carbon Dioxide Fractional Laser for Acne Scars in Asian Patients
Cho SB, Lee SJ, Kang JM, et al (Yonsei Univ College of Medicine, Seoul, Korea; Yonsei Star Skin and Laser Clinic, Seoul, Korea)
Dermatol Surg 35:1955-1961, 2009

Background.—The nonablative 1,550-nm erbium-doped fractional photothermolysis system (FPS) has been effectively used for scar treatments, but it seems that several sessions of treatment must be delivered to achieve satisfactory improvement.

Objectives.—To evaluate the efficacy and safety of the combined use of two treatment modes of an ablative 10,600-nm carbon dioxide fractional laser system (CO_2 FS) on acne scars.

Methods.—Twenty Korean patients with atrophic acne scars treated with a single session of Ultrapulse Encore laser (Lumenis Inc., Santa Clara, CA) were enrolled. The laser fluences were delivered to the scars using the Deep FX mode. Additional treatment using the Active FX mode was performed throughout the entire face.

Results.—Follow-up results revealed that one patient had clinical improvement of 76% to 100%, nine had improvements of 51% to 75%, seven had moderate improvements of 26% to 50%, and three had minimal to no improvements. The mean duration of post-therapy crusting or scaling was 6.3 ± 3.0 days, and post-therapy erythema lasted 2.8 ± 4.6 days.

Conclusion.—We suggest that CO_2 FS used with a combination of two different treatment modes may provide a new treatment algorithm for acne scars in Asians.

▶ Although carbon dioxide (CO_2) or erbium-doped yttrium aluminum garnet (Er: YAG) is a well-accepted treatment for acneiform scarring and facial rejuvenation, many dermatologists are reluctant to use them in Asian patients because of risk of long recovery time, dyschromia, and scarring in this population. Recently, an ablative 10 600-nm CO_2 fractional laser (CO_2FS) was introduced to minimize the side effects of fractional laser technology. This is an investigator-blinded study of 20 patients (Fitzpartrick skin type IV) with mild to severe atrophic acne scars treated using CO_2FS in 2 different modes, Deep FX and Active FX combined. Deep FX mode is used to deliver laser energy to deeper scar tissue to induce thermal stimulation, realignment of thick collagen bundles, and abnormal fibrous anchoring located in deeper portions of the scar. The Active FX mode allows broader treatment zone and penetration into the epidermal-dermal junction. The combination of these 2 modes helps with broader treatment zones. Photographs were taken at baseline and 3 months after treatment with 2 dermatologists comparing before and after photos for clinical assessment. Follow-up results revealed that 1 patient had clinical improvement of 76% to 100%, 9 had improvements of 51% to 75%, 7 had moderate improvements of 26% to 50%, and 3 had minimal to no improvements. However, statistical improvement in atrophic lesion counts compared with baseline for patients was not mentioned. Patient assessment of overall satisfaction revealed that 12 of 20 patients (60.0%) were very satisfied or satisfied, 5 (25.0%) were slightly satisfied, and 3 (15.0%) were unsatisfied. Mean duration of limited daily activities, such as going outdoors and working, was 4.9 ± 2.1 days, which correlated with posttherapy appearance of crusting or scaling ($P = .02$) but not with posttherapy erythema. Only 1 of 20 patients developed transient posttherapy hyperpigmentation resolving after 3 months, and this did not affect patient satisfaction. Neither immediate nor posttherapy hypopigmentation was demonstrated in this study. Limitations of this study included lack of a control or split face design and nonrandomization. Also, this study was only done on Korean patients with skin type IV. It is not safe to assume that this device may be used in all Asians because skin type can vary widely within any ethnic group. In fact, Asian skin encompasses a broad range of skin types. The authors suggest that CO_2FS used with a combination of 2 different treatment modes may be an option for Asians with skin type IV with mild to severe atrophic acne scars.

J. Q. Del Rosso, DO

G. K. Kim, DO

The Spectrum of Adverse Reactions After Treatment with Injectable Fillers in the Glabellar Region: Results from the Injectable Filler Safety Study
Bachmann F, Erdmann R, Hartmann V, et al (Charité-Universitätsmedizin Berlin, Germany; et al)
Dermatol Surg 35:1629-1634, 2009

Background.—For the glabellar region, severe partly vascular adverse events have been reported after treatment with injectable fillers.

Methods and Materials.—For this study, data from the Injectable Filler Safety Study, a German-based registry for those reactions, was analyzed to characterize adverse events seen in the glabellar region. Patients were analyzed descriptively.

Results.—Forty of 139 registered patients reported adverse events in the glabellar region. All patients were female, with an average age of 52.3.

Nineteen patients with adverse reactions to hydroxyethylmethacrylate (HEMA) and ethylmethacrylate (EMA) in a fixed combination with hyaluronic acid (HA) and 10 patients with adverse reactions to different hyaluronic acid products were reported; five patients reacted to poly-L-lactic acid (PLA). The most common adverse reactions to HEMA/EMA in HA and PLA were nodules and hardening. In HA-treated patients, erythema and inflammation, swelling, and pain were most frequent. The adverse reactions to HEMA/EMA in HA were severe in 50% of the patients. Severe adverse reactions were found to a lesser extent in patients treated with HA and PLA. Potential vascular complications were documented in only two patients.

Conclusion.—Adverse reactions seen in the glabella are overwhelmingly product associated and to a lesser extent location associated. Vascular complications with necrosis and ulceration were rare.

▶ In recent years, the use of dermal injectable fillers and botulinum toxin injections has gained increased popularity in the field of facial rejuvenation. Never before has there been such an impressive array of soft tissue filler options available for patients. These include autologous implants, collagens, hyaluronic acids, and biosynthetic polymers. In general, dermal fillers are considered safe when administered by skilled and experienced practitioners; however, there is always a potential for adverse side effects. Moreover, the glabellar region is especially at risk for vascular necrosis possibly because of intra-arterial injection and compression of small vessels in the region. This study investigated the risk of adverse events through the utilization of a German-based registry for injectable filler safety. Researchers found that the most commonly documented adverse reactions in the glabellar region were nodules and hardening followed by erythema and inflammation. These findings were similar to injections in other areas of the face. Vascular necrosis was a rare event occurring in 2 of the 40 patients who reported side effects. In summary, although the risk of injection site necrosis is rare, the possibility for disfigurement from scarring has led to several recommendations in the prevention of this serious side effect. Clinicians can minimize the risk of necrosis by injecting superficially and medially to avoid the supratrochlear vessels, aspirating before injecting to assure that the needle tip is not within a vessel, and avoid overcorrection by using low volumes in multiple treatment sessions.[1] Patients should be observed frequently to monitor progress, and if necrosis does occur, it should be identified and treated promptly.

S. Bellew, DO

J. Q. Del Rosso, DO

Reference

1. Glaich AS, Cohen JL, Goldberg LH. Injection necrosis of the glabella: protocol for prevention and treatment after use of dermal fillers. *Dermatol Surg.* 2006;32:276-281.

Treatment of trichostasis spinulosa with a 755-nm long-pulsed alexandrite laser

Toosi S, Ehsani AH, Noormohammadpoor P, et al (Tehran Univ of Med Sciences, Iran)
J Eur Acad Dermatol Venereol 24:470-473, 2010

Background.—Trichostasis spinulosa (TS) is a common disorder of hair follicle, characterized by spinous plugs. Topical treatments offer temporary relief but permanent removal of the abnormal follicles using hair removal lasers may result in a definite cure.

Objective.—To evaluate the safety and efficacy of 755-nm alexandrite laser for the treatment of TS lesions.

Patients and Methods.—Two consecutive 755-nm alexandrite laser treatments were performed one month apart. The clinical response and adverse effects were assessed four weeks after the first and second treatments and 20 weeks after the second treatment.

Results.—Thirty one patients with skin phototypes II to IV completed the study. At the last follow up visit, a decrease in dark-plug density of greater than 50% was noted in 16 patients (51.3%), while only three patients (9.7%) had an improvement of greater than 75%. Ten of the 21 patients (47.6%) with skin type III and six of the seven patients (85.7%) with skin type IV achieved at least 50% improvement in lesions at the last follow up visit ($P = 0.1$).

Conclusion.—The 755-nm alexandrite laser can safely and effectively reduce TS lesions lasting for a relatively long time in patients with skin types III–IV.

▶ This study suggests that the alexandrite laser at the short pulse duration of 3 ms with cooling is an effective treatment of trichostasis spinulosa. The only question is the longevity of response.

E. A. Tanghetti, MD

Long-term follow-up of photodynamic therapy with a self-adhesive 5-aminolaevulinic acid patch: 12 months data

Szeimies R-M, Stockfleth E, Popp G, et al (Regensburg Univ Hosp, Franz Josef Strauss Allee, Germany; Skin Cancer Ctr Charité Berlin, Germany; Hofackerstraße 19, Augsburg, Germany; et al)
Br J Dermatol 162:410-414, 2010

Background.—Photodynamic therapy with a self-adhesive 5-aminolaevulinic acid (5-ALA) patch shows high efficacy rates in the treatment of mild to moderate actinic keratosis (AK) in short term trials.

Objectives.—The purpose of the trial was to follow up patients after successful 5-ALA patch-PDT at 3 month intervals over a total period of

12 months. Patients who had received placebo-PDT or cryosurgery served for comparison.

Patients/Methods.—Three months after therapy, 360 patients from two separate randomized parallel group phase III studies (one superiority trial vs. placebo-PDT, one noninferiority trial vs. cryosurgery) were suitable for the follow-up study. Patients had to show at least one successfully treated AK lesion after initial therapy. A total of 316 patients completed the follow-up.

Results.—Twelve months after a single treatment, 5-ALA patch-PDT still proved superior to placebo-PDT and cryosurgery ($P < 0.001$ for all tests). On a lesion basis, efficacy rates were 63% and 79% for PDT, 63% for cryosurgery and 9% and 25% for placebo-PDT. Recurrence rates of patch-PDT proved superior to those of cryosurgery (per protocol set: $P = 0.011$, full analysis set: $P = 0.049$). While 31% of cryosurgery lesions were still hypopigmented after 1 year, the 5-ALA patch-PDT groups showed hypopigmentation in 0% (superiority trial) and 3% (noninferiority trial) of the treated lesions.

Conclusion.—Twelve months after a single 5-ALA patch-PDT the majority of lesions were still cleared with an excellent cosmetic outcome. 5-ALA patch-PDT proved to be superior to cryosurgery in the noninferiority study setting.

▶ The use of a novel patch delivery system for 5-aminolevulinic acid (ALA) photodynamic therapy (PDT) in this well-controlled phase III study proved to have superior efficacy and cosmetic results when treating actinic keratoses compared with cryotherapy. The efficacy of a single treatment was similar to previous ALA studies, which often required 2 treatments. Based on these observations, there are several features of the ALA patch that make it attractive: ease of patch application; lack of a need for pretreatment, that is, no curettage of scale was required; and short incubation time (4 hours) prior to irradiation with red light source allowing for a 1 day in-office treatment. All of these make it a viable, efficacious, and nonhypopigmenting alternative to cryotherapy. However, the utility of the ALA patch in daily clinical practice has some obvious limitations when compared with current Food and Drug Administration—approved ALA PDT and methyl aminolevulinate PDT field therapies, which include difficulty in conforming the patch to curved surfaces, such as the nose and ears, and the surface area of the patch ($4\,cm^2$) limits its use as a broad area field therapy. All of the PDT modalities have faced the same requirement of additional personnel and a designated space to perform PDT, which has slowed penetration into most practices. This coupled with third party reimbursement issues will make it difficult for clinicians to put down their liquid nitrogen canisters. Despite these limitations, the patch will hopefully become one more safe and effective tool in the PDT tool chest.

G. Martin, MD

Topical photodynamic therapy is immunosuppressive in humans
Matthews YJ, Damian DL (The Univ of Sydney at Royal Prince Alfred Hosp, Sydney, Australia)
Br J Dermatol 162:637-641, 2010

Background.—Visible light irradiation after application of a photosensitizer (topical photodynamic therapy; PDT) is increasingly used to treat nonmelanoma skin cancers and premalignant actinic keratoses. PDT can provide a cosmetically superior alternative to surgery, but carries failure rates of 10–40%. While some murine studies have suggested immune enhancement by PDT, others reported immunosuppressive effects, which may indicate impaired antitumour immunity and thus compromised tumour clearance.
Objectives.—This study aimed to determine the in vivo immune effects of PDT in humans.
Methods.—Using healthy, Mantoux-positive volunteers, we irradiated discrete areas of the back with narrowband red light (630 nm; 37 J cm^{-2}), with and without prior application of 5-aminolaevulinic acid (ALA) or methyl aminolaevulinate (MAL). Adjacent, untreated areas served as immunologically intact control sites. Delayed-type hypersensitivity responses to tuberculin purified protein derivative (Mantoux reactions) were then elicited in each of the irradiated, unirradiated and control sites, and the intensity of the reactions was quantitated with an erythema meter and by measurement of Mantoux diameter. By comparing Mantoux intensity at treated and control sites, immunosuppression was determined in each volunteer for each intervention.
Results.—We found that both MAL-PDT and ALA-PDT significantly suppressed Mantoux erythema (by 30% and 50%, respectively) and diameter (41% and 38%). Red light alone significantly suppressed diameter (22%) but not erythema (13%).
Conclusions.—Topical PDT induced significant immune suppression, which could impair local antitumour immune responses and may thus contribute to treatment failure.

▶ Photodynamic therapy (PDT) using topical aminolevulinic acid (ALA) and methylaminolevulinic acid (MAL) to treat actinic keratoses (AKs) and nonmelanoma skin cancers (NMSCs) has a significant treatment failure rate (10%-40%). PDT research to date has largely focused on the many variables that affect its targeted cytotoxicity. These variables include ALA and MAL epidermal penetration and target tissue uptake; selective accumulation of the photosensitizing molecule protoporphyrin IX (PpIX) in the target tissue; and optimization of the rate and total amount of activating light energy delivered to the target tissue. The role of skin immunity following PDT has received little attention. The few small studies published in this area have been performed in animal models and have conflicting results. This study examines the effect of PDT on the delayed-type hypersensitivity response in vivo on human skin. It clearly demonstrates that local immune suppression as measured by skin anergy testing takes place following PDT. There is supporting evidence that PDT affects normal immunoregulatory keratinocytes and T cells to some degree, although PDT is more selective for cancerous keratinocytes and T cells. The findings in this study provide a plausible mechanism for impaired immune responses following PDT as a cause for treatment failures. However, a few critical questions remain: how long does the local immune suppression following PDT last beyond the 72-hour measurement? Is this local immune suppression at 72 hours clinically relevant to the final clinical outcome? We are aware that immune surveillance plays a critical role in the treatment efficacy and sustained tumor clearance. This has been proven in the case of imiquimod therapy for AKs and NMSC. Further studies evaluating the immune system's role in PDT are warranted.

G. Martin, MD

Ultrasound tightening of facial and neck skin: A rater-blinded prospective cohort study
Alam M, White LE, Martin N, et al (Northwestern Univ, Chicago, IL)
J Am Acad Dermatol 62:262-269, 2010

Background.—Nonablative skin tightening technologies offer the prospect of reduction of wrinkles and skin sagging with minimal downtime, discomfort, and risk of adverse events. The excellent safety profile is mitigated by the limited efficacy of such procedures.

Objective.—We sought to assess the efficacy of ultrasound skin tightening for brow-lift in the context of a procedure treating the full face and neck.

Methods.—This was a rater-blinded, prospective cohort study at a dermatology clinic in an urban academic medical center. Subjects were medicated with topical anesthetic and then treated with an investigational focused intense ultrasound tightening device to the forehead, temples, cheeks, submental region, and side of neck using the following probes: 4 MHz, 4.5-mm focal depth; 7 MHz, 4.5-mm focal depth; and 7 MHz, 3.0-mm focal depth. Standardized photographs of front and side views were obtained at 2, 7, 28, 60, and 90 days; rating scales of pain, adverse events, physical findings, and patient satisfaction were also completed. Primary outcome measure was detection of improvement in paired comparison of pretreatment and posttreatment (day 90) photographs by 3 masked expert physician assessors, cosmetic and laser dermatologists, and plastic surgeons who were not authors. Second primary outcome measure was objective brow elevation as quantitated by a standard procedure using fixed landmarks. Secondary outcomes measure was patient satisfaction as measured by a questionnaire.

Results.—A total of 36 subjects (34 female) were enrolled, one subject dropped out, and 35 subjects were evaluated. Median age was 44 years (range 32-62). On the first primary outcome measure, 30 of 35 subjects (86%) were judged by the 3 masked experienced clinician raters to show clinically significant brow-lift 90 days after treatment ($P = .00001$). On the second primary outcome measure, mean value of average change in eyebrow height as assessed by measurement of photographs at 90 days was 1.7 mm.

Limitations.—Limitations of this study include the inability to quantitatively measure lower face tightening because of the lack of fixed anatomic landmarks in this area.

Conclusion.—Ultrasound appears to be a safe and effective modality for facial skin tightening. A single ultrasound treatment of the forehead produced on average brow height elevation of slightly less than 2 mm. Most treated individuals responded, commonly with accompanying transitory mild erythema and edema.

▶ This clinical study reviews the first human clinical trial of a new ultrasound technology for skin tightening—specifically looking at a brow-lift in the context of a full face and neck procedure. Ultrasound technologies have been studied for a number of years in laser medicine, and clinical trials that are designed to look at fat reduction are equipped with several high-frequency devices. This device, which is akin to fractional ultrasound, has been shown to be successful in raising eyebrow height from 1.7 to 1.9 mm, which may not seem significant but is in the context of eyebrow elevation by more aggressive means. This was a well-performed, thoughtful clinical evaluation that will pave the way for other ultrasound devices to be used for facial, and perhaps, body contouring. This work is important.

M. H. Gold, MD

17 Miscellaneous Topics in Dermatologic Surgery and Cutaneous Oncology

A Direct Comparison of Visual Inspection, Curettage, and Epiluminescence Microscopy in Determining Tumor Extent Before the Initial Margins are Determined for Mohs Micrographic Surgery
Guardiano RA, Grande DJ (Mystic Valley Dermatology Associates, Stoneham, MA)
Dermatol Surg 36:1240-1244, 2010

Background.—Mohs micrographic surgery (MMS) is a tissue-sparing technique for the removal of cutaneous malignancies. There is no standardized procedure for determining tumor extent before taking the initial margins during the first stage of Mohs.

Objective.—To compare visual inspection, curettage, and dermoscopy in determining tumor extent before initial margins are taken for MMS.

Methods.—Fifty-four patients were randomized into three groups (visual inspection, curettage, or dermoscopy) before MMS for basal cell carcinomas on the nose. One of these three methods was used to delineate the biopsy site or residual tumor. The final number of stages and postoperative defect sizes were recorded.

Results.—There was no statistically significant differences for the final number of stages ($p = .20$) or the final defect sizes ($p = .47$) between the three arms.

Conclusion.—There has been controversy as to whether presurgical curettage is appropriate before MMS. Some feel that curettage better delineates the tumor, leading to fewer stages, whereas others feel that curettage may falsely increase the final defect size, negating any tissue-sparing advantages of the procedure. Our study did not demonstrate any differences in the final number of stages or postoperative defect sizes between the three test groups.

▶ Mohs micrographic surgery (MMS) is tissue sparing and determination of tumor extent is critical when planning the first stage. The authors compared

3 modalities in determining the tumor extent: visual, curettage, and dermoscopy. The study size was small with 54 patients. There was no statistically significant difference in the final defect size and the final number of stages between the 3 arms. As the authors stated, the major limitations of this study included the small study size and the location of the skin cancer.

It is the strong opinion of one of the reviewers (JDR) that curettage prior to completion of MMS is extremely valuable with regard to each individual case, with its value not properly assessed by studies that look at collective results, differences in number of stages, etc. The major value of pre-MMS curettage is assessment of depth and sometimes radial extension, of that specific tumor at hand, prior to determining the anatomic depth and width of the first layer. It clearly is of assistance in some cases. Studies do not evaluate this case-by-case benefit and are misleading in this regard. With pre-MMS curettage, it is important not to haphazardly curette away superficially around the body of the tumor, as this removes skin edge unnecessarily and confounds slide interpretation later.

S. Bhambri, DO

J. Q. Del Rosso, DO

Academic Productivity and Affiliation of Dermatologic Surgeons
Tierney EP, Hanke CW, Kimball AB (Boston Univ School of Medicine, MA; Laser and Skin Surgery Ctr of Indiana, Carmel; Harvard Med School, Boston, MA)
Dermatol Surg 35:1886-1892, 2009

Background.—Because Mohs fellowship training typically incorporates a research component, as required by the Mohs College for fellowship certification, we evaluated whether Mohs microscopic surgery fellowship-trained (MMSFT) dermatologic surgeons were more likely to join academic institutions and demonstrate greater activity in teaching, research, and scientific writing than non-fellowship-trained surgeons (NMMSFT).

Methods.—Responses to the 2002 and 2005 American Academy of Dermatology Practice Profile survey comparing practice settings, proportion of time spent in various practice settings, and professional roles were compared between the two groups.

Results.—MMSFT dermatologic surgeons were 5 times as likely to be in full-time academic practice and 3 times as likely to be in part-time academia as NMMSFT dermatologic surgeons. Consistent with their greater presence in academia, in 2004, 47% of MMSFT dermatologist surgeons participated in teaching, compared with 19% of NMMSFT surgeons ($p = .001$) and 16% of all dermatologists ($p = .001$). Twenty-two percent of MMSFT dermatologic surgeons were involved in research, compared with only 4% of NMMSFT dermatologic surgeons ($p = .001$) and 8% of all dermatologists ($p < .05$).

Conclusions.—Academic productivity of dermatologic surgeons appears to be associated with Mohs fellowship training. The level of teaching and research was significant even in MMSFT surgeons who were not in full- or part-time academic faculty positions. This suggests a strong tradition of academic productivity for dermatologic surgeons outside traditional academic institutions.

▶ The premise of the article raises interesting questions for the practice of medicine, not only for dermatology but also for all of medicine, specialized or not. The reader must infer that practitioners inclined to advanced training are also inclined to research and participate to a greater degree in academic pursuits.

The authors conclude that academic productivity and Mohs micrographic surgery fellowship-trained (MMSFT) dermatologic surgeons co-exist. It is not possible to quantify whether MMSFT dermatologic surgeons are triggered by a desire to pursue further academic pursuits or whether the MMSFT dermatologic surgeons are predisposed to academia.

Although limited, the data presented raises a possible concern for academic institutions in the future. In 2005 only 47% of MMSFT dermatologic surgeons engaged in part-time teaching in an academic institution, and more fellowship positions exist in private practice than in academic institutions. This evidence suggests that in the future it may be harder to attract MMSFT dermatologic surgeons into a traditional academic setting, thus putting them at a decided disadvantage in recruiting the most trained surgeons.

This article displays numerous self-admitted flaws in its methods and conclusions. The data used to support this article are limited (less than 33% response rate) and based solely on self-reported data, which is typically unreliable due to its inability to be peer reviewed. Self-reported data sets also tend to be biased and self-serving by those reporting.

The findings challenge the notion that academic careers must be limited to traditional academic settings. They also provide encouragement for private practice dermatologists to continue to be involved in teaching and research. It will be interesting to see what impact the new ACGME Procedural Dermatology fellowships with increased emphasis on cosmetic dermatology will have. Practice in academic institutions may be even less attractive to these fellowship-trained practitioners.

R. I. Ceilley, MD

Evaluation of a New Wound Closure Device for Linear Surgical Incisions: 3M Steri-Strip S Surgical Skin Closure versus Subcuticular Closure
Kerrigan CL, Homa K (Dartmouth Hitchcock Med Ctr, Lebanon, NH)
Plast Reconstr Surg 125:186-194, 2010

Background.—Technological innovations are often adopted before scientific comparison to an accepted standard. The authors' study compared suture with a new coaptive film device, 3M Steri-Strip S Surgical Skin Closure, on linear incisions.

Methods.—Patients undergoing Wise-pattern breast reduction or abdominal procedures had paired incisions randomly assigned to Steri-Strip S or suture closure. Key outcome measures were closure time, patient comfort, and scar quality at 6 months by patients and surgeons using a new scar evaluation tool, visual assessment of linear scars. Statistical differences between the two closure techniques were assessed by Wilcoxon signed rank test.

Results.—Of 59 patients, eight were excluded from randomization (a surgeon judged Steri-Strip S to be a nonviable closure technique for mismatched wound edges). Fifty-one patients (breast, $n = 24$; abdomen, $n = 27$) were randomized. Operative time with Steri-Strip S for breast was 2.0 minutes (SD = 1.1) versus suture closure at 4.6 minutes (SD = 1.5; $p < 0.001$). Similarly, Steri-Strip S versus suture for the abdomen was faster ($p < 0.001$; 4.9 minutes, SD = 2.3 versus 10.1 minutes, SD = 3.4). Comfort scores did not differ between closures [5.8 (SD = 2.7) versus 6.9 (SD = 2.0), respectively, on breast ($p = 0.142$) and 7.7 (SD = 1.8) versus 7.7 (SD = 2.3) on abdomen ($p = 0.903$)]. Complication rates did not differ between closure types. Patients' visual assessment of linear scars rating of breasts was 3.8 (SD = 2.9) for Steri-Strip S and better at 2.6 (SD = 2.9) for suture ($p = 0.008$). One surgeon rated breast Steri-Strip S scars worse than suture scars (4.3 versus 3.7; $p = 0.014$). For abdominal scars, there was no difference in the patient or surgeon ratings.

Conclusions.—Steri-Strip S permits faster wound closure than suture. On the basis of patient reports of comfort and scar quality, surgeons increase efficiency and maintain quality with the use of Steri-Strip S on abdominal wounds but not on breast wounds.

▶ The objective of this article is to compare the use of 3M closure device for a linear surgical incision with that of a subcuticular closure. This was organized in a study of 59 patients who were undergoing abdominoplasty or a breast surgery. The results appeared to be valid, and the conclusion was valid. It was referenced with a research article with the comparison of the closure quality, speed, efficiency, and appearance as well as comfort on the patient's part. The conclusions appear to be valid based on the data collected during the procedure.

The strength of the article is investigation of this medical device in terms of its assistance in surgery. The weakness of the article is that as dermatologists, we seldom are involved in breast surgery or abdominoplasty but do frequently make large incisions to remove skin cancers, and these would have validity in closures of these defects.

The clinical relevance as mentioned is that as dermatologists we perform routinely large surgical incisions, and assistance and efficiency of closure is certainly a factor. The quality and the patient satisfaction are more major criteria. Not explained in this article were the economics and the cost of the device as compared with the suture. Among the 59 patients who were recruited, 8 were excluded, so in a total of 51 patients, 24 underwent breast surgery and 27 underwent abdominoplasty. The operation time for S-plasty in breast surgery was 2 minutes versus a suture closure time of 4.6 minutes, and the abdominoplasty was faster as well with 4.9 minutes for S-plasty versus 10.1 minutes for suture closure. These scores indicate significant improvement in the speed of closure. Of concern would be the complication rates that did not differ between the closure types, and the patient visual assessment of the linear scar was slightly better for the suture wound. The surgeon's rating of the sterile S scars was worse than the suture wound as well. For abdominal scarring, there was little difference between the patient and surgical ratings.

The overall conclusion is that this is a medical device that may enhance the efficiency of large linear incisions but also may cost more from an economic standpoint. The breast surgery has a less visual assessment score and has less patient satisfaction. Consideration for a revised S-plasty closure was raised. The authors of this article noted that there was a possible bias that the patients knew their closure technique. That is a difficult bias to remove because of the nature of the study. The possibility of the modification of the Steri-Strip S certainly could be done with individual steri strips without the pattern, which should be studied in further studies. This study is of limited use for practicing dermatologists.

L. Cleaver, DO

Improved diagnosis and treatment of soft tissue sarcoma patients after implementation of national guidelines: A population-based study
Jansen-Landheer MLEA, Krijnen P, Oostindiër MJ, et al (Leiden Cancer Registry, The Netherlands; et al)
Eur J Surg Oncol 35:1326-1332, 2009

Aim.—The majority of clinicians, radiologists and pathologists have limited experience with soft tissue sarcomas. In 2004, national guidelines were established in The Netherlands to improve the quality of diagnosis and treatment of these rare tumours. This study evaluates the compliance with the guidelines over time.

Patients.—Population-based series of 119 operated patients with a soft tissue sarcoma (STS) diagnosed in 1998—1999 (79 before implementation of new guidelines) and in 2006 (40 after implementation).

Methods.—Coded information regarding patient and tumour character-istics as well as (the results of) pathology review was collected from the medical patient file by two experienced data-managers.

Results.—Diagnostic imaging of the tumour was performed according to the guidelines in 75—100% depending on the site of the tumour (abdominal versus non-abdominal) as well as the time of diagnosis.

Adherence to the guidelines with respect to invasive diagnostic proce-dures in patients with non-abdominal STS improved over time. A pre-operative histological diagnosis was obtained in 42% of the patients in 1998—1999 and in 72% of the patients in 2006 ($p < 0.001$). The guidelines for reporting on pathology were increasingly adhered to. In 2006, (nearly) all pathology reports mentioned tumour size, morphology, tumour grade, resection margins and radicality. This represents a major improvement compared to the pathology reports in 1998−1999, where these aspects were not mentioned in 14−40% of the cases. The proportion of prospective pathology reviews by (a member of) the expert panel increased from 60% in 1998−1999 to 90% in 2006 ($p = 0.001$).

Discussion.—The compliance with the guidelines has been optimised by the increased attention to this group of patients. Most important factors have been the reporting of the results of the first evaluation and (discussions about) the centralisation of treatment. Further improvements could be reached by the prospective web based registry monitoring logistic aspects as well as parameters useful for the evaluation of the quality of care.

▶ Jansen-Landheer et al performed a population-based study to determine if there was improvement by practitioners in compliance with a set of national guidelines in the Netherlands over time and thus improvement in the diagnosis and treatment of soft tissue sarcomas according to the guidelines. More than 60% of the soft tissue sarcomas in the study were either myogenic sarcomas, myxofibrosarcomas, or liposarcomas. According to the study, experience from clinical trials indicates that diagnosis and treatment according to recommended guidelines affect clinical outcome and patient survival. Based on the results, the study found that there was, in fact, increased adherence to the guidelines. The guidelines provided recommendations for issues such as the diagnostic workup for soft tissue sarcomas and the review of all histologic material by a regional expert panel (a panel made up of at least 5 pathologists from regional hospitals with a special interest in soft tissue tumors). While not an aim of the study, the information contained within the report certainly provides information for further discussion for other countries in setting diagnostic and treatment parameters for soft tissue sarcomas. However, the ease of ability for another country to implement such guidelines may not prove to be as practical as it has proven to be in the Netherlands. For example, implementing guidelines for a regional expert panel to review all histologic material may prove to be more difficult to do in a larger country such as the United States, where the volume burden of health care is much larger. Regardless, the study ultimately achieves its objective in emphasizing the importance of established guidelines for the diagnosis and management of soft tissue sarcomas by highlighting not only its compliance of practitioners within the Netherlands but also the effectiveness of guidelines in optimizing outcomes.

B. D. Michaels, DO

J. Q. Del Rosso, DO

Lack of Complications in Skin Surgery of Patients Receiving Clopidogrel as Compared with Patients Taking Aspirin, Warfarin, and Controls

Kramer E, Hadad E, Westreich M, et al (Assaf Harofeh Med Ctr, Zerifin, Israel; Tel Aviv Univ, Ramat Aviv, Israel)
Am Surg 76:11-14, 2010

Clopidogrel, a new antiplatelet agent that irreversibly inhibits platelet aggregation, is widely used today. This prospective work was conducted to evaluate the safety of performing skin surgery on patients taking clopidogrel. Patients undergoing surgery for excision of skin or subcutaneous lesions under local anesthesia taking clopidogrel were the study group. The control group comprised 2073 historical patients who had undergone a similar procedure. Data collected included: age, sex, past medical history, medications, and late complications. Follow-up was done at 1 to 2 weeks and 3 to 6 months. There were 32 patients on clopidogrel, having 38 lesions removed. Of these, seven patients were on aspirin and clopidogrel combined. The groups taking clopidogrel, aspirin, and warfarin had significantly more males, were older, and had significantly more comorbid medical conditions. There was no significant difference in the incidence of any of the complications in any of the groups. This study shows that patients taking clopidogrel before skin surgery, though older and with more associated medical conditions, do not experience a greater rate of complications. We conclude that patients undergoing minor excisional cutaneous surgery should continue taking clopidogrel because there is no apparent risk for increased complications when good meticulous surgical techniques are used.

▶ Dermatologists are increasingly faced with the dilemma of how to manage patients who are taking anticoagulants or drugs that inhibit platelet aggregation. Numerous studies have shown that the risk of stopping these drugs may be far greater than continuous therapy.

Even minor procedures such as skin biopsy may result in postoperative bleeding. Intraoperative bleeding certainly prolongs and may complicate surgical procedures. This may influence the choice of surgical procedures when one considers the risk/benefit ratio of excessive bleeding.

This is a well-done article that further reinforces that we do not need to stop platelet inhibitors or anticoagulants before skin and subcutaneous surgery. Patients who take these medications tend to be older with more comorbid conditions, especially cardiovascular and peripheral vascular disease. They are at high risk for stroke, pulmonary embolus, and myocardial infarction. There was not any increased risk in any of the groups for complications related to continuing the medication(s). They did find that patients taking clopidogrel had more oozing during the procedure.

Our current approach is to have patients discontinue vitamin and herbal supplements along with any nonprescribed platelet aggregation inhibitors such as aspirin and nonsteroidal anti-inflammatory drugs. Meticulous attention is given to intraoperative hemostatis, postoperative pressure dressings, ice packing, and postsurgical activity restrictions have helped reduce postoperative bleeding. All patients at increased risk of postoperative bleeding or bleeding from minor trauma are given advice on wound care. The only negative critique of the study is its small sample size. Despite this, the conclusions clearly show the safety of continuing platelet inhibitors and anticoagulants for skin surgery. With an aging population, these medications will be increasingly common, and we need studies such as this to confirm the very low risk of serious complications resulting from their continuation.

R. I. Ceilley, MD

B. A. Kopitzki, DO

Nail Matrix Phenolization for Treatment of Ingrowing Nail: Technique Report and Recurrence Rate of 267 Surgeries

Di Chiacchio N, Belda W Jr, Di Chiacchio NG, et al (Hospital do Servidor Público Municipal de São Paulo, Brazil; Univ of São Paulo, Brazil; Univ of Taubaté, São Paulo, Brazil; et al)
Dermatol Surg 36:534-537, 2010

Background.—Common in adolescents and young adults, ingrowing toenail (onychocryptosis) usually affects the lateral side of the great toe. The most effective treatment is phenolization of the nail matrix, which has a lower recurrence rate than surgical matricectomy. Many studies that assess the recurrence rate after phenolization do not include the surgical technique or the experience level of the surgeon. A description of the technique was undertaken.

Methods.—Two hundred sixty-seven nail matrix phenolization procedures were done for ingrowing toenail treatment in 172 patients, mean age 38.5 years. The matrix phenolization technique was performed by the same highly experienced dermatologic surgeon in all cases; follow-up assessments and results were reported.

Technique and Results.—The great toe was disinfected using alcohol, then distal block anesthesia was performed using 2 mL of lidocaine 2% without epinephrine. A tourniquet was applied and the granulation tissue curetted away. A nail elevator was used to detach the lateral nail plate from the lateral and proximal nail fold. A cut was made down the long axis from the free edge of the nail plate to the nail matrix, which was then removed using mosquito forceps rotationally. Gentle curettage was carried out on the nail matrix, nail bed, and lateral nail fold. Dry cotton swabs kept the field free of blood. A cotton swab soaked in phenol solution 88% was strongly rubbed on the nail matrix and nail bed, then the wound was cleaned using alcohol and dried with sterile gauze. The tourniquet was removed and the wound dressed; antibiotic ointment was applied.

The patient was given pain medication and told to keep the foot elevated for 24 hours, then return for a wound check. At this visit the dressing was removed, the wound cleaned with water and antiseptic soaks, and antibiotic ointment applied. Patients were to repeat this procedure twice a day until healing was complete, about 2 to 4 weeks. Postoperative evaluations were done after 10, 30, and 60 days. Follow-up lasted 6 to 33 months. No complications developed postoperatively, but five ingrowing nails recurred, all within 2 to 4 months of surgery, for a success rate of 1.9%.

Conclusions.—Surgical matricectomy for ingrowing toenail is accompanied by considerable morbidity, postoperative pain, and undesirable cosmetic results. With phenolization of the nail matrix, the patient is relatively painfree postoperatively and recurrence rates are low. The fact that an expert dermatologic surgeon performed all the procedures probably contributed to the low recurrence rate.

▶ This large study of 267 ingrown toenails surgically treated with phenol matricectomy beautifully illustrates the technique of partial chemical matricectomy in great detail and discusses the potential complications and recurrence rate for these patients. These authors had an impressive recurrence rate of 1.9%, which is much less than the rate of other previously published series. Their low side effect profile was excellent. This method of partial chemical matricectomy with phenol is standard care, and this article discusses the details of how to perform this procedure and the efficacy and safety. Photographic details of the procedure are very helpful for the novice.

P. Rich, MD

The accuracy of the sentinel lymph node concept in early stage squamous cell vulvar carcinoma

Radziszewski J, Kowalewska M, Jedrzejczak T, et al (The Maria Sklodowska-Curie Memorial Cancer Centre and Inst of Oncology, Roentgena, Warsaw, Poland; et al)
Gynecol Oncol 116:473-477, 2010

Objective.—The purpose of the study was to determine the feasibility and accuracy of the sentinel lymph node (SLN) identification in vulvar carcinoma patients.

Methods.—Sixty-two patients with clinical early stage vulvar cancer underwent SLN detection procedure, followed by a complete inguinofemoral lymphadenectomy. The SLN was identified intraoperatively using lymphoscintigraphy with technetium-99m as well as patent blue V staining. The resected lymph nodes (LN) were submitted for histological examination by hematoxylin—eosin staining (H—E) and cytokeratin immunohistochemistry (IHC) and examined by the reverse transcriptase-polymerase chain reaction (RT-PCR) assay.

Results.—A total of 109 inguinal LN were dissected in 56 patients. SLNs were identified in 76% groins with patent blue V and in 99% with the use of Tc-99 m. The accuracy differed significantly ($p < 0.0001$).

An H—E examination combined with IHC revealed 7 false-negative SLNs. The sensitivity of this method was 73% (95% CI, 64% to 81%) and the negative predictive value for a negative SLN finding was 92% (95% CI, 87% to 97%). The RT-PCR assay showed 8 false-negative SLNs. The sensitivity of the RT-PCR-based assay was 83% (95% CI, 75% to 90%) and the negative predictive value for a negative SLN was 88% (95% CI, 82% to 94%). The two diagnostic methods were found not to differ significantly.

Conclusions.—In SLN mapping, the Tc-99m colloid lymphoscintigraphy is superior to the blue dye staining. Our data do not support the concept of the SLN identification as a highly accurate procedure in predicting the inguinofemoral LN status in patients with early stage vulvar cancer.

▶ This study out of Poland has the objective to determine the feasibility and accuracy of the sentinel node biopsy technique for lymph node involvement in vulvar cancer patients. The study seems to be a valid study for the identification of inguinal lymph nodes in patients presenting with advanced vulvar carcinoma. Sixty-two patients were identified and underwent sentinel node discovery followed by a complete inguinofemoral lymphadenopathy. The sentinel node technique was identified interoperatively using lymphoscintigraphy with technetium-99 m as well as patient blue V staining. Lymph nodes were submitted for histological evaluation with hematoxylin and eisin (H&E) staining and cytokeratin immunohistochemistry, and examined by reverse transcriptase-polymerase chain reaction (RT-PCT). Of the 109 inguinal lymph nodes that were dissected in 56 patients, sentinel nodes were identified in 76% of the groins with blue V and 99% with the use of Tc-99 m. The accuracy differed significantly with p values less than 0.0001.

Dermatologists do not regularly confront patients with vulvar squamous cell carcinoma (SCC), but at times they certainly do. In general, more aggressive treatment is usually handled by an oncologic surgeon or gynecologic surgeon. The patient presenting with early stage 1 and 2 vulvar SCC has a probability of a positive lymph node finding is only 10-26% of cases. Approximately 86% of patients with stage 1 and 2 vulvar SCC undergo unnecessary lymphadenectomy. Further complicating this picture is that 24% of patients with clinically normal lymph nodes have metastasis, and more than 20% of patients with enlarged lymph nodes in clinical examinations are found metastatis-free upon histologic examination. The sentinel node evaluation, which has been utilized in the management of penile cancer, melanoma, and breast cancer, is a method to improve the standard for regional lymph node detection. This study showed that in the 62% patients with stage 1 and 2 vulvar SCC, that utilization of lymphoscintigraphy revealed that the isotope-based method showed a higher identification rate (99%) as compared to the blue dye method (76%). The difference was statistically significant.

The conclusion is that the most accurate determination of the sentinel lymph node in patients with vulvar SCC is preoperative lymphoscintigraphy (administration of Tc-99 m) and intraoperative biopsy under gamma probe.

The blue dye staining alone is not sufficient for sentinel lymph node identification. The RT-PCR detection of CA9 can be recommended for further systematic evaluation for detection of vulvar SCC cells in lymph nodes but is not recommended as a reliable procedure to avoid radical inguinofemoral lymphadenectomy. Safety is certainly important. A 75% sensitivity for the sentinel lymph node examination with routine H&E combined with immunohistochemistry means that 1 of 4 of patients with existing metastasis were not detected, and such patients may not receive optimal therapy. The sentinel lymph node evaluation cannot be recommended overall as a reliable procedure to avoid radical inguinofemoral lymphadenectomy in early stages of vulvar SCC because of the high false negative sentinel lymph node rate. Further evaluation and surgical expertise in the performance of sentinel lymph node evaluation in these patients may improve numbers and make it more of an acceptable procedure.

L. Cleaver, DO

The Effect of Calcium Channel Blockers on Smoking-Induced Skin Flap Necrosis

Rinker B, Fink BF, Barry NG, et al (Univ of Kentucky, Lexington)
Plast Reconstr Surg 125:866-871, 2010

Background.—Calcium channel blockers have been shown experimentally to reverse many of the effects of nicotine. The purpose of this study was to assess the effect of calcium channel blockers on smoking-induced skin flap necrosis.

Methods.—Forty male albino Wistar rats were divided into four groups. Groups A, B, and C were treated in a controlled smoking chamber for 20 minutes daily for 21 days. On day 14, caudally based dorsal skin flaps (3 × 10 cm) were created. On days 14 through 21, group B animals received verapamil (20 mg/kg/day) by gavage. Group C received nifedipine (10 mg/kg/day). On day 21, standardized photographs were taken and flap survival areas determined. Urine cotinine concentrations were measured on days 14 and 21.

Results.—The mean cotinine level at surgery was 161 ng/ml in group A (smoking), 149 ng/ml in group B (verapamil), and 168 ng/ml in group C (nifedipine). These differences were not statistically significant. Cotinine concentration at surgery for group D (no smoking) was less than 10 ng/ml. The mean flap survival in group D was 79.1 percent, compared with 63.7 percent in group A ($p = 0.003$). The mean flap survival in group B (verapamil) was 72.8 percent, compared with 73.7 percent in group C (nifedipine). Both values were significantly greater than in group A ($p = 0.04$ and $p = 0.008$, respectively).

Conclusions.—In this study, enteral calcium channel blockers were associated with a statistically significant improvement in flap survival compared with untreated animals with an equivalent smoke exposure.

Calcium channel blockers may reduce perioperative risk in active smokers who require skin flap surgery.

▶ Flap necrosis and wound dehiscence are 2 of the most dreaded complications in dermatologic surgery. Dermatologic surgeons are faced with a substantial number of patients, who are both smokers and have multiple skin cancer risk factors. Attempts to have such patients cease smoking before surgery are often unsuccessful and may result in delayed surgery for certain malignancies.

Calcium channel blockers have long been used in dermatology for vasospastic conditions such as Raynaud disease. The results of this study showing their value in reducing the perioperative risk in acute smokers requiring skin flap surgery is reassuring. It will be interesting to see if they will be of benefit for other instances where flap ischemia develops or is anticipated.

This article is important because it sets the stage for future studies regarding calcium channel blockers and their use for skin flaps in smokers. It is always disheartening to have a well-executed flap suffer necrosis or dehiscence in a smoker. Additional studies will need to be done in humans before calcium channel blockers can be recommended for smokers who will require a flap. This is a well-done initial study that clearly shows significant improvement in flap survival in rats exposed to smoke that are given calcium channel blockers. We look forward to additional studies that will determine the ideal dose, timing, and reproducible benefit in human subjects.

R. I. Ceilley, MD

B. A. Kopitski, DO

The Influence of Surgical Excision Margins on Keloid Prognosis
Tan KT, Shah N, Pritchard SA, et al (Univ of Manchester, UK; Univ Hosp of South Manchester NHS Foundation Trust, Manchester, UK)
Ann Plast Surg 64:55-58, 2010

Keloid disease is known to have variable clinical behavior in response to therapy and there is no clinicopathologic classification that predicts such varied behavior. The aim of this study was to study the effect of excision margins and other histopathologic characteristics on keloid prognosis.

Seventy-five multiethnic patients presenting with keloid scars at a department of plastic and reconstructive surgery during an 11-year period were included in this study. Clinical data was collected and detailed histologic analyses using light microscopy were carried out on archived patient specimens.

A detailed histopathologic examination of all tissue samples identified keloid border or margin characteristics which were classified into "circumscribed" (borders clearly-demarcated) and "infiltrative" (borders not clearly-demarcated and not easily-definable). The specific histologic findings were correlated with keloid recurrence which revealed that incomplete peripheral $(P < 0.001)$ and deep excision margins $(P < 0.001)$, as well as infiltrative borders ($P < 0.05$) were associated with higher 1-year reported recurrence rates.

This study has given evidence that incomplete surgical excision are associated with higher recurrence and this may justify the practice of routine histopathologic reporting of keloid excision margins.

► Tan et al performed a study reviewing factors that may have a consequence on keloid recurrence prognosis. It was found that surgical methods and keloid border characteristics have an outcome on keloid recurrence. Namely, complete excision of a keloid at both its peripheral and deep margins resulted in a statistically significant decreased recurrence rate at the 3-month, 6-month, and 1-year postexcision intervals versus incomplete excisional margins. The determination of completeness of the excision margins was reviewed by histopathological examinations. In addition, 2 keloid border characteristics were also reviewed: infiltrative borders versus circumscribed borders. Keloids with circumscribed borders, as determined by histopathological techniques, also revealed a decreased recurrence rate versus infiltrative borders that also proved statistically significant. Interestingly, ethnicity was correlated to the type of keloid border that may be encountered, noting that whites were less likely to have infiltrative keloidal borders than Afro-Caribbeans, Asians, and other ethnic groups.

Ultimately, in application to the dermatologist, this article provides useful information for 2 reasons: one, there is now at least some supporting evidence that extralesional versus intralesional excision may be the preferred technique for keloidal removal, as complete excision margins are associated with a decrease in reported recurrence rates for up to 1 year (although the article notes that a further prospective trial is needed to further review extralesional vs intralesional excision of keloid scars) and two, histological reports of surgical margins and the nature of the involved border characteristics may be a useful tool to the clinician, as it may help better assess keloid recurrence and prognosis after excision.

B. D. Michaels, DO

J. Q. Del Rosso, DO

Treatment of Earlobe Keloids by Extralesional Excision Combined with Preoperative and Postoperative "Sandwich" Radiotherapy
Stahl S, Barnea Y, Weiss J, et al (Tel-Aviv Sourasky Med Ctr, Israel; Tel-Aviv Univ, Israel)
Plast Reconstr Surg 125:135-141, 2010

Background.—Earlobe keloids can form after cosmetic ear piercing, trauma, infection, or burns, or spontaneously. These keloids are highly resistant for treatment and are followed by severe cosmetic implications. There are various surgical and nonsurgical treatment modalities for earlobe keloids, with no universally accepted treatment policy and a wide range of reported recurrence rates. The authors present their experience of treating earlobe keloids using the "sandwich" technique protocol;

extralesional excision and external-beam radiotherapy are given a day before and a day after the operation.

Methods.—The authors retrospectively reviewed all patients with earlobe keloids treated by the "sandwich" technique between the years 1996 and 2005. Patients were categorized into two groups: a high-risk group for previously treated patients and patients with a tendency for hypertrophic scars and keloids, and a low-risk group for the others. All patients underwent extralesional excision of the keloid and local radiotherapy before the excision and following it. Follow-up was a minimum of half a year and included a patient satisfaction questionnaire and documentation of keloid recurrence or cure.

Results.—A total of 23 patients were treated by this protocol; 57 percent were male. Patients had an average age of 24 years. The most common keloid etiology was earlobe piercing. Recurrence rates for the low-risk and high-risk groups were 25 and 27 percent [percent of the patients], respectively. Overall patient satisfaction was high.

Conclusion.—The combined excision and "sandwich" radiotherapy technique is a simple and effective method for treating earlobe keloids, with high patient satisfaction and low recurrence and complication rates.

▶ This study does not show improved efficacy of sandwich therapy (pre- and postsurgical radiation) over simple postsurgical radiation. Subjects are stratified into 2 groups; those with keloids who have not had prior treatment (n = 9) and those with recurrent keloids (n = 11). The cure rates for sandwich therapy were 73% and 62.5%, respectively, for the 2 groups. The author goes on to mention 3 previous studies done on excision with postsurgical radiation only that had better cure rates than this study's sandwich therapy. Furthermore, the small sample sizes of the sandwich study would question the power of its data if it had proved to be superior.

In addition, it would have been helpful to add in the numbers of patients and posttreatment follow-up time frames for all of the comparative studies to help give improved perspective. Perhaps those studies were done with small sample sizes too? Then, at least the author could convey that their modality could possibly be on par or better than the others and that a larger scale study should be done to help define which is truly a better treatment.

B. P. Glick, DO, MPH

Wound edge biopsy sites in chronic wounds heal rapidly and do not result in delayed overall healing of the wounds
Panuncialman J, Hammerman S, Carson P, et al (Roger Williams Med Ctr, Providence, RI)
Wound Rep Reg 18:21-25, 2010

Wound biopsies are an essential diagnostic component in the management of chronic wounds. First, the possibility of malignancy or infection in the wound often requires sampling of the wound edge and its bed. Secondly, several practice guidelines recommend biopsying wounds that have not responded to treatment after 2—6 weeks. However, there has always been a concern that the biopsy may worsen the wound and delay overall healing. In this report, we investigated the safety and effects of wound biopsies on overall chronic wound healing rates (advance of the wound edge per week toward the center) before and after the biopsy was performed. In a cohort of 14 consecutive patients with chronic wounds of the lower extremity, we found that postbiopsy chronic wound healing rates (0.99 ± 1.18 mm/week; mean ± SD) were not decreased and were actually higher than prebiopsy chronic wound healing rates (0.49 ± 0.85 mm/week; mean ± SD, $p < 0.05$). In addition, we documented that healing of the biopsy sites up to the original wound edge occurred within 6 weeks in 11 of the 14 subjects. Therefore, we conclude that chronic wounds do not worsen after being biopsied and that wound biopsies are a safe procedure that does not delay overall healing of the chronic wound.

▶ Chronic cutaneous ulcers or nonhealing wounds can often be a sign for malignant skin changes. The most common etiologies for chronic skin ulcers, especially of the lower extremities, are diabetic ulcers, venous stasis ulcers, and pressure ulcers. However, patients with nonhealing wounds of any etiology may warrant biopsies of the margins to exclude possible malignancy. Nevertheless, there are concerns that biopsies may worsen wound healing and lead to further deterioration of the wound site. Therefore, this article investigates the effect of performing a biopsy of chronic wound edges in 14 patients. Investigators found that overall wound healing rates were in fact greater following a full-thickness wedge biopsy than those obtained prebiopsy. In fact, 11 out of 14 patients had complete healing of biopsy sites up to the original wound edge by week 6. One theory is that biopsying a wound edge may produce local acute injury by the removal of the abnormal cells in the nonhealing edge and subsequently resetting the healing process. Clearly, a larger sample study is needed; however, these results do support the idea that biopsies are a safe procedure in chronic ulcers, and clinicians should consider biopsying suspicious nonhealing wounds that do not respond to appropriate treatment.

S. Bellew, DO

J. Q. Del Rosso, DO

Dermatoscopy of basal cell carcinoma: Morphologic variability of global and local features and accuracy of diagnosis
Altamura D, Menzies SW, Argenziano G, et al (Univ of L'Aquila, Italy; Univ of Sydney, Australia; Second Univ of Naples, Italy)
J Am Acad Dermatol 62:67-75, 2010

Background.—Early detection of basal cell carcinoma (BCC) is crucial to reduce the morbidity of this tumor.

Objective.—We sought to investigate the variability and diagnostic significance of dermatoscopic features of BCCs.

Methods.—We conducted retrospective dermatoscopic analysis of 609 BCCs and 200 melanocytic and nonmelanocytic lesions, and assessment of interrater reliability of dermatoscopic BCC criteria.

Results.—Lesions included nonpigmented (15.1%), lightly pigmented (33.2%), pigmented (42.7%), and heavily pigmented (9%) BCCs. Classic BCC patterns including arborizing telangiectasia (57.1%), blue/gray ovoid nests (47.5%), ulceration (39.2%), multiple blue/gray globules (26.1%), leaflike areas (15.9%), and spoke-wheel areas (9%) were significantly increased in pigmented BCCs compared with nonpigmented and heavily pigmented BCCs ($P = .0001$). Among nonclassic BCC patterns, we detected short fine superficial telangiectasia (10%) and multiple small erosions (8.5%), and described two new patterns named "concentric structures" (7.6%) and "multiple in-focus blue/gray dots" (5.1%). Dermatoscopic features suggestive of melanocytic lesions (eg, multiple brown to black dots/globules, blue/white veillike structures, and nonarborizing vessels) were observed in 40.6% BCCs and significantly increased in heavily pigmented BCCs ($P < .0001$). Expert observers provided an accurate (sensitivity: 97%) and reliable (K: 87%) dermatoscopic diagnosis of BCC, although a significant difference in terms of specificity ($P = .0002$) and positive predictive value ($P = .0004$) was found. Arborizing telangiectasia, leaflike areas, and large blue/gray ovoid nests represented reliable and robust diagnostic parameters.

Limitation.—The study was retrospective.

Conclusion.—BCCs show a large spectrum of global and local dermatoscopic features; heavily pigmented BCCs show the most challenging combinations of dermatoscopic features.

▶ This is a great article describing the dermatoscopic features seen in basal cell carcinoma (BCC) to help in early detection. The goals of this retrospective study were to describe the morphologic variability of the dermatoscopic features in BCCs, define the distribution of different dermatoscopic features in specific types of BCC, and evaluate the accuracy and reliability of dermatoscopic diagnosis and the diagnostic significance of BCC-specific patterns. The dermatoscopic model for the diagnosis of pigmented BCC is based on the absence of a pigment network and presence of at least 1 positive feature, including ulceration, multiple blue/gray globules, leaf-like areas, large blue/gray ovoid nests, spoke wheel areas, and arborizing telengectasia. Three observers experienced in dermatoscopic evaluation scored the images without any knowledge of clinical or histopathological data. Observers were asked to make the diagnosis of BCC versus not BCC for each lesion, and then they reported the dermatoscopic features for the BCC lesions and categorized as classic and nonclassic BCC patterns. The most common pattern was the arborizing telengectasia. Classic BCC patterns were significantly more frequent in lightly pigmented and pigmented types of BCC than in nonpigmented and heavily pigmented BCCs. Melanocytic patterns were significantly more frequent in heavily pigmented BCCs as compared with the other variants. The frequency of melanocytic patterns significantly increased linearly with the increasing rate of the pigment in BCC. This study also showed consistency with reported dermatoscopic features for superficial BCC, which included short, fine telengectasia and multiple small ulcerations randomly located in a shiny white to red structureless background. The nonclassic BCC patterns can be used to further support the diagnosis of BCC, especially in early lesions that may lack the classic patterns.

S. B. Momin, DO

J. Q. Del Rosso, DO

Effect of tissue shrinkage on histological tumour-free margin after excision of basal cell carcinoma
Blasdale C, Charlton FG, Weatherhead SC, et al (Royal Victoria Infirmary, Newcastle upon Tyne, UK)
Br J Dermatol 162:607-610, 2010

Background.—Histology reports of skin tumour excisions frequently describe a histological margin significantly less than the planned surgical excision margin.

Objectives.—A novel method of marking visible tumour margin was devised. This allowed us to evaluate the accuracy of tumour detection and to compare tissue contraction of the clinically normal perilesional skin with that of tumour tissue following excision and fixation.

Methods.—Forty-four well-defined basal cell carcinomas were excised from 42 patients. The visible tumour edge was marked by scoring with a blade around its circumference prior to excision. This allowed comparison of visible and true histological tumour margin. The excision margin was carefully measured from the scored line and the tumour excised. After tissue fixation and processing the histological dimensions of tumour and perilesional margin skin were compared with the pre-excision measurements.

Results.—The tumour edge was accurately identified to within 1 mm in 67% of margins and was underestimated in only 4%. The whole specimen contracted by a mean of 14%. Skin containing tumour contracted by a mean of 11% but adjacent tumour-free skin in the same plane contracted by a mean of 19%. There was no significant effect of age and site on difference in percentage shrinkage between tumour and margin.

Conclusions.—We underestimated tumour extent at only 4% of margins. Tissue shrinkage was the most important factor affecting eventual histological margin. Our novel technique allowed us to demonstrate that this shrinkage is not uniform across the specimen, but is disproportionately high in the tumour-free margin. This suggests that previous estimates of margin shrinkage, based on whole-specimen contraction measurements, may have been erroneously low.

▶ The excision of malignant cutaneous neoplasms often engenders considerable concern regarding the generosity of the surgical margin. Whenever a margin seems less than that desired, it may be because either the subclinical extent of the process was not fully appreciated or the tissue has contracted upon extirpation.

Admittedly, varying degrees of concern may be manifested, either by the dermatopathologist or the surgeon. For example, some giants in dermatopathology used to extol, on occasion, that the correct margin is one cell—"it is in or it is out." However, by the same token, typical bread loaf sectioning allows for the inspection of less than 1% of the total margin. Furthermore, the inflammatory process must be considered to potentially eradicate tumor left behind, particularly with regard to basal cell carcinoma.

In this article, the authors suggest that on average a 19% loss of the clinical margin can be explained by tissue shrinkage occurring after extirpation. This is certainly not incompatible with a similar recent investigation that highlighted mean shrinkage of about 21% in length and 12% in width, but a range suggesting in some cases shrinkage might even be on the order of 38% to 42%.[1]

Clearly, the concept of shrinkage must always be considered when evaluating apparent discrepancies between the clinical and histologic record.

W. A. High, MD, JD, MEng

Reference

1. Kerns MJ, Darst MA, Olsen TG, Fenster M, Hall P, Grevey S. Shrinkage of cutaneous specimens: formalin or other factors involved? *J Cutan Pathol*. 2008;35: 1093-1096.

Eruptive Keratoacanthoma-Type Squamous Cell Carcinomas in Patients Taking Sorafenib for the Treatment of Solid Tumors
Smith KJ, Haley H, Hamza S, et al (Quest Diagnostics, Tucker, GA; Haley Dermatology, Fairhope, AL; Health Sciences Centre, Winnipeg, Manitoba, Canada)
Dermatol Surg 35:1766-1770, 2009

Background.—Protein kinases (PKs) are indispensable for most cellular processes, and deregulation of PKs can lead to activation of oncogenic and anti-apoptotic pathways and immune dysregulation.

Objective.—To report the development of keratoacanthoma (KA)-type squamous cell carcinomas (SCCs) in patients treated with the multikinase inhibitor sorafenib for the treatment of solid tumors, to present the possible mechanisms for induction of these SCCs, and to discuss the implications for discontinuation of therapy and possible cotherapies to decrease this side effect.

Participants.—Fifteen patients taking the multikinase inhibitor sorafenib for the treatment of solid tumors who developed multiple KA-type SCCs, which continued to develop while the patients were undergoing therapy but stopped with discontinuation of sorafenib.

Limitations.—This report is limited because it is a retrospective study that included only patients who developed multiple KA-type SCCs.

Conclusions.—Development of cutaneous SCCs appears to be a side effect limited to sorafenib, a multikinase inhibitor that inhibits not only multiple tyrosine kinases (TKs), but also the serine–threonine kinase Raf. The incidence of cutaneous SCCs does not appear greater with multikinase inhibitors that inhibit only TKs.

▶ Sorafenib is a multiple tyrosine kinase (TK) inhibitor with activity against platelet-derived growth factor receptor, c-kit, RET, and vascular endothelial growth factor receptor II and II signaling. Sorafenib also inhibits signaling through the serine-threonine kinase Raf pathway with inhibition of Raf-1 and Braf pathways. Actinic keratosis (AK) and keratoacanthoma (KA)-type squamous cell carcinomas (SCC) have been reported in patients taking sorafenib. This article further supports that patients on sorafenib are at high risk of developing skin cancers. Although the sample size is small, the study reported that all patients had at least 2 SCCs and the SCCs developed within 3 to 7 weeks of starting therapy with sorafenib 400 mg BID. Six of the 11 patients who were seen in follow-up from 6 weeks to 14 months continued to develop SCCs while on sorafenib. Two patients who were switched to sunitinib, a multiple kinase inhibitor with no activity against Raf signaling, stopped developing SCCs. Three patients who discontinued sorafenib also stopped developing SCCs. Reports of KAs and SCCs have also been described in patients receiving suramin for solid tumors, which reversibly inhibits protein-tyrosinase phosphatase and serine-threonine kinase (Ser/Thr kinase) Raf. This supports the conclusion that Raf inhibition may be related to the development of cutaneous SCCs. The article recommends that for treatment of solid tumors, it may be best to start/switch patients on medication that is only a tyrosine kinase inhibitor as long as the underlying tumor is equally responsive compared with a medication that inhibits tyrosine kinase and Raf pathway.

S. B. Momin, DO

J. Q. Del Rosso, DO

Preoperative skin and nail preparation of the foot: Comparison of the efficacy of 4 different methods in reducing bacterial load
Becerro de Bengoa Vallejo R, Losa Iglesias ME, Cervera LA, et al (Universidad Complutense de Madrid, Spain; Universidad Rey Juan Carlos, Madrid, Spain)
J Am Acad Dermatol 61:986-992, 2009

Background.—Orthopedic surgical procedures involving the foot and ankle are associated with high rates of infection. The optimal method of preparing the skin and nails for foot and ankle surgery remains unknown.

Objective.—This study was conducted to compare the efficacy of 4 different methods of skin and nail preparation of the foot using various antiseptic solutions.

Methods.—In this prospective, randomized study, 4 methods of skin and nail preparation were compared in terms of their efficacy in eliminating bacteria from the hallux nailfold and first web space of the normal foot in 28 healthy adult volunteers. Efficacy was determined by evaluating the difference in the total bacterial load before and after skin preparation. The foot-preparation solutions evaluated were 4% chlorhexidine gluconate, 70% isopropyl alcohol, and 7.5% to 10% povidone-iodine.

Results.—The addition of alcohol to povidone-iodine was found to increase the efficacy of the preparation method. The nailfold remained contaminated after any of the preoperative skin- and nail-preparation methods studied.

Limitations.—This study did not measure clinically relevant infections, and the results may not correlate with decreased rates of infection after surgery.

Conclusion.—Incorporation of alcohol and povidone-iodine into the preoperative skin- and nail-preparation process may help reduce the bacterial load. Every effort should be made to lower the risk of contamination from the nail.

▶ Toenail procedures are clean but not sterile and do not require hospital operating room sterility because of the native immunity of the nail unit in healthy people. Even so, nail surgical technique should attempt to provide optimal disinfection of the periungual and subungual tissue; however, the optimal method of preparing the skin around the nail before surgery is unclear. These authors compared the efficacy of 4 different methods of skin and nail preparation of the foot using various antiseptic solutions in a prospective randomized study, and then evaluated the efficacy in eliminating bacteria from the nailfold and first web space of the normal foot in 28 healthy subjects. Evaluation of the bacteria load before and after scrubbing was performed with foot preparation solutions: 4% chlorhexidine gluconate, 70% isopropyl alcohol, and 7.5% to 10% povidone-iodine. The results showed that the nailfold remained contaminated with all of the preparations, but the combination of alcohol and iodine was the most effective in reducing bacteria load. This article does not address the relevance of the bacteria found after the scrub and the potential pathogenicity of these organisms in relation to perioperative infection.

P. Rich, MD

Unit cost of Mohs and Dermasurgery Unit
Wanitphakdeedecha R, Nguyen TH, Chen TM (Mahidol Univ, Bangkok, Thailand; Univ of Texas — MD Anderson Cancer Ctr, Houston)
J Eur Acad Dermatol Venereol 24:445-448, 2010

Background.—Appropriate pricing for medical services of not-for-profit hospital is necessary. The prices should be fair to the public and should be high enough to cover the operative costs of the organization.

Objective.—The purpose of this study was to determine the cost and unit cost of medical services performed at the Mohs and Dermasurgery

Unit (MDU), Department of Dermatology, The University of Texas — MD Anderson Cancer Center, Houston, TX from the healthcare provider's perspective.

Methods.—MDU costs were retrieved from the Financial Department for fiscal year 2006. The patients' statistics were acquired from medical records for the same period. Unit cost calculation was based on the official method of hospital accounting.

Results.—The overall unit cost for each patient visit was $673.99 United States dollar (USD). The detailed unit cost of nurse visit, new patient visit, follow-up visit, consultation, Mohs and non-Mohs procedure were, respectively, $368.27, $580.09, $477.82, $585.52, $1,086.12 and $858.23 USD. With respect to a Mohs visit, the unit cost per lesion and unit cost per stage were $867.89 and $242.30 USD respectively.

Conclusions.—Results from this retrospective study provide information that may be used for pricing strategy and resource allocation by the administrative board of MDU.

▶ This is an interesting article that focuses on the financial aspect of Mohs and dermasurgery unit at a major US hospital (MD Anderson Cancer Center, Houston, Texas). Knowledge of cost data is beneficial both for practicing dermatologists and to dermatologists starting a new practice. Direct cost of the Mohs surgery unit was 80% ($1 503 564.27), and the indirect cost was 20% ($300 712.85). The unit cost of Mohs micrographic surgery was $1086.12 per patient. Awareness of cost can lead the surgeon to curtail cost while providing high-quality care.

S. Bhambri, DO

Dermoscopy of Kaposi's sarcoma: Areas exhibiting the multicoloured 'rainbow pattern'
Hu SC-S, Ke C-LK, Lee C-H, et al (Kaohsiung Med Univ Hosp, Taiwan)
J Eur Acad Dermatol Venereol 23:1128-1132, 2009

Background.—Kaposi's sarcoma is a vascular tumour characterized by a proliferation of spindle cells and endothelial cells to form closely arranged slit-like vascular spaces. Currently, the definitive diagnosis of Kaposi's sarcoma relies on histology. The dermoscopic features of Kaposi's sarcoma are not clearly defined in the scientific literature.

Objectives.—We seek to evaluate the dermoscopic features of Kaposi's sarcoma and compare them with other vascular tumours.

Methods.—One hundred forty-one lesions from seven patients with histologically proven Kaposi's sarcoma were evaluated using polarized light dermoscopy for the presence of various dermoscopic features. Twenty patients with other vascular tumours were also examined.

Results.—Dermoscopic examination revealed bluish-reddish coloration (84% of lesions), multicoloured areas showing various colours of the rainbow spectrum (36%), scaly surface (29%), and small brown globules (15%). The 'rainbow pattern' was found in six out of seven patients with Kaposi's sarcoma and was not observed in other vascular tumours. In addition, there was an absence of dermoscopic features specific for other vascular and non-vascular skin tumours, such as well-defined lacunae or structured vascular pattern, in most of the Kaposi's sarcoma lesions.

Conclusions.—The most frequent dermoscopic patterns in Kaposi's sarcoma were found to be bluish-reddish coloration, the 'rainbow pattern', and scaly surface. The rainbow pattern is a dermoscopic feature which has not been previously described. We propose that dermoscopy, as an adjunct to clinical examination, may enhance accuracy in the preoperative diagnosis of Kaposi's sarcoma.

▶ We commend the authors for taking the time to characterize Kaposi sarcoma (KS) via dermoscopy; yet, at the same time, I question the importance of dermoscopy in diagnosing KS. The dermoscope has become an important tool for increasing the accuracy of diagnosing pigmented and some nonpigmented lesions, and the clinical features seen by dermoscopy are already influencing us as to whether to biopsy or not biopsy. The question that I would have liked the authors of this article to answer is, "Can characterizing KS by dermoscopy change the need for histopathologic evaluation for all lesions resembling KS in the affected patient?"

In reviewing the results of this article, the lack of conformity of lesions of KS under the dermoscope was surprising. The most common characteristic of KS under the dermoscope is the bluish-reddish color (84% of 141 KS lesions), which most of the time can be assessed without the aid of a dermoscope. The characteristic rainbow pattern was seen only in 36% of KS lesions, suggesting that the dermoscope may not be actually helpful in diagnosing KS before histopathologic evaluation in most cases.

J. Levin, DO

Article Index

Chapter 1: Urticarial and Eczematous Disorders

5-Methoxypsoralen plus ultraviolet (UV) A is superior to medium-dose UVA1 in the treatment of severe atopic dermatitis: a randomized crossover trial — 49

A 6-month follow-up study of 1048 patients diagnosed with an occupational skin disease — 50

A randomized controlled trial in children with eczema: nurse practitioner vs. dermatologist — 51

A study of matrix metalloproteinase expression and activity in atopic dermatitis using a novel skin wash sampling assay for functional biomarker analysis — 53

Allergenic potential of *Arnica*-containing formulations in *Arnica*-allergic patients — 55

Association of the *toll-like receptor 2* A-16934T promoter polymorphism with severe atopic dermatitis — 56

Contact allergy to allergens of the TRUE-test (panels 1 and 2) has decreased modestly in the general population — 57

Delay in medical attention to hand eczema: a follow-up study — 58

Effects of nonsedative antihistamines on productivity of patients with pruritic skin diseases — 59

Fragrance contact allergic patients: strategies for use of cosmetic products and perceived impact on life situation — 60

Hairdressers with dermatitis should always be patch tested regardless of atopy status — 61

Histamine H_4 receptor antagonist ameliorates chronic allergic contact dermatitis induced by repeated challenge — 62

Impaired TLR-2 expression and TLR-2-mediated cytokine secretion in macrophages from patients with atopic dermatitis — 63

Increased expression of glucocorticoid receptor β in lymphocytes of patients with severe atopic dermatitis unresponsive to topical corticosteroid — 65

Low-dose cyclosporine A therapy increases the regulatory T cell population in patients with atopic dermatitis — 66

Maternal Asthma, its Control and Severity in Pregnancy, and the Incidence of Atopic Dermatitis and Allergic Rhinitis in the Offspring — 68

Methotrexate: a useful steroid-sparing agent in recalcitrant chronic urticaria — 69

Nickel allergy in patch-tested female hairdressers and assessment of nickel release from hairdressers' scissors and crochet hooks — 70

Patch testing in patients treated with systemic immunosuppression and cytokine inhibitors — 72

Patch testing with benzoyl peroxide: reaction profile and interpretation of positive patch test reactions — 73

Predicting risk for early infantile atopic dermatitis by hereditary and environmental factors — 74

Prevalence of nickel and cobalt allergy among female patients with dermatitis before and after Danish government regulation: A 23-year retrospective study   76

Shoe contact dermatitis from dimethyl fumarate: clinical manifestations, patch test results, chemical analysis, and source of exposure   77

Sites of dermatitis in a patch test population: hand dermatitis is associated with polysensitization   78

Staphylococcus aureus and hand eczema severity   79

Th17/Tc17 infiltration and associated cytokine gene expression in elicitation phase of allergic contact dermatitis   81

The additive value of patch testing with patients' own products at an occupational dermatology clinic   82

The association between hand eczema and nickel allergy has weakened among young women in the general population following the Danish nickel regulation: results from two cross-sectional studies   83

The effectiveness of levocetirizine and desloratadine in up to 4 times conventional doses in difficult-to-treat urticaria   84

The Histamine H_4 Receptor Mediates Inflammation and Pruritus in Th2-Dependent Dermal Inflammation   85

The importance of propolis in patch testing–a multicentre survey   86

Therapeutic Hotline: Treatment of prurigo nodularis and lichen simplex chronicus with gabapentin   87

Topical treatment of perianal eczema with tacrolimus $0 \cdot 1\%$ 88

Treatment with a barrier-strengthening moisturizing cream delays relapse of atopic dermatitis: a prospective and randomized controlled clinical trial   89

A pilot study of emollient therapy for the primary prevention of atopic dermatitis   91

Prednisolone vs. ciclosporin for severe adult eczema. An investigator-initiated double-blind placebo-controlled multicentre trial   92

Effectiveness of skin protection measures in prevention of occupational hand eczema: results of a prospective randomized controlled trial over a follow-up period of 1 year   93

Natural moisturizing factor components in the stratum corneum as biomarkers of filaggrin genotype: evaluation of minimally invasive methods   94

Treatment of episodes of hereditary angioedema with C1 inhibitor: serial assessment of observed abnormalities of the plasma bradykinin-forming pathway and fibrinolysis   96

Antibiotic use in infancy and symptoms of asthma, rhinoconjunctivitis, and eczema in children 6 and 7 years old: International Study of Asthma and Allergies in Childhood Phase III   98

Chapter 2: Psoriasis and Other Papulosquamous Disorders

Antinuclear antibodies associate with loss of response to antitumour necrosis factor-α therapy in psoriasis: a retrospective, observational study   101

Comparison of two etanercept regimens for treatment of psoriasis and psoriatic arthritis: PRESTA randomised double blind multicentre trial   102

Early skin biopsy is helpful for the diagnosis and management of neonatal and infantile erythrodermas — 104

Effective treatment of psoriasis with etanercept is linked to suppression of IL-17 signaling, not immediate response TNF genes — 105

Effectiveness and retention rates of methotrexate in psoriatic arthritis in comparison with methotrexate-treated patients with rheumatoid arthritis — 106

Effectiveness of adalimumab in treating patients with active psoriatic arthritis and predictors of good clinical responses for arthritis, skin and nail lesions — 108

Efficacy and safety of mycophenolate mofetil for lichen planopilaris — 110

Epidemiology and comorbidity of psoriasis in children — 111

Extent and Clinical Consequences of Antibody Formation Against Adalimumab in Patients With Plaque Psoriasis — 112

Guidelines of care for the management of psoriasis and psoriatic arthritis: Section 5. Guidelines of care for the treatment of psoriasis with phototherapy and photochemotherapy — 113

Inverse relationship between contact allergy and psoriasis: results from a patient- and a population-based study — 114

Narrowband ultraviolet B therapy in psoriasis: randomized double-blind comparison of high-dose and low-dose irradiation regimens — 116

No Increased Risk of Cancer after Coal Tar Treatment in Patients with Psoriasis or Eczema — 117

Once-Weekly Administration of Etanercept 50 mg Improves Patient-Reported Outcomes in Patients with Moderate-to-Severe Plaque Psoriasis — 118

Patients with moderate-to-severe psoriasis recapture clinical response during re-treatment with etanercept — 120

Predictive Factors of Eczema-Like Eruptions among Patients without Cutaneous Psoriasis Receiving Infliximab: A Cohort Study of 92 Patients — 121

Prurigo nodularis: systematic analysis of 58 histological criteria in 136 patients — 122

Randomized, double-blind, placebo-controlled evaluation of the efficacy of oral psoralen plus ultraviolet A for the treatment of plaque-type psoriasis using the Psoriasis Area Severity Index score (improvement of 75% or greater) at 12 weeks — 123

Recent Trends in Systemic Psoriasis Treatment Costs — 124

Paediatric psoriasis - narrowband UVB treatment — 125

Standards for genital protection in phototherapy units — 125

The Risk of Stroke in Patients with Psoriasis — 126

Treatment of scalp psoriasis with clobetasol-17 propionate 0.05% shampoo: a study on daily clinical practice — 127

Treatment of severe, recalcitrant, chronic plaque psoriasis with fumaric acid esters: a prospective study — 129

Ustekinumab improves health-related quality of life in patients with moderate-to-severe psoriasis: results from the PHOENIX 1 trial — 131

Chapter 3: Bacterial and Fungal Infections

A double-blind, randomized, placebo-controlled, dose-finding study of oral
pramiconazole in the treatment of pityriasis versicolor — 133

Antibody-mediated enhancement of community-acquired methicillin-resistant
Staphylococcus aureus infection — 134

Bacterial colonization of chronic leg ulcers: current results compared with data
5 years ago in a specialized dermatology department — 135

Borrelia in granuloma annulare, morphea and lichen sclerosus: a PCR-based study
and review of the literature — 137

Clinical Importance of Purulence in Methicillin-Resistant *Staphylococcus aureus*
Skin and Soft Tissue Infections — 138

Clinical Management of Rapidly Growing Mycobacterial Cutaneous Infections in
Patients after Mesotherapy — 140

Sexually Transmitted Infections and Prostate Cancer among Men in the U.S.
Military — 141

Deep cutaneous fungal infections in immunocompromised children — 142

Emergency Management of Pediatric Skin and Soft Tissue Infections in the
Community-associated Methicillin-resistant *Staphylococcus aureus* Era — 144

Epidemiology and Susceptibilities of Methicillin-Resistant *Staphylococcus aureus*
in Northeastern Ohio — 146

Erysipelas: Rare but Important Cause of Malar Rash — 147

Extensive Neonatal Dermatophytoses — 149

Frequency of detection of methicillin-resistant *Staphylococcus aureus* from
rectovaginal swabs in pregnant women — 150

Inpatient treatment patterns, outcomes, and costs of skin and skin structure
infections because of *Staphylococcus aureus* — 151

Nonrandom Distribution of *Pseudomonas aeruginosa* and *Staphylococcus aureus*
in Chronic Wounds — 153

Primary Skin Abscesses Are Mainly Caused by Panton-Valentine Leukocidin-
Positive *Staphylococcus aureus* Strains — 154

Onychomycosis Insensitive to Systemic Terbinafine and Azole Treatments Reveals
Non-Dermatophyte Moulds as Infectious Agents — 155

Recent Microbiological Shifts in Perianal Bacterial Dermatitis: *Staphylococcus
aureus* Predominance — 156

Skin and soft tissue infections caused by community-associated methicillin-
resistant *staphylococcus aureus* among children in China — 158

Subclinical onychomycosis is associated with tinea pedis — 159

Tinea Capitis: Predictive Value of Symptoms and Time to Cure With Griseofulvin
Treatment — 160

Transmission of Methicillin-Resistant *Staphylococcus aureus* to Household
Contacts — 162

Twelve hundred abscesses operatively drained: An antibiotic conundrum? — 164

Tinea capitis in early infancy treated with itraconazole: a pilot study   165

Using a Longitudinal Model to Estimate the Effect of Methicillin-resistant
Staphylococcus aureus Infection on Length of Stay in an Intensive Care Unit   166

Presence of Genes Encoding the Panton-Valentine Leukocidin Exotoxin is not the
Primary Determinant of Outcome in Patients with Complicated Skin and Skin
Structure Infections Due to Methicillin-Resistant *Staphylococcus aureus*: Results of
a Multinational Trial   167

Chapter 4: Viral Infections (Excluding HIV Infection)

Comparative Study on the Efficacy, Safety, and Acceptability of Imiquimod 5%
Cream versus Cryotherapy for Molluscum Contagiosum in Children   169

Cutaneotropic Human β-/γ-Papillomaviruses are Rarely Shared between Family
Members   170

Diversity of human papillomavirus types in periungual squamous cell carcinoma   171

Effectiveness of Pulsed Dye Laser in the Treatment of Recalcitrant Warts in Children   173

Herpes Zoster and Exposure to the Varicella Zoster Virus in an Era of Varicella
Vaccination   174

Parental Refusal of Varicella Vaccination and the Associated Risk of Varicella
Infection in Children   175

Risk Factors for Cutaneous Human Papillomavirus Seroreactivity among Patients
Undergoing Skin Cancer Screening in Florida   176

Chapter 5: Parasitic Infections, Bites, and Infestations

The Clinical Trials Supporting Benzyl Alcohol Lotion 5% (Ulesfia™): A Safe and
Effective Topical Treatment for Head Lice (Pediculosis Humanus Capitis)   179

Chapter 6: Disorders of the Pilosebaceous Apparatus

Trichothiodystrophy and fragile hair: the distinction between diagnostic signs and
diagnostic labels in childhood hair disease   181

Five-year experience in the treatment of alopecia areata with DPC   182

3 Cases of Dissecting Cellulitis of the Scalp Treated With Adalimumab: Control of
Inflammation Within Residual Structural Disease   184

Alefacept for Severe Alopecia Areata: A Randomized, Double-blind, Placebo-
Controlled Study   185

Antimicrobial Property of Lauric Acid Against *Propionibacterium Acnes*: Its
Therapeutic Potential for Inflammatory Acne Vulgaris   186

Psychiatric reactions to isotretinoin in patients with bipolar disorder   188

The Effect of Aminolevulinic Acid Photodynamic Therapy on Microcomedones
and Macrocomedones   189

Dermabrasion for Acne Scars During Treatment with Oral Isotretinoin   189

Hydroxychloroquine and lichen planopilaris: Efficacy and introduction of Lichen
Planopilaris Activity Index scoring system   191

Inter-observer agreement on acne severity based on facial photographs 192

Isotretinoin Is Not Associated With Inflammatory Bowel Disease: A Population-Based Case–Control Study 193

Practical Guidelines for Evaluation of Loose Anagen Hair Syndrome 194

Refractory Acne and 21-Hydroxylase Deficiency in a Selected Group of Female Patients 195

'Relaxers' damage hair: Evidence from amino acid analysis 196

Specific dermatologic features of the polycystic ovary syndrome and its association with biochemical markers of the metabolic syndrome and hyperandrogenism 197

Adapalene–benzoyl peroxide, a unique fixed-dose combination topical gel for the treatment of acne vulgaris: a transatlantic, randomized, double-blind, controlled study in 1670 patients 198

Depressive symptoms and suicidal ideation during isotretinoin treatment: a 12-week follow-up study of male Finnish military conscripts 200

Diet and acne 201

Infliximab therapy for patients with moderate to severe hidradenitis suppurativa: A randomized, double-blind, placebo-controlled crossover trial 202

Photodynamic therapy of acne vulgaris using 5-aminolevulinic acid 0.5% liposomal spray and intense pulsed light in combination with topical keratolytic agents 203

Effect of Smooth Pulsed Light at 400 to 700 and 870 to 1,200 nm for Acne Vulgaris in Asian Skin 205

Chapter 7: Photobiology

A 20-year analysis of previous and emerging allergens that elicit photoallergic contact dermatitis 207

Contact and photocontact sensitization in chronic actinic dermatitis: a changing picture 208

The relation between the amount of sunscreen applied and the sun protection factor in Asian skin 209

Topical aminolaevulinic acid- and aminolaevulinic acid methyl ester-based photodynamic therapy with red and violet light: influence of wavelength on pain and erythema 211

Treatment of Angiofibromas of Tuberous Sclerosis with 5-Aminolevulinic Acid Blue Light Photodynamic Therapy Followed by Immediate Pulsed Dye Laser 212

Chapter 8: Collagen Vascular and Related Disorders

A rare case of frontal linear scleroderma (*en coup de sabre*) with intra-oral and dental involvement 213

Scar classification in cutaneous lupus erythematosus: morphological description 214

Histopathology and immunohistochemistry of depigmented lesions in lupus erythematosus 216

Immune-mediated skin lesions in patients treated with anti-tumour necrosis factor alpha inhibitors 217

Interstitial Lung Disease in Classic and Skin-Predominant Dermatomyositis:
A Retrospective Study With Screening Recommendations 218

Lupus erythematosus tumidus is a separate subtype of cutaneous lupus
erythematosus 220

Rituximab in diffuse cutaneous systemic sclerosis: an open-label clinical and
histopathological study 221

Successful Immunosuppressive Treatment of Dermatomyositis: A Nailfold
Capillaroscopy Survey 222

The Localized Scleroderma Skin Severity Index and Physician Global Assessment
of Disease Activity: A Work in Progress Toward Development of Localized
Scleroderma Outcome Measures 224

B Cell-Targeted Therapies for Systemic Lupus Erythematosus: An Update on
Clinical Trial Data 225

A randomized controlled trial of R-salbutamol for topical treatment of discoid
lupus erythematosus 226

Treatment of Pediatric Localized Scleroderma: Results of a Survey of North
American Pediatric Rheumatologists 228

Chapter 9: Blistering Disorders

A population-based study of acute medical conditions associated with bullous
pemphigoid 231

Anti–Bullous Pemphigoid 180 and 230 Antibodies in a Sample of Unaffected
Subjects 232

Bacteremia in Stevens-Johnson Syndrome and Toxic Epidermal Necrolysis:
Epidemiology, Risk Factors, and Predictive Value of Skin Cultures 233

Common Wound Colonizers in Patients with Epidermolysis Bullosa 235

Pulsed intravenous cyclophosphamide and methylprednisolone therapy in
refractory pemphigus 236

Stevens-Johnson syndrome and toxic epidermal necrolysis in Asian children 238

Elevation of serum prolactin levels in patients with pemphigus vulgaris: A novel
finding with practical implications 239

Chapter 10: Drug Actions, Reactions, and Interactions

Cetuximab-induced cutaneous toxicity 241

Cutaneous adverse effects in patients treated with the multitargeted kinase
inhibitors sorafenib and sunitinib 242

Cutaneous Adverse Reactions to Psychotropic Drugs: Data From a Multicenter
Surveillance Program 243

Dermatologic Infections in Cancer Patients Treated With Epidermal Growth
Factor Receptor Inhibitor Therapy 245

Epicutaneous patch testing in drug hypersensitivity syndrome (DRESS) 247

High Prevalence of Potential Drug-Drug Interactions for Psoriasis Patients
Prescribed Methotrexate or Cyclosporine for Psoriasis: Associated Clinical and
Economic Outcomes in Real-World Practice — 248

Investigation of papulopustular eruptions caused by cetuximab treatment shows
altered differentiation markers and increases in inflammatory cytokines — 249

Management of cutaneous side-effects of cetuximab therapy in patients with
metastatic colorectal cancer — 251

The Safety and Efficacy of Pimecrolimus, 1%, Cream for the Treatment of
Netherton Syndrome: Results From an Exploratory Study — 252

Phenytoin-induced acute generalized exanthemous pustulosis — 253

Role of minor determinants of amoxicillin in the diagnosis of immediate allergic
reactions to amoxicillin — 255

Chapter 11: Drug Development and Promotion

A randomized, controlled comparative study of the wrinkle reduction benefits of
a cosmetic niacinamide/peptide/retinyl propionate product regimen vs.
a prescription 0·02% tretinoin product regimen — 257

Hydrosoluble medicated nail lacquers: *in vitro* drug permeation and corresponding
antimycotic activity — 259

Predicting Migraine Responsiveness to Botulinum Toxin Type A Injections — 260

Reduction in the appearance of facial hyperpigmentation after use of moisturizers
with a combination of topical niacinamide and N-acetyl glucosamine: results of
a randomized, double-blind, vehicle-controlled trial — 261

Chapter 12: Miscellaneous Topics in Clinical Dermatology

A double-blind, randomized study to assess the effectiveness of different
moisturizers in preventing dermatitis induced by hand washing to simulate
healthcare use — 265

A global survey of the role of ultraviolet radiation and hormonal influences in the
development of melasma — 266

Over-the-counter scar products for postsurgical patients: Disparities between
online advertised benefits and evidence regarding efficacy — 268

Acitretin for Severe Lichen Sclerosus of Male Genitalia: A Randomized, Placebo
Controlled Study — 269

Addiction to Indoor Tanning: Relation to Anxiety, Depression, and Substance Use — 270

Aggressive Fibromatosis in Children and Adolescents: The Italian Experience — 272

Chemical Matricectomy with 10% Sodium Hydroxide for the Treatment of
Ingrown Toenails in People with Diabetes — 273

Control of negative emotions and its implication for illness perception among
psoriasis and vitiligo patients — 274

Cutaneous Manifestations in Renal Transplant Recipients of Santiago, Chile — 275

Topical Calcipotriol for Preventive Treatment of Hypertrophic Scars:
A Randomized, Double-Blind, Placebo-Controlled Trial — 277

Early high-dose immunosuppression in Henoch–Schönlein nephrotic syndrome may improve outcome   278

Sun-Protection Behaviors Among African Americans   279

Pulsed High-Dose Corticosteroids Combined With Low-Dose Methotrexate Treatment in Patients With Refractory Generalized Extragenital Lichen Sclerosus   280

Gadolinium deposition in nephrogenic systemic fibrosis: An examination of tissue using synchrotron x-ray fluorescence spectroscopy   281

Growth rate of human fingernails and toenails in healthy American young adults   282

Haematological deficiencies in patients with recurrent aphthosis   284

Hypoglycemia in Children Taking Propranolol for the Treatment of Infantile Hemangioma   285

Lip and oral mucosal lesions in 100 renal transplant recipients   286

Malignancies associated with dermatomyositis and polymyositis in Taiwan: a nationwide population-based study   287

Measurement of skin texture through polarization imaging   289

Nail changes in kidney transplant recipients   290

Narrowband ultraviolet B course improves vitamin D balance in women in winter   291

Neonatal and Early Infantile Cutaneous Langerhans Cell Histiocytosis: Comparison of Self-regressive and Non–Self-regressive Forms   292

Pediatric Mastocytosis Is a Clonal Disease Associated with $D^{816}V$ and Other Activating c-*KIT* Mutations   294

Prevalence and distribution of solitary oral pigmented lesions: a prospective study   295

Recurrent erythema multiforme: Clinical characteristics, etiologic associations, and treatment in a series of 48 patients at Mayo Clinic, 2000 to 2007   296

School-Based Condom Education and Its Relations With Diagnoses of and Testing for Sexually Transmitted Infections Among Men in the United States   297

Seborrhoeic keratoses in patients with internal malignancies: a case–control study with prospective accrual of patients   298

Significant upregulation of antimicrobial peptides and proteins in lichen sclerosus   299

Studying Regression of Seborrheic Keratosis in Lichenoid Keratosis with Sequential Dermoscopy Imaging   300

The 5-D itch scale: a new measure of pruritus   301

The effects of topical isoflavones on postmenopausal skin: Double-blind and randomized clinical trial of efficacy   302

The impact of obesity on skin disease and epidermal permeability barrier status   304

Trends of skin diseases in organ-transplant recipients transplanted between 1966 and 2006: a cohort study with follow-up between 1994 and 2006   305

Truncal Pruritus of Unknown Origin May Be a Symptom of Diabetic Polyneuropathy   307

Visual and Pathologic Analyses of Keloid Growth Patterns   308

Chapter 13: Nonmelanoma Skin Cancer

A basal-cell-like compartment in head and neck squamous cell carcinomas
represents the invasive front of the tumor and is expressing MMP-9   313

A Randomized Trial of Tailored Skin Cancer Prevention Messages for Adults:
Project SCAPE   314

A study of mitochondrial DNA D-loop mutations and p53 status in nonmelanoma
skin cancer   316

Agreement on the Clinical Diagnosis and Management of Cutaneous Squamous
Neoplasms   317

Basal cell carcinoma with perineural invasion: reexcision perineural invasion?   318

Effect of dosing frequency on the safety and efficacy of imiquimod 5% cream for
treatment of actinic keratosis on the forearms and hands: a phase II, randomized
placebo-controlled trial   319

Topical 3.0% diclofenac in 2.5% hyaluronic acid gel induces regression of
cancerous transformation in actinic keratoses   321

Combination Therapy with Imiquimod, 5-Fluorouracil, and Tazarotene in the
Treatment of Extensive Radiation-Induced Bowen's Disease of the Hands   322

Current pathology work-up of extremity soft tissue sarcomas, evaluation of the
validity of different techniques   325

Dermatofibrosarcoma Protuberans of the Vulva: A Clinicopathologic and
Immunohistochemical Study of 13 Cases   326

Dermatofibrosarcoma protuberans: Recurrence is related to the adequacy of
surgical margins   328

Detection of Merkel cell polyomavirus DNA in Merkel cell carcinomas   329

Diagnostic imaging in Merkel cell carcinoma: Lessons to learn from 16 cases with
correlation of sonography, CT, MRI and PET   330

Diameter of Involved Nerves Predicts Outcomes in Cutaneous Squamous Cell
Carcinoma with Perineural Invasion: An Investigator-Blinded Retrospective
Cohort Study   331

Distinct progression-associated expression of tumor and stromal MMPs in HaCaT
skin SCCs correlates with onset of invasion   333

Epidermotropic Merkel cell carcinoma: A case series with histopathologic
examination   334

Expression of hedgehog signaling molecules in Merkel cell carcinoma   335

Expression of p53 and p16 in actinic keratosis, bowenoid actinic keratosis and
Bowen's disease   336

Factors Contributing to Incomplete Excision of Nonmelanoma Skin Cancer by
Australian General Practitioners   337

Follow-up of actinic keratoses after shave biopsy by *in-vivo* reflectance confocal
microscopy – a pilot study   339

Fractional Cryosurgery for Skin Cancer   340

Guidelines for practical use of MAL-PDT in non-melanoma skin cancer   340

Imiquimod 2.5% and 3.75% for the treatment of actinic keratoses: Results of two placebo-controlled studies of daily application to the face and balding scalp for two 2-week cycles
341

Imiquimod 2.5% and 3.75% for the treatment of actinic keratoses: Results of two placebo-controlled studies of daily application to the face and balding scalp for two 3-week cycles
343

Imiquimod Enhances IFN-γ Production and Effector Function of T Cells Infiltrating Human Squamous Cell Carcinomas of the Skin
345

Incidence and Clinical Predictors of a Subsequent Nonmelanoma Skin Cancer in Solid Organ Transplant Recipients With a First Nonmelanoma Skin Cancer: A Multicenter Cohort Study
346

Incidence Estimate of Nonmelanoma Skin Cancer in the United States, 2006
347

Incidence of Merkel cell carcinoma in renal transplant recipients
348

Mechanisms of Inactivation of *PTCH1* Gene in Nevoid Basal Cell Carcinoma Syndrome: Modification of the Two-Hit Hypothesis
350

Merkel cell polyomavirus DNA detection in lesional and nonlesional skin from patients with Merkel cell carcinoma or other skin diseases
351

Merkel Cell Polyomavirus: A Specific Marker for Merkel Cell Carcinoma in Histologically Similar Tumors
353

Organ transplant recipients and skin cancer: assessment of risk factors with focus on sun exposure
354

Patients With Merkel Cell Carcinoma Tumors ≤ 1.0 cm in Diameter Are Unlikely to Harbor Regional Lymph Node Metastasis
355

Prevalence of a History of Skin Cancer in 2007: Results of an Incidence-Based Model
357

Primary cutaneous myxoid spindle cell squamous cell carcinoma: a clinicopathologic study and review of the literature
359

Reflectance Confocal Microscopy for Noninvasive Monitoring of Therapy and Detection of Subclinical Actinic Keratoses
360

Single-Institution Series of Early-Stage Merkel Cell Carcinoma: Long-Term Outcomes in 95 Patients Managed with Surgery Alone
361

Skin cancer: preventive photodynamic therapy in patients with face and scalp cancerization. A randomized placebo-controlled study
362

Skin cancers associated with HIV infection and solid-organ transplantation among elderly adults
363

Sunburns, Sun Protection and Indoor Tanning Behaviors, and Attitudes Regarding Sun Protection Benefits and Tan Appeal among Parents of U.S. Adolescents—1998 Compared to 2004
365

Topical nicotinamide modulates cellular energy metabolism and provides broad-spectrum protection against ultraviolet radiation-induced immunosuppression in humans
366

Viral DNA detection and *RAS* mutations in actinic keratosis and nonmelanoma skin cancers
367

Photodynamic therapy with BF-200 ALA for the treatment of actinic keratosis: results of a prospective, randomized, double-blind, placebo-controlled phase III study
369

Chapter 14: Nevi and Melanoma

A Multimarker Prognostic Assay for Primary Cutaneous Melanoma 371

Accuracy of teledermatology for pigmented neoplasms 372

Characteristics Associated With Early and Late Melanoma Metastases 374

Classifying ambiguous melanocytic lesions with FISH and correlation with clinical long-term follow up 375

Clinical responses observed with imatinib or sorafenib in melanoma patients expressing mutations in *KIT* 376

Dermoscopy of pigmented lesions on mucocutaneous junction and mucous membrane 377

Discordance in the histopathologic diagnosis of melanoma at a melanoma referral center 378

Disparity in Melanoma: A Trend Analysis of Melanoma Incidence and Stage at Diagnosis Among Whites, Hispanics, and Blacks in Florida 380

Efficacy of Skin Self-Examination Practices for Early Melanoma Detection 381

Factors Associated with False-Negative Sentinel Lymph Node Biopsy in Melanoma Patients 382

Histological regression in primary melanoma: not a predictor of sentinel lymph node metastasis in a cohort of 397 patients 384

Increased Melanoma Risk in Parkinson Disease: A Prospective Clinicopathological Study 385

Is There a Benefit to Sentinel Lymph Node Biopsy in Patients With T4 Melanoma? 386

Large congenital melanocytic nevi and neurocutaneous melanocytosis: One pediatric center's experience 387

Low rates of clinical recurrence after biopsy of benign to moderately dysplastic melanocytic nevi 388

Melanoma and Melanocytic Tumors of Uncertain Malignant Potential in Children, Adolescents and Young Adults—The Stanford Experience 1995–2008 390

Melanoma Thickness Trends in the United States, 1988–2006 391

Non-Steroidal Anti-Inflammatory Drugs and Melanoma Risk: Large Dutch Population-Based Case–Control Study 392

Plantar Melanoma: Is the Prognosis Always Bad? 393

Predictors of Occult Nodal Metastasis in Patients With Thin Melanoma 394

Predictors of sentinel lymph node metastasis in melanoma 396

Prevalence and distribution of melanocytic naevi on the scalp: a prospective study 397

Prognostic Significance of a Positive Nonsentinel Lymph Node in Cutaneous Melanoma 398

Reflectance Confocal Microscopy and Features of Melanocytic Lesions: An Internet-Based Study of the Reproducibility of Terminology 400

Reflectance confocal microscopy of facial lentigo maligna and lentigo maligna melanoma: a preliminary study — 401

Sentinel Lymph Node Biopsy in Pediatric and Adolescent Cutaneous Melanoma Patients — 402

Sentinel Lymph Node Dissection in Primary Melanoma Reduces Subsequent Regional Lymph Node Metastasis as Well as Distant Metastasis After Nodal Involvement — 403

Serum 25-Hydroxyvitamin D_3 Levels Are Associated With Breslow Thickness at Presentation and Survival From Melanoma — 404

Should All Patients With Melanoma Between 1 and 2 mm Breslow Thickness Undergo Sentinel Lymph Node Biopsy? — 405

Small and Medium-Sized Congenital Nevi in Children: A Comparison of the Costs of Excision and Long-Term Follow-Up — 407

Staged Excision of Lentigo Maligna and Lentigo Maligna Melanoma: A 10-Year Experience — 408

Sun and Solarium Exposure and Melanoma Risk: Effects of Age, Pigmentary Characteristics, and Nevi — 410

The Importance of Attached Nail Plate Epithelium in the Diagnosis of Nail Apparatus Melanoma — 411

Targeted High-Resolution Ultrasound Is Not an Effective Substitute for Sentinel Lymph Node Biopsy in Patients With Primary Cutaneous Melanoma — 412

The impact of dermoscopy on the management of pigmented lesions in everyday clinical practice of general dermatologists: a prospective study — 413

The Impact of Partial Biopsy on Histopathologic Diagnosis of Cutaneous Melanoma: Experience of an Australian Tertiary Referral Service — 414

The Nodal Location of Metastases in Melanoma Sentinel Lymph Nodes — 416

The Role of Circumstances of Diagnosis and Access to Dermatological Care in Early Diagnosis of Cutaneous Melanoma: A Population-Based Study in France — 418

The Use of High-Resolution Ultrasonography for Preoperative Detection of Metastases in Sentinel Lymph Nodes of Patients with Cutaneous Melanoma — 419

Thick Melanoma: Prognostic Value of Positive Sentinel Nodes — 421

Chapter 15: Lymphoproliferative Disorders

Drug-associated reversible granulomatous T cell dyscrasia: a distinct subset of the interstitial granulomatous drug reaction — 423

Paucity of intraepidermal FoxP3-positive T cells in cutaneous T-cell lymphoma in contrast with spongiotic and lichenoid dermatitis — 424

T-cell receptor γ gene rearrangement in cutaneous T-cell lymphoma: comparative study of polymerase chain reaction with denaturing gradient gel electrophoresis and GeneScan analysis — 426

Cutaneous type adult T-cell leukemia/lymphoma is a characteristic subtype and includes erythema/papule and nodule/tumor subgroups — 427

Chapter 16: Miscellaneous Topics in Cosmetic and Laser Surgery

A Comparative Study of Topical 5-Aminolevulinic Acid Incubation Times in
Photodynamic Therapy with Intense Pulsed Light for the Treatment of
Inflammatory Acne — 429

A Five-Patient Satisfaction Pilot Study of Calcium Hydroxylapatite Injection for
Treatment of Aging Hands — 430

A Retrospective Review of Calcium Hydroxylapatite for Correction of Volume
Loss in the Infraorbital Region — 431

A Safety and Feasibility Study of a Novel Radiofrequency-Assisted Liposuction
Technique — 432

Advanced Laser Techniques for Filler-Induced Complications — 433

Ageing appearance in China: biophysical profile of facial skin and its relationship
to perceived age — 434

Anatomic Concepts for Brow Lift Procedures — 436

Changes in Eyebrow Position and Shape with Aging — 437

Clinical Experience in the Treatment of Different Vascular Lesions Using
a Neodymium-Doped Yttrium Aluminum Garnet Laser — 438

Enhanced Efficacy of Photodynamic Therapy with Methyl 5-Aminolevulinic Acid
in Recalcitrant Periungual Warts After Ablative Carbon Dioxide Fractional Laser:
A Pilot Study — 439

Low-Fluence Q-Switched Neodymium-Doped Yttrium Aluminum Garnet
(1,064 nm) Laser for the Treatment of Facial Melasma in Asians — 440

Needle Preference in Patients Receiving Cosmetic Botulinum Toxin Type A — 441

Outcomes of Childhood Hemangiomas Treated with the Pulsed-Dye Laser with
Dynamic Cooling: A Retrospective Chart Analysis — 442

Perioral Wrinkles: Histologic Differences Between Men and Women — 443

Photorejuvenation with Topical Methyl Aminolevulinate and Red Light:
A Randomized, Prospective, Clinical, Histopathologic, and Morphometric Study — 444

Pulsed Dye Laser in the Treatment of Nail Psoriasis — 445

Randomized, Placebo-Controlled Study of a New Botulinum Toxin Type A for
Treatment of Glabellar Lines: Efficacy and Safety — 445

Reduced Pain with Use of Proprietary Hyaluronic Acid with Lidocaine for
Correction of Nasolabial Folds: A Patient-Blinded, Prospective, Randomized
Controlled Trial — 447

Skin Tightening Effect Using Fractional Laser Treatment: I. A Randomized Half-
Side Pilot Study on Faces of Patients with Acne — 448

Successful Treatment of Atrophic Postoperative and Traumatic Scarring With
Carbon Dioxide Ablative Fractional Resurfacing: Quantitative Volumetric Scar
Improvement — 449

The Efficacy and Safety of 10,600-nm Carbon Dioxide Fractional Laser for Acne
Scars in Asian Patients — 450

The Spectrum of Adverse Reactions After Treatment with Injectable Fillers in the
Glabellar Region: Results from the Injectable Filler Safety Study — 451

Treatment of trichostasis spinulosa with a 755-nm long-pulsed alexandrite laser   453

Long-term follow-up of photodynamic therapy with a self-adhesive
5-aminolaevulinic acid patch: 12 months data   453

Topical photodynamic therapy is immunosuppressive in humans   455

Ultrasound tightening of facial and neck skin: A rater-blinded prospective cohort
study   456

Chapter 17: Miscellaneous Topics in Dermatologic Surgery and Cutaneous Oncology

A Direct Comparison of Visual Inspection, Curettage, and Epiluminescence
Microscopy in Determining Tumor Extent Before the Initial Margins are
Determined for Mohs Micrographic Surgery   459

Academic Productivity and Affiliation of Dermatologic Surgeons   460

Evaluation of a New Wound Closure Device for Linear Surgical Incisions: 3M
Steri-Strip S Surgical Skin Closure versus Subcuticular Closure   461

Improved diagnosis and treatment of soft tissue sarcoma patients after
implementation of national guidelines: A population-based study   463

Lack of Complications in Skin Surgery of Patients Receiving Clopidogrel as
Compared with Patients Taking Aspirin, Warfarin, and Controls   465

Nail Matrix Phenolization for Treatment of Ingrowing Nail: Technique Report and
Recurrence Rate of 267 Surgeries   466

The accuracy of the sentinel lymph node concept in early stage squamous cell
vulvar carcinoma   467

The Effect of Calcium Channel Blockers on Smoking-Induced Skin Flap Necrosis   469

The Influence of Surgical Excision Margins on Keloid Prognosis   470

Treatment of Earlobe Keloids by Extralesional Excision Combined with
Preoperative and Postoperative "Sandwich" Radiotherapy   471

Wound edge biopsy sites in chronic wounds heal rapidly and do not result in
delayed overall healing of the wounds   472

Dermatoscopy of basal cell carcinoma: Morphologic variability of global and local
features and accuracy of diagnosis   473

Effect of tissue shrinkage on histological tumour-free margin after excision of basal
cell carcinoma   475

Eruptive Keratoacanthoma-Type Squamous Cell Carcinomas in Patients Taking
Sorafenib for the Treatment of Solid Tumors   476

Preoperative skin and nail preparation of the foot: Comparison of the efficacy of
4 different methods in reducing bacterial load   477

Unit cost of Mohs and Dermasurgery Unit   478

Dermoscopy of Kaposi's sarcoma: Areas exhibiting the multicoloured 'rainbow
pattern'   479

Author Index

A

Abdelaziz AM, 290
Abdulla FR, 125
Aben KKH, 117
Abramovits W, 341
Adami H-O, 410
Adams B, 125
Ahlgrimm-Siess V, 339, 401
Airola K, 333
Akaishi S, 308
Aksoy B, 438
Al-Doukhi A, 169
Al-Farag S, 169
Al-Mutairi N, 169
Al Quran H, 430
Al-Refu K, 214
Alam M, 456
Alanko K, 50
Allen G, 380
Allen MH, 101
Altamura D, 473
Amler S, 220
Andersen KE, 78
Andersen RF, 278
anh Duong T, 233
Apalla Z, 269, 362
Arellano I, 266
Argenziano G, 473
Ariza A, 255
Arkachaisri T, 224
Augustin M, 111
Aziz N, 253

B

Bachmann F, 451
Bae I-G, 167
Bagatin E, 189
Bagazgoitia L, 336
Bajetta E, 361
Balato A, 81
Bandi P, 365
Bangsgaard N, 79, 114
Bargo PR, 289
Barnea Y, 471
Barnett AG, 166
Barry NG, 469
Bashir SJ, 208
Bassiouny DA, 182
Bassoli S, 400
Batra R, 166
Battistella M, 292

Baudraz-Rosselet F, 155
Baumann L, 445
Baumeister T, 93
Baumert J, 393
Beauchesne M-F, 68
Becerro de Bengoa
  Vallejo R, 477
Bechert CJ, 318
Beer KR, 343
Behrendt M, 162
Belda W Jr, 466
Bergman W, 413
Berk DR, 390
Berman B, 341
Berneburg M, 266
Bernstein CN, 193
Berry TM, 91
Bertoni JM , 385
Beswick S, 404
Beyer V, 124
Beylot C , 192
Bhogal B, 236
Bierhoff E, 321
Binder B, 165
Bisogno G, 272
Bjarnsholt T, 153
Bjerring P, 203
Blanc V, 154
Blasdale C, 475
Blugerman G, 432
Blumer JL, 160
Bodemer C, 104, 294
Boezeman J, 116
Bogart MM, 260
Bohnenberger K, 403
Bosbous MW, 408
Boschiero L, 346
Boucher KM, 388
Bourdon-Lanoy E, 104
Bovenschen HJ, 127
Bowe WP, 201
Braga JC, 317
Brandling-Bennett HA, 235
Brandt C, 66
Brandt F, 445
Brauer JA, 374
Bregnhøj A, 70
Breneman C, 125
Brightman L, 442, 449
Brooks DR, 381
Brown M, 281
Brown PA, 91
Brunner M, 335
Bruscino N, 295
Buer J, 135

Buettner PG, 403
Burton A, 405

C

Cacciapuoti S, 189
Cadili A, 396
Calkoen F, 94
Calvino F, 284
Cambau E, 140
Campbell RM, 447
Campos M, 125
Cantatore-Francis JL, 194
Caputo V, 195
Carlsen BC, 76, 78
Carroccio A, 284
Carson P, 472
Casparie MK, 392
Cassuto D, 433
Celio L, 361
Cencelj S, 251
Cervera LA, 477
Chang SE, 242
Chapas AM, 442, 449
Charlton FG, 475
Chen P-C, 74
Chen TM, 478
Chen YJ, 287
Cheng S, 181
Chetoni P, 259
Chew A-L, 208
Chiang C, 191
Chiang T-L, 74
Cho BK, 110, 191
Cho SB, 450
Chovarda E, 362
Christensen E, 340
Chwalek J, 110
Cieścińska C, 274
Cinelli C, 334
Civas E, 438
Cohen DE, 207
Cokkinides VE, 365
Comfere NI, 232
Compilato D, 284
Comrov E, 160
Cornillet-Lefebvre P, 426
Corral I, 279
Costagliola D, 363
Coughlin JA, 141
Cowden JM, 85
Cowen PSJ, 319
Crawford SE, 138
Creech CB, 150

Criscione VD, 391
Cruz-Inigo AE, 423
Cuadrado A, 407
Cuevas J, 336
Curiale S, 195

D

Dabbs K, 396
Dadras SS, 390
D'Agostino M, 334
Dainichi T, 448
Dakic B, 313
Damian DL, 455
Danoff-Burg S, 270
Darling MI, 129
David MZ, 138
Davis MDP, 296
de Berker D, 181
Decarie J-C, 387
de Fijter JW, 305
De Giorgi V, 295, 397
de Leeuw J, 203
del Giudice P, 154
Delorme T, 146
Dengel LT, 355
Dennis LK, 141
de Prost N, 233
Dereure O, 351
de Rougemont A, 154
de Sa Earp AP, 430
Desai N, 156
De Santis G, 433
de Souza EM, 216
De Vita V, 189
Díaz C, 275
Di Chiacchio N, 466
Di Chiacchio NG, 466
Dirschka T, 321
Dodge B, 297
Dommasch ED, 126
Donahue JG, 174
Dong Q, 350
dos Santos Guadanhim LR, 189
Dowling JP, 414
Drecoll U, 354
Driessen RJB, 112
Drukker N, 51
Duncavage EJ, 353
Dunford PJ, 85
Durbec F, 418
Durlach A, 426

Dusza SW, 317
Dzwierzynski WW, 408

E

Eberle JY, 419
Edelbroek JRJ, 305
Edelweiss M, 326
Ehsani AH, 453
Eilers RE Jr, 245
Eimpunth S, 440
Elashoff D, 394
Elenitsas R, 331
Elman S, 301
Elmets CA, 113
Elsawy EM, 290
El-Zawahry BM, 182
Endrizzi B, 212
Engels EA, 363
Engkilde K, 114
Erdmann R, 451
Eren C, 273
Esmailzadeh A, 121
Exarchou SA, 217

F

Fabbrocini G, 189
Faergemann J, 133
Fallahzadeh MK, 239
Fang J-Y, 186
Farhi D, 121
Faries MB, 394
Fazli M, 153
Feldman BM, 228
Fernández J, 255
Filz D, 298
Fink A, 298
Fink BF, 469
Fiorella S, 195
Fishelevich R, 81
Fleming K, 231
Florell SR, 388
Foliaki S , 98
Fölster-Holst R, 92
Fonia A, 101
Foulongne V, 351
Fraitag S, 292
França AFEC, 216
Frieden IJ, 285
Frommelt PC, 285
Frowen K, 82

Fu JJJ, 257
Fuentes-Duculan J, 105
Furuya K, 62

G

Gabriel V, 301
Gaifullina R, 280
Gaiser T, 375
Gajdos C, 386
Gambichler T, 171, 299
Gandhi M, 245
Garcia JA, 437
Gargiullo PM, 174
Gattu S, 123
Gebauer K, 319
Gelfand JM, 126
Geller AC, 381
Gencoglan G, 87
Geng W, 158
Ghaferi AA, 398
Gibson LE, 232
Giménez-Arnau A, 77
Giuliano AR, 176
Glaeske G, 111
Glanz JM, 175
Glanz K, 314
Glikman D, 138
Godwin H, 53
Goeldel AL, 426
Göker M, 170
Gollnick HPM , 198
Gonçalo M, 247
Gonçalves JCA, 340
Gonzalez T, 202
Goodfield M, 214, 226
Goodson AG, 388
Görkemli H, 197
Gottschling M, 170
Goupille P, 108
Grande DJ, 459
Granel-Brocard F, 418
Grant A, 202
Grattan CEH, 69
Graves N, 166
Graw KS, 355
Grazzini M, 397
Green A, 53
Griffith KA, 386
Griffiths AP, 316
Grill JP, 372
Grohmann R, 243
Gronchi A, 272

Guérin A, 248
Guardiano RA, 459
Güleç AT, 286
Guida B, 304
Gumedze F, 196
Gunduz K, 87
Gunn DA, 434

H

Haberal M, 286
Hadad E, 465
Hägg PM, 65
Haidar MA, 302
Hald M, 58
Haley H, 476
Halliday GM, 366
Hamann L, 56
Hamilton AL, 376
Hamilton-Dutoit SJ, 416
Hammerman S, 472
Hamza S, 476
Han C, 131
Han EC, 429
Han SS, 249
Handolias D, 376
Hanke CW, 343, 460
Hanley A, 359
Hansen C, 337
Hansen M, 337
Harper JI, 53
Harris AR, 347
Hartmann V, 451
Haslund P, 79
Hawk JLM, 208
Heath C, 156
Herbenick D, 297
Hermine O, 294
Hernando AB, 407
Heuvel ST, 328
Hevia O, 431
Higgins GC, 228
High WA, 281
Hijnen D, 345
Hillebrand GG, 257
Hiremagalore RN, 173
Holland KE, 285
Holzer G, 49
Homa K, 461
Hong J, 123
Honig PJ, 252
Hook KP, 212
Höök-Nikanne J, 200
Hou N, 282

Howman-Giles R, 402
Hu S, 380
Hu SC-S, 479
Huang SJ, 345
Huang YL, 287
Hubbard R, 231
Hunter S, 188
Hurskainen T, 65
Hyakusoku H, 308
Hynan LS, 301

I

Iani V, 211
Iannacone MR, 176
Inanir I, 87
Ingen-Housz-Oro S, 233
Ioannides D, 269
Issa MCA, 444

J

Jacobs AA, 322
Jacobs XE, 277
Jafarian F, 142
Jansen-Landheer
    MLEA, 463
Jarløv JO, 79
Jaszewska J, 274
Jedrzejczak T, 467
Jemec GBE, 226
Jespersen B, 278
Jocher A, 55
Johansen JD, 60, 76
Johnson TM, 398
Jolanki R, 50
Joncas V, 142
Joosse A, 392
Joseph K, 96
Joshi A, 149
Joshi SS, 201
Juarranz Á, 336
Juzeniene A, 211

K

Kaczvinsky JR, 261
Kamali-Sarvestani E, 239
Kammeyer A, 94
Kanellou P, 367
Kang JM, 450
Kao MC, 186

Kaplan AP, 96
Karincaoğlu Y, 445
Kashani-Sabet M, 371, 378
Kato T, 205
Kautiainen H, 291
Kawaguchi A, 448
Kawana S, 205
Ke C-LK, 479
Kerrigan CL, 461
Kezic S, 94
Khella A, 182
Khumalo NP, 196
Kieke BA, 174
Kim BJ, 439
Kim CC, 260
Kim MN, 439
Kim SM, 209
Kimball AB, 261, 460
King CM, 86
Kirketerp-Møller K, 153
Kirkham B, 102
Kiss M, 329
Kitaba S, 59
Kittler H, 49
Kleinpenning MM, 116
Kluger N, 351
Knize DM, 436
Koc E, 438
Koga H, 377
Koh MJ-A, 238
Köhler A, 170
Körber A, 135
Kohoutek M, 241
Koljonen V, 348
Koller S, 339
Kollias N, 289
Koomen ER, 392
Koop WA, 443
Korman NJ, 113
Kossakowska MM, 274
Kowalewska M, 467
Koyuncu E, 445
Krajnik G, 298
Kralimarkova T, 84
Kramer E, 465
Kreider ME, 218
Kreuter A, 171, 280
Krijnen P, 463
Kroon S, 340
Krueger-Corcoran D, 360
Kukko H, 348
Kukutsch NA, 413
Kulle C, 313
Kunte C, 393, 419
Kütting B, 93
Kutzner H, 375

L

Labuz E, 390
Lamant L, 384
Landrine H, 279
Langan SM, 231
Lange-Asschenfeldt B, 243
Lange-Asschenfeldt C, 243
Lanoy E, 363
Lashkarizadeh H, 239
Lauwers-Cances V, 384
Lazaridou E, 269
Le B-M, 353
Lebwohl M, 131
Leclerc-Mercier S, 104
Lecluse LLA, 112
Lederle FA, 372
Lederle W, 333
Lee C-H, 479
Lee JL, 242
Lee M, 249
Lee SJ, 450
Lee WJ, 242
Lee YW, 209
Leiter U, 403
Lessmann H, 73
Lewis PD, 316
Li J, 261
Li SC, 228
Lie E, 106
Lin J, 377
Lin MW, 287
Linneberg A, 57, 83
Litzner B, 150
Longobardi T, 193
Looney RJ, 225
Lorch Dauk KC, 160
Losa Iglesias ME, 477
Lovett A, 387
Lund E, 410
Lurati M, 155
Lutat C, 63
Lysdal SH, 60

M

Maari C, 387
Macri V, 222
Magid DJ, 175
Magro CM, 423
Mahmoud KM, 290
Mälkönen T, 50
Malo J-L, 68
Malpica A, 326
Manger B, 108

Marangoni O, 433
Marcoux D, 142
Markatseli TE, 217
Marmur ES, 430
Martel M-J, 68
Martin N, 456
Martin RCG, 382, 405
Marton JP, 151
Massone C, 401
Matros E, 437
Matthews YJ, 455
Mayes AE, 434
Mays MP, 405
McCalmont TH, 411
McClure DL, 175
Mc Fadden JP, 61
McFadden JP, 72
McKinnon BC, 141
McMichael A, 185
McShane P, 265
Meazza C, 272
Meinking TL, 179
Meningaud J-P, 140
Menné T, 57, 78, 83
Menon K, 185
Menter A, 113
Menzies SW, 473
Menzin J, 151
Mercader P, 77
Meririnne E, 200
Mertz KD, 137
Metkar A, 149
Metze D, 122
Meuth AM, 220
Meyers JL, 151
Michael KM, 176
Mikolajewska P, 211
Miller C, 268
Miller Whalen F, 331
Milting K, 70
Ming ME, 252
Mistry RD, 144
Miyata T, 427
Modi G, 322
Mollema FPN, 162
Moncrieff M, 412
Monheit GD, 447
Montgomery MO, 202
Monti D, 259
Moraes AB, 302
Morel KD, 235
Morganroth PA, 218, 268
Mornchan R, 440
Mosher CE, 270
Muller-Mang C, 330
Murota H, 59

Murphy GF, 345
Murray PG, 434

N

Nakatsuji T, 186
Naldi L, 346
Navarini AA, 184
Neuburg M, 408
Neugent H, 447
Newton-Bishop JA, 404
Ng JC, 414
Nguyen TH, 478
Niebuhr M, 63
Nigra T, 253
Nino M, 304
Nist G, 55
Nohlgård C, 89
Noormohammadpoor P, 453
Nosrati M, 371
Novotny C, 330
Nugent Z, 193
Nyberg F, 89
Nyengaard JR, 416

O

O'Connell RL, 61
O'Connor K, 147
Ockenfels H-M, 73
Ocvirk J, 251
Ogawa R, 308
Oh BH, 209
Oh D-Y, 56
Oh SH, 429
Okawa J, 218
Oldenhof UTH, 117
Omura M, 62
Oostindiër MJ, 463
Oram Y, 445
Orengo IF, 322
Orlow SJ, 194
Ormerod AD, 120
Ortiz M, 275
Ortonne J-P, 102, 120
Ortonne JP, 266
Özdemir M, 197
Özdemir S, 197

P

Paauw D, 147
Pace A, 213

Pace C, 213
Paes EC, 443
Palatsi R, 65
Palmérini F, 294
Palmedo G, 375
Pammer J, 335
Pan S, 350
Panuncialman J, 472
Papp K, 131
Park GH, 249
Parmet Y, 380
Patel JD, 245
Pather S, 133
Paul MD, 432
Pavlovic V, 66
Pellacani G, 400
Peloschek P, 330
Perez A, 69
Perrino NR, 304
Pfister H, 171
Pflugfelder A, 321
Piñeiro-Maceira J, 444
Pichon LC, 279
Pier GB, 134
Pink AE, 101
Platania M, 361
Pleass RD, 129
Pollitt RA, 381
Popov TA, 84
Popp G, 453
Powell A-M, 236
Pras E, 328
Price KM, 441
Prior SL, 316
Pritchard SA, 470

R

Radbruch A, 66
Radny P, 369
Radtke MA, 111
Radziszewski J, 467
Rajpara S, 86
Raleigh P, 257
Randerson-Moor J, 404
Ranville JF, 281
Reece M, 297
Regnier S, 140
Rehn LMH, 200
Reich K, 118
Riber-Hansen R, 416
Riccieri V, 222
Richards KA, 173
Richardus JH, 162
Richtig E, 165, 339

Rinker B, 469
Rizzo C, 442
Roelofzen JHJ, 117
Roewert-Huber J, 360
Rogers HW, 347
Roldán FA, 407
Rose S, 146
Ross AS, 331
Ross MI, 382
Rubak S, 278
Ruben BS, 411
Ruffieux C, 155
Ruzicka T, 88
Ryu DJ, 429

S

Saccomani L, 259
Sagebiel RW, 378
Sah D, 110, 191
Saha M, 236
Salemi R, 376
Salsench E, 300
Sandoval M, 275
Sanki A, 412
Santiago F, 247
Sasaki H, 307
Sastrowijoto PSH, 421
Saurat J-H, 248
Schäkel K, 92
Schaffer CB, 188
Schaffer LC, 188
Schauber J, 88
Schavelzon D, 432
Schmid EN, 135
Schmid M, 137
Schmidt M, 393
Schmitt J, 92
Schmitt V, 220
Schoenfeld ER, 314
Schuh T, 419
Schumann RR, 56
Schuttelaar MLA, 51
Scoggins CR, 382
Scolyer RA, 402
Scope A, 401
Scott HF, 144
Sebastian M, 369
Segaert S, 118
Seike M, 62
Senita J, 146
Serrano P, 300
Sestini S, 295, 397
Sethuraman G, 173
Shah N, 470

Shalita AR, 201
Shaw HM, 402
Shin DB, 126
Shoo BA, 378
Shumack S, 319
Sigel S, 63
Silverberg NB, 156
Silvestre JF, 77
Simpson EL, 91
Sivanesan SP, 123
Sivapirabu G, 366
Skrygan M, 299
Slining MM, 282
Slodownik D, 82
Smith KJ, 476
Smith V, 221
Smits T, 116
Soares Júnior JM, 302
Socrier Y, 384
Soter NA, 207
Sotiriou E, 362
Spandidos DA, 367
Spuls PI, 112
Ständer S, 122
Staevska M, 84
Stahl S, 471
Steffen A, 314
Stern JB, 318
Stern RS, 357
Sterry W, 102
Sterz CM, 313
Stockfleth E, 343, 354, 453
Stoffan A, 164
Stokes JB, 355
Stone J, 181, 196
Strober BE, 185
Stryjewski ME, 167
Suárez-Fariñas M, 105
Sun L-S, 350
Suurmeijer A, 328
Swain S, 414
Swanson N, 341, 445
Szabó K, 329
Szeimies R-M, 369, 453

T

Tachihara R, 205
Takata M, 377
Talbot TR, 150
Tan KT, 470
Tani M, 59
Tatlican S, 273
Taïeb A, 120
Tay Y-K, 238

Teepen HJLJM, 443
Teillac DH, 292
Terhorst D, 354
Terushkin V, 317
Tessari G, 346
Tholanikunnel TE, 96
Thurnher D, 335
Thyssen JP, 57, 70, 76, 83, 114
Tierney EP, 460
Tigges C, 280, 299
Todd G, 133
Toerge S, 253
Tomková H, 241
Tonthat GT, 167
Toosi S, 453
Torres MJ, 255
Trüeb RM, 184
Troxel AB, 374
Tukiainen E, 348
Tyburski JG, 164
Tzaneva S, 49

U

Ueda S, 448
Uhlig T, 106
Ullman S, 226
Ulrich M, 360
Uren RF, 412
Uter W, 73
Utsunomiya A, 427

V

Vähävihu K, 291
Van de Kerkhof P, 118
Van de Kerkhof PCM, 127
Van den Bosch F, 108
van der Beek N, 203
van der Ent FWC, 421
van der Heijde D, 106
van der Rhee JI, 413
van der Veer WM, 277
van Gorp J, 325
Vandooren B, 221
Van Praet JT, 221
Varga E, 329
Vasile M, 222
Veierød MB, 410

Velázquez D, 125
Velazquez EF, 359
Venna S, 371
Verheijen P, 325
Vermeeren L, 421
Vermeulen KM, 51
Vicaria M, 179
Victor FC, 207
Vieira MTC, 444
Vieira R, 247
Villar ME, 179
Vinceti M, 400
Vishalakshi V, 149
Vitry F, 418
Vosseler S, 333
Votava H, 423
Voulgari PV, 217

W

Waardenburg IE, 277
Wada DA, 424
Wain EM, 129
Walling HW, 159
Wanek LA, 394
Wang C, 158
Wang D, 353
Wanitphakdeedecha R, 478
Ward SE, 213
Warloe T, 340
Warshaw EM, 372
Wattanakrai P, 440
Weatherhead SC, 475
Wee JS, 72
Wee SA, 260
Weenig RH, 424
Weger W, 165
Weigelt N, 122
Weinberger CH, 212
Weinstock MA, 347, 365, 391
Weisenseel P, 88
Weiss ET, 449
Weiss JM, 55, 471
Weistenhöfer W, 93
Weisz K, 144
Wen H-J, 74
Westreich M, 465
Wetter DA, 296
White IR, 61
White JML, 72

White LE, 456
Wieland CN, 232
Wilcox RA, 424
Wilkinson D, 337
Wilkinson MS, 86
Wilkinson SM, 265
Willard R, 334
Williams C, 265
Williams J, 82
Williams ZY, 441
Wilmot AC, 268
Wirén K, 89
Wisgerhof HC, 305
Witjes H, 325
Wolverton SE, 124
Wong SL, 386, 398
Woods A, 69
Woodward JA, 441
Wriston CC, 374

Y

Yaemsiri S, 282
Yamangokturk B, 273
Yamaoka H, 307
Yamasaki H, 307
Yan AC, 252
Yang A, 359
Yang Y, 158
Yarak S, 189
Yaremchuk MJ, 437
Yiasemides E, 366
Ylianttila L, 291
Yonekura K, 427
Yoo KH, 439
Yoong P, 134
Yousefi P, 121
Yu AP, 248

Z

Zaba LC, 105
Zaballos P, 300
Zábojníková M, 241
Zamberk P, 125
Zaravinos A, 367
Zhang M, 85
Zhao Y, 81
Zimmerman LH, 164
Zollinger T, 137

Printed and bound by CPI Group (UK) Ltd, Croydon, CR0 4YY

08/05/2025

01864677-0018